Inhalation Aerosols

Lung Biology in Health and Disease

Series Editors: Peter Calverley, Fernando Martinez, Anthony Newman-Taylor and Jadwiga Wedzicha

Series formerly edited by: Claude Lenfant, Former Director, National Heart, Lung, and Blood Institute, National Institutes of Health, Bethesda, Maryland

Recent Titles

Inhalation Aerosols: Physical and Biological Basis for Therapy, Third Edition
Edited by Anthony J. Hickey and Heidi M. Mansour

Respiratory Infections
Edited by Sanjay Sethi

Sleep Apnea: Implications in Cardiovascular and Cerebrovascular Disease, Second Edition
Edited by T. Douglas Bradley and John S. Floras

Interventional Pulmonary Medicine, Second Edition
Edited by John F. Beamis, Jr., Praveen Mathur, and Atul C. Mehta

Pleural Disease, Second Edition
Edited by Demosthenes Bouros

Chronic Obstructive Pulmonary Disease Exacerbations
Edited by Jadwiga A. Wedzicha and Fernando J. Martinez

Interstitial Pulmonary and Bronchiolar Disorders
Edited by Joseph P. Lynch III

Diagnostic Pulmonary Pathology, Second Edition
Edited by Philip T. Cagle, Timothy C. Allen, and Mary Beth Beasley

Ventilatory Support for Chronic Respiratory Failure
Edited by Nicolino Ambrosino and Roger S. Goldstein

Sleep and Breathing in Children, Second Edition: Developmental Changes in Breathing During Sleep
Edited by Carole L. Marcus, John L. Carroll, David F. Donnelly, and Gerald M. Loughlin

Sleep in Children, Second Edition: Developmental Changes in Sleep Patterns
Edited by Carole L. Marcus, John L. Carroll, David F. Donnelly, and Gerald M. Loughlin

The opinions expressed in these volumes do not necessarily represent the views of the National Institutes of Health.

For more information about this series, please visit: [https://www.crcpress.com/Lung-Biology-in-Health-and-Disease/book-series/IHCLUBIHEDIS]

Inhalation Aerosols

Physical and Biological Basis for Therapy

THIRD EDITION

Edited by

Anthony J. Hickey

Heidi M. Mansour

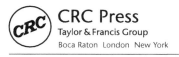

CRC Press
Taylor & Francis Group
Boca Raton London New York

CRC Press is an imprint of the
Taylor & Francis Group, an **informa** business

CRC Press
Taylor & Francis Group
6000 Broken Sound Parkway NW, Suite 300
Boca Raton, FL 33487-2742

First issued in paperback 2020

ISBN 13: 978-0-367-73148-9 (pbk)
ISBN 13: 978-1-138-06479-9 (hbk)

Library of Congress Cataloging-in-Publication Data

Names: Hickey, Anthony J., 1955- editor. | Mansour, Heidi M., editor.
Title: Inhalation aerosols : physical and biological basis for therapy /
[edited by] Anthony J. Hickey, Heidi M. Mansour.
Description: Third edition. | New York, NY : CRC Press, [2019] | Includes
bibliographical references and index.
Identifiers: LCCN 2018043533| ISBN 9781138064799 (hardback : alk. paper) |
ISBN 9781315159768 (ebook)
Subjects: | MESH: Aerosols--therapeutic use | Aerosols--pharmacology |
Nebulizers and Vaporizers | Pulmonary Ventilation--physiology
Classification: LCC RM161 | NLM WB 342 | DDC 615.8/36--dc23
LC record available at https://lccn.loc.gov/2018043533

Visit the Taylor & Francis Web site at
http://www.taylorandfrancis.com

and the CRC Press Web site at
http://www.crcpress.com

Contents

Preface   vii

Editors   ix

Contributors   xi

Introduction   xv

PART I   FUNDAMENTALS   1

1   Physicochemical properties of respiratory particles and formulations   3
     Boris Shekunov
2   Particle deposition in the respiratory tract and the effect of respiratory disease   31
     William D. Bennett
3   Mathematical modeling of inhaled therapeutic aerosol deposition in the respiratory tract   41
     Jeffry Schroeter, Bahman Asgharian, and Julia Kimbell
4   Lung transporters and absorption mechanisms in the lungs   57
     Mohammed Ali Selo, Hassan H.A. Al-Alak, and Carsten Ehrhardt
5   Bioavailability of inhaled compounds   71
     Lucila Garcia-Contreras
6   3D models as tools for inhaled drug development   107
     Sally-Ann Cryan, Jennifer Lorigan, and Cian O'Leary
7   Overview of the delivery technologies for inhalation aerosols   123
     Daniel F. Moraga-Espinoza, Ashlee D. Brunaugh, Silvia Ferrati, Lara A. Heersema, Matthew J. Herpin,
     Patricia P. Martins, Hairui Zhang, and Hugh D.C. Smyth

PART II   APPLICATIONS, INFLUENCE OF LUNG DISEASE PATHOPHYSIOLOGY ON AEROSOL DEPOSITION,
          INHALER DEVICE TECHNIQUE IN RESPIRATORY DISEASE, AND CLINICAL OUTCOMES IN DRUG
          PERFORMANCE ASSESSMENT   145

8   Neonatal and pediatric inhalation drug delivery   147
     Ariel Berlinski
9   Asthma   161
     Omar S. Usmani
10   Drug delivery in pulmonary aspergillosis   167
     Sawittree Sahakijpijarn, Jay I. Peters, and Robert O. Williams, III
11   Lung cancer inhalation therapeutics   187
     Rajiv Dhand
12   Inhaled therapeutics in chronic obstructive pulmonary disease   215
     Tejas Sinha, Paul Dejulio, and Philip Diaz
13   Cystic fibrosis infection and biofilm busters   223
     Jennifer Fiegel and Sachin Gharse
14   Current and future CFTR therapeutics   239
     Marne C. Hagemeijer, Gimano D. Amatngalim, and Jeffrey M. Beekman

15 Innate and adaptive barrier properties of airway mucus   257
    Alison Schaefer and Samuel K. Lai

16 Nontuberculous mycobacteria   275
    M. Ghadiri, P.M. Young, and D. Traini

17 Inhalational therapies for non-cystic fibrosis bronchiectasis   291
    Ashvini Damodaran, Dustin R. Fraidenburg, and Israel Rubinstein

18 Pulmonary fibrosis   303
    Priya Muralidharan, Don Hayes, Jr., and Heidi M. Mansour

19 Therapeutics in pulmonary hypertension   313
    Maria F. Acosta, Don Hayes, Jr., Jeffrey R. Fineman, Jason X.-J. Yuan, Stephen M. Black, and Heidi M. Mansour

20 Overview of lung surfactant and respiratory distress syndrome   323
    Heidi M. Mansour, Debra Droopad, and Julie G. Ledford

21 Surfactant aerosol therapy for nRDS and ARDS   327
    Donovan B. Yeates

22 Fundamentals in nasal drug delivery   343
    Zachary Warnken, Yu Jin Kim, Heidi M. Mansour, Robert O. Williams, III, and Hugh D.C. Smyth

23 Inhaled therapeutics against TB: The promise of pulmonary treatment and prevention strategies in the clinic   361
    Dominique N. Price, Nitesh K. Kunda, Elliott K. Miller, and Pavan Muttil

PART III   INTEGRATED STRATEGIES (REFLECTING COMBINED ELEMENTS FROM CHAPTERS 8 THROUGH 23)   377

24 Inhaled medication: Factors that affect lung deposition   379
    Joy H. Conway

25 A critical perspective on future developments based on the knowledge we have now   389
    Tania F. Bahamondez-Canas, Jasmim Leal, and Hugh D.C. Smyth

26 Ensuring effectiveness and reproducibility of inhaled drug treatment   397
    Anthony J. Hickey

27 Conclusion   405
    Anthony J. Hickey and Heidi M. Mansour

Index   409

Preface

Inhalation aerosols continue to be the basis for successful lung therapy for a variety of diseases. Since the turn of the millennium, many new products have been approved. Arguably the most substantial have been the first approved inhaled drugs and drug combinations for the treatment of chronic obstructive pulmonary disease (COPD). More recently, the development of drugs to treat pulmonary infection and diabetes has continued the translation of drug therapy to aerosol technology. With this background, it is evident that technological advancements and therapeutic strategies have evolved since the first two editions of this book were published. The original focus on asthma as the most significant target of inhaled therapy has broadened to include numerous local and systemic diseases. And the range of technology forming the basis for novel inhaler design has expanded significantly.

In this text, rather than simply expand and update the original two editions, we decided to address the close integration of technology with its application. An introductory section (Part I) on the fundamental science acts as a transition from past volumes to the present text by presenting briefly the general considerations that apply to physical chemistry, device technology, aerosol physics, lung deposition, clearance, physiology, and pharmacology. Part II represents a new approach in which a disease and therapeutic agent focus is employed to illustrate the application of a technology. It is evident from the number of chapters in this section (13) that the opportunities for the application of aerosol drug delivery have increased dramatically in recent years. Finally, an integrated strategies section (Part III) draws the major points from the applications regarding disease targets and drug products in the form of generalizations that may be valuable to readers.

In modifying the approach to the structure of the book, we are aligning with the translational imperative that has emerged in the last decade. In addition, this third edition is aligned with the latest scientific initiatives on precision medicine that has been gaining much attention recently. This approach encompasses precision pulmonary medicine. The ability to extract knowledge rapidly and effectively from study data and apply it in a therapeutically relevant manner is considered an urgent demand of the scientific and clinical research community. In presenting the content as described in this preface, we hope that relevance to development and clinical evaluation can be established.

Anthony J. Hickey
Chapel Hill, North Carolina

Heidi M. Mansour
Tucson, Arizona

Editors

Anthony J. Hickey, PhD, DSc, is Distinguished RTI Fellow at the Research Triangle Institute (2010–present), Emeritus Professor of Molecular Pharmaceutics of the Eshelman School of Pharmacy (1993–2010), and Adjunct Professor Biomedical Engineering in the School of Medicine at the University of North Carolina at Chapel Hill. He obtained PhD (1984) and DSc (2003) degrees in pharmaceutical sciences from Aston University, Birmingham, United Kingdom, following postdoctoral positions at the University of Kentucky (1984–1988). Dr. Hickey then joined the faculty at the University of Illinois at Chicago (1988–1993). In 1990, he received the American Association of Pharmaceutical Scientists (AAPS) Young Investigator Award in Pharmaceutics and Pharmaceutical Technology. He is a Fellow of the Royal Society of Biology (2000), the American Association of Pharmaceutical Scientists (2003), the American Association for the Advancement of Science (2005), and the Royal Society of Biology (2017). He received the Research Achievement Award of the Particulate Presentations and Design Division of the Powder Technology Society of Japan (2012), the Distinguished Scientist Award of the American Association of Indian Pharmaceutical Scientists (2013), the David W. Grant Award in Physical Pharmacy of the American Association of Pharmaceutical Scientists (2015), the Thomas T. Mercer Joint Prize for Excellence in Inhaled Medicines and Pharmaceutical Aerosols of the American Association for Aerosol Research and the International Society for Aerosols in Medicine (2017). He has published numerous papers and chapters (over 250) in the pharmaceutical and biomedical literature, one of which received the AAPS Meritorious Manuscript Award in 2001. He has edited five texts on pharmaceutical inhalation aerosols and co-authored three others on pharmaceutical process engineering, pharmaceutical particulate science, and pharmaco complexity. He holds 25 U.S. patents on a variety of inhaler device technologies, and pulmonary and oral drug delivery formulation technologies. He is founder (1997, and formerly president and CEO, 1997–2013) of Cirrus Pharmaceuticals, Inc., which was acquired by Kemwell Pharma in 2013; founder (2001, and formerly CSO, 2002–2007) of Oriel Therapeutics, Inc., which was acquired by Sandoz in 2010; and founder and CEO of Astartein, Inc. (2013–present). He is a member of the Pharmaceutical Dosage Forms Expert Committee of the United States Pharmacopeia (USP, 2010–2015, Chair of the Subcommittee on Aerosols), and formerly Chair of the Aerosols Expert Committee of the USP (2005–2010). Dr. Hickey conducts a multidisciplinary research program in the field of pulmonary drug and vaccine delivery for treatment and prevention of a variety of diseases.

Heidi M. Mansour, PhD, RPh, is a tenured Associate Professor of Pharmaceutical Sciences in the College of Pharmacy with joint faculty appointments in the BIO5 Research Institute and the College of Medicine in the Division of Translational and Regenerative Medicine at The University of Arizona (UA) in Tucson, Arizona. Dr. Mansour has faculty member affiliations in the UA Institute of the Environment, and the UA NCI Comprehensive Cancer Center. She lectures in the BS Pharmaceutical Sciences undergraduate program, the Pharm. D. professional program and in the Pharmaceutics and Pharmacokinetics track of the graduate program at The University of Arizona. In addition to teaching, Dr. Mansour serves as Faculty Advisor in the Pharm. D./PhD Dual Degree Joint Program and Director of the Pharmaceutics and Pharmacokinetics track in the Pharmaceutical Sciences graduate program in The UA College of Pharmacy. Dr. Mansour has published over 80 peer-reviewed scientific journal papers, 9 book chapters, 2 edited books, and over 100 scientific conference abstracts. She serves on the editorial advisory boards of the Royal Society of Chemistry *Molecular Systems Design & Engineering*, APhA/FIP *Journal of Pharmaceutical Sciences*, and *Pharmaceutical Technology*.

Dr. Mansour is an annual Faculty Instructor at International Society of Aerosols in Medicine (ISAM) Aerosol School, instructor in two online webinars on inhalation aerosol drug delivery, and instructor in Buchi Advanced Spray Drying short courses. She was recently Co-Chair of the Drug Delivery: New Devices & Emerging Therapies Group in ISAM, and has been an expert member of the National Institutes of Health (NIH) NICHD U.S. Pediatric Formulations Initiative New Drug Delivery Systems Aerosols Working Group for several years. Dr. Mansour currently serves on the Drug/Device Discovery and Development (DDDD) Committee of the American Thoracic Society (ATS). She regularly serves as an expert reviewer for scientific journals and grant funding agencies, including NIH study sections; Department of Defense (DOD) study panels; National Science Foundation (NSF) study panels; American Association for the Advancement of Science (AAAS); Catalent Drug Delivery Institute; and international funding agencies such as the German–Israeli Foundation, German International Exchange Service (DAAD), Cochrane Airways Group of the National Health Service (London, United Kingdom), Engineering and Physical Sciences Research Council (London, United Kingdom), PRESTIGE Postdoc Fellowship Programme of the European Commission (Paris, France), and the Biomedical Innovation Program of the French National Research Agency (Paris, France).

In addition to serving on NSF study panels, NIH study sections, and international study panels in the European Union and Great Britain, her innovative research program continuously attracts competitive funding awards from federal sources (NIH, NSF, FDA, DOD) and the pharmaceutical industry. In addition to lecturing in the BS Pharmaceutical Sciences undergraduate, PhD graduate, and Pharm. D. professional programs, Dr. Mansour leads her research labs where she trains postdoctoral scholars, visiting scholars, visiting professors, graduate students, Pharm. D. student researchers, and physician-scientist (MD/PhD) fellows. As Major Professor and mentor, her research program has successfully graduated several PhDs. Her innovative research program has produced assistant professors employed at research universities in the United States and in the Republic of South Korea, and senior research scientists employed at major pharmaceutical companies in the United States.

Dr. Mansour is an active, long-time member of several scientific organizations and elected member to honor societies, including the Sigma Xi Scientific Research Honor Society, Rho Chi Pharmaceutical Honor Society, and Golden Key International Honor Society. A registered pharmacist for over 20 years, she earned her BS in pharmacy with honors and distinction, a PhD minor in advanced physical and interfacial chemistry (Department of Chemistry), and a PhD major in drug delivery/pharmaceutics (School of Pharmacy) from the University of Wisconsin–Madison. Also at the University of Wisconsin–Madison, she was a clinical instructor for a few years. Having completed postdoctoral fellowships at the University of Wisconsin–Madison and at the University of North Carolina–Chapel Hill, she was awarded the University of North Carolina–Chapel Hill Postdoctoral Award for Research Excellence from the Office of the Vice-Chancellor, the AAPS Postdoctoral Fellow Award in Research Excellence, and the PhRMA Foundation Postdoctoral Fellowship Award. As an instructor, she served on the Graduate Faculty at the University of North Carolina–Chapel Hill.

Contributors

Maria F. Acosta
College of Pharmacy
The University of Arizona
Tucson, Arizona

Hassan H.A. Al-Alak
School of Chemistry
University of Kufa
Kufa, Iraq

Mohammed Ali Selo
School of Pharmacy and Pharmaceutical Sciences
Trinity College Dublin
Dublin, Ireland
and
Faculty of Pharmacy
University of Kufa
Kufa, Iraq

Gimano D. Amatngalim
Department of Pediatric Pulmonology
Wilhelmina Children's Hospital
and
Regenerative Medicine Center Utrecht
University Medical Center Utrecht
Utrecht, The Netherlands

Bahman Asgharian
Applied Research Associates
Raleigh, North Carolina

Tania F. Bahamondez-Canas
Division of Molecular Pharmaceutics and Drug Delivery
College of Pharmacy
University of Texas–Austin
Austin, Texas

Jeffrey M. Beekman
Department of Pediatric Pulmonology
Wilhelmina Children's Hospital
and
Regenerative Medicine Center Utrecht
University Medical Center Utrecht
Utrecht, The Netherlands

William D. Bennett
School of Medicine
University of North Carolina–Chapel Hill
Chapel Hill, North Carolina

Ariel Berlinski
Pediatric Aerosol Research Laboratory
Arkansas Children's Research Institute
University of Arkansas for Medical Sciences
Little Rock, Arkansas

Stephen M. Black
College of Medicine
The University of Arizona
Tucson, Arizona

Ashlee D. Brunaugh
College of Pharmacy
University of Texas
Austin, Texas

Joy H. Conway
Faculty of Health Sciences
University of Southampton
Southampton, United Kingdom

Sally-Ann Cryan
School of Pharmacy
Royal College of Surgeons of Ireland
Dublin, Ireland

Ashvini Damodaran
Division of Pulmonary, Critical Care, Sleep and Allergy Medicine
Department of Medicine
University of Illinois–Chicago
and
Jesse Brown Veterans Administration Medical Center
Chicago, Illinois

Paul Dejulio
Department of Internal Medicine, Pulmonary, Critical Care and Sleep Medicine
The Ohio State University
Columbus, Ohio

Rajiv Dhand
School of Medicine
University of Tennessee Graduate School of Medicine
Knoxville, Tennessee

Philip Diaz
Department of Internal Medicine, Pulmonary, Critical Care
and Sleep Medicine
The Ohio State University
Columbus, Ohio

Debra Droopad
College of Pharmacy
The University of Arizona
Tucson, Arizona

Carsten Ehrhardt
School of Pharmacy and Pharmaceutical Sciences
Trinity College Dublin
Dublin, Ireland

Silvia Ferrati
College of Pharmacy
University of Texas
Austin, Texas

Jennifer Fiegel
Department of Chemical and Biochemical Engineering
and
Department of Pharmaceutical Sciences and Experimental
Therapeutics
The University of Iowa
Iowa City, Iowa

Jeffrey R. Fineman
School of Medicine
University of California–San Francisco
San Francisco, California

Dustin R. Fraidenburg
Division of Pulmonary, Critical Care, Sleep and Allergy
Medicine
Department of Medicine
University of Illinois–Chicago
and
Jesse Brown Veterans Administration Medical Center
Chicago, Illinois

Lucila Garcia-Contreras
College of Pharmacy
University of Oklahoma Health Sciences
Oklahoma City, Oklahoma

M. Ghadiri
Woolcock Respiratory Research Institute
Sydney, New South Wales, Australia

Sachin Gharse
Department of Pharmaceutical Sciences and Experimental
Therapeutics
The University of Iowa
Iowa City, Iowa

Marne C. Hagemeijer
Department of Pediatric Pulmonology
Wilhelmina Children's Hospital
and
Regenerative Medicine Center Utrecht
University Medical Center Utrecht
Utrecht, The Netherlands

Don Hayes, Jr.
College of Medicine
The Ohio State University
and
Nationwide Children's Hospital
Columbus, Ohio

Lara A. Heersema
College of Pharmacy
University of Texas
Austin, Texas

Matthew J. Herpin
College of Pharmacy
University of Texas
Austin, Texas

Anthony J. Hickey
RTI International, RTP
Durham, North Carolina

Yu Jin Kim
College of Pharmacy
and
Center for Innovation in Brain Science
The University of Arizona
Tucson, Arizona

Julia Kimbell
School of Medicine
University of North Carolina–Chapel Hill
Chapel Hill, North Carolina

Nitesh K. Kunda
Department of Pharmaceutical Sciences
College of Pharmacy
University of New Mexico
Albuquerque, New Mexico
and
Industrial Pharmacy & Pharmaceutics
Department of Pharmaceutical Sciences
College of Pharmacy and Health Sciences
St. John's University
Queens, New York

Samuel K. Lai
Division of Pharmacoengineering and Molecular
    Pharmaceutics
Eshelman School of Pharmacy
and
UNC/NCSU Joint Department of Biomedical Engineering
and
Department of Microbiology and Immunology
University of North Carolina–Chapel Hill
Chapel Hill, North Carolina

Jasmim Leal
Division of Molecular Pharmaceutics and Drug Delivery
College of Pharmacy
University of Texas
Austin, Texas

Julie G. Ledford
College of Medicine
The University of Arizona
Tucson, Arizona

Jennifer Lorigan
School of Pharmacy
and
Tissue Engineering Research Group
Department of Anatomy
and
Centre for Research in Medical Devices (CURAM)
Royal College of Surgeons in Ireland
Dublin, Ireland

Heidi M. Mansour
College of Pharmacy
and
Division of Translational and Regenerative Medicine
Department of Medicine
College of Medicine
and
The BIO5 Research Institute
and
Institute of the Environment
The University of Arizona
Tucson, Arizona

Patricia P. Martins
College of Pharmacy
University of Texas
Austin, Texas

Elliott K. Miller
Department of Pharmaceutical Sciences
College of Pharmacy
University of New Mexico
Albuquerque, New Mexico

Daniel F. Moraga-Espinoza
Division of Molecular Pharmaceutics and Drug Delivery
College of Pharmacy
The University of Texas at Austin
Austin, Texas

and

Escuela de Química y Farmacia Facultad de Farmacia
and
Centro de Investigación Farmacopea Chilena
Universidad de Valparaíso
Valparaíso, Chile

Priya Muralidharan
College of Pharmacy
The University of Arizona
Tucson, Arizona

Pavan Muttil
Department of Pharmaceutical Sciences
College of Pharmacy
University of New Mexico
Albuquerque, New Mexico

Cian O'Leary
School of Pharmacy
and
Tissue Engineering Research Group
Department of Anatomy
and
Centre for Research in Medical Devices (CURAM)
Royal College of Surgeons in Ireland
and
Advanced Materials and Bioengineering Research
    (AMBER) Centre
Royal College of Surgeons in Ireland and Trinity College
    Dublin
Dublin, Ireland

Jay I. Peters
Division of Pulmonary Diseases/Critical Care Medicine
Department of Medicine
University of Texas Health Science Center at San Antonio
San Antonio, Texas

Dominique N. Price
Department of Pharmaceutical Sciences
College of Pharmacy
University of New Mexico
Albuquerque, New Mexico

Israel Rubinstein
Division of Pulmonary, Critical Care, Sleep and Allergy
    Medicine
Department of Medicine
University of Illinois–Chicago
and
Jesse Brown Veterans Administration Medical Center
Chicago, Illinois

Sawittree Sahakijpijarn
Department of Molecular Pharmaceutics and Drug
    Delivery
College of Pharmacy
University of Texas–Austin
Austin, Texas

Alison Schaefer
UNC/NCSU Joint Department of Biomedical Engineering
University of North Carolina–Chapel Hill
Raleigh, North Carolina

Jeffry Schroeter
Applied Research Associates
Raleigh, North Carolina

Boris Shekunov
Shire Pharmaceuticals
Exton, Pennsylvania

Tejas Sinha
Department of Internal Medicine, Pulmonary, Critical Care
    and Sleep Medicine
The Ohio State University
Columbus, Ohio

Hugh D.C. Smyth
College of Pharmacy
University of Texas
Austin, Texas

D. Traini
Woolcock Respiratory Research Institute
Sydney, New South Wales, Australia

Omar S. Usmani
National Heart and Lung Institute
Imperial College London
and
Royal Brompton Hospital
London, United Kingdom

Zachary Warnken
College of Pharmacy
University of Texas–Austin
Austin, Texas

Robert O. Williams, III
Department of Molecular Pharmaceutics and Drug
    Delivery
College of Pharmacy
University of Texas–Austin
Austin, Texas

Donovan B. Yeates
KAER Biotherapeutics
Escondido, California

P.M. Young
Woolcock Respiratory Research Institute
Sydney, New South Wales, Australia

Jason X.-J. Yuan
College of Medicine
The University of Arizona
Tucson, Arizona

Hairui Zhang
College of Pharmacy
University of Texas–Austin
Austin, Texas

Introduction

ANTHONY J. HICKEY AND HEIDI M. MANSOUR

The evolution of inhalation aerosol technology over the last half-century has created unique opportunities to treat disease. The fundamentals of pharmaceutical aerosol generation and delivery are well established and require the consideration of physical pharmacy, aerosol physics, device technology, process and product engineering, and pulmonary biology. The latter includes knowledge of lung deposition, clearance, and local and systemic pharmacology of delivered drugs.

As the use of aerosols in the treatment of disease has been explored, a greater understanding of the best therapeutic approaches has been developed. The nature of questions regarding selection of technologies has progressed from a desire to be informed about performance specifications to greater curiosity about the suitability of the technology for a specific disease therapy. The facility with which particular technologies can be adapted for use allows the optimization of all elements of the inhaled drug product to meet the needs of the biological and therapeutic endpoints.

A number of outstanding texts on the subject of aerosols and aerosol technology have been published (1–7). In the field of inhalation aerosols, the focus varies from fundamental science (8,9) and technology (10–15), and expands to clinical application (16–18) and the entire topic of drug delivery and translation to the clinic (19). The present text is arranged to cover some basic principles and then to focus extensively on translation of pharmaceutical inhalation aerosol technology into the clinic to treat specific diseases. Figure I.1 indicates the sequence of topics this volume covers.

The fundamental aspects of medicinal aerosol delivery may be considered as a sequence of events that first involve the formation of the aerosol from a variety of formulations and devices, each of which is optimized for a specific application. Once the aerosol is formed, the physicochemical properties and airborne behavior of the aerosol interacts with the pulmonary physiology to dictate deposition and disposition of drugs from the lungs. These properties and parameters can be modeled to predict deposition of particles and droplets in the lungs, and these predictions can be supplemented with experimental measures of deposition achieved by radiological imaging. After deposition, disposition can be followed by considering local transport and metabolism in the context of the systemic appearance of drugs in pharmacokinetic studies. Each of the common therapeutic aerosol systems can be evaluated for its potential to serve the needs of particular diseases.

A major debilitating lung disease, asthma has been the primary focus of aerosol treatment since the 1950s. As the understanding of key elements of effectiveness was identified, aerosol treatment has been expanded to include a wide range of diseases. Chronic obstructive pulmonary disease (COPD) was a logical target for treatment as manifestations of this disease are similar to asthma. As the vision of aerosol therapy broadened and new drug and biochemical targets were identified, other areas such as genetic disorders, airway remodeling, vascular disease, and infectious disease have received considerable attention, from which new products have been developed.

As in other areas of human endeavor, the discoveries that have occurred in the parallel field of research serve to inform each other in a manner that synergistically moves the field in a sometime discontinuous or disruptive manner. Several recent events have promoted discoveries and inventions. The most substantial was the implication of chlorofluorocarbon (CFC) propellants in ozone depletion and their subsequent phase-out, which resulted in the development of hydrofluoroalkane (HFA) alternatives. A similar phenomenon is now occurring as the role of HFAs in global warming is evident and the desire for potential alternatives is driving new developments. A second event of arguably similar magnitude to the propellant replacement was the desire for methods to deliver the products of biotechnology that were difficult to prepare as stable formulations, that were difficult to deliver by other routes of administration, or that would simply benefit from the characteristic disposition from the lungs. The need for a stable formulation and dose considerations resulted in a focus on dry powder inhalers (DPIs), which were until the late 1980s were poorly designed and inefficient systems with respect to the needs for macromolecule delivery. The innovations arising from the research of the following twenty years, particularly that focused on insulin delivery, elevated the field significantly and positioned the technology for the many successes that have occurred since 2000. Finally, the same drivers in the context of aqueous solution aerosol delivery resulted in an evolution from the dominant theme of air jet and ultrasonic

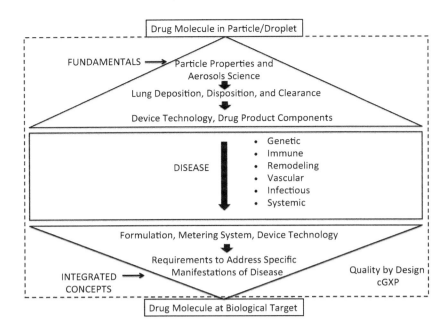

Figure I.1 The sequence of topics addressed in this text. Fundamental considerations are the foundation for the adoption of technologies to treat specific diseases. Knowledge gained from these experiences can be integrated to establish general principles that may be used prospectively in transferring the drug molecule from its starting environment to the proximity of its biological target. Many of the intervening steps are controlled either in manufacturing or in patient training.

nebulizers to smaller, more efficient vibrating mesh nebulizers and ultimately to handheld soft mist inhalers (SMIs).

As progress has been made to apply the fundamental understanding of the dosage forms and the route of administration to the context of specific diseases, an integrated body of knowledge can now be drawn together to make general observations about the foundation of technology available and its impact on certain aspects of disease.

The complexity of inhaled products and the multitude of factors that affect their performance requires a quality by design (QbD) approach if overall quality is to be ensured. The spatial (chemical and physical structure) and temporal (motion and disposition) behaviors of the product are subject to change by a range of variables, and each variable requires sufficient monitoring and control to meet product specifications and regulatory approval. The efficacy and safety of the product are linked to quality metrics, since the characteristic therapeutic needs of each disease are matched to the performance of the drug product.

Subsequent chapters of the book will guide the reader through the fundamentals (Part I) into specific disease considerations with translation to precision pulmonary medicine (Part II) from which integrated expositions on the nature of technology and the impact of disease considerations will be concluded. The importance of developing products in a controlled environment and the ways in which this might be translated into a uniform therapeutic outcome are discussed (Part III).

This systematic method ideally accounts for the drug molecule from its starting environment, accounting for adjacencies, to its presentation to the molecular therapeutic target, controlling as many of the intervening variables as possible.

REFERENCES

1. Fuchs N. *The Mechanics of Aerosols*. Mineola, NY: Dover Press, 1989.
2. Davies C. *Aerosol Science*. New York: Academic Press, 1966.
3. Mercer T. *Aerosol Technology in Hazard Evaluation*. New York: Academic Press, 1973.
4. Reist PC. *Aerosol, Science and Technology*. New York: McGraw-Hill, 1993.
5. Hinds W. *Aerosol Technology. Properties, Behavior and Measurement of Airborne Particles*, 2nd ed. New York: John Wiley & Sons, 1999.
6. Kulkarni P, Baron P, Willeke K. *Aerosol Measurement: Principles, Techniques, and Applications*, 3rd ed. New York: John Wiley & Sons, 2011.
7. Ruzer L, Hartley N. *Aerosols Handbook: Measurement Dosimetry and Health Effects*, 2nd ed. Boca Raton, FL: CRC Press, 2012.
8. Finlay W. *The Mechanics of Inhaled Pharmaceutical Aerosols. An Introduction*. New York: Academic Press, 2001.

9. Tougas T, Mitchell J, Lyapustina S, Eds. *Good Cascade Impactor Practices, AIM and EDA for Orally Inhaled Products.* New York: Springer, 2013.

10. Purewal T, Grant D. *Metered Dose Inhaler Technology.* Boca Raton, FL: CRC Press, 1997.

11. Srichana T. *Dry Powder Inhalers. Formulation, Device and Characterization.* Hauppauge, NJ: Nova Science Publishers, 2016.

12. Zeng X, Martin G, Marriott C. *Particulate Interactions in Dry Powder Formulations for Inhalation.* New York: CRC Press, 2000.

13. Hickey A. *Pharmaceutical Inhalation Aerosol Technology,* 2nd ed. New York: Marcel Dekker, 2004.

14. Smyth H, Hickey A. *Controlled Pulmonary Drug Delivery.* New York: Springer, 2011.

15. Colombo P, Traini D, Buttini F. *Inhaled Drug Delivery: Techniques and Products.* New York: Wiley-Blackwell, 2013.

16. Newman S. *Respiratory Drug Delivery: Essential Theory and Practice.* Richmond, VA: RDD Online, 2009.

17. Jacob B, O'Driscoll B, Dennis J. *Practical Handbook of Nebulizer Therapy.* Boca Raton, FL: CRC Press, 2003.

18. Gradon L, Marijnisson J. *Optimization of Aerosol Drug Delivery.* New York: Springer, 2003.

19. Dhand R, Rothen-Rutishauser B, Hickey A. *ISAM Textbook of Aerosol Medicine.* New Rochelle, NY: ISAM-Mary Ann Liebert, 2015.

PART I

Fundamentals

1 Physicochemical properties of respiratory particles and formulations   3
   Boris Shekunov
2 Particle deposition in the respiratory tract and the effect of respiratory disease   31
   William D. Bennett
3 Mathematical modeling of inhaled therapeutic aerosol deposition in the respiratory tract   41
   Jeffry Schroeter, Bahman Asgharian, and Julia Kimbell
4 Lung transporters and absorption mechanisms in the lungs   57
   Mohammed Ali Selo, Hassan H.A. Al-Alak, and Carsten Ehrhardt
5 Bioavailability of inhaled compounds   71
   Lucila Garcia-Contreras
6 3D models as tools for inhaled drug development   107
   Sally-Ann Cryan, Jennifer Lorigan, and Cian O'Leary
7 Overview of the delivery technologies for inhalation aerosols   123
   Daniel F. Moraga-Espinoza, Ashlee D. Brunaugh, Silvia Ferrati, Lara A. Heersema, Matthew J. Herpin,
   Patricia P. Martins, Hairui Zhang, and Hugh D.C. Smyth

Physicochemical properties of respiratory particles and formulations

BORIS SHEKUNOV

Introduction: Physicochemical particle properties and inhaler performance 3
Major factors affecting particle aerosolization 5
    Aerodynamic diameter and Stokes number 5
    Particle aggregate strength 7
    Modeling of dry powder dispersion 9
    Atomization of droplets 13
Drug solubility and mechanism of particle dissolution 14
Formulation aspects of respiratory drug delivery 15

Solid-state chemistry of crystalline and amorphous materials 15
    Lactose carriers and adhesive blends 18
    Engineered solid particles 19
    Liposomes 23
    pMDI solutions and suspensions 24
Conclusions and future perspective 25
Nomenclature 27
References 28

INTRODUCTION: PHYSICOCHEMICAL PARTICLE PROPERTIES AND INHALER PERFORMANCE

Drug delivery by inhalation can be considered as a sequence of three equally important stages: particle aerosolization within an inhaler device (as solid particles or liquid droplets); particle deposition/distribution in the airways and, finally, drug release/particle uptake/clearance at the site of action. The anatomy of respiratory tract presents a natural barrier to any particulate matter and, if particles penetrate into the deeper lungs, they tend to be rapidly removed by one of the physiological defense mechanisms (1,2). Consequently a major goal of respiratory drug delivery is to optimize physicochemical particle properties in order to achieve the maximum efficacy and safety of these dosage forms. The physicochemical properties of respiratory formulations can also be classified in accordance with their material characterization level and in relationship with their biopharmaceutical effects as illustrated in Table 1.1. This table also contains information pertinent to regulatory considerations during development, quality control and bioequivalence studies of inhalation drug products (3–6). Particle size distribution, in combination with the particle density and shape factor, is the most important critical attribute for any respiratory formulation and at each drug delivery stage: it determines the ability of formulation to be efficiently aerosolized at predefined inspiratory flow rates, controls the particle deposition profile, drug dissolution and particle uptake rates. Particle inertial deposition is typically associated with the fine particle fraction (FPF) between 1 and 5 μm in terms of the aerodynamic diameter, d_A, with maximum deposition in alveoli region between 1 and 2 μm. It is also known that particles with $d_A \approx 100$ nm also exhibit a peak related to the deposition by Brownian diffusion mechanism (1), although generating such nanosize aerosols is rather hypothetical. Particles in the micron, and especially the submicron, range are very cohesive. Small variations in size, surface and morphology, and some environmental conditions can significantly affect the powder aerosolization leading to low or, even worse, inconsistent FPF. Particles that deposit into the alveolar region are removed by phagocytosis, which may influence the efficacy of drug formulation (2,7). For this uptake, the volume-weighted particle diameter, d, and surface-to-volume shape factor, α_{sv}, are important: for example, spherical particles 1–5 μm are taken at a greater extent than smaller or larger particles, or particles of acicular shape, or those with modified surface and charge. By using different means of particle engineering it is therefore theoretically possible to optimize most drug delivery characteristics. There are, however, very significant practical limitations to that imposed by the inherent material properties of active pharmaceutical ingredients (APIs) and carriers, their toxicology, the inhaler design, the patient variability, as well as by the stringent requirements of drug product manufacturing and pharmaceutical quality control.

Table 1.1 Different levels of physicochemical functionality in relationship to major biopharmaceutical and drug delivery characteristics, combined with its regulatory considerations for development, bioequivalence, and quality control of inhalation drug products

Physicochemical characteristics	Affected biopharmaceutical parameters	Related regulatory considerations
Solid State		
Molecular structure, impurities; crystal form/crystallinity/amorphous content; equilibrium solubility, intrinsic dissolution rate; hygroscopicity / moisture content	Physical and chemical stability, potency, safety; systemic bioavailability and/or local drug concentration; bioequivalence (for generics)	Physicochemical characterization of API(s) and excipients relevant to their functionality in drug product; compatibility with diluents[c]; effects of environmental moisture[a,b], low temperature[b]; temperature cycling[b,d]; moisture content[a,b]; sameness/therapeutic equivalence of API (generics).
Particulate and Surface		
Volume or mass-weighted particle size distribution (PSD); shape factor and specific surface area; porosity/density; rugosity/asperity and rigidity; specific surface free energy, work of cohesion and adhesion; electrostatic charge or zeta potential; dissolution rate; dose delivered (emitted dose); fine particle dose/mass (FPD); aerodynamic particle size distribution (APSD): MMAD/GSD; FPF	*In vivo* regional deposition profiles; dose delivered; dose uniformity/consistency; rate of particle uptake/clearance and toxicity; systemic bioavailability (AUC/C_{max}) and/or local drug concentration; bioequivalence (for generics)	PSD (for APIs and carriers); ASPD; single actuation FPD[a,b,d]; (delivered) dose content uniformity (DCU)[a,b,d] (containers intra- and inter-batch) or uniformity of dosage units[a,c,d]; DCU and FPD at various flow rates[a] and at various lifestages (i.e., beginning, middle, end)[a,b,d]; FPD with spacer[b]; actuator/mouthpiece deposition[a,b,d]; shaking requirements; drug delivery rate and total drug delivered[c]; foreign particulate matter.
Formulation		
Type of formulation, dosage form and packaging presentation; carrier(s)[a,b], composition and coating[a,b]; dispersion media[b,c,d]; powder triboelectric charge, bulk and tapped density[a]; aggregate structure, density and strength; impact of processing/mixing; bulk flow properties/powder handling/filling[a].	Mode of administration; immediate, sustained or controlled drug delivery; dose metering, devise retention; dose uniformity/consistency; systemic bioavailability and/or local drug concentration; therapeutic efficacy and therapeutic index; ADME; safety/toxicology/ irritability; storage stability/shelf life; bioequivalence (for generics).	Assay, mean delivered dose vs. label claim[a,b,d]; DCU[a,b,d]; dose proportionality (for different strengths and/or APIs); formulation/inhaler robustness; drug product stability; qualitative (Q1) sameness and quantitative (Q2) equivalence of excipients and media physicochemical similarity[c] (generics).

[a] DPIs.
[b] pMDIs.
[c] Nebulizers.
[d] Non-pressurized metered-dose inhalers; otherwise generally applicable.

The medical science of respiratory drug delivery is discussed in the following chapters of this book. The present chapter is concerned with material science—physicochemical particle properties that directly impact formulation and inhaler design, especially for dry powder inhalers (DPIs). Although other type of devices such as pressurized metered-dose inhalers (pMDIs), nebulizers and non-pressurized metered-dose inhalers/soft mist inhalers are very important; the range of material science issues with them is much narrower. The fundamental reasons for this observation will also be discussed.

DPIs certainly belong to the cutting technological edge, due to the wide range of different active ingredients, doses, formulations as well as current and potential therapeutic applications (8). They also present the greatest challenges in pharmaceutical development, and from the regulatory viewpoint, are considered one of the most complex drug products (4). Since the early application of DPIs in the 1960s, there has been a great body of work done and literature accumulated for this technology, but there are still many unresolved fundamental issues. In recent reviews, for example, it has been pointed out that lack of understanding of powder dispersion mechanisms is a major obstacle to improved inhaler performance (9). Several misconceptions are highlighted in relationship to optimal inhaler performance with the air-flow independent therapy (8), device resistance and application of high-resistance devices by patients with reduced lung function (8,10). It was noted that surprisingly little attention has been given to the improvement of inhaler designs and new integrated device-formulation systems, with most modern inhalers still delivering only 20%–30% FPF of the label claim (10). For the carrier-based formulations, the consensus is that the relationship between properties of the starting materials, the mixing process, and dispersion performance is not well understood and constitutes a mostly empirical endeavor (11). This list of misconceptions can further be extended to other areas of inhalation material science including, for example, mechanisms of interparticle interaction, dispersion, particle dissolution and solid-state stability of amorphous formulations, as discussed in this chapter.

Although the complexity of interactions within the triad "formulation—airflow—inhaler design" should not be underestimated, in the author's opinion many of these gaps are methodological. For instance, one may consider independence of FPF from the airflow as a desirable characteristic for any respiratory formulation, but this point needs to be clarified in conjunction with a specific inhaler design. If formulation is readily fluidizable and dispersible at any flow rate, this implies a low "threshold energy" (or, more precisely, minimal stresses required for powder disaggregation, see the section called "Major factors affecting particle aerosolization") with very high FPF approaching the ideal 100%. Also for such particles, the inertial impaction parameter is sufficiently small to bypass deposition in the upper respiratory tract resulting in low *in vivo* variability (12). In practice, however, neither formulation nor inhaler are perfect, so if FPF increases steadily with flow or pressure drop, this most likely indicates a cohesive formulation and variable dispersion mechanism, whereas a steady but low FPF value may suggest a problem with either formulation or inherent inhaler design and may, in fact, be attributed to the fundamental properties of turbulent flow, as shown below. A significant issue here is that flow rate, pressure drop and inhaler resistance are usually not related quantitatively to the material characteristics of the formulation (e.g., particle adhesion/cohesion and aggregate strength), flow regime (character and intensity of turbulence) or the inhaler performance in terms of FPF or other measurable aerosolization parameters. Indeed, the most widely used approach consists of an array of empirical studies, oriented towards proving how certain formulation properties are important for better inhaler performance. Even when supported by the design of experiments (DoE), these studies often lead to contradictory conclusions and, by their nature, cannot result in generalized models (13). Of course, such studies may solve some short-term problems of industrial development or commercial production. On the other hand, more recent applications of computational fluid dynamics (CFD) predominantly concentrate on the description of aerodynamic flow fields, but usually do not contain principal closure equations of particle aerosolization and dispersion. Understanding of these mechanisms, in turn, requires a purposeful experimental methodology to determine the key material and fluid dynamic parameters, rather than statistical correlations.

The major objective of this chapter is not to review previous developments of inhalation particle technology or formulations, an extensive topic already covered by multiple recent publications (e.g., 1,8,10,11,14–17). Although a comprehensive assessment is also difficult to accomplish in a single chapter, the main intention here is to provide the reader with a systematic quantitative description of the key physicochemical parameters and, when possible, relate these parameters to the inhaler performance using analytical concepts developed for this work. In what follows, the definitions are introduced and mechanisms discussed by which the physicochemical properties of solid particles and liquid drops are translated into the drug delivery characteristics of pharmaceutical aerosols, most important, the FPF. This is concluded with a brief review of different formulation approaches and optimization strategies, and future perspectives in this important and fast-growing therapeutic field.

MAJOR FACTORS AFFECTING PARTICLE AEROSOLIZATION

Aerodynamic diameter and Stokes number

Particles for inhalation may not only have different geometric size (usually defined through the volume-equivalent diameter, d, [18]) but also exhibit different shape, density/porosity and aggregate structure. In order to standardize the fluid dynamic equations for different kinds of particles, the concept of aerodynamic diameter, d_A, is introduced. It is defined as the diameter of spheres of unit density, which undergo the same acceleration in the air stream as non-spherical particles of arbitrary density, therefore moving along the same streamlines. Following this definition, the general dynamic equation leads to the following relationship:

$$d_A = d \frac{\rho}{\rho_1} \frac{1}{\alpha_{sv}} \frac{C_d(Re_A)}{C_d(Re)} \frac{C_c(Re)}{C_c(Re_A)} \qquad (1.1)$$

where ρ_1 is the unit density (e.g., 1 g/cm^3) and ρ is the particle density. C_d is the particle drag coefficient which is a function of the particle Reynolds number, $Re = ud/v$, where v is the air kinematic viscosity, u is the particle (slip) velocity relative to the air stream. Re_A and Re denote numbers for particles with diameters d_A and d, respectively. C_c is the Cunningham slip correction factor dependent on the particle diameter (18,19). Experimentally, the aerodynamic particle size distribution (APSD) is typically measured using cascade impactor devices such as Andersen cascade impactor, next generation cascade impactor (NGI) and muti-stage liquid impinger (MSLI), all of which operate on the principle of particle classification by using a series of jets and collection plates with different Stokes numbers (see below). APSD can also be measured using time-of-flight (TOF) techniques (18).

Surface-to-volume shape factor, α_{sv}, is the ratio of the characteristic particle cross-section with equivalent diameter, d_s, to that of the particle with volume-equivalent diameter, d:

$$\alpha_{sv} = \left(\frac{d_s}{d} \right)^2 \qquad (1.2)$$

Equations (1.1) and (1.2) define this shape factor through the particle geometry, whereas the drag coefficients are written for the spherical particles, thus decoupling these quantities. This definition is different from the dynamic shape factor considered elsewhere (18,19). The advantage is that it can be determined experimentally from microscopic image analysis, or from other measurements given independent assessment of both d and d_s. These parameters are usually measured through a combination of laser diffraction and microscopic imaging studies. For solid particles with density ρ_p, it is useful to define α_{sv} (for randomly oriented particles) through the specific surface area (SSA) which are related through the well-known Cauchy theorem stipulating that the mean projected area is equal to quarter of the surface area, leading to the following expression:

$$\alpha_{sv} = \frac{1}{6} SSA \rho_p d \qquad (1.3)$$

whereby SSA can be determined from the Brunauer–Emmett–Teller (BET) gas adsorption measurements.

The general equation (1.1) is solved numerically and equally applicable to droplets, solid particles, porous particles and aggregates provided that the particle density (or void fraction for aggregates) and particle shape factor are known. The flow regimes applicable to respiratory delivery or measurements can be defined as Stokesian ($Re < 0.1$) and ultra-Stokesian ($0.5 < Re < 100$). For the spherical particles in the Stokesian flow regime, the drag coefficient assumes the well-known relationship: $C_d = 24/Re$. Also, taking $C_c \approx 1$ for the micron particle size range (the estimated error <10% for particles approximately 2 μm in size [19]), Eq. (1.1) leads to the simplified expression for Stokes aerodynamic diameter widely used in the aerosol literature:

$$d_A(Stokes) = d \left(\frac{\rho}{\alpha_{sv}\rho_1} \right)^{1/2} \qquad (1.4)$$

Thus non-spherical particles and porous particles have a smaller aerodynamic diameter than solid spherical particles of the same mass. For liquid aerosols, such as nebulizer and pMDIs sprays, the droplet particle shape is also not completely spherical due to deformation by air stresses, as will be discussed in the following sections.

The dimensionless Stokes number (given here as the generalized effective Stokes number, Stk_e), can be viewed as

the ratio of the characteristic particle relaxation time under the drag, to the characteristic flow time around the obstacle (20). At small $Stk_e \ll 1$, a particle follows the fluid streamlines whereas at $Stk_e \gg 1$, particle follows its initial trajectory and impact the obstacle. This definition depends on the particle Re number (20,21):

$$Stk_e = \psi \left(Re \right) Stk \qquad (1.5)$$

where Stk is this number in the Stokesian flow regime ($\psi = 1$):

$$Stk = \frac{\rho d_A^2 u}{18 \mu L} \qquad (1.6)$$

$\mu = \upsilon \rho_0$ is the dynamic air viscosity and L is the characteristic dimension of an obstacle. The non-Stokesian particle drag correction factor, ψ, can be calculated numerically (21). The importance of the Stokes number is that it can describe at least three categories of events:

1. Deposition by inertial impaction in the upper airways defining the fine particle dose (FPD) delivered to the lungs. The "inertial impaction parameter," $d_A^2 Q$ (according to Eq. [1.6]), is often used to describe the mouth-throat deposition (12).
2. Measurements of the aerodynamic particle diameters (e.g., mass-median aerodynamic diameter [MMAD]) and fine particle fraction (FPF) with different cascade impactors or liquid impingers, typically used for in vitro R&D studies and industrial quality control of different inhalers; and applied for recalibration of impactor cut-off diameters at different flow rates Q (18).
3. Efficiency of particle deaggregation within the DPIs, in particular those purposely designed for particle impaction.

One may consider possible deviations introduced in Eqs. (1.1) and (1.5) in the ultra—Stokesian flow regime. Although the particle Re is much smaller than corresponding numbers for airflow within both the human respiratory system and inhalation devices, it can reach levels sufficiently high to introduce non-Stokesian corrections. For example, for a turbulent flow (at least at the peak airflow rate) in the mouth-throat, $Re \approx 1$, for particles below 10 μm, which give the value of $\psi \approx 0.9$, so the effect on the throat deposition is likely to be minimal. However, for the turbulent flow within the inhaler itself, and for larger aggregates, Re may reach one or two orders of magnitude higher (see the section called "Modelling of dry powder dispersion"), thus $\psi \approx 0.4-0.8$, introducing a significant correction, for example, in assessing the particle impaction on an inhaler grid. Similarly, calculations of the precise cut-off diameters in the cascade impactors may require application of complete Eqs. (1.1) and (1.5) (18).

Particle aggregate strength

Particle aggregates are always present in dry powder respiratory formulations, and in most suspension formulations, necessitating their dispersion into primary particles for efficient delivery. In other words, the aggregate strength should be sufficiently low compared to the mean dispersion stresses within the inhalation device. The assessment of this strength is a major formulation task. Much of the aerosol literature considers cohesive interparticulate forces and cohesive-adhesive force balances between the drug- and drug-carrier particles (8,11,22–24). However, quantitative analysis of these forces, although important, is quite insufficient for realistic description of the dispersion mechanism. Most particles in respiratory formulations have a non-spherical irregular shape and microscopically rough surfaces, forming aggregates with a wide spectrum of contact areas and separation distances and thus making determination of such forces ambiguous or, at best, very time consuming in both theory and practice. Perhaps more important, such an approach neglects powerful factors associated with the aggregate structure itself, that is, packing characteristics, coordination numbers, shape, density, porosity and defects/flaws as well as the fact that dispersion of aggregates is governed by the applied stress, not by the force. For example, it is well known that particles with high adhesion can form loose aggregates of reduced strength. Unfortunately, the structure of aggregates in respiratory formulations is rarely considered and, apart from the particle size distribution, poorly described in quantitative terms. Nevertheless, aggregate structures have been investigated for other materials (25–28) for which several models of packing, fractal dimension and tensile strength have been developed since the definitive work by Rumpf (29). In this chapter, an alternative model is proposed which describes the aggregate strength considering their size and surface effects, which is of importance for respiratory formulations. As will be shown below, this is also essential for understanding of the mechanism of particle "erosion" which occurs on the periphery of the aggregate close to its surface (27,28). In contrast, the aggregate "rupture" or fragmentation occurs within the aggregate bulk and is typically associated with the tensile strength.

Figure 1.1 illustrates the present model for quantifying the aggregate structure and strength. The primary particles compose a pseudo-lattice with vacancies which mainly define the aggregate density and strength. Such pseudo-lattice does not imply a long-range space ordering, like in crystal structure, but is an indication of the most probable packing with the maximum coordination number, K, whereas major defects affecting this number are attributed to vacancies. The structure without vacancies corresponds to the highest coordinated packing with powder density, ρ_{max}, achievable for particles of a given shape but, in practice, can only be observed locally. Both parameters, K and ρ_{max}, can be calculated for simple packing geometries, such as spheres within cubic or hexagonal structures; however, no general

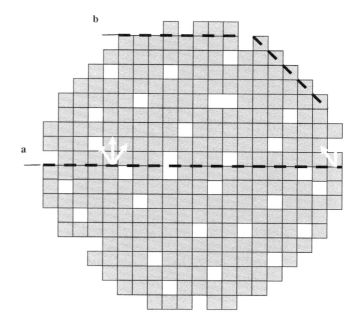

Figure 1.1 Structure of aggregate composed of pseudo-lattice of primary particles: ■—position of a particle, □—vacancy) with arrows depicting the coordination number across the fracture cross-section. Dashed lines represent: **(a)** tensile fracture surface and **(b)** erosion surfaces. Although this schematic shows a simple cubic lattice, the particles (and vacancies) may have a different shape and 3D coordination number.

relationship between the packing fraction and coordination number is assumed here, unlike that in the semi-empirical relationships developed by Kendell or Rumpf (25,29). In the present model, the probability of finding a particle in its lattice position is ρ/ρ_{max} where ρ is the aggregate density. Assuming the isotropic structure (no preferred orientation) for primary particles and considering the hypothetical fracture cross-sections (Figure 1.1), it can be written for the tensile strength, σ_T:

$$\sigma_T = K\left(\frac{\rho}{\rho_{max}}\right)^2 \frac{F}{d_0^2} \qquad (1.7)$$

where d_0 is the characteristic lattice parameter which is related to the volume mean diameter, d_p, and density, ρ_{max}, of primary particles through the following expression:

$$d_0 = d_p\left(\frac{\pi\rho_p}{6\rho_{max}}\right)^{\frac{1}{3}} \qquad (1.8)$$

K is the mean coordination number of primary particles (or vacancies), with each pair connected by interparticulate bonding force, F, intersecting the fracture cross-section. Only such bonds contribute to the work of adhesion, W. Furthermore, considering any fracture cross-section of characteristic dimension, d, it can be seen (Figure 1.1) that coordination number on the edges, K_e, is generally smaller that coordination number, K_b, in the bulk, whereas the mean coordination number for the entire cross-section can be calculated as:

$$K = K_e + \frac{(K_b - K_e)}{\left(1 + \dfrac{d_0}{d}\right)^2} \qquad (1.9)$$

The mean interparticle cohesive force, F, depends on several factors, including the particle shape and surface roughness; however the analytical equations are only available for smooth elastic spheres under attractive (usually van-der-Waals) contact forces. For example, a well-accepted Johnson-Kendall-Roberts (JKR) (30) relationship reads:

$$F = -\frac{3}{8}\pi W d_p \qquad (1.10)$$

In case of particles of different diameters, d_{p1} and d_{p2}, the interactive diameter can be taken as the harmonic mean:

$$\frac{2}{d_p} = \frac{1}{d_{p1}} + \frac{1}{d_{p2}} \qquad (1.11)$$

Eqs. (1.7) through (1.11) are sufficient to describe practically all effects related to interactions of particles in aggregates and also to make a quantitative assessment of the aggregate tensile strength:

1. The aggregate strength is inversely proportional to d_p, although the magnitude of interparticulate bonds is directly proportional to d_p according to Eq. (1.10). This comes from the fact that tensile strength is defined by the force per unit area of cross-section in Eq. (1.7). In particular larger "porous" particles of the same aerodynamic diameter form weaker aggregates than solid particles.

2. Small surface irregularities (also called asperities or corrugated surfaces [22]) can significantly decrease both the interparticle bond and aggregate strength (by a factor $\sim 2y/d_p$ where y is the diameter of asperity for a single contact). For multiple contacts with number, q, the mean interparticulate bond increases to $\sim 2qy/d_p$, but may still be below the value for smooth particles if $y \ll d_p$. This effect can be calculated based on geometry for specific packing.

3. For binary mixtures consisting of nanoparticles, the same applies as for asperities. The mean interparticulate bond and aggregate strength both decrease with increasing concentration of nanoparticles, reaching a minimum at a certain surface coverage corresponding to approximately a single particle-nanoparticle-particle contact within the entire lattice, after which the aggregate strength increases again due to increasing number of such contacts.

4. For binary mixtures consisting large carrier particles, such as lactose crystals, the aggregates mostly consist of a carrier with adhered drug particles. According to Eqs. (1.10) through (1.11), the carrier-drug bond increases by a factor of 2, given the same W and contact cross-section, compared to the bond between drug particles themselves. However, the balance of strength for such aggregates depends on the drug-carrier surface coverage and packing order of drug particles.

5. Both parameters, K and σ_T, become dependent on the aggregate (or cross-section) size when they are comparable to the size of primary particles. In particular, K has a smaller value for the fracture cross-sections close to the aggregate surface (Eq. 1.9).

Note that the current model does not assume an increase of aggregate porosity with their size, as in the fractal description (26,28), because there is no physical basis by which this porosity should increase with size given that all aggregates are produced from the same powder bed.

The magnitude of aggregate strength can be assessed as follows, taking typical parameters: $d_p = 2\ \mu m$; $\rho = 0.3\ g/cm^3$; $\rho_{max} = 1\ g/cm^3$; $\rho_p = 1.4\ g/cm^3$; $K_b = 3$; $W = 20\ mJ/m^2$ (22). One then obtains: $\sigma_T = 3.2\ kPa$ for large aggregates, $\sigma_T = 1.6\ kPa$ for small aggregates according to this model; whereas the computation using other models gives: $\sigma_T = 3.6\ kPa$ (29); $\sigma_T = 0.3\ kPa$ (25). Thus, the present model suggests the aggregate strength just below that predicted by Rumpf but significantly above that following from the model by Kendell. One should also consider rather unreliable predictions of the bonding force, F, based on the assumption of idealized geometry of smooth elastic spheres, which is used in the JKR model, as well as in all other similar models of particle interactions. In reality the rough particle surface and non-spherical morphology ensure that the effective contact area would be significantly reduced below that for the smooth sphere in most cases but flat contacts. Also, these models assume uniform distribution of particle defects, whereas the breakup would first occur in planes with the weakest σ_T, as observed experimentally (27). Practically that means that Eq. (1.10) would have a significantly smaller numerical coefficient dependent on the particle shape, albeit the dependence on volume diameter and work of adhesion in this equation would likely hold from the fundamental considerations, at least for the mean values of these parameters. In this connection, it should also be mentioned that the work of adhesion, W, is often confused in literature with the surface energy (or, more precisely, with the specific surface free energy) of a solid, γ_s. W is defined by the minimum of energy per unit area required to separate two surfaces in mechanical contact (25), whereas the surface energy is defined thermodynamically as the specific free energy created by the new solid surface, for example, in the processes of crystal nucleation, growth or cleavage (31) (the analogue for liquids is surface tension). Both definitions are only equivalent for a perfect contact between similar and ideally smooth (on the atomic level) surfaces, which is never the case for particles, although these quantities relate to each other progressively.

From the experimental viewpoint, the value of pull-off force, F, can be determined using atomic force microscopy (AFM) (22–24). Such experiments may involve acquisition of large sets of data, statistically representative of different particle orientations, geometries and contact areas. Estimations of W from such measurements are much less reliable because of the ambiguity of determining the curvature and contact areas of interacting particles. In addition, flat substrates often used in such studies may exhibit a different nature of chemical bonds, making contributions of two contacting surfaces to W convoluted and ill-defined. This problem is well known in inverse gas chromatography (IGC), which also has been applied to measure the surface energetics of inhalable particles (32–35). The dispersive component of the surface free energy can be considered representative of the non-polar interactions associated with the van der Waals forces; but it does not account for specific polar interactions such as permanent dipole forces and hydrogen bonding. These polar interactions often make significant contributions to the overall specific surface energy and interparticulate forces, but they are difficult to discriminate quantitatively. Thus although a priori assessment of the aggregate strength based entirely on material properties is possible in theory, the principal difficulties involved, as well as extensive time and efforts required, pose a question if the same can be accomplished more efficiently by direct and relatively fast measurements of aggregate dispersion by aerodynamic forces under controlled conditions. This concept is explored in the next section.

Finally, it should be noted that assessment of the mechanical aggregate strength, σ_A, is typically based on the tensile strength, σ_T, (25–29) which can be explained by a relative simplicity of calculating separation forces as originally proposed by Rumpf (29). However, the fluid dynamics and mechanical stresses considered in the following section may act either on compression or shear. The strength to shear can be considered close to the magnitude of tensile strength, whereas the compression strength has a more complex mechanism and usually exceeds both the shear and tensile strengths as was determined experimentally (26,27). This difference should be taken into account if more precise description of the breakage mechanism is desired.

Modeling of dry powder dispersion

The major goal of any dispersion model for respiratory drug delivery is to define how the aerosol parameters (e.g., FPF, FPD, MMAD) relate to the formulation physicochemical properties, airflow rate and inhaler design. Presented in Figure 1.2 is a "black-box" approach in which an aerodynamic dispersion device (DPI, standardized entrainment tubes (36) or dry powder dispersion unit for particle size measurements) transforms a powder characterized by the initial fine particle fraction, FPF_0 (mass fraction of particles already dispersed at time 0), into an aerosol with the FPF dependent on the airflow rate, Q. The macroscopic parameters describing the device itself are the pressure drop, ΔP,

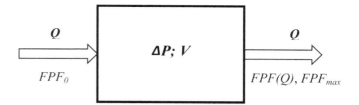

Figure 1.2 A generalized model of aerodynamic particle dispersion in which a steady-state flow, Q, passes through a device which is characterized by the pressure differential, ΔP, and volume of the active dispersing zone, V. The input-output parameters include the initial fine particle fraction, FPF_0, the fine particle fraction, FPF (as a function of Q) and the maximum achievable fine particle fraction, FPF_{max}.

and volume of the effective turbulent dispersion zone, V. This description can also incorporate fine particle fraction, FPF_{max}, which is the maximum limit achievable for a given formulation. This limit follows from a practical consideration that no formulation can realistically achieve 100% FPF even at the highest possible flow rate. The major reasons for such an effect may include presence of hard agglomerates of primary drug particles or strongly adhesive drug-carrier agglomerates, or an existence of "dead zones" which allow some particles to bypass dispersion. The most important parameter for calculating the extent of dispersion is the relative mass of unbroken aggregates, m_A, remaining after dispersion for which an exponential decay function can be written:

$$m_A = e^{-\Gamma\tau} \tag{1.12}$$

Here τ is the mean residence time of aggregates within the device and Γ (1/s) is the relative rate of breakage (also called the breakage kernel [28]). The quantity $(1 - m_A)$ in Eq. (1.12) can be considered as the probability of an aggregate to be dispersed within the device. An exponential term with breakup frequency linked to Weibull statistics has been considered (37). The similarity, however, ends there because Eq. (1.12) does not postulate an exponential dependence between the probability of breakup and impact energy (37). Such dependence can be more complex, as shown below. Also, a dimensionless parameter named "non-dimensional specific dissipation (NDSD)" was discussed by Longest et al. (38) for which a strong empirical correlation with both FPF and MMAD was observed. Although NSDS and $\Gamma\tau$ are related to each other in Kolmogorov theory, because NSDS was not connected to any specific dispersion model in this work, it was assigned to the kinetic energy available for breakup on a certain scale multiplied by time, whereas $\Gamma\tau$ is simply the number of turbulent fluctuations, and therefore these parameters have completely different physical interpretation. The frequency of turbulent fluctuations, Γ, increases for small-scale turbulent eddies, whereas the eddy turbulent energy decreases with the scale. The dispersion of aggregates is not directly governed by the turbulent energy but, in addition to the turbulent fluctuation rate and residence time, requires an independent assessment of the aerodynamic stress, σ.

Considering the mass balance of breakable aggregates, unbreakable agglomerates and fine particles before and after dispersion process:

$$m_A = \frac{(FPF_{max} - FPF)}{(FPF_{max} - FPF_0)} \qquad (1.13)$$

and therefore the breakage parameter is related to the FPF as follows:

$$\Gamma\tau = ln\frac{(FPF_{max} - FPF_0)}{(FPF_{max} - FPF)} \qquad (1.14)$$

with the following simple relationship between the FPF and mass-weighted momentum of aerodynamic particle size distribution, $d_{4,3}$:

$$d_{4,3} = d_A(1 - FPF) + d_{Ap}FPF \qquad (1.15)$$

where d_A and d_{Ap} are the mean (mass-weighted) aerodynamic diameters of the aggregates and fine particles correspondingly. Such a relationship is simple for a bimodal distribution consisting only one kind of aggregates and fine (primary) particles but in general can be applied to any distribution if the diameters d_A and d_{Ap} are known; $d_{4,3}$ has a somewhat larger, although usually close value to the *MMAD*, which is commonly used in all aerosol literature. For the purposes of quantitative modeling, however, $d_{4,3}$ is a better-defined parameter.

The breakage kernel, Γ, in Eq. (1.12) is determined by the dominant mechanism (or in some cases several parallel mechanisms) of particle disaggregation within the device. In what follows, it is assumed that breakage occurs stepwise according to the scheme in Figure 1.1, when the stresses exerted on particles within the device exceed the mechanical strength of agglomerates: $\sigma > \sigma_A$, otherwise no breakage. The airflow within DPIs and SETs devices, at least within their active dispersion zone and typical flow rates, occur at Reynold numbers sufficient for turbulence flow regime under the rough entry conditions. The developed turbulent flow was also confirmed in several CFD computations done for specific devices (37–41). Thus type of dispersion stresses can be defined in terms of the isotropic turbulence theory below and above the Kolmogorov scale, λ_K:

$$\lambda_K = \frac{\upsilon^{3/4}}{\varepsilon^{1/4}} \qquad (1.16)$$

1. Stress defined by the viscous shear:

$$d \le \lambda_K; \Gamma = C_b\left(\frac{\varepsilon}{\upsilon}\right)^{1/2} \quad if \ \mu\left(\frac{\varepsilon}{\upsilon}\right)^{1/2} > \sigma_A \qquad (1.17)$$

where υ and μ are the kinematic and dynamic air viscosities, ε is the average rate of energy dissipation per

unit mass (m^2/s^3) and C_b is the proportionality constant in this breakage kernel (28).

2. Stress defined by the inertial forces above λ_K, whereby:

$$d > \lambda_K; \Gamma = C_b\varepsilon^{1/3}\left(\frac{C_d\alpha_{sv}\rho_0}{4\rho d}\right)^{2/3} if \ 0.3C_d^{1/3}\rho_0^{1/3}\rho^{2/3}\left(\frac{\varepsilon d}{\alpha_{sv}}\right)^{2/3} > \sigma_A \qquad (1.18)$$

where ρ and ρ_0 are the densities of particles and airflow. This stress is generated by the difference in densities between the particle and turbulent airflow according to Levich (42) and acted for particle compression. The magnitude of such stress is greater, by a factor of $(\rho/\rho_0)^{2/3}$, than shear stress caused by the gradient of turbulent eddy velocity over the distance of particle diameter, important for liquids (28,42). It should be noted here that the drag coefficient C_d in this assessment is related to the aggregate particle size, d. However, for the erosion mechanism, which concerns the shear stress acting on aggregate surface, a correction factor of C_d'/C_d, should be introduced, where C_d' is the drag coefficient of a primary particle or very small secondary aggregate close to the surface. The magnitude of this factor is approximately 2–6, which may create a significant increase of this shear stress for the erosion process.

3. Stress related to the re-entrainment process caused by air-shearing near a stationary powder surface (41) which can be defined as follows:

$$\Gamma = C_b\left(\frac{\varepsilon}{L^2}\right)^{1/3} \quad if \ \frac{1}{2}C_d\rho_0(\varepsilon L)^{2/3} > \sigma_A \qquad (1.19)$$

where L is the integral scale of turbulent fluctuations, which corresponds to the characteristic dimension of the dispersing zone. Similar to the aerodynamic stress (2), the drag coefficient of a primary particle or very small secondary aggregate can be significantly larger (by a factor of approximately 2–6) for erosion of small surface particles than disintegration of large agglomerates.

4. Stress generated during mechanical impaction of an aggregate on a device surface, for example, wall or grid. Such an impaction has been considered, for example, in CFD simulations (38–40), although without defining this mechanism quantitatively. This compression stress is of a different nature from the fluid dynamic stresses (1–3) considered above. A simple estimate of conversion between kinetic and elastic energies on impact (not presented here) leads to the following relationship for the volume-mean maximum mechanical stress generated within agglomerates:

$$\Gamma = C_i\left(\frac{\varepsilon}{L^2}\right)^{1/3} \quad if \ A\left(\rho\frac{EE_s}{(E+E_s)}\right)^{1/2}(\varepsilon L)^{1/3} > \sigma_A \qquad (1.20)$$

where C_i is the proportionality constant for impaction, A is the coefficient defining the normal component (i.e., angle and relative magnitude) of the particle impact velocity related to the large-scale turbulent eddies; E and E_s are Young's modulus for the aggregates and surface (typically $E << E_s$).

5. Stress created during collisions between aggregates or between aggregates and primary particles. The rate of such collisions is defined by the relative velocity of particles caused by the gradient of turbulent velocities over distance $(d_1 + d_2)/2$, where d_1 and d_2 are the particles' diameters, as discussed in work (43). These authors considered collision of drops below λ_K. For solid particles, the mechanical stresses generated are of the same nature as discussed in (4). The following estimate can be written for aggregates of the same size:

$$d \leq \lambda_K; \Gamma = C_k \left(\frac{\varepsilon}{\upsilon}\right)^{1/2} \quad if \; 0.3 \left(\rho E\right)^{1/2} \left(\frac{\varepsilon}{\upsilon}\right)^{1/2} d > \sigma_A \quad (1.21)$$

Here, C_k is the proportionality constant for successful collisions leading to breakage, which depends on the particle cross-section and squire of number concentration according to reference (43). The numerical coefficient comes from the expression for the velocity gradient below the Kolmogorov scale.

6. Similarly, for the inertial range, collisions for larger particles are defined by the gradient of turbulent eddy velocity in the inertial subrange over the distance d:

$$d > \lambda_K; \Gamma = C_k \left(\frac{\varepsilon}{d^2}\right)^{1/3} \quad if \left(\frac{\rho E}{2}\right)^{1/2} \left(\varepsilon d\right)^{1/3} > \sigma_A \quad (1.22)$$

Overall it can be said that the breakage frequency, Γ, in Eqs. (1.17) through (1.22) is directly related to the characteristic frequency of turbulent fluctuations at an appropriate length scale, whereas the minimal breakage stress is related to fluid velocities on the same scale, expressed through the rate of turbulent energy dissipation. Furthermore, assuming the superposition of breakage mechanisms (28), for the overall breakage kernel it can be written:

$$\Gamma = \sum_{i}^{n} \Gamma_i \quad (1.23)$$

Thus a superposition of different kernels, particularly as a result of changing ε (or flow rates), may lead to a rather complex breakage mechanism. However, it is likely that one or two major mechanisms may dominate the disaggregation process depending on the type of device used.

Since in a typical inhalation device the particle breakage occurs within a small volume, V, defined by geometry of restricted passage, or possibly chamber with baffles or grid, the energy is dissipated mainly within this volume:

$$\varepsilon = \frac{\Delta P Q}{\rho_0 V} \quad (1.24)$$

$$\tau = \frac{V}{Q} \quad (1.25)$$

where Eq. (1.25) represents the definition of residence time. The following proportionalities can be written for the flow parameters:

$$\varepsilon \sim \frac{U^3}{L}; Q \sim UL^2; V \sim L^3 \quad (1.26)$$

where L is the characteristic dimension of the inhaler restriction or dispersing chamber. Eqs. (1.26) yields the following definition of device resistance, R_D:

$$\Delta P^{1/2} = R_D Q; R_D = Z \frac{\rho_0^{1/2}}{L^2} \quad (1.27)$$

where U is the mean airflow velocity and the dimensionless constant, Z, is mainly defined by the inhaler type/geometry and can be determined experimentally. For instance, for the SET devices (36) within the resistance range $R_D = 0.007 - 0.044 \, kPa^{1/2} min/L$, $Z = 2.3 \times 10^3 - 2.6 \times 10^3$, practically independent of the inner inlet tube diameter. For a dispersing device (41), consisting of a rectangular duct and inserts with $R_D = 0.019 - 0.04 \, kPa^{1/2} min/L$, $Z \approx 5.5 \times 10^3$ also weakly dependent on the type of insert used. Thus, Z is practically independent of L, as indeed follows from Eqs. (1.27). The dispersing volume can be assessed on the basis of device type/geometry, CFD simulations or experimental data, and typically vary between ~1–30 cm^3 for different devices (36,38,40,41). For most commercial DPIs, R_D falls within the range 0.01–0.07 kPa$^{1/2}$ min/L (12). An inhaler with typical resistance 0.04 kPa$^{1/2}$ min/L, flow rate 45 L/min, and $V = 10$ cm^3 results in $\varepsilon = 2 \times 10^5$ m^2/s^3 which corresponds to the Kolmogorov scale $\lambda_k = 11$ μm. Thus, all mechanisms (1–6) are theoretically possible for aggregates but can be limited by the magnitude of aerodynamic stresses developed. Given typical values: $d = 50$ μm (or 5 μm at $d < \lambda_k$); $\rho = 0.3$ g/cm^3; $E = 0.1$ GPa (25,26), the following relationship between σ for different regimes (1–6) can be written:

$$\sigma_1 (10^{-3}) << \sigma_2 (10^{-1}) \approx \sigma_3 (10^{-1}) < \sigma'_{2,3} (10^0) << \sigma_5 (10^1)$$
$$< \sigma_6 (10^2) < \sigma_4 (10^2) \quad (1.28)$$

Here $\sigma'_{2,3}$ denotes the shear aerodynamic stresses during erosion from the aggregate surface. The order of magnitude is given in kPa. Perhaps not surprisingly, the stresses generated by mechanical impact on surfaces and, to a lesser extent, particle collisions have the highest magnitude, although lower breakage frequency. The aerodynamic stress (2) has the highest breakage frequency. Viscous stresses (1) have the lowest value, only sufficient for dispersing the weakest and smallest aggregates. Both aerodynamic stresses generated during powder re-entrainment and dispersion by turbulence in the inertial range are below the mean estimated agglomerate strength (see previous section). This is in line with the experimental results (27) and can be explained by overestimation of interparticulate forces within the aggregate discussed in the section called "Particle aggregate strength," particularly taking into account that the stresses required for the mechanisms of surface erosion are significantly lower than for the aggregate rupture. However, this also indicates that there is some theoretical discrepancy between the amplitude of aerodynamic stresses and the aggregate strength, and more research in this area is indicated.

Following the considerations above, the dispersion mechanism can be described as follows: the large aggregates are efficiently ruptured by mechanical forces of collision and simultaneously eroded by smaller but faster fluid dynamic stresses from the aggregate surfaces, whereas large fluffy aggregates may also be ruptured into denser fragments by fluid dynamic stresses, as illustrated in Figure 1.3. This process cascades down to smaller particle sizes until a certain population is reached on the exit from dispersion zone.

The superimposed breakage kernel in Eq. (1.23) may have a dependency on the turbulent energy dissipation rate approximated by function $\Gamma \sim \varepsilon^x$ where the power $x \approx 1/3 - 1/2$. Consequently, the following relationship can be anticipated from Eqs. (1.14) and (1.24) through (1.27) between the FPF and airflow rate:

$$log\left(ln\frac{(FPF_{max} - FPF_0)}{(FPF_{max} - FPF)} \right) = A + (3x - 1)logQ \quad (1.29)$$

or for the powders entirely consisting of dispersible aggregates:

$$log(-\ln(1 - FPF)) = A + (3x - 1)logQ \quad (1.30)$$

where parameter A depends on the device design (R_D and V), but not on the airflow rate.

Equations (1.29) and (1.30) show that most valuable data on the dispersion mechanism may come from measuring FPF (or corresponding particle size distributions) within a wide dynamic range of Q. Unfortunately, such data are difficult to come by because most of the experimental studies focus on changing a few formulation parameters, or type of device, but only for two or three different flow rates. Figure 1.4 shows data recalculated from the mechanistic study by Gac et al. (41) and for this device and different inserts used, the average value $x \approx 0.4$. More precise data, however, are required to distinguish between different dispersion regimes versus flow rate. It should be noted that at $x = 1/3$, FPF becomes independent of Q (or ΔP). This seeming

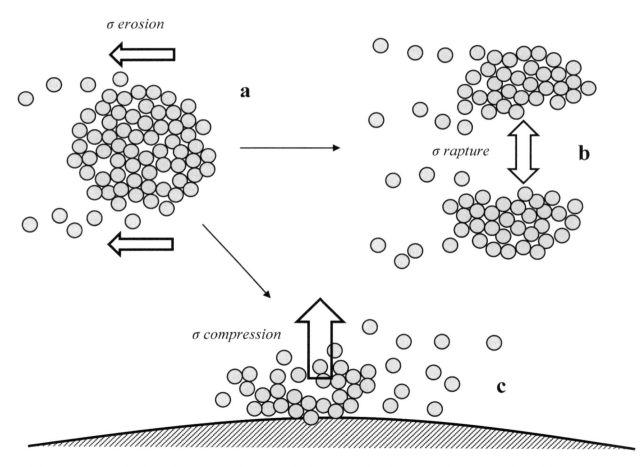

Figure 1.3 Proposed mechanism of aggregate dispersion in dry powder inhalers: (a) Surface erosion by fluid stresses; (b) rupture of large aggregates into denser fragments by fluid stresses followed by erosion; and (c) rupture by an impact on the surface.

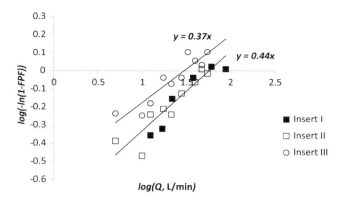

Figure 1.4 Relationship between the parameter − ln(1 − FPF) and airflow rate, Q (L/min), in logarithmic coordinates according to Eq. (1.30). FPF was recalculated from the particle size data of a dispersing device with different inserts according to Gac et al. (From Gac, J. et al., *Aerosol Sci.*, 39, 113–126, 2008.)

paradox originates from the fact that the increase in the breakage rate is exactly compensated by the reduction in residence time. Such a phenomenon can be expected as the majority of kernels (1–6) exhibit $\varepsilon^{1/3}$ dependency. If only one such dispersion mechanism persists, the FPF would change as a step-wise function. There is evidence that this behavior is indeed observed for some devices above a certain flow rate (36,38,39), or even perhaps commonly for some formulations (8). In this case, an optimization of inhaler design is necessary to increase its efficiency. This effect needs to be differentiated from the limitations imposed by the properties of formulation itself, as expressed through the parameter FPF_{max} in Eq. (1.13). In addition, Eq. (1.30) is derived under the assumption that all aggregates break at the same threshold level of σ_A. In reality, some distribution of tensile strengths is expected and may mask the dispersion mechanism. If such tensile strengths distribution is known, it can be introduced numerically in the above model, together with corrections related to the particle size distribution of aggregates. Alternatively, the formalism of moment balance equations (28) can be used in such a description.

Finally, it should be noted that, although the considerations above are based on the concept of isotropic turbulence, some of the most important conclusions also apply to the transitional and laminar flow regimes, which may exist at relatively low airflow rates and/or for devices with very low resistance. In such case, the major dispersion mechanisms described by Eqs. (1.19) and (1.20) (i.e., flow entrainment and particle-surface collision) dominate and remain practically unchanged when rewritten in terms of the air or particle velocity.

Atomization of droplets

Although the range of different dispersion mechanisms applicable to nebulizers, soft mist inhalers, and pMDIs can be greater than that for DPIs, the fundamental difference which makes the discussion of liquid droplet breakup much simpler is that droplet diameter can be directly related to and, in practice, efficiently controlled by the atomization stresses. The parameter analog to the aggregate strength, σ_A, for liquids is the surface (Laplace) pressure, σ_L:

$$\sigma_L = \frac{4\gamma_L}{d} \tag{1.31}$$

where γ_L is the surface tension. $\sigma_L \approx 5.8$ kPa, calculated for 50 μm diameter droplet of water without surfactants, is above the typical strength of solid aggregates. Smaller droplets or droplets of higher viscosity are even more difficult to disperse; however, more powerful dispersion stresses available for these devices compensate for this.

The maximum stable droplet size, d_{max}, in turbulent airflow can be found by assuming a balance between the turbulent stresses in Eqs. (1.18) and (1.19) and σ_L:

$$d_{max} = 4.5 \frac{\gamma_L^{3/5}}{C_d^{1/5} \rho_0^{1/5} (\rho\varepsilon)^{2/5}} \tag{1.32}$$

$$d_{max} = \frac{8\gamma_L}{C_d \rho_0 u^2} \tag{1.33}$$

Equation (1.32) is similar to the original expression derived by Kolmogorov (42) for droplet breakup under turbulent stresses but contains a factor $(\rho/\rho_0)^{2/3}$ responsible for the particle inertial effects. Equation (1.33) is rewritten from Eq. (1.19) to account for the particle slip velocity, u, and responsible for droplet breakup during acceleration stage, for example, immediately after introduction of liquid into a twin-fluid nebulizer nozzle. This gives the critical Weber number, $We_c = \rho_0 u^2 d/\gamma_L$, for the droplet breakup about 12 under the typical $C_d = 0.7$ ($Re \approx 300$) in accordance with the Taylor criterion (13). Although further inroads can be made to estimate the complete droplet size distribution, from the practical viewpoint, diameter d_{max} is sufficient in most cases to assess the inhaler performance in terms of the FPF.

Equations (1.32) and (1.33) are directly relevant to the mechanism of dispersion in twin fluid-nozzles or jet nebulizers as well as for propellant breakup by interactions with air in the MDIs sprays. For small $We \ll 1$, that is, for relatively low jet velocities (but still sufficient for jet formation) and/or small nozzle diameters, such as the case of liquid jets atomized through capillary channels or micron-sized orifices, the dispersion mechanism proceeds in the Rayleigh regime due to liquid surface instabilities and the theory predicts the following droplet diameter (13):

$$d = 1.89 d_j (1 + 3Oh)^{1/2} \tag{1.34}$$

where d_j is the jet diameter and Ohnesorge number for liquid jet is defined as:

$$Oh = \frac{\mu_L}{\sqrt{\gamma_L \rho d_j}} = \frac{\sqrt{We}}{Re} \qquad (1.35)$$

Oh can also be defined for drops and describes the impact of liquid viscosity on droplet dispersion, although it can be seen that for most diluted aqueous solutions and suspensions, $Oh < 0.1$, so the liquid can be considered non-viscous; therefore for low-viscosity jets, the droplet size can be directly related to the jet diameter: $d = 1.89 d_j$. This represents a convenient way to produce monodispersed droplets, a practice used for small-scale spray-drying or printing applications. With growing We number, the kinetics of droplet breakup becomes more complex and involves interactions with air through drop deformations and Rayleigh-Taylor surface instabilities, as discussed in more detail elsewhere (13). There are several other important atomization mechanisms applicable to liquid formulations such as ultrasonic dispersion and cavitation (28), expansion/cavitation within pMDI propellants, droplet collision with baffles usually integrated into the jet nebulizer design, collision between jets/droplets in soft mist inhaler: for all, breakup stresses can be assessed and the parameters d_{max} and FPF determined based on the liquid surface tension and viscosity. Droplets may also precipitate and evaporate during atomization. These tasks may be considered in future publications.

DRUG SOLUBILITY AND MECHANISM OF PARTICLE DISSOLUTION

In vivo dissolution of inhaled particles in the lungs occurs in competition with particle clearance, adsorption and metabolism and therefore knowledge and control of dissolution parameters are of high importance for respiratory drug delivery. In vitro dissolution is sometimes used as a development tool and quality control test (44) and can be determined using compendial methods, such as USP Apparatuses 2 or 4, or customer-made systems of suitable design. Due to the small size and often hydrophobic character of inhalable particles, care should be taken to avoid artifacts introduced by poor wetting, floating and cohesion/aggregation. These artifacts may distort the dissolution measurements, particularly during its initial and most important stage. The most common simulated lung fluids (SLFs) are listed in reference (45). As will be shown below, steering speed or through-flow rate have little effect on the dissolution of small particles; thus, both drug solubility and intrinsic dissolution rate (i.e., dissolution rate per unit surface area) are largely defined by the solid-state particle properties, which can be assigned to a specific crystal or salt form, or manipulated through use of different excipients in composite particles for potential sustained or controlled drug delivery applications. Particle size and shape define the overall dissolution or drug release rate. The equilibrium solubility is not significantly affected

by the particle size down to nanoparticles <0.1 μm, which can be demonstrated on the basis of characteristic values for the specific surface energy of organic solids (46). This phenomenon is also related to the effect known as Oswald ripening: crystal growth (and change with particle shape) in liquid formulations driven by the differences in solubilities due to surface curvature. Oswald ripening is pronounced for submicron particles and highly anisotropic micron particles (large shape factor) and proportional to the absolute value of the equilibrium solubility (31).

Often dissolution process has been described by the Noyes-Whitney diffusion equation, which can be written as:

$$\frac{dm}{dt} = \frac{D}{\delta} SSA (c_0 - c) \qquad (1.36)$$

where dm/dt is the relative (to the total mass remained) dissolution rate, D is the diffusion coefficient in solution, δ is the thickness of diffusion boundary layer, c_0 is the equilibrium solubility and c is the bulk solution concentration. It has been shown however (47) that a more general dissolution equation is:

$$\frac{dm}{dt} = k \, SSA (c_0 - c) \qquad (1.37)$$

$$\frac{1}{k} = \frac{1}{k_i} + \frac{1}{k_s} + \frac{\theta}{k_D} \qquad (1.38)$$

k describes the combined coefficient of mass transfer defined though the coefficients k_i, k_s, k_D which are assigned to the internal, surface and solution mass transfer correspondingly. θ denotes the solute distribution (partition) coefficient, only applicable for particles where the active ingredient is distributed or encapsulated, for example, particles designed for sustained or controlled drug release, whereas for solid particles $\theta = 1$. Furthermore, for small particles (i.e., within and below the micron size range of inhalation particles) the following approximations are valid (47):

$$k_i = \frac{2 D_i}{d} \qquad (1.39)$$

$$k_D = \frac{2 D}{d} \qquad (1.40)$$

where D_i and D are the diffusion coefficients within and outside the particles; the surface kinetic coefficient k_s is independent of diffusion being defined by the solid state and sometimes by the properties of the surface absorption layer (47). Equation (1.40) is the limiting case of diffusion equation for small particles when the Sherwood number, $Sh = k_D d / D \rightarrow 2$ and the nominal thickness of diffusion layer is equal to the particle radius. Clearly in the case of composite particles $k_i << k_D / \theta$, so that drug release is defined by a smaller (by several orders of magnitude) diffusion coefficient within an insoluble carrier matrix. Less obvious is the fact that even for immediate release formulations, given the typical experimental parameters for most pharmaceutical substances: $D \approx 10^{-5}$ cm^2/s and $k_s \approx 10^{-3}$–10^{-2} cm/s (48), the ratio $k_s/k_D < 0.1$, and therefore the dissolution process is mainly controlled by the surface kinetic step. Application of the diffusion Eq. (1.36) instead of the complete mass transfer Eq. (1.37) for particles can result in very significant error (47). Another limitation of the Noyes-Whitney diffusion equation, more applicable to the determination of intrinsic dissolution rate (47,48), is that diffusion of ionizable drugs, as well as micelle-mediated drug diffusion, cannot be described by a single value of diffusion boundary thickness, δ, but requires a more detailed analysis of interactions between different dissolving species. Thus Noyes-Whitney equation represents only a special case of either very fast surface kinetics and/or slow diffusion of non-dissociated molecules, which is rarely applicable to dissolution of small inhalable particles. The drug dissolution rate is also directly proportional to the SSA, which is, in turn, proportional to the surface-to-volume shape coefficient and inversely proportional to the particle diameter. However, if particles form aggregates during dissolution, this may significantly decrease the dissolution rate.

The dissolution profile of solid drug particles under sink conditions ($c = 0$) can be considered when particles dissolve isomorphically, that is, when the shape factor, α_{sv}, does not change with dissolution time. It can also be concluded from the considerations above that the kinetic coefficient $k \approx const$. In such cases, Eq. (1.37) can be easily integrated, leading to the following relationship for the fraction of particle mass dissolved, m:

$$m(t) = 1 - \left(1 - \frac{t}{t_0}\right)^3 \qquad (1.41)$$

$$t_0 = \frac{d\rho_p}{2\alpha_{sv}kc_0} \qquad (1.42)$$

Here t_0 is the time constant of complete dissolution. When particles have a size distribution:

$$m(t) = \sum_i^n m_i(t) \qquad (1.43)$$

where m_i is the weight fraction dissolved for each particle class of size d_i.

FORMULATION ASPECTS OF RESPIRATORY DRUG DELIVERY

Solid-state chemistry of crystalline and amorphous materials

Most currently marketed respiratory drug products, similar to other solid dosage forms, contain crystalline drug substances. The molecules usually have several functional groups and significant conformational mobility and are thus likely to have multiple polymorphic forms or solvates. Screening, identification and characterization of different crystal forms are described in detail elsewhere (49). As with any other formulations consisting of solid particles, the most desirable form for pharmaceutical development of inhalation drug products is typically the most thermodynamically stable (under ambient conditions) crystal form. A higher solubility or superior powder properties of some metastable forms normally do not justify the risks associated with their lower physicochemical stability during processing, production or shelf life (49). However, some crystal forms such as monotropic polymorphs and desolvates may prove to be exceptionally stable in their solid formulations, at the same time providing advantages of higher solubility, purity, or perhaps better dispersability compared to the crystals of the thermodynamically more stable form. This is also helped by stringent requirements for the container-closure system and foil blister packaging, which are designed to prevent the moisture ingress that is detrimental for the dry powder inhaler performance. Many inhalation drugs have very low aqueous solubility, which limits both their therapeutic efficacy and therapeutic index; therefore some solid-state engineering may be required. This, first, includes synthesis of salts of ionizable drug molecules, potentially formation of cocrystals and, for more complex formulations, generating amorphous materials. In addition to enhanced solubility and bioavailability, composite amorphous particles may offer the benefits of superior dispersion, aerodynamic characteristics and dose uniformity. For example, both the "large-" and "small-" porous particles considered later in this chapter are normally amorphous, as are most of the particles with "open" and "corrugated" surface morphology that are typically produced using different spray-drying techniques (8,10,15). Solid and porous particles explored for sustained and controlled drug release options are usually also amorphous.

Stability of amorphous drugs alone or in the form of solid solution (molecular dispersion) with excipients is one of the most discussed and at the same time least understood topics of solid-state chemistry. It has been said that stabilization of amorphous formulations is often an empirical exercise (8,50). For small molecules, the amorphous state can result in manifold increase of equilibrium solubility and dissolution rate but at the expense of lower physicochemical stability, whereas for biological molecules, the glassy excipient matrix is necessary for their stability. The prevailing approach to describe these phenomena is centered on the concepts of "molecular mobility" and "structural relaxation" in the vicinity of the glass transition temperature, T_g. These concepts (and also the related terms "glass-forming ability" and "fragility") originate from the vitrification theories for inorganic glasses and polymers (51–53) which relate the cooperative molecular motions (α—relaxations) to certain measurable thermodynamic quantities such as the Kauzmann temperature, T_K, and configurational entropy, ΔS_c. The molecular mobility should be understood here as a parameter associated with the dynamic-mechanical or dielectric relaxation (51), directly responsible for the viscoelastic behavior during glass transition. For example, it can account for stickiness and irreversible sintering of inhalation particles (8). However, in terms of physicochemical stability as relevant to both recrystallization behavior of active ingredients for small drug molecules or stabilizing excipients for proteins, or most solid-state chemical reactions, these concepts alone proved to be inadequate. For some molecules, the temperatures just below T_g are shown to be sufficient for long-term stability, whereas others may undergo transitions even below the Kauzmann temperature (e.g., at temperature approximately T_g–50K which is usually considered a safe rule of thumb (8,50,54,55). Thus a growing body of experimental evidence suggests the importance of the higher frequency β-relaxations attributed to the localized molecular motions (see the detailed review in [56]). Other experimental evidence comes from studying thermal relaxations between different glass states (annealing) leading to changes with their thermodynamic functions (54,55,57,58). The activation energies, E_A, of these transitions, as measured using differential scanning calorimetry (DSC), isothermal calorimetry/thermal activity monitoring (TAM) or thermally stimulated current (TSC), can be classified in accordance with the α- and β-relaxations and are shown to be consistent with the same energies measured using dielectric relaxation spectroscopy (DRS) (54,55). However, a significant methodological issue with most of these descriptions is that the relationship between the critical thermodynamic and kinetic parameters responsible for physicochemical stability is predominantly sought in the form of empirical correlations or "couplings" with molecular mobility, but not from the kinetic mechanism for a specific transition. For example, α-relaxations were intuitively considered a precursor for crystallization (52,53); however, the elemental mechanism of crystallization for small molecules (31,59) does not include cooperative molecular motions, but requires localized rotational and short-order translational (approximate scale of intermolecular distance) motions. In addition, as shown below, a continuous Arrhenius-type dependence of crystallization times is expected for temperature ranges both below and above T_g. Thus, this process is more consistent with the characteristics of β-relaxations involving entire molecules, sometimes referred to as Johari-Goldstein relaxations (56), although the mechanistic relationship between the two, to the author's best knowledge, has not been established. This mechanism is considered below.

The kinetic equations for crystallization in supersaturated solutions and supercooled melts can be written as follows (31,59):

$$V_s \simeq f\Omega n e^{\frac{-\left(\Delta H^* - T\Delta S^*\right)}{RT}} \left(c - c_0\right)/\rho c \qquad (1.44)$$

$$V_m \simeq f\Omega n \frac{-\Delta S^*}{RT} e^{\frac{-\left(\Delta H^* - T\Delta S^*\right)}{RT}} \left(T_m - T\right) \qquad (1.45)$$

where V_s and V_m (cm/s) are the growth rates of crystal phase in solution or supercooled melt (or glass); c_0 and c (g/cm³) define the solute surface concentrations (the activity coefficients neglected) in the saturated (equilibrium) and supersaturated states at given temperature T; T_m is the melting temperature. ΔH^* and ΔS^* are correspondingly the enthalpy and entropy barriers for transitional complexes between solution (or melt/glass) and crystalline phases and thus define the kinetic rate of transition between the amorphous and crystalline states. For the pre-exponential parameters: f is the frequency of activation in the order of 10^{12}–10^{13} s⁻¹ (31); Ω is the molecular volume in crystal phase and n is the surface density of active molecular sites which depends on the specific crystallization mechanism (31,59). These pre-exponential multipliers play little role in the present discussion, but they are shown here to indicate that they may also depend on temperature.

Equations (1.44) and (1.45) are derived based on the absolute rate theory of chemical reactions (31) and therefore should be applicable to both liquid ($T > T_g$) and glass ($T < T_g$) crystallization. $\Delta c = (c - c_0)$ is absolute supersaturation and $\Delta T = (T_m - T)$ is supercooling, representing the crystallization driving forces. Deviation from this linearity occurs at large values of these parameters far from equilibrium; however, Eqs. (1.44) and (1.45) represent the most important attributes of crystallization kinetics in therms of both activation and thermodynamic functions. Diffusion may introduce an additional barrier in solid solutions (similar to liquid solutions [31]) but this would be manifested by a gradual decrease in the parameter Δc with crystallization time and does not alter the mechanism itself. For melts the mass-transfer is not limited by diffusion. Proportionality between the diffusion coefficient and crystal growth rate in amorphous state is coincidental because both of these quantities depend similarly on the activation energies, which should be considered the cause. It is possible that, if densities of the crystalline and glassy amorphous states are significantly different, this may cause mechanical stresses affecting the equilibrium and, as a result, change the thermodynamic driving force expressed through ΔT. The observations of crystal morphology and growth kinetics close to T_g, reported in (60), point to another effect which is well known for melt crystallization (59). It is related to changes of surface crystallization mechanism due to a surface kinetic transition (31,59), which is essentially a step-wise increase of the parameter n in Eqs. (1.44) and (1.45) and, correspondingly, an increase in the growth rate with increasing ΔT or Δc. This is particularly common for supercooled melts where specific interface energies are low and temperatures are high. On the other hand, transition of the crystallization front to the "fiber-like" morphology (60) can be associated with surface instabilities caused by non-uniform temperature gradients from the heat of crystallization combined with insufficient heat conductivity, leading to the surface perturbations growing with higher values of supercooling, ΔT, around fibers (59). Thus all of these phenomena can be explained within the context of classical crystallization theory. For more mechanistic details, refer to the monograph by Chernov (59).

The nucleation step may not be the limiting stage for crystallization for several reasons. Very low values of interfacial surface energy tend to reduce the critical nuclei size to a few nanometers. Such nuclei (or structures close to them) are also likely to be present after the glass annealing that inevitably occurs during the cooling stages. Even more important, the crystal growth rate or conversion rate are the actual experimental parameters usually measured in such systems, even when the lag-time, onset or induction time of crystallization are observed (57,58,61). Thus the major physicochemical parameters involved in the amorphous-to-crystalline stability can be associated with the growth of crystal phase. The characteristic time of growth in solution and melt are defined as follows (13):

$$\tau_s = \frac{(c - c_0)}{\rho_c \, SSA' V_s} \tag{1.46}$$

$$\tau_m = \frac{\rho_m}{\rho_c \, SSA' V_m} \tag{1.47}$$

where ρ_c and ρ_m are the crystal and melt densities, and SSA' defines the mean specific surface area of the crystal phase per unit volume of solution or melt, whereas V_s and V_m should be taken as the average growth rates during the time of conversion.

The enthalpy of activation complexes, ΔH^*, in Eqs. (1.44) and (1.45) is formally similar to the activation energy, E_A, describing the relaxation time:

$$\tau = \frac{1}{f} e^{\frac{E_A}{RT}} \tag{1.48}$$

Since the elemental molecular crystallization step includes a local molecular motion in the amorphous state, it can be written:

$$\Delta H^* = E_A + \Delta H' \tag{1.49}$$

where $\Delta H'$ is an additional activation enthalpy part responsible for incorporation into the crystal lattice. Equations (1.44) and (1.45) and (1.46) through (1.49) result in the following proportionality between the crystallization time, relaxation time, temperature and activation parameters:

$$\tau_s = \frac{\tau}{SSA'\Omega n} e^{\frac{-\Delta S^*}{R}} e^{\frac{\Delta H'}{RT}} \tag{1.50}$$

$$\tau_m = \frac{\tau \rho_m}{\rho_c \, SSA'\Omega n} \frac{R}{(-\Delta S^*)} e^{\frac{-\Delta S^*}{R}} e^{\frac{\Delta H'}{RT}} \frac{T}{\Delta T} \tag{1.51}$$

These equations indicate a linear relationship between the β-relaxation molecular mobility and crystallization time. For example, using the data provided in (61), the following value can be determined for a proprietary drug substance labeled there as SSR: $\Delta H^* = 79$ kJ/mol, $E_A = 52$ kJ/mol and $\Delta H' = 27$ kJ/mol. However, such quantitative data are very rare. For studies on β-relaxations, the crystallization data are usually missing, whereas in others the data on β-relaxations are absent and correlations are sought between crystallization time and α-relaxations. As explained above, the latter is not justified by the crystallization theory, although such correlations can certainly be built because both the crystallization time and time for α-relaxations increase progressively (or even linearly in log coordinates) versus $1/T$ within a narrow temperature interval around T_m.

From Eq. (1.51), the Arrhenius plot for crystallization in melt or glass is:

$$\ln\left(\tau_m \frac{\Delta T}{T}\right) \sim \frac{\Delta H^*}{RT} \tag{1.52}$$

The contribution of activation entropy cannot be determined from this plot; however, it can be estimated by the melting entropy at T_m:

$$\Delta S^* \approx \Delta S_m = \Delta H_m / T_m \tag{1.53}$$

For solid solutions the Arrhenius dependence of crystallization time versus inverse temperature holds as the crystallization time in terms of Eqs. (1.44) and (1.46) and is independent of solute concentration, but the data are very scarce for such systems. Contributions of different parameters can be assessed between two different amorphous glasses or melts at the same temperature assuming that their pre-exponential factors in Eq. (1.45) are similar:

$$\frac{\tau_{m1}}{\tau_{m2}} = \frac{\Delta S^*_2}{\Delta S^*_1} e^{\frac{-\Delta\Delta S^*}{R}} e^{\frac{\Delta\Delta H^*}{RT}} \frac{\Delta T_2}{\Delta T_1} \tag{1.54}$$

This relationship suggests that the activation enthalpy and entropy are the most essential parameters defining recrystallization time. For example, according to (58,62), for the two structurally related drugs investigated, nifedipine crystallizes much faster than felodipine, despite having very similar T_g values. The Arrhenius dependence Eq. (1.52) applied to data (58) gives the following values of the activation enthalpies around T_g: ΔH^* (nifedipine) = 28 kJ/mol; ΔH^* (felodipine) = 42 kJ/mol (the difference in these values is also confirmed by the data in [62]). Similar difference can be found by calculating data from reference (62). According to Eq. (1.54), $\Delta\Delta H^*$ provides by far the greatest differentiator for the crystallization time ratio ($\simeq 6 \times 10^{-3}$), with the next largest contribution from $\Delta\Delta S^{*}$ ($\simeq 6$) and smaller contributions from the configurational entropies and temperature, both at about 0.8. The product of all these contributions gives an order of approximately 10^2 faster crystallization times for nifedipine, which can be confirmed by the experimental values for their induction times (58).

As follows from the above considerations, the molecular relaxation/mobility constitutes only a partial descriptor of the phase transitions in amorphous systems. A more precise measure of these transitions involves definition of the activation energy and thermodynamic functions between the crystal and amorphous states. Although most amorphous systems are physically unstable, there is a possibility to kinetically control solid dispersions with appropriate choice of excipient matrixes for a sufficiently long shelf life. This choice is rather limited for melts, as their stability is defined by the inherent properties of the amorphous glasses. The chemical transformations, such as configurational stability of biological molecules, protein aggregation and some degradation reactions are also controlled by the activation energies of an amorphous matrix and would exhibit similar kinetic relationships to Eqs. (1.50) and (1.51). Unfortunately the energy landscape in the amorphous systems of pharmaceutical interest has not been sufficiently studied, perhaps due to the lack of robust experimental and theoretical methodologies to monitor kinetics of the solid state below T_g.

Lactose carriers and adhesive blends

With the notable exception of the original Turbuhaler® device utilizing spherical pellets of micronized drug, most currently marketed DPIs use blends with coarse crystalline lactose and designed for the high-potent Chronic Obstructive Pulmonary Disease (COPD) and asthma medications (10). Two main reasons for introducing any adhesive blend formulation are usually named as, first, diluting low drug doses to facilitate reproducible dose measuring and smaller device retention (for both prefilled single-dose units and multidose containers) and, second, improving the dispersability of highly cohesive micronized drug particles, potentially increasing the FPF and FPD for DPIs. It can be seen, however, that these formulation goals are somewhat contradictory in nature: stronger adhesion to carrier is necessary to break drug aggregates but, at the same time, it may require more aerodynamic or mechanical stresses to dislodge drug particles from the carrier surface than to disperse drug aggregates themselves. It can be noticed from many reviewed studies that measured FPFs are typically low, with most being within the 10%–30% interval. In addition, the mean interpatient variability in lung delivery was reported to be high at 30%–50% (8). These numbers indicate inefficiency of many blend formulations, since very similar FPFs can be achieved by using micronized drug powders alone (14,19). Perhaps not surprisingly, different studies on the effects of carrier particle size, coarse and fine particle fractions and lactose surface rugosity met with little success in obtaining conclusive results, with trends dependent on the carrier grade and device used (11). This ambiguity becomes even greater for a fixed dose combination of two or more drugs where the complexity of interactions leads to differences in the aerosol performance compared to the monotherapy, as well as to batch-to-batch variability (8,63). Some of these challenges come from the discussed methodological limitations in the formulation studies, where the surface and particulate powder properties or device aerosolization mechanism are not well defined. However there are indeed fundamental limitations for using such carriers.

An "ordered" mixture with carrier is envisaged as a single particulate drug layer on the carrier surface. The maximum theoretical drug weight fraction (or loading), m_d/m_c, to obtain such idealized coverage can be estimated using the following simplified relationship, which originates from the comparison between the specific surface areas, SSA (for drug) and SSA_c (for carrier) and Eq. (1.3):

$$\frac{m_d}{m_c} \simeq \Phi \frac{4 SSA_c}{SSA} = \Phi \frac{4\rho d \alpha_{svc}}{\rho_c d_c \alpha_{sv}} \qquad (1.55)$$

where α_{sv}, α_{svc}, d and d_c are the surface-to-volume shape coefficients and volume diameters for the active and carrier, correspondingly. Φ is the packing factor which is equal to approximately 0.9 for the ideal hexagonal packing of spheres, giving the maximum loading with perfect order at about 7.2% for diameters $d = 2$ μm and $d_l = 100$ μm, but, in reality, it is much lower because of disorder, defects and multilayers. Predictably, when the size of a coarse carrier increases at constant m/m_l, this leads to a competing effect between ordered mixtures and separation into drug aggregates. Loadings for such formulations are known to be between 0.1% and 4% (8,11). Assuming the same work of adhesion 20 mJ/ m² (see the section called "Particle aggregate strength"), an estimated strength of adhesion of these drug particles to the carrier particles is about 29 kPa, whereas a 10 μm aggregate composed of the same particles has strength 2.5 kPa. The absolute numbers here are less significant than the order of magnitude difference between them, which is related to the high adhesion strength of ordered layer. Large particles generally move with higher relative velocity to the airflow; thus, stresses increase approximately $(C_d d^2)^{1/3}$ (see the section called "Modeling of dry powder dispersion"). This factor leads to an increase of compression aerodynamic stress by a factor of 2, and shear stress for erosion mechanism by a factor of 5 for the carrier particles. Also the larger carrier particles have a greater Stk number and thus are more likely to collide with inhaler surfaces. All these effects may, at least partially, compensate for higher adhesion of drug particles to the carriers; however, in order to make use of the aerodynamic factors, the adhesive and cohesive aggregate strengths need to be balanced in a relatively small window of opportunity. Therefore, it is unlikely that carriers may lead to a higher FPF unless both the particle adhesion and cohesion are significantly reduced. It appears that, in general, ordered mixtures are not beneficial for deagglomeration and perhaps a mixture containing bulk excipient with uniformly dispersed small drug aggregates may be a better option in this case.

There are many different grades of lactose available commercially that vary by their particle size distribution (coarse and fine particle fractions), particle shape as well as by their surface and solid-state properties. Alpha-lactose monohydrate crystals are the original and still prevailing form used in DPIs, although other physical forms, for example, anhydrous beta-lactose, spray-dried amorphous lactose, and roller-dried anhydrous beta-lactose have been tried in R&D and may work better for some drug molecules (15). However, there is no well-defined strategy for selecting a specific type of lactose. It is clear from considerations in the section called "Particle aggregate strength" that, if lactose surfaces are rough on the scale smaller than characteristic size of primary drug particles, this would enhance dispersion, whereas larger defects may lead to an opposite effect. Reduction of the specific surface energy (and work of adhesion) reduces the adhesion to carrier and thus has a positive effect on dispersion, provided that uniform mixing can be achieved. Furthermore, the lactose surface can be modified by various techniques including surface smoothing with aqueous ethanol solvents, and wet coating with magnesium stearate or amino acids (64) or hydrophilic polymers, for example, hydroxypropyl methylcellulose (15). Most of the industrially oriented applications, however, focus on ternary mixtures with fine lactose particles and use of dry coating with hydrophobic "force control agents" (8,10,11,64,65).

Mixtures with fine lactose (roughly with median diameter between 2 and 10 μm) are the most accepted way of modifying dispersability of these formulations, although its effect on dispersion performance has also been inconsistent (11). A well-known mechanism proposed to explain a better dispersion is that fine lactose may occupy "active" strong bonding sites on carrier surface, thus reducing adhesion of drug particles. It should be said, however, that undamaged crystal surfaces or even surfaces of spray-dried particles are very uniform on this scale, both in terms of the surface morphology and specific surface energy. Of course, large mechanical defects and milling may create preferable adhesion sites. On the other hand, fine lactose is likely to create additional aggregates with drug particles. As seen from the calculations above, the strength of such aggregates is usually much smaller than that of ordered layers on large lactose carriers. The fine lactose-drug aggregation therefore may facilitate dispersion, but only when such aggregates are formed in significant quantity because they compete with both formations of coarse lactose-drug and drug–drug aggregates. Another possibility should be noted here: if large carrier particles are coated with fine lactose, this would disrupt the ordered layer of drug particles on the same surface, leading to reduction in this layer strength at least by a factor of 2 or greater (see the section called "Particle aggregate strength"). This fact has nothing to do with the "active sites," however, but with a statistical competition between fine lactose and drug particles within the layer, which may also lead to formation of fine lactose-drug aggregates.

An "ideal" adhesive mixture would have both cohesive and adhesive interactions reduced to a minimum. Such a task can be accomplished using either a coating with material of low adhesion or a coating reducing the particle contact area, or both. Magnesium stearate, a very common hydrophobic lubricant for oral dosage forms, has been tried extensively for adhesive respiratory blends, typically in concentrations 0.5%–3% w/w. Uniform coatings have been reported for lactose carriers as well as micronized drugs utilizing different high-energy shear mixing (64). Such intensive mechanical treatment also changes the particle surface morphology and possibly the particle size distribution, which need to be taken into account. Significant improvement of powder dispersability has been reported for coated materials in several studies (FPF about 50%) (64), presumably by reduction of adhesion and also moisture uptake by such coated powders. Other excipients tried as force-controlled agents in blends include leucine and lecithin, which are known for their surface-active properties. Although coatings can improve such formulations, the safety of the hydrophobic excipients (e.g., magnesium stearate) for use in the lungs has yet to be established at the concentrations used for dry powder formulations because their clearance mechanisms from the lungs are not well understood. More about different surface-active agents suitable for inhalable engineered particles will be discussed in the next section.

Although lactose has historically been employed in DPI formulation, it is not a universal drug carrier, as it can be chemically incompatible with certain drugs such as formoterol, and peptides or proteins through the Maillard reactions (15). Inter-batch variability of inhalation-grade lactose is known and, since it is a critical formulation ingredient, the precise grade and manufacturer of lactose has to be specified for regulatory applications and continuously monitored in the cGMP environment. Mannitol, a non-reducing sugar alcohol, has been extensively investigated as an alternative carrier, sometimes demonstrating a higher respirable fraction than standard lactose carrier (15) as well as improved physicochemical stability (being more crystalline and less hydroscopic than lactose); thus, it is particularly suitable for blend formulations with biological molecules (66). Ternary mixtures with jet-milled fine mannitol have also been investigated, so all mechanistic principles highlighted above for lactose formulations can also be applied to this carrier. Mannitol is currently on the list of regulatory-approved (by the FDA and EMA) excipients for inhalation.

Engineered solid particles

The greatest potential to manipulate aerodynamic and dispersive properties lies in formulation of uniform particles with controlled size, shape, density and surface characteristics (rugosity and work of cohesion/adhesion). In parallel, engineering such particles may achieve goals related to their solid-state structural stability; dissolution and drug release functionality, including fixed-dose drug combination; potential for sustained or controlled release; and site-specific drug targeting.

One of the most significant advancements in powder technologies for respiratory drug delivery was the application of spray drying to inhalable forms of insulin conducted in 1990s. Although the marketing strategy for these products failed, extensive physicochemical and manufacturing developments in this area have had a large impact, leading to other opportunities. "Small" low-density ($d < 5$ μm) particles are produced by the PulmoSphere® process, involving spraying an emulsion of fluorocarbon (perfluorooctyl bromide) in water stabilized by phospholipid, where the drug is dissolved or dispersed in the external aqueous phase, which also contains excipients. The fluorocarbon serves as a blowing agent at high temperature to produce porous or hollow structures with a powder tapped density <0.1 g/cm³ (3,15). Further progress has been achieved in the use of these particles to deliver inhaled antibiotics to treat lung infections, resulting in the TOBI Podhaler® product (8). The AIR® inhaled insulin system was based on "large" porous particles (67) ($d > 5$ μm, tapped powder density <0.4 g/cm³) comprised of dipalmitoyl phosphatidylcholine (DPPC) with a characteristic "crumpled" particle morphology (16). This morphology reduces the effective particle density and aerodynamic diameter with a contribution from the particle shape factor. Presumably, a similar process is used to make formulations for inhaled levodopa (marketing application for Inbrija® [CVT-301]). In parallel with these commercial developments, a number of approved drugs, including those for asthma and COPD, pulmonary infections, and some peptides and proteins for systemic delivery, have been reformulated using the porous particles approach and evaluated in animal studies or even investigated in human trials, but none yet have reached the market. More information on different lipid formulations and animal and clinical studies can be found in (16).

In addition to the optimized aerodynamic diameter combined with a larger geometric diameter, spray-dried particles often exhibit higher particle rugosity (surface asperities), which is also advantageous for reducing the aggregates strength. All of these factors lead to the possibility of high emitted dose, low device retention, and high FPF which may be between 65% and 95% (15,16). Here the effect of surface morphology on the aggregate packing can be more important than the reduction of interparticulate forces: the asperities and low particle density both lead to formation of loose aggregates desired for better fluidization and dispersion in DPIs. On the other hand, reduced flowability of such powders compared with the engineered blends has necessitated the use of more advanced filling machines (8,16). Another very important approach is the incorporation of force-control agents into the particle shell, which can be applied to both low-density particles and particles with relatively

high density ($\rho_p > 1$ g/cm³) (35). Phosphatidylcholines such as distearoyl phosphatidylcholine (DSPC) and dipalmitoyl phosphatidylcholine (DPPC) can serve this purpose, with the very significant advantage of being endogenous surfactants present in the lungs. In addition, DPPC has been shown to enhance the permeation (absorption) of some active ingredients (15). DSPC is approved as a shell-forming excipient in TOBI Podhaler with a nominal daily dose of more than 50 mg (8). These surfactant molecules tend to accumulate on particle surfaces during spray drying, thus enhancing their surface modification effect. Another extensively studied group of compounds include hydrophobic amino acids, from which leucine has shown an exceptional dispersion enhancing effect for a number of spray-dried pulmonary formulations (15,35). For instance, in the case of disodium cromoglycate (DSCG) (35), the relatively strong cohesion characteristic of the pure drug resulted in a strong dependence of FPF on the inhalers type and the airflow rate, but leucine-containing powders exhibited a significant increase in FPF and a reduction of FPF dependence on the flow rate and inhaler type. It was proposed that this effect can be correlated with the different polarity of intermolecular interactions between DSCG and leucine at the particle surface, expressed by the difference in their component Hansen solubility parameters measured by IGC. In this work it was also suggested that higher segregation of leucine on the particle surfaces, even for dense particles, may lead to increased particle rugosity.

Porous particles or hollow particles can be obtained by a variety of different processing techniques, including spray drying, spray freezing, emulsion and some supercritical fluid (SCF) methods (see Table 1.2 and Figure 1.5). From the currently marketed formulations, one needs to mention fast-acting inhalable insulin drug product (Afrezza®) which is composed of aggregates (2–3 μm) of fumaryl diketopiperazine (FDKP) nanosize platelet crystals, providing a high SSA with insulin absorbed on or otherwise distributed within these aggregates. The bioavailability of insulin is significantly enhanced with FDKP, also leading to a fast onset of action for this formulation. This method can be classified in a group where carriers are produced by crystallization or coacervation in liquid solutions (15).

Crystallization in supercritical carbon dioxide with very rapid mixing (13) tends to produce highly crystalline materials of controlled size, which have been extensively studied for small-molecule anti-asthmatic compounds such as salmeterol xinafoate, albuterol sulfate, terbutaline sulfate and fenoterol hydrobromide (14,15,68). The advantages of particle engineering in this case relate mostly to a reduction in specific surface energy, combined with relatively large surface-to-volume shape factor for these single crystals. As described previously (13,15), all direct crystallization techniques, including the SCF crystallization, are subject to limitations in their lowest particle size by the fundamental parameters of nucleation and growth. Thus, they have to be optimized to obtain

MMAD within a desired respirable range. In some cases, this requires a very significant process modification so that such SCF technology is not universal, which is also true for any other technology. Considering the high-pressure equipment, there are also restrictions imposed by the manufacturing scale and higher complexity compared to spray drying, which up-to-date has prevented this technology from being used commercially.

From the other potential techniques for solid particle engineering (see Table 1.2), spray-freeze-drying in various modifications (15,69,70) holds promise, notwithstanding its manufacturing complexity, because of the ability to produce

Table 1.2 Different types of engineered particles for inhalation, therapeutic areas of application (current or potential), and particle formation techniques used

Particle type	Products or potential therapeutic applications	Particle formation techniques
Lipid microparticles (1,8,16,63,74)	Exubera® (insulin), TOBI Podhaler (tobramycin), Inbrija (levodopa); APIs for asthma and COPD, antibiotics; candidates for systemic delivery, carriers for fixed-dose therapy	Spray drying (PulmoSphere; AIR/Arcus® platforms)
Liposomes (1,16)	Arikayce® (amikacin), Lipoquin®/Pulmaquin® (Linhaliq™) (ciprofloxacin) antibiotics, antifungals, pain medication, hormones, therapeutic proteins, oligonucleotides, cyclosporine, asthma and oncology drugs	Liquid dispersion/separation/encapsulation/osmosis, combined with lyophilization, spray- or freeze-drying (for dry powder formulations)
Engineered microcrystals (14,15,19)	Candidates for asthma and COPD, antibiotics and other drugs for systemic delivery	SCF crystallization; direct solution crystallization, emulsion-based crystallization
Composite microparticles (8,15,35) (including amorphous porous structures and shells)	Stabilized therapeutic proteins, peptides, vaccines, candidates for asthma and COPD	Spray drying, spray freeze drying, coacervation
Nanocrystals/nanosuspensions (15,46,79)	Candidates for asthma and COPD	High-pressure homogenization, wet (ball) milling, emulsion-based precipitation, SCF extraction of emulsions
Nanoaggregates (15,77,79)	Afrezza® (insulin), antibiotics, asthma and COPD compounds, immune-suppressants, contrast agents, anticancer agents	Precipitation, coacervation, spray drying, spray freeze drying (of emulsions, nanosuspensions)
Polymeric micro- and nanospheres or capsules (1,71,78)	Antibiotics, anticancer drugs, therapeutic proteins, peptides, plasmid DNA, for sustained/controlled-release or targeting	Emulsion-based precipitation, SCF extraction of emulsions
Solid lipid nanoparticles (16,74)	Antiasthmatics, antibiotics, anticancer compounds, peptides, DNA, siRNA for targeting and controlled release	High-pressure homogenization, emulsion-based precipitation, SCF extraction of emulsions
Surface-modified micelles (1,7)	Anticancer, antiasthmatic, antigen compounds for solubilization, sustained/controlled release	Self-assembly
Exploratory miscellaneous: dendrimers, polymer conjugates, carbon nanotubes, mesoporous silica, surface-modified colloidal gold, microfabricated shapes (1,7,8)	Anticancer compounds, various model compounds	Surface reactions, grafting, solution impregnation, templating/lithography

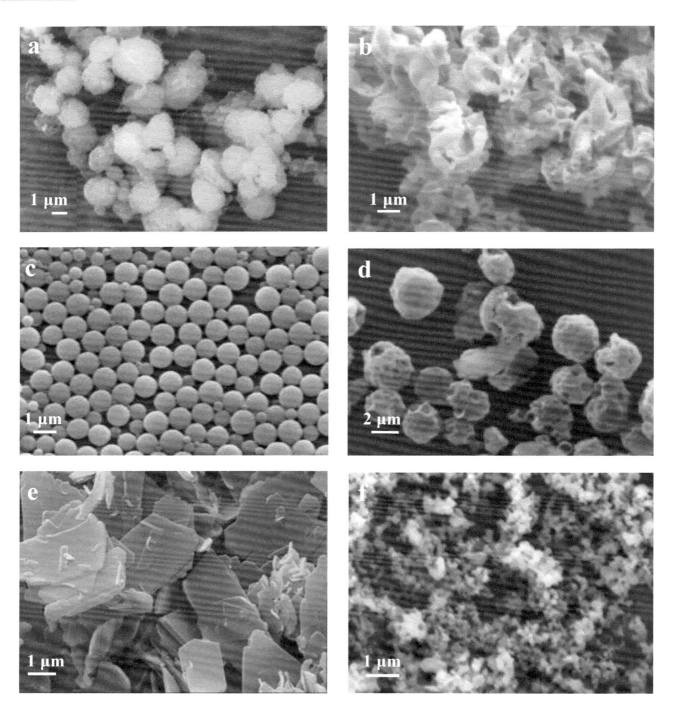

Figure 1.5 Scanning electron microscopy images of: (a) Spray freeze-dried insulin/trehalose formulation; (b) spray freeze-dried vaccine formulation; (c) solid PLGA microparticles fabricated using SCF extraction of emulsions; (d) porous deslorelin-PLGA microparticles prepared by SCF expansion; (e) crystals of salmeterol xinafoate; and (f) nanoparticles of a new drug candidate for respiratory delivery, both prepared by SCF crystallization. Previously published photos are reproduced with permission. ([c] From Chattopadhyay, P. et al., *J. Pharm. Sci.*, 95, 667–680, 2006; [d] From Koushik, K., and Kompella, U.B., *Pharm. Res.*, 21, 524–535, 2004; [e] From Shekunov, B.Y. et al., *J. Aerosol Sci.*, 34, 553–568, 2003.)

porous respirable particles of stabilized biological entities, including peptides, proteins and vaccines (see Figure 1.5), which is also supported by an extensive formulation research and development already done in the area of lyophilization. Nanoaggregates consisting of solid nanoparticles in a format of larger respirable microparticles may possess some advantages, from the perspective of either improved dissolution or modified uptake mechanism in the lungs, when formulated to disintegrate into primary nanoparticles *in vivo*.

On the other end of the drug delivery spectrum, polymeric and lipid micro- and nanocarriers can be used to improve efficacy and reduce systemic toxicity in many potential respiratory applications (1,7,16,46,71–79). For nanoparticles, the volume-equivalent particle diameter where distinct quantitative changes occur with particles' solid-state thermodynamic/surface properties and biological responses (e.g., translocation and endocytosis) is approximately 100 nm (16), and this unique advantage can be utilized for transfection into the lung cells (Figure 1.6). Nanoparticles are typically produced by different emulsion-, self-assembly, or homogenization-based methods and showed some promise during *in vitro* and in animal studies. Polymers exploited for respiratory drug delivery included natural molecules such as albumin and polysaccharides carrageenan, chitosan, gelatin, and hyaluronic acid; certain synthetic biocompatible and biodegradable polymers such as poly(lactic) acid (PLA), poly(lactic-co-glycolide acid) (PLGA), poly(vinyl) alcohol (PVA); and block polymers such as PLA-PEG-PLA.

One of the major obstacles to employing many excipients is their safety profiles, especially for chronic indications. On the other hand, solid lipid nanoparticles (16) offer a higher biocompatibility and lower potential (acute and chronic) toxicity than polymeric nanoparticles or any other synthetic nano-constructs, as well as a relatively streamlined manufacturing process, which ideally is a high-pressure homogenization from low-temperature melts. The actives are usually incorporated within the lipid core matrix but may also be physically or chemically absorbed onto the surface (e.g., biomolecules) or form lipid-drug conjugates. These formulations typically contain between 0.1% and 30% w/w of lipid phase (a combination of triglycerides, acylglycerols, fatty acids, steroids, and sometimes waxes or paraffins) stabilized in an aqueous suspension with 0.5%–5% w/w of suitable surfactants. The challenges with these systems are typically related to their relatively low drug loading capacity (likely <1% w/w relative to the lipid phase) limited by the solubility of most drugs in solid lipids, which may also lead to insufficient drug release characteristics (16). Micelles (5–100 nm size range), formed from amphiphilic block copolymers or polyethylene-glycol- (PEG-)modified lung surfactants, can overcome many of these disadvantages and currently represent a somewhat underexplored area of nano-formulations. The feasibility of all these systems for sustained/controlled respiratory drug delivery has yet to be proven, however, in clinic trials and on an industrial scale.

Liposomes

Liposomes are vesicles usually comprised of different phosphatidylcholine (PC) derivatives (e.g., egg or soy PC, DPPC, DSPC) which are biocompatible and biodegradable in the lung. These natural surfactants form structures varying in size from less than 50 nm for unilamellar liposomes to several microns for multilamellar liposomes. The hydrophilic drugs may be encapsulated within the aqueous interior or lipophilic drugs incorporated within the lipid bilayers, which may also include cholesterol to increase the vesicle rigidity, surface modification with PEG, or agents for targeting liposomes to specific receptors. The physicochemical properties of liposomes and their drug release profile can be modified through the liposomal composition, size, membrane thickness, charge and drug loading characteristics, and other factors including osmolarity, pH, and choice of buffer and excipients. Thus, in principle, liposomes represent a versatile drug delivery platform for small molecules, nucleic acids, and peptides, with the rationale of modifying the pharmacokinetic profile in the lung, typically to treat lung diseases (16). These systems have been investigated for their potential as a pulmonary drug delivery vehicle since the mid-1980s, with a number of inhaled liposomal formulations for asthma and oncology applications investigated in the clinic; however, the most active areas of current clinical research involve liposomal formulations of the antifungals and antibiotics. Inhaled liposomal formulation Arikayce (amikacin) has been approved by FDA, and another antibiotic formulation Linhaliq™ (ciprofloxacin) is still under development after receiving complete response letter from FDA in January 2018. In terms of the excipient safety profile, several different formulations containing synthetic or animal-derived lung surfactants, mainly DPPC (e.g., Exosurf® and Curosurf®), have already been used for treatment of neonatal respiratory distress syndrome.

Despite the fact that liposomes have a long R&D history, including more than ten approved liposomal products in other therapeutic areas, their formulation and

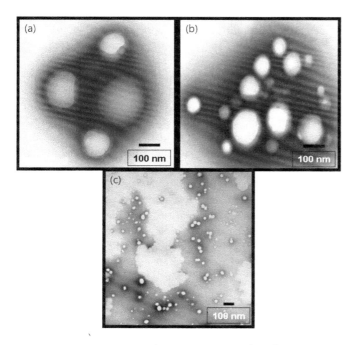

Figure 1.6 Transmission electron micrographs of nanoparticles a plasmid DNA (pFlt23K or pEGFP) encapsulated into PLGA using supercritical fluid extraction of emulsions and used for studies of *in vitro* transfection into human lung alveolar epithelial cells (A549). (a) PLGA (85:15)-placebo nanoparticles, (b) pFlt23K-PLGA (2%, w/w, loaded) nanoparticles, and (c) pEGFP-PLGA (20% w/w, loaded) nanoparticles. (Reproduced from Mayo, A.S. et al., *Int. J. Pharmaceutics*, 387, 278–285, 2010. With permission.)

manufacturing still present some challenges, which may serve as an example for other nanoparticulate drug delivery systems. Liposomes spontaneously form when lipid layers are hydrated under shear. However, the industrial processes can be quite sophisticated, involving lipid dissolution and removal of organic solvent, concentration, homogenization or extrusion through a membrane, whereas drug loading can occur during liposome formation, or after formation using a pH or ion gradient for ionizable drugs. The quality control requirements include physicochemical stability of both drug and critical excipients. The lipids are known to undergo degradation via acid or base catalyzed lipid hydrolysis or oxidation reactions. This problem, prevalent earlier for impure and inhomogeneous lipids, is now dramatically reduced by using well-controlled cGMP supply sources and use of high-purity semisynthetic lipids (16). Liposomes must also maintain physical stability to provide the desired drug release characteristics, which include vesicle lamellarity, size distribution and charge/zeta potential, membrane permeability and the drug encapsulation state. These parameters have to be sustained during manufacturing, shelf life (presumably with acceptable stability at least 18 months), and product use, which includes aerosolization and possible reconstitution from lyophilized state. Although significant progress has been achieved, stability still represents an issue for most inhalable formulations. For liquid formulations, more robust to dispersion stresses are small unilamellar liposomes with hydrophobic drugs incorporated into the lipid layer, as was confirmed by experimental studies (16). For dry powder formulations, liposomes are protected during dehydration (e.g., by spray drying or freeze drying) by glass-forming excipients such as sucrose or trehalose (8,15), which also help maintaining integrity of liposomes during rehydration. Several dry powder liposome formulations have been explored for respiratory drug delivery of small molecules and macromolecules (8).

pMDI solutions and suspensions

The formulations for pressurized metered-dose inhalers (pMDIs) contain drugs either suspended or solubilized in a propellant, with the help of stabilizing excipients and/or cosolvents. In their original design, pMDIs were based on chlorofluorocarbon (CFC) propellants, which were later phased-out due to their detrimental environmental impact (formalized in the 1989 Montreal Protocol). The introduction of hydrofluoroalkane (HFA) propellants as replacements necessitated reformulation of several compounds (as well as some canister changes) because of their different physicochemical properties. Although both HFAs 134a and 227 have similar boiling point and vapor pressure as CFC 12 (17), generally enabling filling under similar manufacturing conditions, there are significant differences in their molecular properties such as decreased polarizability, increased dipole moment, higher hydrogen bonding propensity and higher water solubility for HFAs, leading typically to

lower solubility of non-polar solutes and higher solubility of hydrogen-bonding polar solutes in HFAs (17). For example, beclomethasone dipropionate (BDP) is partially soluble in HFA134a, which results in an unstable dispersion and particle growth of this compound (80). Other excipient groups used include co-solvents (typically ethanol with possible addition of glycerol or PEG), surfactants/suspending aids and different preservatives (for a detailed list see [17]). It seems that the initial droplet velocity of CMC was much greater (>30 m/s) for CFCs than for HFAs (2–8.4 m/s) (63). This is likely related to the thermodynamic properties (i.e., enthalpy of evaporation, viscosity, surface tension) of these propellants during atomization. In this case, the low velocity is more advantageous for lower mouth-throat deposition but may potentially affect the particle dispersability in suspensions or primary particle size in solution formulations.

If the drug is completely dissolved in the formulation, then particle formation may proceed in sequence: propellant atomization—formation of less volatile drops (e.g., ethanol cosolvent, non-volatile cosolvent and excipients)—formation of solid drug particles (possibly also in combination with supersaturated solution). For suspension formulations, this sequence is: propellant atomization—dispersion of solid drug particles (possibly in combination with carriers/excipients). In the first instance, formation of drug particles occurs in situ by drop evaporation at relatively low temperatures, affected by concentration of the cosolvents and the drug. The droplets may not entirely dry and increase deposition in the mouth and throat. Conversely, the same factors may affect the precipitation mechanism, leading to the structures that are often observed during the spray-drying process such as porous/hollow and amorphous particles (81). The process may also result in significant changes with the solid-state chemistry and dissolution, including formation of different solvates or hydrates dependent on the formulation characteristics, in particular, on the ethanol content and co-drugs concentrations (e.g., BDP and formoterol fumarate) (80). For suspension formulations, the major concerns are related to physicochemical stability of such particles (i.e., particle growth, agglomeration, flocculation, sedimentation or phase separation) directly affecting the dose uniformity. MMAD is largely defined by the primary particle size (given low particle number concentration), although this may also be affected by the particle aggregation before atomization, as well as the size, density and viscosity of the suspension droplets during evaporation, which depends on many formulation characteristics (17).

Particle engineering techniques used for the DPI formulations can also in general be applied to pMDIs, provided that the propellant does not affect the particles' physicochemical stability and the particle concentration is sufficiently small for proper functioning of the valve-metering system. It is likely that specific surface energy in propellants is reduced compared to that at the particle-air interface, by as much as an order of magnitude judging by the corresponding values for crystals in different media (31), further reducing propensity for particle aggregation in propellants (see the section called "Particle aggregate strength"). This effect can be pronounced for both solid and porous particles, although perhaps the experimental evidence in this respect is lacking. The original rationale for use of porous lipid microparticles in pMDI formulations was the ability to provide better control over particle size with improved FPF, which might lead to both higher lung doses and reduced dose variability. This superior aerosol performance was indeed confirmed in the laboratory for three PulmoSphere pMDI formulations of cromolyn, albuterol and formoterol and in the clinic for the albuterol PulmoSphere formulation compared to a conventional micronized pMDI formulation (16), although currently there are no pMDI drug products based on such engineered particles. For drugs that are soluble in the pMDI propellant (e.g., glycopyrrolate) or have poor long-term stability in the form of single engineered particles, there are other options. Several studies have been conducted on use of bulking agents (such as lactose and leucine) to improve suspension stability (and dose uniformity) by employing different grades of micron- and submicron size excipient particles to form drug-excipient coflocculated matrix (17).

From a different perspective, advanced carrier-drug mixtures can be beneficial for fixed-dose drug combinations. Such formulations may represent significant challenges for any inhaler type due to chemical incompatibility of drugs, different drug solubilities in a single solvent system but more often because of the difficulty to deliver the required fixed dose as solid particles, for a range of drug loadings, and for individual drugs as required for comparative clinical studies. For DPIs there is also a potential dependency on the airflow rate. If different micronized drug particles are suspended in a pMDI, they may form separate aggregates/flocculates of different composition, producing different FPFs for individual drugs, thus not allowing for dose proportionality. This problem can be solved in different ways, but one of the most developed approaches consists of using standard micronized drug powders co-suspended with porous lipid microparticles (17,63). These excipient particles provide a bulk dilution for the drug, with the possibility of reducing interparticle interactions between carrier-drug aggregates and increasing physical stability for such suspensions. A fixed-dose pMDI combination product containing glycopyrrolate and formoterol fumarate has been commercially approved in the United States as Bevespi Aerosphere™. Recent investigations of triple-drug combinations with the Co-Suspension® technology have shown that the three major drug classes for treating asthma and COPD (i.e., long-acting beta-agonist [LABA], long-acting muscarinic antagonist [LAMA] and bronchodilator inhaled corticosteroid [ICS]), each with differing pharmacological and physicochemical properties) can be consistently delivered with the same FPF and MMAD by single pMDI, compared with giving each component individually, or as a one- or two-drug combination (63). The principal difference between this type of formulation and those containing standard lactose blends is that porous lipid microparticles may be delivered into the lung together with the drug load, thus eliminating the need to separate them from the carrier surfaces. As discussed above, the capacity of engineered blends to accept drug load is inversely proportional to both the carrier particle diameter and density, so for porous particles of 3–5 μm geometric diameter, this capacity is increased by about two orders of magnitude compared to lactose carriers. Measurements of the aggregate strength between drug crystals and porous microparticles in such systems have not been reported, but most likely such associations are reduced compared to the ordered lactose mixtures. More important, the large excess of the surface area available in such formulations physically separate drug crystals from each other so that there is a reduced probability for the drug-to-drug particle interactions.

CONCLUSIONS AND FUTURE PERSPECTIVE

The major goal of this chapter was to define different critical parameters and quality attributes that govern performance of respiratory formulations. Special emphasis was placed on quantitative description of mechanisms that present challenges or are identified as knowledge gaps in the current development of respiratory drug delivery technology. These topics include particle dispersion and flow rate dependence, interparticle interactions and aggregate strength, the relationship between aerodynamic dispersion and inhaler design, the performance of carrier-based formulations and engineered particles, and fundamental and practically important subjects such as particle dissolution and solid-state stability of amorphous materials.

Clearly, understanding physicochemical particle properties is paramount for designing efficient and robust inhalation products. In this relationship, the first-principles systematic approach may represent a more time- and cost-efficient strategy than empirically driven statistical DoE studies, which dominate current research and development. Within the remits of this chapter, the following points are discussed:

- Particle aerodynamic diameter and Stokes number can be defined a priori for any airflow regime of inhaler device, cascade impactor or mouth-throat deposition using experimentally determined geometric particle diameter, density, surface-to-volume shape factor and drag coefficients (see the section called "Aerodynamic diameter and Stokes number").
- Particle aggregate strength, the major parameter of dispersability, can be calculated on the basis of the model proposed, taking into account the aggregates size structure and particle rugosity, but within the limitations imposed by the undefined interparticulate contact area (see the section called "Particle aggregate strength").
- The model of aerodynamic dispersion enables the relationship between FPF and airflow rate to be determined based on different deaggregation kernels that are classified and ranked according to the magnitude

of aerodynamic or mechanical stresses involved. In addition, quantitative relationship is established between the inhaler parameters in terms of the device resistance, residence time, characteristic dispersion volume/dimensions and the average rate of energy dissipation which is a fundamental property of turbulence (see the section called "Modeling of dry powder dispersion").

- Atomization of droplets for different liquid formulations can be adequately described by the maximum stable droplet size, which can also be linked to the dispersion mechanisms for such formulations and devices (see the section called "Atomization of droplets").
- Dissolution of inhalable particles is largely determined by their solid-state properties rather than by solution diffusion or agitation. The dissolution profile in case of immediate release is defined through the particle size distribution, shape factor, surface kinetic coefficient and equilibrium solubility by a cubic polynomial function (see the section called "Drug solubility and mechanism of particle dissolution").
- It is proposed that the activation enthalpy and entropy associated with non-cooperative molecular (rotational and translational) motions are the most essential fundamental parameters defining the different types of transitions in amorphous state. The contribution of these activation parameters, together with contributions from supersaturation (or supercooling) and configurational entropy can be assessed in experimental studies, although challenged by the long times required for such measurements below the glass transition temperature (see the section called "Solid-state chemistry of crystalline and amorphous materials").
- Quantitative analysis of interactions in the carrier blends indicated that ordered mixtures are often undesirable for efficient deagglomeration, whereas the engineering of such blends requires reduction in both drug–drug and drug-carrier interactions. Such a task can be achieved, in principle, using ternary mixtures with micro- and nanoparticles or surface coatings (see the section called "Lactose carriers and adhesive blends").
- Solid engineered particles currently represent the most advanced (and commercially proven) approach to achieving superior aerodynamic characteristics, dose uniformity and potentially drug-release functionality. This approach can be used for both DPI and pMDI systems. Liposomes also represent commercially viable and potentially versatile drug delivery systems, when their physicochemical stability can be controlled in the liquid or solid formulation. Other particle engineering techniques offer an array of possibilities to modify particles properties and drug release characteristics, but their clinical/industrial potentials have yet to be determined (see the sections called "Engineered solid particles," "Liposomes," and "pMDI solutions and suspensions").

These points represent only a brief overview of the most important, from the author's perspective, physicochemical properties and mechanisms involved in the material science of respiratory drug delivery. The optimistic intention here is to show that most issues or limitations can be resolved rationally by using an integral approach to the formulation/inhaler design and to particle technology, and in relationship to the device-patient interface. Some factors, however, are beyond pure technical feasibility. Although encouraging, the use of solid engineered particles or liposomes in several currently approved (or close to the marketing authorization) products has to be cautiously considered in the light of over 25 years industrial development in this area. The current products with advanced formulations are based on well-known active ingredients, such as antibiotics or fixed dose combination asthma medicines, rather than new chemical or biological entities. There is also a very little current interest in developing inhalation products for systemic delivery or sustained release. Although there are many potential possibilities in this area, the more delicate biology of the lungs imposes more risks and requires more subtle approaches compared to delivery through the gastrointestinal tract. Thus, it would be premature to say that particle engineering has become an accepted approach to formulation of new drugs, although there are clear and distinct advantages for these particles in terms of high efficiency and dose uniformity.

In this connection, it is worthwhile to consider parallels with nanotechnology platforms previously discussed in our review on lipid inhalable formulations (16). Nanomedicine has been one of the most speculative areas after decades of research and development with little practical success until now. The main reason seems to be in the lack of clinical justification for biopharmaceutical mode of action and drug targeting of nanoparticles compared to more traditional formulations, also with uncertainties associated with long-term toxicity or immunogenicity, particularly for formulations using new excipients. These conceptual issues are combined with very significant industrial difficulties in optimizing and controlling physicochemical properties of nanocarriers on a relatively large and complex manufacturing scale, thus creating additional (either psychological or real) hurdles for the industrial development.

The industrial perspective is often missed in academic studies, particularly considering certain aspects of product developability such as short- and long-term physicochemical stability, cGMP manufacturing scalability, process control and robustness, and increased complexity/challenges with the regulatory submissions. Although theoretically the number of possibilities for different technologies and formulations is endless, one has to take into account that full-scale industrial applications dramatically restrict this choice, mostly on the basis of available, regulatory accepted and cGMP-controlled excipients as well as natural gravitation to simple manufacturing procedures and proven formulation strategies. The major concerns of any pharmaceutical company are finding the fastest, risk-controlled development path to a viable pharmaceutical product and, second, creating its reliable supply to patients. The area of inhalation products is not different. If a new particle formulation or engineering technology cannot offer substantial and clear benefits for ether biopharmaceutics or industrial manufacturing, it is highly unlikely that such a technology can be successful commercially.

It is inevitable, however, that an increasing range of sophisticated respiratory drug delivery systems will be available to the patient. One of the driving forces is the shift from traditional crystalline drugs to larger synthetic or biological molecules, which necessitates development of stabilized amorphous formulations and engineered particles. Second, there is an introduction of new classes of potent medicines, or their combinations, specifically tailored for the delivery to the lungs and requiring higher efficiency, reproducibility, and higher therapeutic index achievable with an advanced inhaler-formulation design. An additional aspect of advanced formulation strategies that should not be ignored is the ability to generate novel intellectual property and to withstand generic competition, which is important for progressing such systems into commercial development. Eventually, particles will be designed for sustained and targeted delivery for topical applications, or delivery modes in which excipients play a functional role, for example, enhancing drug stability, adsorption, or residence time *in vivo*. The idea of systemic delivery is still viable for classes of drugs that require the rapid onset of action or enhanced bioavailability of pulmonary administration. The current state and potential applications of such therapeutics are discussed in the following chapters of this book.

NOMENCLATURE

C_c Cunningham slip correction factor
C_d particle drag coefficient
c solution concentration
c_0 equilibrium concentration (solubility)
D diffusion coefficient of solute
D_i diffusion coefficient of solute within particles (for sustained release)
d volume-weighted particle diameter
d_0 characteristic interparticle (lattice) parameter in the aggregate model
$d_{4,3}$ mass-weighted momentum of aerodynamic particle size distribution
d_A aerodynamic diameter
d_c volume-weighted diameter of carrier
d_{max} maximum stable droplet diameter
d_p volume-weighted diameter of primary particles
d_s cross-section equivalent diameter
E Young's modulus of aggregate
E_s Young's modulus of impact surface
F interparticulate bonding force
FPD fine particle dose
FPF fine particle fraction
FPF_0 initial *FPF* before dispersion

FPF_{max} maximum achievable *FPF* for given formulation
f frequency of activation of transitional complexes
ΔH^* enthalpy of transitional complexes in amorphous state
$\Delta H'$ enthalpy of activation for incorporation into the crystal lattice
K mean coordination number of particles in aggregate
K_b coordination number in aggregate bulk
K_e coordination number on aggregate surface
k total mass-transfer coefficient
k_i internal mass-transfer coefficient within particles
k_s mass-transfer coefficient on particle surface
k_D diffusion mass-transfer coefficient
L characteristic large-scale dimension in a device
$MMAD$ mass-median aerodynamic diameter
m relative amount of drug dissolved
m_A relative mass of unbroken aggregates
m_d mass of drug in blend
m_c mass of carrier in blend
n density of active molecular sites on crystal interface
Oh Ohnesorge number
ΔP device air pressure drop
Q airflow rate
q number of contacts between particles
Re Reynolds number
R_D device resistance
Sh Sherwood number
SSA specific surface area per unit mass
SSA' specific surface area per unit volume of solution or melt
Stk Stokes number
Stk_e generalized (effective) Stokes number
ΔS_c configurational entropy
ΔS^* configurational entropy of transitional complexes in amorphous state
T temperature
T_g glass transition temperature
T_m melting temperature
U mean airflow velocity
u particle relative (slip) velocity
V_s crystal growth rate in solid solution
V_m crystal growth rate in melt (glass)
V volume of effective dispersion zone
W work of adhesion
We Weber number
x power of ε in the breakage kernel
y diameter of asperity
α_{sv} surface-to-volume shape factor
Γ relative rate of aggregate breakage (breakage kernel)
γ_L droplet surface tension
γ_s specific surface free energy
δ thickness of the diffusion boundary layer
ε average rate of energy dissipation per unit mass
θ equilibrium distribution (partition) coefficient of solute
λ_K Kolmogorov scale of turbulence
μ dynamic air viscosity

μ_L dynamic liquid viscosity
ν kinematic viscosity of air
ρ particle (aggregate) density
ρ_0 air density
ρ_c crystal density
ρ_m melt density
ρ_{max} powder density at the maximum coordination number
ρ_p primary particle density
ρ_1 unit density
σ aerodynamic stress
σ_A aggregate strength
σ_L surface tension pressure
σ_T aggregate tensile strength
τ mean residence time of aggregates during dispersion
τ_s characteristic time of growth in solution
τ_m characteristic time of growth in melt
Φ packing factor of ordered layer in blends
ψ non-Stokesian particle drag correction factor
Ω molecular volume in crystal phase

REFERENCES

1. Loira-Pastoriza C, Todorof J, Vanbever R. Delivery strategies for sustained drug release in the lungs. *Adv Drug Deliv Rev.* 2014;75:81–91.
2. Patel B, Gupta N, Ahsan F. Particle engineering to enhance or lessen particle uptake by alveolar macrophages and to influence the therapeutic outcome. *Eur J Pharm Biopharm.* 2015;89:163–174.
3. Guidance for industry. Nasal spray and inhalation solution, suspension, and spray drug products-chemistry, manufacturing, and controls documentation. U.S. Department of Health and Human Services Food and Drug Administration Center for Drug Evaluation and Research (CDER); 2002.
4. Guidance for industry. Metered dose inhaler (MDI) and dry powder inhaler (DPI) drug products. U.S. Department of Health and Human Services Food and Drug Administration Center for Drug Evaluation and Research (CDER); 1998.
5. Guideline on the pharmaceutical quality of inhalation and nasal products. European Medicines Agency. Committee for Medical Products for Human Use (CHMP); 2006.
6. Lee SL, Saluja B, García-Arieta A et al. Regulatory considerations for approval of generic inhalation drug products in the US, EU, Brazil, China, and India. *AAPS J.* 2015;17:1285–1303.
7. Van Rijt SH, Bein T, Meiners S. Medical nanoparticles for next generation drug delivery to the lungs. *Eur Respir J.* 2014;44:765–774.
8. Weers JG, Miller DP. Formulation design of dry powders for inhalation. *J Pharm Sci.* 2015;104:3259–3288.
9. Tong ZB, Zheng B, Yang RY et al. CFD-DEM investigation of the dispersion mechanisms in commercial dry powder inhalers. *Powder Technol.* 2013;240:19–24.
10. Hoppentocht M, Hagedoorn P, Frijlink HW et al. Technological and practical challenges of dry powder inhalers and formulations. *Adv Drug Deliv Rev.* 2014;75:18–31.
11. Grasmeijer F, Grasmeijer N, Hagedoorn P et al. Recent advances in the fundamental understanding of adhesive mixtures for inhalation. *Curr Pharm Des.* 2015;21:5900–5914.
12. Weers J, Clark A. The impact of inspiratory flow rate on drug delivery to the lungs with dry powder inhalers. *Pharm Res.* 2017;34:507–528.
13. Baldyga J, Henczka M, Shekunov BY. Fluid dynamics, mass transfer, and particle formation in supercritical fluids. In: York P, Kompella UB, Shekunov BY, editors. *Supercritical Fluid Technology for Drug Product Development.* New York: Marcel Dekker; Drugs and the Pharmaceutical Sciences; vol. 138; 2004. pp. 91–157.
14. Shekunov BY. Production of powders for respiratory drug delivery. In: York P, Kompella UB, Shekunov BY, editors. *Supercritical Fluid Technology for Drug Product Development.* New York: Marcel Dekker; Drugs and the Pharmaceutical Sciences; vol. 138; 2004. pp. 247–282.
15. Chow AHL, Tong HHY, Chattopadhyay P et al. Particle engineering for pulmonary delivery. *Pharm Res.* 2007;24:411–437.
16. Cipolla D, Shekunov B, Blanchard J et al. Lipid-based carriers for pulmonary products: Preclinical development and case studies in humans. *Adv Drug Deliv Rev.* 2014;75:53–80.
17. Myrdal PB, Sheth P, Stein SW. Advances in metered dose inhaler technology: Formulation development. *AAPS PharmSciTech.* 2014;15:434–453.
18. Shekunov BY, Chattopadhyay P, Tong HHY et al. Particle size analysis in pharmaceutics: Principles, methods and applications. *Pharm Res.* 2007;24:203–227.
19. Shekunov BY, Feeley JC, Chow AHL et al. Aerosolisation behaviour of micronised and supercritically-processed powders. *J Aerosol Sci.* 2003;34:553–568.
20. Israel R, Rosner DE. Use of a generalized Stokes number to determine the aerodynamic capture efficiency of non-Stokesian particles from a compressible gas flow. *Aerosol Sci Technol.* 1983;2:45–51.
21. Wessel RA, Righi J. Generalized correlations for inertial impaction of particles on a circular cylinder. *Aerosol Sci Technol.* 1988;9:29–60.
22. Weiler C, Egen M, Trunk M et al. Force control and powder dispersibility of spray dried particles for inhalation. *J Pharm Sci.* 2010;99:303–316.
23. Begat P, Morton DAV, Staniforth JN et al. The cohesive-adhesive balances in dry powder inhaler formulations I: Direct quantification by atomic force microscopy. *Pharm Res.* 2004;21:1591–1597.
24. Davies M, Brindley A, Chen X et al. Characterization of drug particle surface energetics and Young's modulus by atomic force microscopy and inverse gas chromatography. *Pharm Res.* 2005;22:1158–1166.

25. Kendall K, Stainton C. Adhesion and aggregation of fine particles. *Powder Tech.* 2001;121:223–229.

26. Tang S, Ma Y, Shiu C. Modelling the mechanical strength of fractal aggregates. *Colloids Surf A Physicochem Eng Asp.* 2001;180:7–16.

27. Rwei SP, Manas-Zloczower I, Feke DL. Observation of carbon black agglomerate dispersion in simple shear flows. *Polymer Eng Sci.* 1990;30:701–706.

28. Bałdyga J, Makowski Ł, Orciuch W et al. Deagglomeration processes in high-shear devices. *Chem Eng Res Des.* 2008;86:1369–1381.

29. Rumpf H. The strength of granules and agglomerates. In: *Agglomeration.* New York: Interscience; 1962. pp. 379–413.

30. Johnson KL, Kendall K, Roberts AD. Surface energy and the contact of elastic solids. *Proc R Soc Lond A Math Phys Sci.* 1971;324:301–313.

31. Shekunov B, Lai C. Crystallization: General principles and significance in product development. In: Swarbrick J, editor. *Encyclopedia of Pharmaceutical Science and Technology,* 4th ed. Boca Raton, FL: CRC Press; 2013. pp. 760–784.

32. Tong HHY, Shekunov BY, York P et al. Predicting the aerosol performance of dry powder inhalation formulations by interparticulate interaction analysis using inverse gas chromatography. *J Pharm Sci.* 2006;95:228–233.

33. Tong HHY, Shekunov BY, York P et al. Influence of polymorphism on the surface energetics of salmeterol xinafoate crystallized from supercritical fluids. *Pharm Res.* 2002;19:640–648.

34. Chow AHL, Tong HY, Shekunov BY. Control of physical form of pharmaceutical substances. In: York P, Kompella UB, Shekunov BY, editors. *Supercritical Fluid Technology for Drug Product Development.* New York: Marcel Dekker; Drugs and the Pharmaceutical Sciences; vol. 138; 2004. pp. 283–342.

35. Chew NYK, Shekunov BY, Tong HHY et al. Effect of amino acids on the dispersion of disodium cromoglycate powders. *J Pharm Sci.* 2005;94:2289–2301.

36. Louey MD, Van Oort M, Hickey AJ. Standardized entrainment tubes for the evaluation of pharmaceutical dry powder dispersion. *Aerosol Sci.* 2006;37:1520–1531.

37. Suwandecha T, Wongpoowara W, Maliwan K et al. Effect of turbulent kinetic energy on dry powder inhaler performance. *Powder Tech.* 2014;267:381–391.

38. Longest PW, Son YJ, Holbrook L et al. Aerodynamic factors responsible for the deaggregation of carrier-free drug powders to form micrometer and submicrometer aerosols. *Pharm Res.* 2013;30:1608–1627.

39. Coates MS, Chan HK, Fletcher DF et al. Influence of airflow on the performance of a dry powder inhaler using computational and experimental analyses. *Pharm Res.* 2005;22:1445–1453.

40. Wong W, Fletcher D, Traini D et al. Particle aerosolisation and break-up in dry powder inhalers: Evaluation and modelling of the influence of grid structures for agglomerated systems. *J Pharm Sci.* 2011;100:4710–4721.

41. Gac J, Sosnowski TR, Gradon L. Turbulent flow energy for aerosolization of powder particles. *Aerosol Sci.* 2008;39:113–126.

42. Levich VG. *Physicochemical Hydrodynamics.* New York: Prentice-Hall; 1962, p. 464.

43. Saffman PG, Turner JS. On the collision of drops in turbulent clouds. *J Fluid Mech.* 1956;1:16–30.

44. Son YJ, McConville JT. Development of a standardized dissolution test method for inhaled pharmaceutical formulations. *Int J Pharm.* 2009;382:15–22.

45. Margues MRC, Loebenberg R, Almukainzi M. Simulated biological fluids with possible application in dissolution testing. *Dissolution Tech.* 2011;8:15–28.

46. Shekunov BY, Chattopadhyay P, Seitzinger J et al. Nanoparticles of poorly water-soluble drugs prepared by supercritical fluid extraction of emulsions. *Pharm Res.* 2006;23:196–204.

47. Shekunov B. Theoretical analysis of drug dissolution in micellar media. *J Pharm Sci.* 2017;106:248–257.

48. Shekunov B, Montgomery ER. Theoretical analysis of drug dissolution: I. Solubility and intrinsic dissolution rate. *J Pharm Sci.* 2016;105:2685–2689.

49. Shekunov B, Sarsfield B. Form analysis of drug substances. In: Swarbrick J, editor. *Encyclopedia of Pharmaceutical Science and Technology,* 4th ed. Boca Raton, FL: CRC Press; 2013. pp. 723–741.

50. Laitinen R, Löbmann K, Strachan CJ et al. Emerging trends in the stabilization of amorphous drugs. *Int J Pharm.* 2013;453:65–79.

51. Adam G, Gibbs JH. On the temperature dependence of cooperative relaxation properties in glass-forming liquids. *J Chem Phys.* 1965;43:139–146.

52. Zhou D, Zhang GGZ, Law D et al. Physical stability of amorphous pharmaceuticals: Importance of configurational thermodynamic quantities and molecular mobility. *J Pharm Sci.* 2002;91:1863–1872.

53. Graeser KA, Patterson JE, Zeitler JA et al. Correlating thermodynamic and kinetic parameters with amorphous stability. *Eur J Pharm Sci.* 2009;37:492–498.

54. Vyazovkin S, Dranca I. Effect of physical aging on nucleation of amorphous indomethacin. *J Phys Chem B.* 2007;111:7283–7287.

55. Vyazovkin S, Dranca I. Comparative relaxation dynamics of glucose and maltitol. *Pharm Res.* 2006;23:2158–2164.

56. Bhattacharya S, Suryanaraynan R. Local mobility in amorphous pharmaceuticals-characterization and implications on stability. *J Pharm Sci.* 2009;98:2935–2953.

57. Bhugra CN, Rambhatla S, Bakri A et al. Prediction of the onset of crystallization of amorphous sucrose below the calorimetric glass transition temperature from correlations with mobility. *J Pharm Sci.* 2007;96:1258–1269.

58. Bhugra CN, Shmeis R, Krill SL et al. Prediction of onset of crystallization from experimental relaxation times. II. Comparison between predicted and experimental onset times. *J Pharm Sci*. 2008;97:455–472.

59. Chernov AA. Crystal growth. In: *Modern Crystallography III*: Berlin, Germany: Springer, 1984.

60. Sun Y, Xi H, Ediger MD et al. Diffusionless crystal growth from glass has precursor in equilibrium liquid. *J Phys Chem B*. 2008;112:5594–5601.

61. Alie J, Menegotto J, Cardon P et al. Dielectric study of the molecular mobility and the isothermal crystallization kinetics of an amorphous pharmaceutical drug substance. *J Pharm Sci*. 2004;93:218–233.

62. Marsac PJ, Konno H, Taylor LS. A comparison of the physical stability of amorphous felodipine and nifedipine systems. *Pharm Res*. 2006;23:2306–2316.

63. Ferguson GT, Hickey AJ, Dwivedi S. Co-suspension® delivery technology in pressurized metered-dose inhalers for multidrug dosing in the treatment of respiratory diseases. *Respir Med*. 2018;134:16–23.

64. Zhou Q, Morton DAV. Drug-lactose binding aspects in adhesive mixtures: Controlling performance in dry powder inhaler formulations by altering lactose carrier surfaces. *Adv Drug Deliv Rev*. 2012;64:275–284.

65. Pilcer G, Wauthoz N, Amighi K. Lactose characteristics and the generation of the aerosol. *Adv Drug Deliv Rev*. 2012;64:233–256.

66. Mönckedieck M, Kamplade J, Fakner P et al. Dry powder inhaler performance of spray dried mannitol with tailored surface morphologies as carrier and salbutamol sulphate. *Int J Pharm*. 2017;524:351–363.

67. Edwards DA., Ben-Jebria A, Langer R. Recent advances in pulmonary drug delivery using large, porous inhaled particles. *J Appl Physiol*. 1998;85:379–385.

68. Rehman M, Shekunov BY, York P et al. Optimization of powders for pulmonary delivery using supercritical fluid technology. *Eur J Pharm Sci*. 2004;22:1–18.

69. Shekunov BY, Chattopadhyay P, Seitzinger J. Production of respirable particles using spray-freeze-drying with compressed CO_2. In: *Proceedings of the Conference on Respiratory Drug Delivery*, Palm Springs, CA. vol. IX; 2004. pp. 489–492.

70. Henczka M, Baldyga J, Shekunov BY. Modelling of spray-freezing with compressed carbon dioxide. *Chem Eng Sci*. 2006;61:2880–2888.

71. Chattopadhyay P, Shekunov BY, Huff R. Drug encapsulation using supercritical fluid extraction of emulsions. *J Pharm Sci*. 2006;95:667–680.

72. Shekunov BY, Chattopadhyay P, Seitzinger J. Engineering of composite particles for drug delivery using supercritical fluid technology. In: Svenson S, editor. *Polymeric Drug Delivery Vol. II - Polymeric Matrices and Drug Particle Engineering*. Washington DC: ACS Symposium Series; vol. 924; 2006. pp. 234–249.

73. Yim D, Cipolla D, Shekunov BY et al. Feasibility of pulmonary delivery of nano-suspension formulations using the AERx system. *J Aerosol Med*. 2005;18:101–102.

74. Chattopadhyay P, Shekunov BY, Yim D et al. Preparation of drug-lipid nanosuspensions for pulmonary delivery using supercritical fluid extraction of emulsions (SFEE). *Adv Drug Deliv Rev*. 2007;59:444–453.

75. Mayo AS, Ambatic BK, Kompella UB. Gene delivery nanoparticles fabricated by supercritical fluid extraction of emulsions. *Int J Pharmaceutics*. 2010;387:278–285.

76. Koushik K, Kompella UB. Preparation of large porous deslorelin–PLGA microparticles with reduced residual solvent and cellular uptake using a supercritical carbon dioxide process. *Pharm Res*. 2004;21:524–535.

77. Muralidharan P, Malapit M, Mallory E et al. Inhalable nanoparticulate powders for respiratory delivery. *Nanomedicine*. 2015;11:1189–1199.

78. Menon JU, Ravikumar P, Pise A et al. Polymeric nanoparticles for pulmonary protein and DNA delivery. *Acta Biomaterialia*. 2014;10:2643–2652.

79. Zhang J, Wu L, Chan HK et al. Formation, characterization, and fate of inhaled drug nanoparticles. *Adv Drug Deliv Rev*. 2011;63:441–455.

80. Buttini F, Miozzi M, Balducci AG et al. Differences in physical chemistry and dissolution rate of solid particle aerosols from solution pressurised inhalers. *Int J Pharm*. 2014;465:42–51.

81. Zhu B, Traini D, Lewis DA et al. The solid-state and morphological characteristics of particles generated from solution-based metered dose inhalers: Influence of ethanol concentration and intrinsic drug properties. *Colloids Surf A Physicochem Eng Asp*. 2014;443:345–355.

Particle deposition in the respiratory tract and the effect of respiratory disease

WILLIAM D. BENNETT

Introduction   31
Particle deposition mechanisms   31
Experimental measurement of total and regional
deposition in the respiratory tract   32
    Total deposition   33
Regional deposition   33
Effect of respiratory tract disease on total and
regional particle deposition   34
Conclusion   37
References   38

INTRODUCTION

Total and regional particle deposition of inhaled therapeutic aerosols in the respiratory tract depends on factors related to both the inhaled particles and the patient being treated. The mechanisms of deposition are, in large part, determined by the physical (size, shape, and density) and chemical (hygroscopicity and charge) characteristics of the inhaled particles (1). The general properties of particles, aerosol distributions, and particle kinetics in air have been the topic of several texts over the years (e.g., Hinds [2]). Biological factors of the patients, including breathing pattern (tidal volume, flow, and rate of breathing), the anatomy of the airways, and regional ventilation, also affect total and regional deposition in an individual's respiratory tract (3).

Understanding regional particle deposition in the respiratory tract is important for targeting aerosolized drugs to their region of interest to maximize the drugs' effect while avoiding delivery to other regions to minimize unwanted side effects (4). An additional reason for targeting drugs to their desired location is to improve the cost-effectiveness of drug delivery. For example, it may simply be important to differentially partition drug delivery between the conducting airways and the alveolar region of the lung. Recent interest to deliver hyperosmolar solutions or other ion channel modulators to airway epithelial cells in cystic fibrosis (CF) (5) may require targeted delivery to the bronchial airways, where the defect in epithelial Cl⁻ ion transport (CFTR) is manifested, in order to obtain maximum effect for improving mucociliary clearance in these patients. As an example of the need for optimal alveolar targeting, the recent development of a_1-antitrypsin therapy for emphysema, a costly drug of limited availability, requires optimal delivery of the drug to the lung periphery (6).

PARTICLE DEPOSITION MECHANISMS

The mechanisms of particle deposition in the respiratory tract have been detailed in numerous publications over the past 40 years, most recently by Darquenne (1). In brief, particle deposition in the respiratory tract occurs primarily by three mechanisms: impaction, sedimentation, and diffusion. Impaction and sedimentation depend on a particle's aerodynamic diameter (d_{ae}), which is the size of a sphere of unit density that has the same terminal settling velocity as the particle of interest. Impaction occurs when a particle, due to its inertia, is unable to follow a change in flow direction, for example, at airway bifurcations, and deposits on an airway surface. Sedimentation occurs by the gravitational settling of particles to an airway wall. The deposition efficiencies for impaction and sedimentation in a region of the respiratory tract region are d_{ae}^2u (where u is the mean linear velocity within an airway) and d_{ae}^2t (where t is the mean residence time within an airway), respectively. Since mean linear velocities are a function of airway cross-sectional area, the deposition efficiency for impaction is generally considered as a function of d_{ae}^2Q (where Q is inspiratory flow). Diffusive deposition takes place when a particle reaches an airway surface by random Brownian movement. Diffusion, or more specifically a particle's diffusion coefficient, D, is a function of the physical diameter (d_p) of a particle. Particle density does not affect the diffusion coefficient. Diffusive deposition efficiency in a region of the respiratory tract is a function of $(Dt)^{0.5}$, where t is time in the region.

The combined processes of diffusive and sedimentary deposition are important for particles in the range of 0.1–1 μm. Impaction and sedimentation predominate above and diffusion predominates below this range (1).

EXPERIMENTAL MEASUREMENT OF TOTAL AND REGIONAL DEPOSITION IN THE RESPIRATORY TRACT

Early experimental studies to characterize total deposition in the respiratory tract employed light-scattering photometry and nonhygroscopic, monodisperse aerosols >0.5 μm (7) to determine fractional deposition at the mouth on a breath-by-breath basis. The total deposition of ultrafine particles was most commonly measured using condensation particle counting techniques (8,9). Besides its use to measure total deposition of inhaled aerosols, the light-scattering method has also been employed with a bolus technique to study regional airway deposition in the human lung (10). The bolus method consists of inserting a small amount of aerosol of the inhaled breath at a predetermined point in the subject's inspiratory volume and measuring the deposition of the aerosol bolus during the subsequent expiration. The methodology assumes that a bolus inserted early in the inspiratory volume probes the lung periphery while a bolus inserted late in the inspiratory volume probes more proximal lung regions. The depth reached by the bolus is usually referred to as the penetration volume (Vp) and is defined as the volume of particle-free air inhaled from the mode of the bolus to the end of inspiration. In normal subjects, for Vp > 100 mL, aerosol bolus deposition has been shown to increase linearly with depth of inhalation of the bolus within the lung (1).

Imaging technologies have been used more recently to assess both total and regional deposition of inhaled drugs (or their surrogates), important for estimating the amount of medication delivered to the lung for new drug delivery devices. Furthermore, these imaging methods allow for assessment of bioequivalence by comparing total and regional lung deposition associated with multiple aerosol devices/products. To standardize the techniques for *in vivo* aerosol deposition assessment of orally inhaled products a supplement to *JAMPDD* was published (11) that provides practical guidance on the methods and techniques for standardizing radiolabel validation (12) and image acquisition/analysis using planar (two-dimensional [2D]), single-photon emission computed tomography (SPECT) and positron emission tomography (PET) imaging modalities. Newman and others (13) detail the methods for quantifying total and regional deposition in the lungs and extrathoracic airways (mouth, throat, pharynx, and larynx) by planar (two-dimensional [2D]) imaging using a single-headed or dual-headed gamma camera, the most widely used and most straightforward of the radionuclide imaging methods used to assess drug deposition (Figure 2.1). A common index available from imaging and region-of-interest

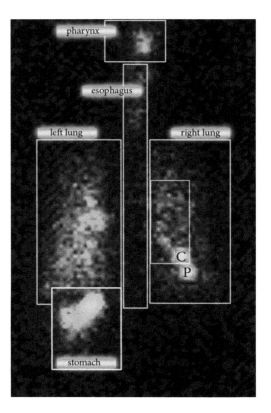

Figure 2.1 2D Gamma scintigraphy posterior deposition image. Areas of deposition increase from dark to light. C and P are the central and peripheral regions, respectively, used for C/P analysis. (From Zeman, K.L. et al., *J. Aerosol. Med. Pulm. Drug Deliv.*, 23, 363–369, 2010.)

analysis is the central-peripheral (C/P) ratio of deposited radioactivity used for assessing conducting airway versus parenchymal deposition (Figure 2.1). The C/P of the deposition image is generally normalized by the C/P of a gas (e.g., Xe133) or transmission (e.g., Co57) scan in the same individual to account for differences in size and thickness of the C versus P region (13). While both the central and peripheral regions overlay alveoli and small airways, the central region also incorporates large, bronchial airways not present in the peripheral region. Thus, increases in C/P to values greater than 1.0 reflect increases in large airway deposition.

Clearance of deposited particles has also been used to assess regional deposition, assuming that the particles in question are removed only by mucociliary clearance, that there is no long-term retention component on the conducting airways, and that the radiotracer is tightly bound. In this case, the percentage cleared by 24 h postdeposition may be taken as an estimate of the percentage of particles depositing in tracheobronchial airways (3,14,15). It is likely, however, that this value is an underestimate of deposited activity in the airways (14), especially in patients who may not clear their airways of particles completely by 24 h postdeposition (16). Twenty-four-hour whole-lung retention in normal lungs has been shown to correlate with the initial aerosol deposition pattern (e.g., C/P) in healthy subjects (17–19) but may not always do so in disease (16).

Total deposition

The effect of particle size on total deposition in the lung was well described by Heyder et al. (20) using light-scattering photometry and particle counting at the mouth methodologies described above. Figure 2.2 illustrates the dependence of total deposition on particle size. All curves show a minimum total deposition for particle sizes around 0.5 μm, a size for which the combined contributions to deposition from impaction, sedimentation, and diffusion are least effective. For particles larger than 0.5 μm, deposition increases with increasing particle size due to increased sedimentation and impaction, while for particles smaller than 0.5 μm in diameter, deposition increases with decreasing particle size due to increased diffusion. Particles in the size range of 0.3–0.7 μm follow convective transport, depositing primarily after mixing with residual air in the lungs.

The effect of breathing pattern on total deposition is also illustrated in Figure 2.2. At a fixed tidal flow consistent with resting breathing (250 mL/min), the increase in tidal volume (1000–2000 mL) results in increased penetration and residence time in the lung, leading to increased total deposition by time dependent mechanisms across all particle sizes (diffusion for <0.5 μm and sedimentation >0.5 μm).

Hydrophilic pharmaceutical particles may grow in size when they enter the respiratory tract where the relative humidity rapidly increases from ambient to near 100%. For example, Heyder et al. (21) showed that solid 0.7-μm salt particles grew 5–6 times by the time they were inhaled and exhaled to 400 mL depth into the airways at a flow of 250 mL/sec. In this case, the increased size increases the particles' probability for deposition (moving up the curve

to the right of 0.7 μm in Figure 2.2). On the other hand, it is also predicted that deposition probability would decrease for hydrophilic salt particles of ≤0.1 μm particles or less (i.e., as deposition moves down the curve to the right of 0.1 μm in Figure 2.2).

Regional deposition

The first obstacle to overcome delivering aerosol to the lungs is to have the airborne droplets or particles escape deposition in the mouth (or nose for transnasal delivery) and the larynx. Early studies by Chan and Lippman (22) showed that mouth deposition of fine and coarse particles is proportional to the square of particle aerodynamic size and flow rate. The use of spacers or holding chambers with metered-dose inhalers (MDIs) has helped decrease particle impaction in the mouth by eliminating the large particles from the inhaled stream and decreasing jet velocities from the MDI (23). An interesting study by Svartengren et al. (24) found that the presence of an external resistance on the inhalation device (such as that associated with many dry powder inhalers) enhanced penetration of particles past the mouth, not merely by slowing flow but by changing the shape of the upper airways to influence flow dynamics and particle deposition. Emmett and Aitken (25) have also shown that most of the extrathoracic deposition of coarse particles during mouth breathing occurs in the larynx. There has been some recent interest in transnasal delivery of aerosols to the lungs (26,27) as they might be delivered via nasal cannula over longer periods of time (e.g., during sleep) or during non-invasive ventilation. The nose, however, is a more effective filter than the mouth for preventing penetration of particles to the lower respiratory tract; for example, Heyder et al. (28) showed that total deposition of 0.5–3 μm particles is greater for nose than mouth breathing.

Most of the available data on tracheobronchial versus alveolar deposition have been acquired using radiolabeled aerosols. As discussed above, the site of deposition has been typically inferred from particle retention at 24-h postinhalation under the assumption that mucus clearance of the bronchial airways is nearly complete by this time (14,16,19). The tracheobronchial region consists of relatively large airways and small airways, that is, the bronchi and bronchioles, respectively. Relative to the bronchioles, linear velocities in the bronchi are high and residence time is short. Deposition of fine and coarse particles in the bronchi occurs mainly by impaction, whereas deposition in the bronchioles occurs due to sedimentation. In general, relative to that aerosol delivered to the trachea, the deposition efficiency of fine and coarse particles in the tracheobronchial (TB) region increases in a sigmoidal fashion with log (dae) from a few percent at dae = 1 μm to nearly 100% at dae = 10 μm (14). Due to deposition in the extrathoracic airways (particularly during nasal breathing), however, the deposition fraction of particles in the TB region relative to that delivered at the mouth begins to decrease above dae = 5 μm, especially for relatively high inspiratory flows. Deposition in the

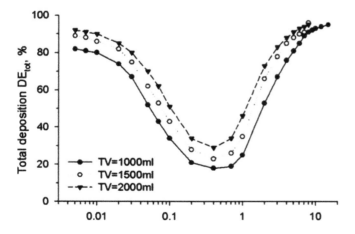

Figure 2.2 Total deposition as a function of particle diameter at a constant flow rate of 250 mL/sec and variable tidal volume (TV) by oral breathing. Data are averaged experimental data obtained in healthy adults by Heyder et al. (From Heyder, J. et al., *J. Aerosol. Sci.*, 17, 811–825, 1986.)

tracheobronchial region is also enhanced with increased flow rate as impaction is increased in the larger airways. Decreased depth of breathing, that is, smaller tidal volumes, also increase the fraction of deposition occurring in the conducting airways by correspondingly reducing the fraction of particles that penetrate into the alveolar region.

The bolus technique with light scattering at the mouth described above was used by Kim et al. (10) to estimate regional deposition within the airways and calculate local surface dose of deposited aerosols for 1, 3, and 5 μm diameter particles in healthy adult subjects (Figure 2.3). By delivering small boli of each aerosol in 50 mL increments to lung depths ranging between 100 and 500 mL, they showed that surface dose was (1) larger at shallow penetration volumes (Vp < 200 mL) compared to deeper lung regions (Vp = 200–500 mL), and (2) that the difference increased with increasing particle size. These findings are important for considering therapeutic effects of inhaled drugs at the tissue level. Even though fractional deposition of inhaled therapeutic aerosols is generally much higher in the alveolar region than in the proximal conducting airways, the markedly smaller surface area in the conducting airways results in a many times higher dose/surface area of deposited drugs, helping to provide an enhanced therapeutic effect for many drugs targeted to the bronchial airway epithelia.

A number of investigators have attempted to take advantage of various combinations of particle size, inhaled flow rates, bolus delivery, and depth of breathing to target delivery of inhaled aerosols to the bronchial airways (15,29–32). Anderson et al. (29) proposed a novel strategy to enhance deposition on the small bronchial airways by using a large particle size of 6 μm while restricting the inhalation to extremely low flow rates (0.04 L/sec). At these low flows,

deposition by impaction in the extrathoracic and oropharyngeal surfaces is reduced, while within the small airways the transit time of the particle becomes longer than the gravitational settling time for the large particle, thereby increasing deposition in this region. Zeman et al. (15) expanded on this proposal by comparing single breaths (10 sec duration) of a nebulized aerosol (9.5 μm mass median aerodynamic diameter [MMAD]) from a modified jet nebulizer inhaled at 0.08 L/sec in healthy subjects to a more typical tidal breathing delivery (30 breaths/min) of 5 μm particles at 0.5 L/sec. Relative to total deposition, they found significantly less oropharyngeal and greater tracheobronchial deposition (based on both 24 h clearance and C/P ratio) for the large particle/slow inhalation method compared to the tidal breathing delivery. While such an approach may seem impractical for aerosolized drug delivery given the extremely slow inhalation required, there are recently developed devices that can control the inhalation flow rate for patients (33). Furthermore, a few single breaths of a very large particle (e.g., 9 μm MMAD) is capable of delivering a much higher drug mass to the airways than the typical tidal inhalation of nebulized particles (e.g., 3 μm MMAD) (i.e., 27-fold by delivered mass in the same inhaled volume).

A number of studies (34–37) have shown that aerosol distribution in the lungs tends to correlate well with ventilation; that is, aerosols are transported to the regions of the lung that receive the greatest ventilation. This is especially true for fine particles that are less likely to deposit by impaction in the conducting airways, but it has also been shown for coarse particles in the healthy lung (34,36). This similarity in aerosol and gas distribution suggests potential approaches for regional targeting aerosols within the lung based on ventilation studies. For example, Sybrecht et al. (38) showed that the ratio of apical to basal Xe133 gas bolus distribution was increased at all flow rates simply by changing body posture from the upright to the supine position. Presumably, the change in gravitational dependence of lung inflation was responsible for this shift. Subsequently, Sa et al. (39) recently studied the regional deposition of coarse particles (5 μm) delivered in the supine versus seated position of healthy adults. No change was observed in the apex-to-base ratio or homogeneity of deposition between seated and supine postures. However, they did find a shift in relative deposition from the alveolar to the bronchial airways for supine versus seated, likely driven by changes in functional residual capacity, and airway size, as well as changes in the regional distribution of ventilation between postures.

EFFECT OF RESPIRATORY TRACT DISEASE ON TOTAL AND REGIONAL PARTICLE DEPOSITION

Both total and regional particle deposition in the lung may be affected by respiratory disease. While the mechanisms of particle deposition in the diseased lung are the same as those in the healthy lung, deposition may be altered by airway

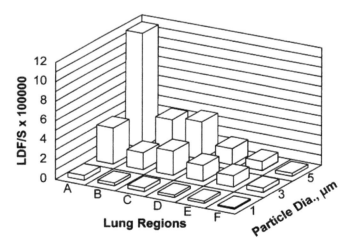

Figure 2.3 Deposition dose per unit surface area, for mouth breathing with tidal volume of 500 mL and flow rate of 250 mL/sec, in local volumetric regions: 50–100 mL (**A**), 100–150 mL (**B**), 150–200 mL (**C**), 200–250 mL (**D**), 250–350 mL (**E**), and 350–500 mL (**F**). LDF, local deposition fraction; S, surface area (cm²) of each region estimated by Weibel's lung model; Dia, diameter. (From Kim, C.S. et al., *J. Appl. Physiol.* (1985), 81, 2203–2213, 1996.)

geometry, breathing patterns, and regional ventilation compared to normal. For example, the bronchial airways of the lungs may be chronically or acutely obstructed in chronic bronchitis or asthma, respectively, leading to enhanced particle impaction at sites of narrowing. On the other hand, the enlargement of peripheral airspaces associated with emphysema may reduce particle deposition by sedimentation and/or diffusion in the deep lung. Heterogeneity of obstruction or emphysema in the lung also modifies regional ventilation and thus regional deposition of particles within the lung.

In general, studies have shown enhanced total particle deposition for all particle sizes in patients with chronic obstructive pulmonary disease (COPD) compared to healthy adults. For example, Schiller-Scotland and coworkers (40) showed total deposition fraction (DF) was increased in chronic obstructive pulmonary disease (COPD) patients compared to normal subjects for 1, 2, and 3 μm particles breathed with controlled tidal flow and volume. However, the relative difference in deposition from normal was greater for fine versus coarse particle size. Kim and Kang (41) also reported 106% greater deposition fractions of 1 μm particles inhaled via the mouth by COPD patients versus healthy adults breathing under the same controlled breathing pattern.

In addition to having altered airway geometry, patients with chronic obstructive pulmonary disease (COPD) use different breathing patterns than individuals with normal lungs (42). Only a few studies have attempted to measure DF in health and COPD with realistic natural breathing conditions for individual subjects in each study group. For example, Bennett et al. (43) found that COPD patients had a 50% larger fractional deposition of fine particles (2 μm) with natural breathing conditions at rest than an age-matched healthy cohort. Furthermore, patients characterized as generally chronically bronchitic, rather than emphysematous, had the greatest increase in deposition. In other words, the enlargement of peripheral airspaces associated with emphysema tended to decrease total deposition efficiency while increased bronchoconstriction increased deposition.

While spontaneous breathing patterns are generally associated with nebulized drug delivery in COPD, controlling inhalation flows and volumes may be useful for both increasing deposition and decreasing inter- and intra-subject variability (33). Brand et al. (44) showed enhanced deposition and decreased variability of particle deposition (3 μm monodisperse) in patients with chronic bronchitis and asthma for controlled versus spontaneous breathing. For controlled inhalation of 1-liter tidal breaths, variability decreased remarkably when inhaled flow rate was decreased to 100 mL/sec (Figure 2.4).

The correlation between increased fractional deposition and airway resistance (43) suggests increased inertial deposition at sites of obstruction in COPD. Dolovich et al. (45), using gamma scintigraphy, found that alveolar deposition of 3 μm particles was decreased and tracheobronchial deposition was increased in patients with COPD compared to normal that correlated with their degree of obstruction. Smaldone and Messina (46) also showed enhanced airway

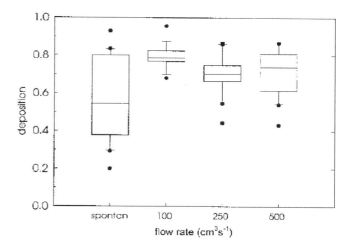

Figure 2.4 Particle deposition in COPD and asthma patients with spontaneous versus controlled breathing patterns. (From Brand, P. et al., *J. Pharm. Sci.*, 89, 724–731, 2000.)

deposition of fine particles in COPD patients with chronic expiratory flow limitation that was further enhanced by coughing in these individuals. Model and animal experiments suggest that this enhancement of particle deposition occurs during expiration and is highly localized to airway surfaces immediately downstream to sites of flow limitation (e.g., segmental and subsegmental bronchi) (47,48). These "hot spots" of particle deposition have been observed in severely obstructed patients by gamma scintigraphy for a variety of particle sizes and breathing patterns (49–52). From a drug delivery perspective, it is clear that hot spots of deposition within the bronchial airways result in very high surface doses of therapy at those sites. However, the question arises as to whether this represents a benefit (that is, these deposition sites are targets for therapy) or a detriment (that is, deposition at these sites prevents targeting regions of the lung that are more likely to benefit from the inhaled therapy).

Most deposition studies in asthma have been used to characterize regional deposition in these patients, especially the relative deposition in the airways versus alveolar region. This is not surprising given that asthma is a disease of the bronchial airways. For example, using the 24-h retention as a measure of alveolar fraction of initial aerosol deposition (monodisperse 3.6 μm) in moderate to severe asthmatics, Svartengren et al. (53) showed a negative correlation between airway resistance and 24-h retention; that is, increased baseline obstruction leads to greater bronchial airway deposition. Backer et al. (54) also found that asthmatics with irregular central distribution of radioaerosol had an increased degree of bronchial responsiveness to inhaled histamine. When bronchoconstriction is induced with methacholine, both fine and coarse particle deposition shifts even more towards proximal airways, away from the lung periphery (55,56). Bennett and coworkers (57,58) have recently shown by gamma scintigraphy that challenge with either dust mite allergen or endotoxin in asthmatics also resulted in an increase in bronchial versus alveolar deposition and frequency of hot spots for inhaled coarse particles (5 µm).

As expected, treatment with bronchodilators in asthma has shown an improved homogeneity of particle deposition in the lungs (i.e., fewer hot spots in the lungs) post-treatment [e.g., early study by Chopra et al. (59)]. A few investigators (60,61) have hypothesized that targeting deposition of bronchodilators to the bronchial airways of asthmatics may improve therapeutic effect of the drug but with mixed results. An early study by Mitchell et al. (60) showed no difference in distribution within the lung or any difference in bronchodilator effect between an aerosol of small (1.4 µm) particle size and an aerosol of 5.5 µm in patients with severe but stable asthma. A more recent study by Usmani et al. (61) altered regional deposition of equivalent doses of radiolabeled, monodisperse aerosols of albuterol, 1.5, 3, and 6 µm, in mild-moderate asthmatics (Figure 2.5). While distal airway penetration and peripheral lung deposition increased with decreasing particle size, the best improvement in forced expiratory volume in 1 second (FEV1) was observed with the largest particle size (and smallest lung deposition), suggesting the importance of regional targeting to the bronchial airways for this drug. One difference between these two studies was in the severity of asthmatics studied, mean FEV1% pred = 47 versus 77 for Mitchell et al. (60) versus Usmani et al. (61), respectively. It may be that, as severity increases, the difference in deposition between airways and alveoli becomes less dependent on particle size; that is, even a 1.4 µm particle deposition is sufficiently deposited in bronchial airways to achieve a maximal therapeutic effect for an inhaled B-adrenergic bronchodilator. The same may not be true for other drugs, however.

Among those individuals with pulmonary disease, patients with cystic fibrosis (CF) probably require the most inhalation aerosol therapy, for example, antibiotics, hydrators, and mucolytics. CF, like chronic bronchitis and asthma,

is associated with increased fine particle deposition in the airways and inhomogeneities of deposition within the lung compared to normal (34,62–64). The poorly ventilated lung regions in CF patients have the least deposition of inhaled therapeutics and consequently are likely to be most affected by infection. Brown et al. (34) found that coarse particle (5 µm) deposition in the peripheral lung regions of CF patients followed ventilation patterns as measured by xenon-133 washout. However, in the same patients, there was increased coarse particle deposition within the bronchial airways of poorly ventilated lung regions. This was in sharp contrast to the association between particle deposition within the airways of healthy subjects, which closely followed regional ventilation. Their results suggest that bronchial airways within poorly ventilated regions may receive a high surface dose of coarse particles, while the deposition in the parenchyma of these regions is diminished compared to that of well-ventilated lung regions. Furthermore, there was a distinct decrease in both ventilation and parenchymal deposition from the base to the apex of the lung in CF, suggesting that these apical regions of the lungs are most affected by disease.

Historically, regional analyses like those of Brown et al. (34) and others (13,46,61) have been assessed by partitioning lung images into multiple, but relatively large, regions of interest. Bennett et al. (63) recently developed new analytical methods that are independent of specific regions of interest to improve localization/quantification of high (hot) and low (cold) regions of inhaled, particle deposition (Figure 2.6) (in this case 5 µm MMAD inhaled under controlled conditions).

They compared these analyses in a group of healthy and CF patients with mild airway disease to determine if they were sensitive at distinguishing differences in regional deposition between these two cohorts. While the standard analyses of C/P and skew of the particle distribution showed no difference between mild CF and normal, the fraction of cold deposition pixels in the lungs was significantly increased in the CF lung (e.g., Figure 2.6), primarily

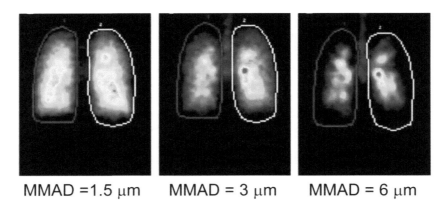

MMAD =1.5 µm   MMAD = 3 µm   MMAD = 6 µm

Figure 2.5 Posterior lung deposition images of 1.5, 3, and 6 µm MAAD 99mTc labeled albuterol aerosol in a patient with asthma. Red areas within the lungs indicate regions of highest radioactivity concentration, and black areas indicate regions with least radioactivity. (From Usmani, O.S. et al., *Am. J. Respir. Crit. Care Med.*, 172, 1497–1504, 2005.)

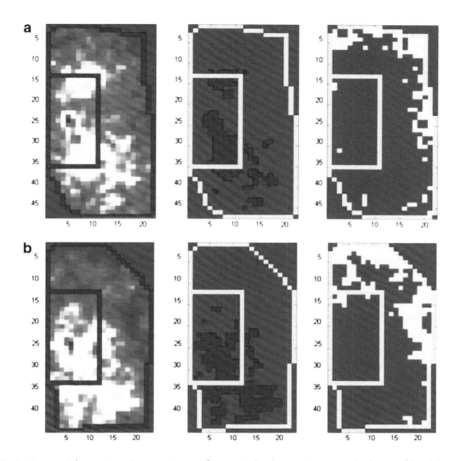

Figure 2.6 **(a)** Left: Ratio image (deposition/transmission) for particle deposition in right lung of healthy subject (%pred FEV1 = 111); Center: Deposition hot spots (red = hot); Right: Deposition cold spots (light blue = cold); **(b)** Left: Ratio image (deposition/transmission) for particle deposition in right lung of CF patient (%pred FEV1 = 64); Center: Deposition hot spots (red = hot); Right: Deposition cold spots(light blue = cold). (From Bennett, W.D. et al., *J. Aerosol. Med. Pulm. Drug Deliv.*, 28, 211–218, 2015.)

occurring in the apical region of the lung. Across all CF patients, the fraction of cold spots significantly increased as lung function declined. Some of these same authors (65) applied this pixel analysis of deposition to the results of a therapeutic intervention in CF, oral ivacaftor (Vertex Pharmaceuticals), a chloride channel (CFTR) potentiator in a small fraction of CF patients. They showed a significant decrease in both cold and hot spots in the lung post- versus pre-drug, despite there being no effect on the traditional regional deposition indices of C/P ratio and skew. These data reflected improved ventilation to the lungs with ivacaftor that in turn may translate into improved distribution of other inhaled, aerosol therapeutics that the patients may be taking, for example, inhaled antibiotics.

CONCLUSION

The primary mechanisms for inhaled particle deposition in the respiratory tract are inertial impaction, gravitational sedimentation, and Brownian diffusion. In general, total deposition increases with particle size >0.5 μm, but as the size increases above >5 μm, the amount depositing in the extrathoracic region increases under normal breathing conditions. Regional deposition also depends on particle size, breathing patterns, and ventilation distribution, and is important for determining both the surface dose of inhaled particles within the bronchial airways versus alveolated lung as well as lobar distribution of deposited particles. In the presence of lung disease, changes from normal airway geometry, breathing patterns, and regional ventilation affect both total and regional deposition of particles in the lungs. Total deposition is increased with obstructive airway disease, while regional deposition of both fine and coarse particles is shifted to more proximal airways. Regional deposition for all inhalable particles also becomes more heterogeneous with development of lung disease. These alterations in total and regional deposition with lung disease may modify therapeutic effects of inhaled particulates in these patients. Understanding the deposition mechanisms and how they are influenced by breathing patterns and regional ventilation in lung disease may allow us to improve targeting of aerosols to lung regions where the greatest benefit may be realized.

REFERENCES

1. Darquenne C. Aerosol deposition in health and disease. *J Aerosol Med Pulm Drug Deliv.* 2012;25(3):140–147. doi:10.1089/jamp.2011.0916.

2. Hinds WC. *Aerosol Technology: Properties, Behavior and Measurement of Airborne Particles.* 2nd ed. New York: John Wiley & Sons; 2012.

3. ICRP model. International Commission on Radiological Protection. Human respiratory tract model for radiological protection. *Ann ICRP.* 1994;24:1–482.

4. Bennett WD, Brown JS, Zeman KL, Hu SC, Scheuch G, Sommerer K. Targeting delivery of aerosols to different lung regions. *J Aerosol Med.* 2002;15(2):179–188. doi:10.1089/089426802320282301.

5. Bennett WD, Henderson AG, Donaldson SH. Hydrator therapies for chronic bronchitis. Lessons from cystic fibrosis. *Ann Am Thorac Soc.* 2016;13 Suppl 2:S186–S190. doi:10.1513/AnnalsATS.201509-652KV.

6. Brand P, Beckmann H, Maas Enriquez M, Meyer T, Mullinger B, Sommerer K, Weber N, Weuthen T, Scheuch G. Peripheral deposition of alpha1-protease inhibitor using commercial inhalation devices. *Eur Respir J.* 2003;22(2):263–267.

7. Gebhart J, Heigwer G, Roth C, Stahlhofen W. The use of light scattering photometry in aerosol medicine. *J Aerosol Med.* 1988;1:89–112.

8. Jaques PA, Kim CS. Measurement of total lung deposition of inhaled ultrafine particles in healthy men and women. *Inhal Toxicol.* 2000;12(8):715–731. doi:10.1080/08958370050085156.

9. Schiller CF, Gebhart J, Heyder J, Rudolf G, Stahlhofen W. Deposition of monodisperse insoluble aerosol particles in the 0.005 to 0.2 µm size range within the human respiratory tract. *Ann Occup Hyg.* 1988;32(suppl 1):41–49.

10. Kim CS, Hu SC, DeWitt P, Gerrity TR. Assessment of regional deposition of inhaled particles in human lungs by serial bolus delivery method. *J Appl Physiol (1985).* 1996;81(5):2203–2213. doi:10.1152/jappl.1996.81.5.2203.

11. Laube BL, Corcoran TE, Devadason SG, Dolovich MB, Fleming J, Newman S. Editorial: Standards for lung imaging techniques. *J Aerosol Med Pulm Drug Deliv.* 2012;25 Suppl 1:S1–S2. doi:10.1089/jamp.2012.1Su1.

12. Devadason SG, Chan HK, Haeussermann S, Kietzig C, Kuehl PJ, Newman S, Sommerer K, Taylor G. Validation of radiolabeling of drug formulations for aerosol deposition assessment of orally inhaled products. *J Aerosol Med Pulm Drug Deliv.* 2012;25 Suppl 1:S6–S9. doi:10.1089/jamp.2012.1Su3.

13. Newman S, Bennett WD, Biddiscombe M, Devadason SG, Dolovich MB, Fleming J, Haeussermann S et al. Standardization of techniques for using planar (2D) imaging for aerosol deposition assessment of orally inhaled products. *J Aerosol Med Pulm Drug Deliv.* 2012;25 Suppl 1:S10–S28. doi:10.1089/jamp.2012.1Su4.

14. Stahlhofen W, Rudolf G, James AC. Intercomparison of experimental regional aerosol deposition data. *J Aerosol Med.* 1989;2(3):285–308.

15. Zeman KL, Wu J, Bennett WD. Targeting aerosolized drugs to the conducting airways using very large particles and extremely slow inhalations. *J Aerosol Med Pulm Drug Deliv.* 2010;23(6):363–369. doi:10.1089/jamp.2008.0711.

16. Smaldone GC, Perry RJ, Bennett WD, Messina MS, Zwang J, Ilowite JS. Interpretation of "24 hour lung retention" in studies of mucociliary clearance. *J Aerosol Med.* 1988;1(1):11–20.

17. Bennett WD, Laube BL, Corcoran T, Zeman K, Sharpless G, Thomas K, Wu J, Mogayzel PJ, Jr., Pilewski J, Donaldson S. Multisite comparison of mucociliary and cough clearance measures using standardized methods. *J Aerosol Med Pulm Drug Deliv.* 2013;26(3):157–164. doi:10.1089/jamp.2011.0909.

18. Clark AR. Understanding penetration index measurements and regional lung targeting. *J Aerosol Med Pulm Drug Deliv.* 2012;25(4):179–187. doi:10.1089/jamp.2011.0899.

19. Ilowite JS, Smaldone GC, Perry RJ, Bennett WD, Foster WM. Relationship between tracheobronchial particle clearance rates and sites of initial deposition in man. *Arch Environ Health.* 1989;44(4):267–273. doi:10.1080/00039896.1989.9935893.

20. Heyder J, Gebhart J, Rudolf G, Schiller C, Stahlhofen W. Deposition of particles in the human respiratory tract in the size range 0.005–15 µm. *J Aerosol Sci.* 1986;17:811–825. doi:10.1016/0021-8502(86)90035-2.

21. Heyder J, Gebhart J, Roth C, Ferron GA. Transport and deposition of hydrophilic drug particles in the lungs. In: Gradon L, Marijnissen J, editors. *Optimization of Aerosol Drug Delivery.* Dordrecht, the Netherlands: Kluwer Academic Publishers; 2003. pp. 139–147.

22. Chan TL, Lippmann M. Experimental measurements and empirical modelling of the regional deposition of inhaled particles in humans. *Am Ind Hyg Assoc J.* 1980;41(6):399–409. doi:10.1080/15298668091424942.

23. Newman SP, Newhouse MT. Effect of add-on devices for aerosol drug delivery: Deposition studies and clinical aspects. *J Aerosol Med.* 1996;9(1):55–70. doi:10.1089/jam.1996.9.55.

24. Svartengren K, Lindestad P, Svartengren M, Philipson K, Bylin G, Camner P. Added external resistance reduces oropharyngeal

deposition and increases lung deposition of aerosol particles in asthmatics. *Am J Respir Crit Care Med.* 1995;152(1):32–37. doi:10.1164/ajrccm.152.1.7599841.

25. Emmett PC, Aitken RJ. Measurements of the total and regional deposition of inhaled particles in the human respiratory tract. *J Aerosol Sci.* 1982;13:549–560.

26. Longest PW, Walenga RL, Son YJ, Hindle M. High-efficiency generation and delivery of aerosols through nasal cannula during noninvasive ventilation. *J Aerosol Med Pulm Drug Deliv.* 2013;26(5):266–279. doi:10.1089/jamp.2012.1006.

27. Zeman KL, Balcazar JR, Fuller F, Donn KH, Boucher RC, Bennett WD, Donaldson SH. A trans-nasal aerosol delivery device for efficient pulmonary deposition. *J Aerosol Med Pulm Drug Deliv.* 2017;30(4):223–229. doi:10.1089/jamp.2016.1333.

28. Heyder J, Armbruster L, Gebhart J. Total deposition of aerosol particles in the human respiratory tract for nose and mouth breathing. *J Aerosol Sci.* 1975;6:311–328.

29. Anderson M, Philipson K, Svartengren M, Camner P. Human deposition and clearance of 6-micron particles inhaled with an extremely low flow rate. *Exp Lung Res.* 1995;21(1):187–195.

30. Bennett WD, Scheuch G, Zeman KL, Brown JS, Kim C, Heyder J, Stahlhofen W. Bronchial airway deposition and retention of particles in inhaled boluses: Effect of anatomic dead space. *J Appl Physiol (1985).* 1998;85(2):685–694. doi:10.1152/jappl.1998.85.2.685.

31. Pavia D, Thomson ML. The fractional deposition of inhaled 2 and 5 μm particles in the alveolar and tracheobronchial regions of the healthy human lung. *Ann Occup Hyg.* 1976;19(2):109–114.

32. Stahlhofen W, Gebhart J, Rudolf G et al. Measurement of lung clearance with pulses of radioactively labelled particles. *J Aerosol Sci.* 1986;17:333–338.

33. Bennett WD. Controlled inhalation of aero-solised therapeutics. *Expert Opin Drug Deliv.* 2005;2(4):763–767. doi:10.1517/17425247.2.4.763.

34. Brown JS, Zeman KL, Bennett WD. Regional deposition of coarse particles and ventilation distribution in healthy subjects and patients with cystic fibrosis. *J Aerosol Med.* 2001;14(4):443–454. doi:10.1089/08942680152744659.

35. Chamberlain MJ, Morgan WK, Vinitski S. Factors influencing the regional deposition of inhaled particles in man. *Clin Sci (Lond).* 1983;64(1):69–78.

36. Sa RC, Zeman KL, Bennett WD, Prisk GK, Darquenne C. Regional ventilation is the main determinant of alveolar deposition of coarse particles in the supine healthy human lung during tidal breathing.

J Aerosol Med Pulm Drug Deliv. 2017;30(5):322–331. doi:10.1089/jamp.2016.1336.

37. Trajan M, Logus JW, Enns EG, Man SF. Relationship between regional ventilation and aerosol deposition in tidal breathing. *Am Rev Respir Dis.* 1984;130(1):64–70. doi:10.1164/arrd.1984.130.1.64.

38. Sybrecht G, Landau L, Murphy BG, Engel LA, Martin RR, Macklem PT. Influence of posture on flow dependence of distribution of inhaled 133Xe boli. *J Appl Physiol.* 1976;41(4):489–496. doi:10.1152/jappl.1976.41.4.489.

39. Sa RC, Zeman KL, Bennett WD, Prisk GK, Darquenne C. Effect of posture on regional deposition of coarse particles in the healthy human lung. *J Aerosol Med Pulm Drug Deliv.* 2015;28(6):423–431. doi:10.1089/jamp.2014.1189.

40. Schiller-Scotland CF, Gebhart J, Hochrainer D, Siekmeier R. Deposition of inspired aerosol particles within the respiratory tract of patients with obstructive lung disease. *Toxicol Lett.* 1996;88(1–3):255–261.

41. Kim CS, Kang TC. Comparative measurement of lung deposition of inhaled fine particles in normal subjects and patients with obstructive airway disease. *Am J Respir Crit Care Med.* 1997;155(3):899–905. doi:10.1164/ajrccm.155.3.9117024.

42. Tobin MJ, Chadha TS, Jenouri G, Birch SJ, Gazeroglu HB, Sackner MA. Breathing patterns. 2. Diseased subjects. *Chest.* 1983;84(3):286–294.

43. Bennett WD, Zeman KL, Kim C, Mascarella J. Enhanced deposition of fine particles in COPD patients spontaneously breathing at rest. *Inh Toxicol.* 1997;9(1):1–14.

44. Brand P, Friemel I, Meyer T, Schulz H, Heyder J, Haubetainger K. Total deposition of therapeutic particles during spontaneous and controlled inhalations. *J Pharm Sci.* 2000;89(6):724–731. doi:10.1002/(SICI)1520-6017(200006)89:6 < 724::AID-JPS3 > 3.0.CO;2-B.

45. Dolovich MB, Sanchis J, Rossman C, Newhouse MT. Aerosol penetrance: A sensitive index of peripheral airways obstruction. *J Appl Physiol.* 1976;40(3):468–471. doi:10.1152/jappl.1976.40.3.468.

46. Smaldone GC, Messina MS. Flow limitation, cough, and patterns of aerosol deposition in humans. *J Appl Physiol.* 1985;59(2):515–520. doi:10.1152/jappl.1985.59.2.515.

47. Christensen WD, Swift DL. Aerosol deposition and flow limitation in a compliant tube. *J Appl Physiol (1985).* 1986;60(2):630–637. doi:10.1152/jappl.1986.60.2.630.

48. Smaldone GC, Itoh H, Swift DL, Wagner HN, Jr. Effect of flow-limiting segments and cough on particle deposition and mucociliary clearance in the lung. *Am Rev Respir Dis.* 1979;120(4):747–758. doi:10.1164/arrd.1979.120.4.747.

49. Isawa T, Wasserman K, Taplin GV. Lung scintigraphy and pulmonary function studies in obstructive airway disease. *Am Rev Respir Dis*. 1970;102(2):161–172. doi:10.1164/arrd.1970.102.2.161.

50. Lin MS, Goodwin DA. Pulmonary distribution of an inhaled radioaerosol in obstructive pulmonary disease. *Radiology*. 1976;118(3):645–651. doi:10.1148/118.3.645.

51. Santolicandro A, Giuntini C. Patterns of deposition of labelled monodispersed aerosols in obstructive lung disease. *J Nucl Med Allied Sci*. 1979;23(3):115–127.

52. Taplin GV, Tashkin DP, Chopra SK, Anselmi OE, Elam D, Calvarese B, Coulson A, Detels R, Rokaw SN. Early detection of chronic obstructive pulmonary disease using radionuclide lung-imaging procedures. *Chest*. 1977;71(5):567–575.

53. Svartengren M, Anderson M, Bylin G, Philipson K, Camner P. Regional deposition of 3.6-micron particles and lung function in asthmatic subjects. *J Appl Physiol* (1985). 1991;71(6):2238–2243. doi:10.1152/jappl.1991.71.6.2238.

54. Backer V, Mortensen J. Distribution of radioactive aerosol in the airways of children and adolescents with bronchial hyper-responsiveness. *Clin Physiol*. 1992;12(5):575–585.

55. O'Riordan TG, Walser L, Smaldone GC. Changing patterns of aerosol deposition during methacholine bronchoprovocation. *Chest*. 1993;103(5):1385–1389.

56. Svartengren M, Philipson K, Camner P. Individual differences in regional deposition of 6-micron particles in humans with induced bronchoconstriction. *Exp Lung Res*. 1989;15(1):139–149.

57. Bennett WD, Herbst M, Alexis NE, Zeman KL, Wu J, Hernandez ML, Peden DB. Effect of inhaled dust mite allergen on regional particle deposition and mucociliary clearance in allergic asthmatics. *Clin Exp Allergy*. 2011;41(12):1719–1728. doi:10.1111/j.1365-2222.2011.03814.x.

58. Bennett WD, Herbst M, Zeman KL, Wu J, Hernandez ML, Peden DB. Effect of inhaled endotoxin on regional particle deposition in patients with mild asthma. *J Allergy Clin Immunol*. 2013;131(3):912–913. doi:10.1016/j.jaci.2012.09.010.

59. Chopra SK, Taplin GV, Tashkin DP, Trevor E, Elam D. Imaging sites of airway obstruction and measuring functional responses to bronchodilator treatment in asthma. *Thorax*. 1979;34(4):493–500.

60. Mitchell DM, Solomon MA, Tolfree SE, Short M, Spiro SG. Effect of particle size of bronchodilator aerosols on lung distribution and pulmonary function in patients with chronic asthma. *Thorax*. 1987;42(6):457–461.

61. Usmani OS, Biddiscombe MF, Barnes PJ. Regional lung deposition and bronchodilator response as a function of beta2-agonist particle size. *Am J Respir Crit Care Med*. 2005;172(12):1497–1504. doi:10.1164/rccm.200410-1414OC.

62. Anderson PJ, Blanchard JD, Brain JD, Feldman HA, McNamara JJ, Heyder J. Effect of cystic fibrosis on inhaled aerosol boluses. *Am Rev Respir Dis*. 1989;140(5):1317–1324. doi:10.1164/ajrccm/140.5.1317.

63. Bennett WD, Xie M, Zeman K, Hurd H, Donaldson S. Heterogeneity of particle deposition by pixel analysis of 2D gamma scintigraphy images. *J Aerosol Med Pulm Drug Deliv*. 2015;28(3):211–218. doi:10.1089/jamp.2013.1095.

64. Laube BL, Links JM, LaFrance ND, Wagner HN, Jr., Rosenstein BJ. Homogeneity of bronchopulmonary distribution of 99mTc aerosol in normal subjects and in cystic fibrosis patients. *Chest*. 1989;95(4):822–830.

65. Bennett WD, Zeman KL, Laube BL, Wu J, Sharpless G, Mogayzel PJ, Jr., Donaldson SH. Homogeneity of aerosol deposition and mucociliary clearance are improved following ivacaftor treatment in cystic fibrosis. *J Aerosol Med Pulm Drug Deliv*. 2017. doi:10.1089/jamp.2017.1388.

3

Mathematical modeling of inhaled therapeutic aerosol deposition in the respiratory tract

JEFFRY SCHROETER, BAHMAN ASGHARIAN, AND JULIA KIMBELL

Introduction	41		Experimental data to confirm nasal models	45
CFD modeling	42		Mouth/throat CFD-particle transport modeling	45
Fundamentals of CFD deposition modeling	42		Lung CFD-particle transport modeling	46
Simulation of airflow	42		Whole-lung particle deposition modeling	47
Simulation of particle transport	42		Future needs and directions for respiratory tract	
Nasal CFD-particle transport modeling	43		model development	48
Recent literature	43		References	49
Features specific to nasal models and applications	43			

INTRODUCTION

The possibility of predicting how particles will behave inside the respiratory tract has fascinated researchers for many years. Experimental measurements are still a gold standard, but they are limited in quantity and scope by cost and respiratory tract access. The advantages of computational modeling, with its ability to extend measurement data beyond these limitations to test ever-broader hypotheses, are compelling.

Mathematical modeling of respiratory particle deposition dates from Findeisen's work in 1935 (1) to the present day. During that time, models have developed from simple systems of one- or two-dimensional equations focused on occupational exposure to dust and fumes, to highly sophisticated, three- and four-dimensional representations of form and function, accounting for effects of disease, surgery, age, and ethnicity, incorporating complex anatomy, particle characteristics, and transport mechanisms from concepts in inhalation toxicology to medicine and rehabilitation.

Today's respiratory deposition models combine several types of mathematical models to achieve this complexity, but a typical central feature is the use of three-dimensional (3D), anatomically accurate, computational fluid dynamics (CFD). CFD is the application of numerical methods to the solution of nonlinear differential equations governing fluid flows (2) and can provide detailed information about flow velocities, pressures, and energy transport through a specific geometry. CFD modeling in 3D used to be too

computationally intensive to conduct outside a supercomputing center. Since the mid-1990s, however, desktop computers have become powerful enough to carry out useful 3D CFD simulations without being prohibitively expensive. A number of companies that commercialize CFD software packages, as well as researchers in numerical simulation, have kept up with these platform changes, and the result is an increasing number of studies being conducted using CFD modeling to study respiratory particle deposition.

Despite this progress in CFD modeling, however, other modeling methods are needed when the respiratory tract as a whole must be considered. Current imaging methods used to provide the anatomical domain for CFD cannot resolve important features of the deep lung, and questions on multiple levels of scale are not amenable to CFD modeling techniques. Multi-scale approaches such as physiologically based pharmacokinetic (PBPK) modeling, cellular transport modeling, multiple-path lung dosimetry modeling, and combined imaging and volume filling methods (3) can address these issues. These approaches have progressed during recent years as well, taking advantage of the increased computational power available on our desktops and benefitting from new cellular and genetic knowledge and advanced imaging techniques.

The purpose of this chapter is to provide a sense of the impact that CFD as well as other modeling approaches in whole lung/respiratory tract modeling have had on therapeutic aerosol research and development by describing the state of the art of human respiratory tract deposition modeling during the past decade. Examples of experimental evidence available for confirmation of model predictions will be given, and needs for future models will be discussed.

CFD MODELING

Fundamentals of CFD deposition modeling

Particles are transported in the respiratory tract by their initial velocity at the entrance and respiratory airflow. To understand the effects of both, the geometry of the airway and a predictive model of the airflow are needed, so airflow simulation using CFD will be discussed briefly first, followed by comments on particle transport modeling. A broad overview on these topics can be found in recent books by Tu and colleagues (4) and Finlay (5).

SIMULATION OF AIRFLOW

Respiratory airflow occurs at velocities for which the air can be considered incompressible (6). Information about airflows can therefore be obtained by solving the Navier-Stokes equations of motion, which are derived from Newton's Second Law (Conservation of Momentum) for fluids such as air and water (2). CFD modeling involves the numerical solution of the Navier-Stokes equations, subject to conditions on the airflow at the start of the flow in time, called initial conditions, and the state of the flow at the inlet, outlet, and walls of the flow domain, called boundary conditions (2). The main components of respiratory CFD models, therefore, are the geometry of the respiratory tract; a numerical method for solving the Navier-Stokes equations; decomposition of the airspace into small, discrete pieces or elements for application of the numerical method; and specification of the initial and boundary conditions. Several recent overviews describe these components in detail (4,7–10), so only brief comments will be made here in the context of 3D, anatomically accurate CFD models.

Respiratory tract geometry for 3D CFD models is generally obtained from digitally processing computed tomography (CT) or magnetic resonance imaging (MRI) images to locate air spaces and creating a surface rendering of the interface between air and tissue. This process is called segmentation and produces a 3D airway reconstruction that depends on the threshold value used to differentiate air from tissue; the algorithms used to create edges and surfaces from the threshold values; editing by hand; and the level of smoothing, if any, that is applied to the reconstructed surfaces (8,11). Changes in these segmentation factors affect the size and shape of the reconstruction, so ideally the segmentation is confirmed by reconstruction of a known phantom imaged at the same time. If concurrent phantom images are not obtainable, a sensitivity analysis to segmentation factors can be conducted, though there is a lack of such studies in the literature (8). Generally, when CFD simulations using the segmentation are compared to experimental measurements, at least a functional assessment of segmentation accuracy can be made.

Once the respiratory tract geometry is in hand, a choice must then be made about the numerical approach to take. This selection depends on whether airflows are likely to be predominantly laminar, transitional, or turbulent since the numerical approaches to the solution of the Navier-Stokes equations are quite different in each case (12). At rest, breathing rates are generally low enough that laminar simulations in the nasal passages are relatively accurate (13–16), but all three flow regimes can co-exist in respiratory flows, at least at higher flow rates (11,17), and there have been nasal CFD studies with confirming experimental measurements for each regime (e.g., 18–20). One recent study comparing laminar and turbulent solvers found that laminar simulations of nasal airflow compared best with flow measurements at low flow rates and turbulent simulations were in better agreement at high flow rates, though interestingly the differences among velocity magnitudes predicted by the different numerical solutions were not especially large (21). For oral inhalation, transitional and turbulent flow regimes may be present and CFD simulations using low Reynolds number turbulence models have proven successful at simulating these different regimes (22).

The next step is to decompose or discretize the airspace into a mesh or grid of elements that need to be small enough for adequate algebraic approximation of derivatives. To determine if mesh elements are small enough, simulations need to be conducted for refinements of the mesh until results are insensitive to further mesh changes (e.g., 23,24), so initial and boundary conditions on the airflow need to be specified. These conditions can take the form of specifying a pressure gradient to drive the flow, or specifying the flow itself at the inlet or outlet, and can be time-dependent to emulate a dynamic breathing state. Airflow rates used in steady-state inspiratory CFD simulations are often taken to be twice the minute-volume, derived by dividing the amount of inspired air (tidal volume) by the estimated time involved in inhalation (half the time a breath takes, or ($\frac{1}{2}$) (1/breathing frequency) (25). A frequently used value of 15 L/min for steady-state inspiratory flows corresponds to a minute volume of 7.5 L/min, which is listed as a reference value for adult men at rest by the International Commission for Radiological Protection (26).

SIMULATION OF PARTICLE TRANSPORT

CFD models of respiratory geometry and airflow can be used with equations describing particle motion to simulate the transport and deposition of inhaled or sprayed aerosols. Particle transport equations can be solved in the computational mesh of the airway using the computed airflow as input, or the particle transport and airflow equations can be solved together if interactions between particles and airflow are substantial. Since delivery devices affect particle transport and deposition as well, CFD modeling has also been conducted for the devices themselves or in conjunction with airway geometry (27). CFD-particle transport models can provide airway deposition predictions throughout the geometry of the model; thus these models can potentially be used to find conditions that minimize loss of therapeutic aerosols in delivery devices while maximizing delivery to specific target sites (28).

The main mechanisms by which particles deposit in the respiratory tract are inertial impaction, sedimentation, and diffusion, with interception if the particle is elongated or fiber-shaped (29). The degree to which each mechanism contributes to particle deposition depends on the geometry of the airway and the airflow passing through it, as well as the characteristics of the particles, including size and shape, density, chemical composition, surface structure, initial velocity, electrical charge, interactions with each other and the surrounding air, and the way they are generated and introduced to the respiratory tract. Sprayers, inhalers, and some nebulizers inject particles with nonzero, often substantial, initial velocities. Initial particle velocity can be zero, as in the cases of ambient air pollutants in still air, or assumed to be zero compared to inspiratory airflow rates in the case of many nebulized products. A recent review describes these factors and their effects on deposition in detail (29).

Since CFD-particle transport models provide a means to test the effects that variations in these characteristics have on target site deposition, clues can be gained as to how these characteristics may be manipulated to help maximize that deposition. A growing number of studies (e.g., 30–33) are focused on this goal.

Nasal CFD-particle transport modeling

RECENT LITERATURE

As the number of studies using respiratory CFD-particle transport modeling has increased over the past 20 years, so has the number of nasal CFD-particle transport modeling studies (Figure 3.1). In the 1990s, the nasal cavity was considered difficult to model due to its complex shape, which was not easily reconstructed in 3D or meshed (34). Since then, significant advances in computer hardware and software have made 3D CFD modeling in the nasal cavity much more accessible, and therefore more useful, as a hypothesis-testing and sensitivity-analysis tool.

The potential impact of this tool to study nasal physiology, pathology, toxicology, and medical and surgical treatment has been well-recognized for some time (35–38), and has generated a number of thoughtful reviews in the past 10 years (Table 3.1). Since these reviews contain extensive literature surveys on nasal CFD-particle transport modeling, an attempt to regenerate that information will not be given here. However, the evolving needs that researchers in this field have described will be summarized.

A decade ago, an overview of the state of the art was presented in a series of critical reviews on the mechanics of nasal airflow (11), nasal air conditioning (39), airflow and particle transport processes (40), and the use of particle image velocimetry to measure nasal airflow (41). At that time, the authors emphasized needs for more data to validate

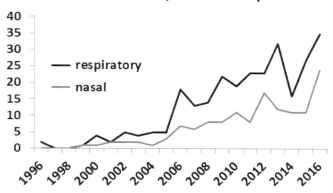

Number of CFD/Particles Papers

Figure 3.1 Literature searches on "computational fluid dynamics" and "particles" with either "nasal" or "respiratory" shows increasing trends between the late 1990s and 2016.

CFD model predictions, reducing the use of oversimplifying assumptions, incorporating unsteady airflow and dynamic geometry (including the nasal cycle), speeding up and improving the creation of patient-specific nasal models, and standardizing modeling methods among researchers. Several years later, most of these concerns were raised again by other reviewers (9,10,27,37,42–44), with additional concerns about postural, gender, and interindividual effects on image-based reconstructions of nasal anatomy (42,44,45); the study of nanoparticles (46,47); and the need for the use of improved transport equations for micron-sized particles (48) and turbulence models (10,27). Since then, improved numerical options for particle transport and turbulent simulation have become available (21), and a large-scale project to compare the results of these options with experimental data in a mouth-throat geometry is underway (49). Other recent reviews (7,49,50) continue to emphasize the need for detailed experimental measurements against which CFD model results can be compared. Further comments on this need are given below.

FEATURES SPECIFIC TO NASAL MODELS AND APPLICATIONS

Since all modeling involves some level of simplification, the application for which a nasal CFD-particle transport model is constructed drives the features and level of detail included in the model (27,34). Some features are common to all applications of nasal CFD-particle transport modeling, such as basic nasal anatomical structure and nasal airflow simulation. Anatomy is usually image-based and therefore patient-specific, but there are also examples in the literature of models that offer these features in a non-subject-specific manner (e.g., 51,52). Additional features are then added to the model as needed by the application of the model. The level of detail included in the model can, of course, be extended to the limits of the computational resources available, but in good modeling practice, only limited extrapolation should

Table 3.1 A list of reviews of nasal CFD-particle transport modeling since 2008

Title	Authors	Year
The Mechanics of Inhaled Pharmaceutical Aerosols: An Introduction	Finlay (5)	2001
Mechanics of airflow in the human nasal airways	Doorly et al. (11)	2008
Air-conditioning in the human nasal cavity	Elad et al. (39)	2008
Modeling airflow and particle transport/deposition in pulmonary airways	Kleinstreuer et al. (40)	2008
Digital particle image velocimetry studies of nasal airflow	Chung, Kim (41)	2008
A review of the implications of computational fluid dynamic studies on nasal airflow and physiology	Leong et al. (37)	2010
Evaluation of continuous and discrete phase models for simulating submicrometer aerosol transport and deposition	Longest, Xi (48)	2011
Review: A critical overview of limitations of CFD modeling in nasal airflow	Zubair et al. (42)	2012
Recent advances and key challenges in investigations of the flow inside human oro-pharyngeal-laryngeal airway	Pollard et al. (43)	2012
In silico models of aerosol delivery to the respiratory tract—Development and applications	Longest, Holbrook (27)	2012
Impacts of fluid dynamics simulation in study of nasal airflow physiology and pathophysiology in realistic human three-dimensional nose models	Wang et al. (44)	2012
Computational fluid dynamics (CFD) applied in the drug delivery design process to the nasal passages: A review	Kleven et al. (10)	2012
Particle transport and deposition: Basic physics of particle kinetics	Tsuda et al. (46)	2013
Patient specific CFD models of nasal airflow: Overview of methods and challenges	Kim et al. (9)	2013
Computational Fluid and Particle Dynamics in the Human Respiratory System	Tu et al. (4)	2013
Mechanisms of pharmaceutical aerosol deposition in the respiratory tract	Cheng (29)	2014
Pediatric *in vitro* and *in silico* models of deposition via oral and nasal inhalation	Carrigy et al. (45)	2014
Review of computational fluid dynamics in the assessment of nasal airflow and analysis of its limitations	Quadrio et al. (8)	2014
The transport and deposition of nanoparticles in respiratory system by inhalation	Qiao et al. (47)	2015
The evolution of inhaled particle dose modeling: A review	Phalen, Raabe (38)	2016
Image-based computational fluid dynamics in the lung: Virtual reality or new clinical practice?	Burrowes et al. (7)	2017
Experimental methods for flow and aerosol measurements in human airways and their replicas	Lizal et al. (50)	2018
Regional aerosol deposition in the human airways: The SimInhale benchmark case and a critical assessment of *in silico* methods	Koullapis et al. (49)	2018

be made in interpreting results past the level of detail in the experimental data used to confirm model predictions.

As noted above, each of the main application areas of nasal CFD-particle transport modeling, nasal physiology, surgical planning, toxicology, and nasal drug delivery has driven interesting and significant advancements in modeling of anatomy, airflow, and particle transport. Since applications of nasal CFD-particle transport modeling have been reviewed extensively by other authors (Table 3.1), only brief summary comments on some of the features that these applications have required for nasal modeling will be given here.

Normal nasal physiology (anatomical form and the functions of olfaction and cleansing, heating, and humidifying air) underlies all nasal modeling studies. We cannot know if surgeries or drug treatments will help patients or if toxic effects affect health if we do not have a baseline for comparison of these effects or a context in which to understand

them. A number of researchers have studied normal nasal structure using CFD models based on imaging of healthy individuals (e.g., 15,53,54), though lengthy model construction methods generally restricted these studies to too few subjects to account for interindividual anatomical effects. Ongoing efforts to speed up the model-building process have resulted more recently in larger studies (e.g., 55,56), indicating that soon there may be statistically sound bounds on normative CFD modeling results for multiple ethnicities. On the functional side, other features that nasal physiology modeling requires in nasal CFD-particle transport models include accounting for nasal cycling (57,58), and large temperature and humidity gradients compared to other areas of the respiratory tract. Modeling heat and water vapor transport is especially important when predicting the deposition of hygroscopic or evaporating particles (59).

Surgical planning for nasal procedures requires explicit rendering of nasal anatomy in normal, abnormal, and surgically altered circumstances. Nasal CFD-particle transport models constructed for surgical planning purposes provide the means to study questions about therapeutic particle deposition to treat practically any diseases or disorder for which imaging exists. Thus, this application requires nasal CFD models to incorporate anatomical detail in the vicinity of the surgical site, and to incorporate methods for digitally altering the model geometry to mimic surgical change. These methods have ranged from hand-editing (e.g., 60–62) to the creation of new software platforms (e.g., 63,64).

Toxicology and nasal drug delivery applications require nasal models to account for widely varying particle characteristics, which are often not relevant for other parts of the respiratory tract, such as deposition of large spray droplets in nasal target sites, and sometimes in ranges that put normally well-protected nasal areas at risk, such as nanoparticle toxicity in olfactory epithelium. In addition to driving deposition modeling, these applications also require models to account for disposition of particulate material in nasal tissues after deposition. Thus, another important feature specific to nasal CFD-particle transport models is the incorporation of particle-specific solubility and reactivity in relation to the uptake and metabolic properties of nasal tissues. Some recent efforts are leading the way in this area of coupling nasal CFD-particle transport and PBPK modeling (65–67).

EXPERIMENTAL DATA TO CONFIRM NASAL MODELS

As noted above, the availability of detailed experimental data against which nasal CFD-particle transport model results can be compared is extremely important. First and foremost, experimental measurements are used to provide credibility for model predictions. With enough detail, measurements can also be used to assess the effects of simplifying assumptions and numerical methods choices on model accuracy. This assessment informs the level of model complexity needed and can be used to generate new hypotheses about the application being studied; in fact, it can be argued that we learn more from disagreement with experimental data than we do from agreement.

In particular, experimental data can help modelers determine the need for laminar or turbulent modeling approaches and even help modelers decide which turbulent model performs best in the given scenario. Experimental measurements can help determine if the level of anatomical detail is sufficient, if the numerical approach has been properly implemented, and if assumptions about boundary conditions adversely affect model predictions. The types and status of experimental data that can be used to confirm nasal CFD-particle transport models have been extensively reviewed in prior literature (e.g., 10,41,43) as well as more recently (50).

In order to gain this much insight about a numerical model, however, the experimental setup must be closely matched with the model scenarios, and such experiments are usually conducted hand-in-hand with the modeling effort. If nasal CFD-particle transport modeling is to be generally useful, detailed experimental confirmation of each modeling scenario cannot be required as the resources needed will not usually be available or affordable. Thus, nasal CFD-particle transport models are needed that are sufficiently validated for the application at hand, for which extrapolation of the prior establishment of model credibility to the present scenario is not excessive. At present, the identification of such models is somewhat elusive, since validation studies often confirm model predictions that are significantly less complex than those produced by model use in a subsequent application (8). It is incumbent on modelers to avoid this situation or at least state clearly when the use of the model exceeds the current level of its validation. In such cases, sensitivity analyses should be conducted on the less-validated components of the model to determine the potential effects of this uncertainty.

Mouth/throat CFD-particle transport modeling

Therapeutic aerosols intended for delivery to the lung must first bypass deposition in the extrathoracic airways. Unlike the nasal airways, where local deposition is needed for topical delivery, deposition must be avoided in the mouth/throat (MT) region. The MT region can be a formidable obstacle to overcome for drug delivery to the lung, however, due to the high velocities that particles possess exiting delivery devices such as metered-dose inhalers (MDIs) and dry powder inhalers (DPIs). Another difficulty in the study of MT deposition is the high degree of variability in MT deposition that is evident from *in vivo* studies using inhaled monodisperse particles (68,69). This variability can then affect downstream deposition and lead to variability in lung deposition of inhaled drugs (70).

Numerous CFD studies have been conducted to better understand the mechanisms that lead to particle deposition in the MT and also to improve device design to minimize deposition in this region. These models have been used to study airflow and particle deposition in various types of MT geometries, including simplified models and models derived directly from imaging data. Simplified models retain the general shape of the oral cavity based on characteristic dimensions and use idealized shapes to simplify the overall geometry for ease of computations. In one of the first CFD oral airway modeling efforts, the k-ε turbulence model was used to simulate airflow through a simplified model of the oral passageway (71). Good predictions with *in vitro* data were observed at low flow rates in the laminar regime, but poor correlations with experimental data were observed at flow rates where one would expect the onset of turbulence. Subsequently, particle image velocimetry (PIV) and several Reynolds-averaged Navier-Stokes (RANS) turbulence models were used to simulate oral cavity airflow and showed areas of separated flow and recirculation at high flow rates (72). The turbulent characteristics of airflow that were identified in the oral cavity promoted the use of turbulence models in CFD simulations that could accurately simulate transitional and turbulent airflows.

Zhang and colleagues (22) used a low-Reynolds-number (LRN) k-ω turbulence model in a model of the oral cavity and trachea to simulate the laminar-to-turbulent flow regimes present in the upper airways and found good agreement with experimental airflow profiles and particle deposition fractions in the upper airways. However, they found that near-wall corrections were needed to overcome the assumption of isotropic near-wall turbulence, which assumes turbulent fluctuations are equal in all directions. Simulation results from multiple turbulence models in locally constricted conduits were compared and it was found that the LRN k-ω model was more suitable to simulate the laminar-transitional-turbulent flow regime that is present in these geometries that are characteristic of respiratory airways (73). The k-ω turbulence model was then used to show the laminar-to-turbulent nature of flows in this region and to study airflow and particle deposition in a simplified MT geometry (74–76). Matida and coworkers (77) used a large eddy simulation (LES) solver to improve deposition predictions in their oral cavity model. CFD predictions of aerosol deposition in the MT region were in good agreement with experimental data, and the LES approach showed improvement over RANS turbulence models without the near-wall corrections that have been found to be necessary. LES is more accurate than standard RANS approaches but is much more computationally expensive. As a result, k-ω approaches with the near-wall correction terms have been more widely used in respiratory dosimetry modeling efforts and have had success when comparing CFD-predicted aerosol deposition to results from experimental deposition studies in replica casts.

The LRN k-ω turbulence models were also applied to models of the oral airway with varying degrees of geometric simplification (78). The level of reduction in model simplification was found to have a substantial impact on deposition patterns of inhaled micro-particles but did not have a significant effect on nanoparticle deposition, highlighting the roles of surface geometry and inertial impaction on aerosol deposition in the MT region (79). This airway model was also used to evaluate the effect of inhaler insertion angle on drug deposition and found that the inhaler angle can significantly affect mouth deposition (80).

CFD studies using idealized MT models have provided valuable insights into aerosol deposition behavior in the upper respiratory tract. In addition, in some cases, cast models were made so that modeling predictions could be compared with experimental particle deposition data in the identical geometry. The collection of studies using idealized MT models has shown that geometry plays a significant role in aerosol deposition behavior in this region. For this reason, CFD studies have also been conducted using patient-specific models derived from imaging data. While these models are not as flexible as idealized MT models and only capture the geometry of a single individual at the moment the scan was taken, they nonetheless do provide more anatomical realism than idealized models. Jayaraju and colleagues (81) developed an oral airway model derived from CT scans and used the LRN k-ω turbulence model; they found good agreement with experimental data for airflow and particle deposition. Patient-specific models of the MT region were also developed by other groups to study oral deposition of micron-sized particles (82) and aerosol drug delivery in air and helium-oxygen mixtures (83,84).

CFD studies have also been conducted to simulate the transport and deposition of droplets and particles from spray inhalers in MT geometries. One of the biggest concerns with aerosolized drug delivery efficiency is impaction at the back of the throat. While an increase in inhalation flow rate can yield better deagglomeration of particles from DPIs, for example (85), the higher flow rates also result in higher impaction efficiencies from the turbulent jet striking the back of the oral cavity. Matida and colleagues (86) changed the size of the inlet of an MT geometry to simulate inlet conditions from DPIs. When RANS turbulence models were used with near-wall corrections, good comparisons were found with experimental data (87). Aerosol momentum was also studied by Longest and coworkers (88) to investigate its effects on deposition in a standard induction port and more realistic MT geometry. They also evaluated the effects of generation time on aerosol deposition in MT geometries to see if extending the generation time would reduce spray momentum (89). Kleinstreuer and colleagues (90) used CFD models to predict aerosol deposition in an MT geometry from chlorofluorocarbon (CFC) and hydrofluoroalkane-134a (HFA) MDIs and to evaluate the effects of propellant, nozzle diameter, and spacer distance on MT deposition. These numerical modeling studies demonstrate the utility of CFD modeling to study how to minimize deposition in the MT region and promote delivery of aerosols to the lung airways for improved efficacy.

Lung CFD-particle transport modeling

The human lung consists of a dichotomously branching network of airways with generally decreasing diameters through, on average, 16 generations, followed by approximately 7 generations of acinar airways where gas exchange occurs (91). For CFD modeling studies of airflow and particle deposition in the lung, segments of the overall airway structure have been modeled as networks of bifurcating tubes. Earlier modeling studies used airway geometries based on several bifurcations (92–97). Good agreement was obtained with in vitro deposition data as long as the inlet velocity and particle profiles were accurately modeled (24). A natural progression from two- or three-bifurcation models was to extend the geometries further down the tracheobronchial tree. Subsequent modeling efforts simulated airflow and particle deposition in the upper tracheobronchial airways consisting of three to six airway generations (79,98,99). Beyond five or six generations, the geometry development process can be quite cumbersome, and models with further airways were developed using automated techniques. Several efforts have been made to develop lung morphological models for lung geometries of the entire tracheobronchial

(TB) tree (100–102). While these models have successfully extended the simulation domain through the TB tree, they nonetheless are typically generated from morphometric data of human airway casts and are based on simplified symmetric (91) or asymmetric structures (103). To incorporate more anatomical realism, Gemci and coworkers (104) developed an airway model of the TB tree based on a digital reference model of the TB airways derived from CT data. The advantages of this approach are that most of the TB airways can be accounted for in the CFD model, but the individual airways are assumed to be cylindrically shaped, so care must be taken to accurately conjoin airways at bifurcations due to the influence of bifurcation shapes on localized deposition hot spots.

Rather than generating complete branching structures, an alternative approach has been to take advantage of the assumed symmetry at airway bifurcations and develop typical-path airway models. In these models, a single path is followed from the trachea through the TB airways and possibly to generation 23, with the opposing pathway at each bifurcation truncated at the daughter airway. In this way, the lung structure from the trachea to the lower airways is represented (105). This modeling approach was used to apply stochastic individual paths extending to the terminal bronchioles in a single lung lobe (106) and was then extended further to all five lobes of the lung by developing stochastic paths into each lobe and using the CFD models to evaluate lung delivery of MDIs and DPIs (107).

CFD lung airway models based on morphometric data have the advantage of being more flexible in terms of generating models for different regions of the lung, but they lack the anatomical realism of real lung airways. Patient-specific CFD models of the upper TB airways based on CT images have been more frequently studied in recent years, with models usually progressing down to the mid-bronchial airways, depending on the resolution of the scanner (e.g., 81,108–110). With current imaging technology, airways can be resolved until approximately generation 7–11 (7). Patient-specific models derived from CT scans can capture finer geometric airway features such as airway curvature and cartilaginous rings that may affect the flow field and particle deposition. Nowak and colleagues (111) reported that CFD studies of airflow and particle deposition in the bronchial tree showed dramatic differences between the Weibel model and those using CT data. Due to artifacts in the CT scan and the airway diameters approaching the resolution of the scanner, decisions must be made about where to truncate the airways and create outlets for CFD calculations. Planar outlets are usually formed at the terminus of each airway branch and boundary conditions applied to each outlet face. The simplest boundary conditions to apply at the outlets are uniform pressure or velocity conditions. While these are easy to implement, they do not capture differences in lobar ventilation that will affect the airflow distribution. DeBacker and coworkers (112) showed that different pressure values applied at the outlets of CFD lung airway models can produce heterogeneous and asymmetric flow patterns, and another DeBacker study (113) showed the effects of outlet

boundary conditions by comparing CFD predictions with single photon emission computed tomography (SPECT)/CT data taken at functional residual capacity and total lung capacity. A hybrid approach to add more realistic boundary conditions has been proposed by coupling 3D CFD models of the upper airways with lower dimensional models of airway resistance and compliance at each outlet to examine the effects of distal lung mechanics on regional airflow (114,115).

In order to use CFD models to study aerosolized drug delivery in the lung, models have to contain the complete upper and lower respiratory tracts. Recent modeling efforts have focused on all-inclusive models that contain the MT region, the pharynx/larynx regions, and bronchial airways. Computer-aided design can also be used to engineer devices at the entrance to the MT region so that the atomization process from the device can be simulated using CFD techniques rather than assuming that delivered drug particles start at the mouth entrance. As with MT geometries, the selection of turbulence model can have a profound influence on airflow and particle deposition predictions. Most researchers continue to implement RANS methods in order to capture the transitional to turbulent airflow characteristics in the upper lung airways; LES approaches are also being more widely implemented as computer power increases, thereby making this approach more accessible.

CFD models of the upper bronchial airways developed from imaging data leave a lot of the lung unresolved. There have been recent efforts to develop airway models from imaging data to the point of resolution, and then to develop the remaining airways using idealized models. For example, Lin and coworkers (116) used a volume-filling method to create a 3D model down to the terminal bronchioles. Yin and colleagues (117) also started with a 3D CFD model of the upper TB airways and then extended the model using a 1D airway tree down to the terminal bronchioles. Another approach has been to develop "whole-airway" CFD models of the respiratory tract (118). In this approach, the complete airway tree is represented through the third bifurcation so that airway paths are directed to each lobe and then stochastic pathway models are applied for the remainder of the bronchial tree in each lobe. This modeling approach was recently used to study deposition of MDIs and DPIs throughout the lung (119). To add realistic breathing scenarios to these models, the alveolar region has been simulated using moving walls to initiate inhalation (120). Kolanjiyil and Kleinstreuer (121) also recently introduced a "whole-lung" modeling approach using wall displacement boundaries in the alveolar region to simulate breathing patterns. These studies demonstrate the progression of CFD models in recent years toward the goal of simulating airflow and particle deposition in the "entire lung."

Whole-lung particle deposition modeling

Whole-lung deposition models recognize the inter-subject variability of experimental deposition measurements and adopt the view that the deposition model represents the "average" behavior in the population considered. Whole-lung dosimetry models range in complexity from semi-empirical models to multiple-path models based on morphometric measurements of lung airways. Semi-empirical models are geometry independent and estimate lung deposition based on fitting equations in terms of analytical parameters to deposition data (122,123). Generally, for particles >1 μm in diameter, the impaction parameter or Stokes number is used, whereas a diffusion parameter is used for submicron particles. Empirical models are useful for quick calculations of overall deposition in the lung, but they lack robustness, cannot enable more site-specific deposition information, and should not be used outside the measurement range of the data upon which they are based. As such, they are limited in usefulness for therapeutic aerosol deposition predictions.

Single-path models assume that all airways in each generation have the same dimensions; thus, each generation can be represented by a single airway with averaged dimensions, leading to a single path through the lung. Some of the earlier examples of single-path models include the national council on radiation protection and measurements (NCRP) (124) and international commission on radiological protection (ICRP) (125) models and models developed by Yeh and Schum (126) and Martonen (127). As noted by Martonen (127), single-path models can be used to predict lung deposition of inhaled pharmaceuticals for therapeutic purposes. These models require definition of lung morphology, ventilatory parameters, and particle deposition processes. These models require definition of lung morphology, ventilatory parameters, and particle deposition processes. Due to their single-path nature, these types of models were naturally set up to use the Weibel model of lung morphology, which assumes symmetric dichotomously branching airways (91). Ventilatory parameters needed in the models consist of the parameters necessary to define the breathing maneuver and consist of the tidal volume, breathing frequency, and/or inhalation/exhalation times. In each airway, particle deposition is calculated due to the processes of inertial impaction, sedimentation, and diffusion. A stochastic approach has also been used to capture variability in lung structure. Stochastic whole-lung models use probability density functions describing airway parameters and parent-daughter correlations to derive airway paths through the entire airway tree (128).

Some of the highlighted findings from these modeling studies include that, for total deposition in the respiratory tract, the dependence on particle diameter predicts minimum deposition at a particle diameter in the 0.1–0.5 μm range. As particle diameter increases, deposition increases due to impactive deposition in the upper respiratory tract and large bronchi, and due to sedimentation in the smaller airways and pulmonary region. As particle diameter increases, the location of deposition shifts to more proximal regions of the respiratory tract where inertial impaction is the dominant deposition mechanism and flow rates are high. For particles smaller than 0.1 μm, the mechanism of particle diffusion becomes important, and the overall deposition

increases with decreasing particle diameter. These modeling results have provided insights for pharmaceutical applications regarding shifts in particle deposition in the lung as breathing rate or particle size changes.

One example of a whole-lung dosimetry model that is used by many researchers in the field is the multiple-path particle dosimetry (MPPD) model (129). The MPPD model is a comprehensive, mechanistic deposition model that was developed based on the physics of airflow and particle transport in lung airways to calculate total or regional deposition and clearance of particles. The MPPD software contains a user-friendly interface and is available to the public (http://www.ara.com/products/mppd.htm).

The MPPD model contains several lung geometries to choose from, including single-path symmetric, asymmetric, stochastic, children of different ages, and geometries for animal species. Particle deposition can be calculated in any geometric structure of the lung. As with single-path models, particle deposition is calculated based on the mechanisms of inertial impaction, sedimentation, and diffusion. Airflow velocity at a location within an airway is assumed uniform and proportional to the lung volume distal to that location. Consequently, airflow rates decrease distally within the lung. At the same time, lung airways expand and contract uniformly during a breathing cycle that includes inhalation, pause, and exhalation. Particle deposition is calculated at a lung volume midway between the lung at rest and end of inhalation. Particle deposition results can be presented in many forms, including deposition fraction or mass deposited in regional, lobar, or total lung. The MPPD model allows investigators to study the effects of lung heterogeneity on particle deposition and is a valuable tool for predicting the required exposure dose of pharmaceutical aerosols and deposition sites in the lung and can also be used for targeting pharmaceutical aerosols to specific locations within the lung. The MPPD model has undergone many improvements and modifications in recent years (130), most notably the inclusion of hygroscopic aerosols (131), nanoparticles (132), and vapors (133).

FUTURE NEEDS AND DIRECTIONS FOR RESPIRATORY TRACT MODEL DEVELOPMENT

One of the most pressing needs for nasal CFD-particle transport modeling continues to be detailed experimental data against which CFD model results can be compared. Regional deposition data measured in a nasal cavity geometry that is publicly available would be very helpful. Such information could be used by individual researchers to simulate the experimental scenario using computational resources available to them, and allow adjustment of simulation parameters until agreement with measurements is achieved.

Another continued need for nasal CFD-particle transport modeling is incorporation of fluid-structure interaction methods that would allow the study of dynamic effects in the nasal valve area and nasopharynx. The static nature of these nasal airway components in most of the modeling approaches currently in use does not allow for accurate study of nasal valve collapse or obstructive sleep apnea. Some researchers have explored this area of research (e.g., 134–137), but more research and validation studies are needed.

Information about localized mucus flow patterns, thickness and composition within the nose, as well as particle size distributions of active pharmaceutical ingredients (APIs) and chemical interactions of APIs with nasal tissues is also needed (138). Continued development of linked CFD-particle transport and PBPK modeling requires uptake and clearance information, which depends on mucus characteristics and dissolution properties of APIs and metabolic activity in order to simulate uptake and systemic circulation. This information is needed for bioavailability studies and comparisons of products among different delivery routes.

Alternative ways to obtain nasal cavity geometry for nasal CFD-particle transport modeling besides CT and MRI are needed. Radiation exposure from CT and lengthy sessions that require sedation in small children for MRI makes these imaging modalities prohibitive in prospective studies. While cone-beam technologies are decreasing CT radiation exposure (139) and there is extensive research into improvements in MRI as well (e.g., 140–142), new imaging techniques are needed that can provide nasal geometry for accurate three-dimensional reconstruction without radiation or sedation. Endoscopic visualization has promise, especially as this modality allows potential quantification of dynamic effects (143,144); use of this approach in conjunction with the development of fluid-structure interaction models (134) will be very powerful.

Validation with experimental data is also a vital need for lung CFD-particle transport modeling. Many studies have compared CFD modeling predictions of specific airway segments with *in vitro* data using replica casts. While these comparisons have proven valuable for validating CFD approaches, the experiments and computational simulations are typically conducted using steady inspiratory flow rates. With lung models now progressing to more distal airways, approaches that account for the natural breathing cycle are more appropriate and will involve *in vivo* imaging studies of deposition. This also ties in with recent efforts at coupling lower dimensional models with 3D CFD models of the bronchial airways in order to obtain more realistic outlet boundary conditions. This will be especially important in order for CFD models to accurately simulate airflow and drug delivery in diseased lungs, where more heterogeneous airflow patterns are expected (145). An intimate coupling of imaging and modeling is needed to achieve these aims (7).

Most respiratory dosimetry modeling studies to date have simulated solid particles, but pharmaceutical aerosols may be composed of particles, liquid droplets, or suspensions. In addition, droplets may contain several constituents such as propellants and excipients. The concentrations of these constituents and their corresponding saturation vapor pressures will dictate how rapidly they evaporate from the liquid droplets. Because particle size is one of the primary determinants of deposition location, accounting for these thermodynamic processes to study the phase change of each constituent is important for accurate quantification of respiratory deposition. A number of studies have simulated hygroscopic growth of inhaled aerosols (131,146,147), and Hindle and Longest (148) have promoted the idea of enhanced condensational growth for aerosol delivery so that small particles delivered through the nose will have low nasal deposition, yet their hygroscopic properties will lead to larger droplets with higher deposition in the lung airways.

Respiratory dosimetry modeling studies, including 3D CFD and whole-lung models, have made significant advances over the last few decades and have provided valuable predictions on the locations of particle deposition in the respiratory tract as a function of geometry, flow rate, and particle size. A natural area to investigate now is what happens to the drug particle after it has deposited. Mucociliary clearance, diffusion, metabolism, and blood perfusion all play important roles. PBPK models are frequently used to investigate tissue disposition of drugs and chemicals, but a linking of PBPK models with respiratory dosimetry models will allow for more advanced predictions of systemic pharmacokinetics (PK) following drug delivery. This approach has been used with success for inhaled chemicals (110,149), and there have been several modeling studies with inhaled drugs (150,151). A close interaction of PBPK models with 3D CFD models of the respiratory tract will bring us closer to being able to predict systemic PK following aerosolized drug delivery to the nose or lungs.

REFERENCES

1. Findeisen W. Über das Absetzen kleiner, in der Luft suspendierter Teilchen in der menschlichen Lunge bei der Atmung. *Pflüger's Archiv für die gesamte Physiologie des Menschen und der Tiere.* 1935;236(1):367–379.

2. Batchelor GK. *An Introduction to Fluid Dynamics.* Cambridge, UK: Cambridge University Press; 1967.

3. Lin CL, Tawhai MH, Hoffman EA. Multiscale image-based modeling and simulation of gas flow and particle transport in the human lungs. *Wiley Interdisciplinary Reviews: Systems Biology and Medicine.* 2013;5(5):643–655.

4. Tu J, Inthavong K, Ahmadi G. *Computational Fluid and Particle Dynamics in the Human Respiratory System.* Greenbaum E, editor. Dordrecht, the Netherlands: Springer Science+Business Media; 2013.

5. Finlay WH. *The Mechanics of Inhaled Pharmaceutical Aerosols: An Introduction.* San Diego, CA: Academic Press; 2001.

6. Kaminski DA, Jensen MK. *Introduction to Thermal and Fluids Engineering.* Hoboken, NJ: Wiley; 2005.

7. Burrowes KS, De Backer J, Kumar H. Image-based computational fluid dynamics in the lung: Virtual reality or new clinical practice? *Wiley Interdisciplinary Reviews: Systems Biology and Medicine.* 2017;9(6).

8. Quadrio M, Pipolo C, Corti S, Lenzi R, Messina F, Pesci C et al. Review of computational fluid dynamics in the assessment of nasal air flow and analysis of its limitations. *European Archives of Oto-Rhino-Laryngology.* 2014;271(9):2349–2354.

9. Kim SK, Na Y, Kim J-I, Chung S-K. Patient specific CFD models of nasal airflow: Overview of methods and challenges. *Journal of Biomechanics.* 2013;46(2):299–306.

10. Kleven M, Melaaen MC, Djupesland PG. Computational fluid dynamics (CFD) applied in the drug delivery design process to the nasal passages: A review. *Journal of Mechanics in Medicine and Biology.* 2012;12(1):1230002.

11. Doorly D, Taylor D, Schroter R. Mechanics of airflow in the human nasal airways. *Respiratory Physiology & Neurobiology.* 2008;163(1–3):100–110.

12. Aref H, Balachandar S. *A First Course in Computational Fluid Dynamics.* Cambridge, UK: Cambridge University Press; 2018.

13. Subramaniam RP, Richardson RB, Morgan KT, Kimbell JS, Guilmette RA. Computational fluid dynamics simulations of inspiratory airflow in the human nose and nasopharynx. *Inhalation Toxicology.* 1998;10(2):91–120.

14. Garcia G, Mitchell G, Bailie N, Thornhill D, Watterson J, Kimbell J, editors. Visualization of nasal airflow patterns in a patient affected with atrophic rhinitis using particle image velocimetry. *Journal of Physics: Conference Series*; 2007;85(1):012032.

15. Segal RA, Kepler GM, Kimbell JS. Effects of differences in nasal anatomy on airflow distribution: A comparison of four individuals at rest. *Annals of Biomedical Engineering.* 2008;36(11):1870–1882.

16. Chung S-K, Son YR, Shin SJ, Kim S-K. Nasal airflow during respiratory cycle. *American Journal of Rhinology.* 2006;20(4):379–384.

17. Xi J, Longest PW. Numerical predictions of submicrometer aerosol deposition in the nasal cavity using a novel drift flux approach. *International Journal of Heat and Mass Transfer.* 2008;51(23–24):5562–5577.

18. Keyhani K, Scherer P, Mozell M. Numerical simulation of airflow in the human nasal cavity. *Journal of Biomechanical Engineering.* 1995;117(4):429–441.

19. Phuong NL, Ito K. Investigation of flow pattern in upper human airway including oral and nasal inhalation by PIV and CFD. *Building and Environment.* 2015;94:504–515.

20. Calmet H, Gambaruto AM, Bates AJ, Vázquez M, Houzeaux G, Doorly DJ. Large-scale CFD simulations of the transitional and turbulent regime for the large human airways during rapid inhalation. *Computers in Biology and Medicine.* 2016;69:166–180.

21. Li C, Jiang J, Dong H, Zhao K. Computational modeling and validation of human nasal airflow under various breathing conditions. *Journal of Biomechanics.* 2017;64:59–68.

22. Zhang Y, Finlay W, Matida E. Particle deposition measurements and numerical simulation in a highly idealized mouth–throat. *Journal of Aerosol Science.* 2004;35(7):789–803.

23. Frank-Ito DO, Wofford M, Schroeter JD, Kimbell JS. Influence of mesh density on airflow and particle deposition in sinonasal airway modeling. *Journal of Aerosol Medicine and Pulmonary Drug Delivery.* 2016;29(1):46–56.

24. Longest PW, Vinchurkar S. Effects of mesh style and grid convergence on particle deposition in bifurcating airway models with comparisons to experimental data. *Medical Engineering and Physics.* 2007;29(3):350–366.

25. Kimbell J, Subramaniam R, Gross E, Schlosser P, Morgan K. Dosimetry modeling of inhaled formaldehyde: Comparisons of local flux predictions in the rat, monkey, and human nasal passages. *Toxicological Sciences.* 2001;64(1):100–110.

26. ICRP. *Human Respiratory Tract Model for Radiological Protection. Annals of the International Commission on Radiological Protection.* Tarrytown, NY: Elsevier Science; 1994.

27. Longest PW, Holbrook LT. In silico models of aerosol delivery to the respiratory tract—development and applications. *Advanced Drug Delivery Reviews.* 2012;64(4):296–311.

28. Longest PW, Hindle M. Quantitative analysis and design of a spray aerosol inhaler. Part 1: Effects of dilution air inlets and flow paths. *Journal of Aerosol Medicine and Pulmonary Drug Delivery.* 2009;22(3):271–283.

29. Cheng YS. Mechanisms of pharmaceutical aerosol deposition in the respiratory tract. *AAPS PharmSciTech.* 2014;15(3):630–640.

30. Tong X, Dong J, Shang Y, Inthavong K, Tu J. Effects of nasal drug delivery device and its orientation on sprayed particle deposition in a realistic human nasal cavity. *Computers in Biology and Medicine.* 2016;77:40–48.

31. Inthavong K, Fung MC, Yang W, Tu J. Measurements of droplet size distribution and analysis of nasal spray atomization from different actuation pressure. *Journal of Aerosol Medicine and Pulmonary Drug Delivery.* 2015;28(1):59–67.

32. Si XA, Xi J, Kim J, Zhou Y, Zhong H. Modeling of release position and ventilation effects on olfactory aerosol drug delivery. *Respiratory Physiology & Neurobiology.* 2013;186(1):22–32.

33. Perkins EL, Basu S, Garcia GJ, Buckmire RA, Shah RN, Kimbell JS. Ideal particle sizes for inhaled steroids targeting vocal granulomas: Preliminary study using computational fluid dynamics. *Otolaryngology–Head and Neck Surgery.* 2018;158(3):511–519.

34. Kimbell J. *Computational Fluid Dynamics of the Extrathoracic Airways.* Southampton, UK: WIT Press; 2001.

35. Bockholt U, Mlynski G, Müller W, Voss G. Rhinosurgical therapy planning via endonasal. *Computer Aided Surgery.* 2000;5(3):175–179.

36. Feron V, Arts J, Kuper C, Slootweg P, Woutersen R. Health risks associated with inhaled nasal toxicants. *Critical Reviews in Toxicology.* 2001;31(3):313–347.

37. Leong S, Chen X, Lee H, Wang D. A review of the implications of computational fluid dynamic studies on nasal airflow and physiology. *Rhinology.* 2010;48(2):139.

38. Phalen R, Raabe O. The evolution of inhaled particle dose modeling: A review. *Journal of Aerosol Science.* 2016;99:7–13.

39. Elad D, Wolf M, Keck T. Air-conditioning in the human nasal cavity. *Respiratory Physiology & Neurobiology.* 2008;163(1–3):121–127.

40. Kleinstreuer C, Zhang Z, Li Z. Modeling airflow and particle transport/deposition in pulmonary airways. *Respiratory Physiology & Neurobiology.* 2008;163(1–3):128–138.

41. Chung S-K, Kim SK. Digital particle image velocimetry studies of nasal airflow. *Respiratory Physiology & Neurobiology.* 2008;163(1–3):111–120.

42. Zubair M, Abdullah MZ, Ismail R, Shuaib IL, Hamid SA, Ahmad KA. A critical overview of limitations of CFD modeling in nasal airflow. *Journal of Medical and Biological Engineering.* 2012;32(2):77–84.

43. Pollard A, Uddin M, Shinneeb A-M, Ball C. Recent advances and key challenges in investigations of the flow inside human oro-pharyngeal-laryngeal airway. *International Journal of Computational Fluid Dynamics.* 2012;26(6–8):363–381.

44. De Yun Wang HPL, Gordon BR. Impacts of fluid dynamics simulation in study of nasal airflow physiology and pathophysiology in realistic human three-dimensional nose models. *Clinical and Experimental Otorhinolaryngology.* 2012;5(4):181.

45. Carrigy NB, Ruzycki CA, Golshahi L, Finlay WH. Pediatric in vitro and in silico models of deposition via oral and nasal inhalation. *Journal of Aerosol Medicine and Pulmonary Drug Delivery.* 2014;27(3):149–169.

46. Tsuda A, Henry FS, Butler JP. Particle transport and deposition: Basic physics of particle kinetics. *Comprehensive Physiology.* 2013;3(4):1437–1471.

47. Qiao H, Liu W, Gu H, Wang D, Wang Y. The transport and deposition of nanoparticles in respiratory system by inhalation. *Journal of Nanomaterials.* 2015;2015:2.

48. Longest PW, Xi J. Evaluation of continuous and discrete phase models for simulating submicrometer aerosol transport and deposition. In: Amano RS, Sunden B, editors. *Computational Fluid Dynamics and Heat Transfer: Emerging Topics.* Southampton, UK: WIT Press; 2011. pp. 425–457.

49. Koullapis P, Kassinos S, Muela J, Perez-Segarra C, Rigola J, Lehmkuhl O et al. Regional aerosol deposition in the human airways: The SimInhale benchmark case and a critical assessment of in silico methods. *European Journal of Pharmaceutical Sciences.* 2018;113:77–94.

50. Lizal F, Jedelsky J, Morgan K, Bauer K, Llop J, Cossio U et al. Experimental methods for flow and aerosol measurements in human airways and their replicas. *European Journal of Pharmaceutical Sciences.* 2018;113:95–131.

51. Liu Y, Johnson MR, Matida EA, Kherani S, Marsan J. Creation of a standardized geometry of the human nasal cavity. *Journal of Applied Physiology.* 2009;106(3):784–795.

52. Javaheri E, Golshahi L, Finlay W. An idealized geometry that mimics average infant nasal airway deposition. *Journal of Aerosol Science.* 2013;55:137–148.

53. Zhu JH, Lee HP, Lim KM, Lee SJ, Wang DY. Evaluation and comparison of nasal airway flow patterns among three subjects from Caucasian, Chinese and Indian ethnic groups using computational fluid dynamics simulation. *Respiratory Physiology & Neurobiology.* 2011;175(1):62–69.

54. Xi J, Berlinski A, Zhou Y, Greenberg B, Ou X. Breathing resistance and ultrafine particle deposition in nasal–laryngeal airways of a newborn, an infant, a child, and an adult. *Annals of Biomedical Engineering.* 2012;40(12):2579–2595.

55. Zhao K, Jiang J, Blacker K, Lyman B, Dalton P, Cowart BJ et al. Regional peak mucosal cooling predicts the perception of nasal patency. *The Laryngoscope.* 2014;124(3):589–595.

56. Keeler JA, Patki A, Woodard CR, Frank-Ito DO. A computational study of nasal spray deposition pattern in four ethnic groups. *Journal of Aerosol Medicine and Pulmonary Drug Delivery.* 2016;29(2):153–166.

57. Hildebrandt T, Heppt WJ, Kertzscher U, Goubergrits L. The concept of rhinorespiratory homeostasis—A new approach to nasal breathing. *Facial Plastic Surgery.* 2013;29(2):85–92.

58. Patel RG, Garcia GJ, Frank-Ito DO, Kimbell JS, Rhee JS. Simulating the nasal cycle with computational fluid dynamics. *Otolaryngology–Head and Neck Surgery.* 2015;152(2):353–360.

59. Schroeter JD, Asgharian B, Price OT, Kimbell JS, Kromidas L, Singal M. Simulation of the phase change and deposition of inhaled semi-volatile liquid droplets in the nasal passages of rats and humans. *Journal of Aerosol Science*. 2016;95:15–29.

60. Wofford M, Kimbell J, Frank-Ito D, Dhandha V, McKinney K, Fleischman G et al. A computational study of functional endoscopic sinus surgery and maxillary sinus drug delivery. *Rhinology*. 2015;53(1):41–48.

61. Frank-Ito DO, Kimbell JS, Laud P, Garcia GJ, Rhee JS. Predicting postsurgery nasal physiology with computational modeling: Current challenges and limitations. *Otolaryngology--Head and Neck Surgery*. 2014;151(5):751–759.

62. Lee H, Garlapati R, Chong V, Wang D. Effects of septal perforation on nasal airflow: Computer simulation study. *The Journal of Laryngology & Otology*. 2010;124(1):48–54.

63. Burgos M, Sanmiguel-Rojas E, Del Pino C, Sevilla-García M, Esteban-Ortega F. New CFD tools to evaluate nasal airflow. *European Archives of Oto-Rhino-Laryngology*. 2017;274(8):3121–3128.

64. Quammen CW, Taylor RM, II PK, Mitran S, Enquobahrie A, Superfine R et al. The virtual pediatric airways workbench. *Studies in Health Technology and Informatics*. 2016;220:295.

65. Rygg A, Longest PW. Absorption and clearance of pharmaceutical aerosols in the human nose: Development of a CFD model. *Journal of Aerosol Medicine and Pulmonary Drug Delivery*. 2016;29(5):416–431.

66. Rygg A, Hindle M, Longest PW. Linking suspension nasal spray drug deposition patterns to pharmacokinetic profiles: A proof-of-concept study using computational fluid dynamics. *Journal of Pharmaceutical Sciences*. 2016;105(6):1995–2004.

67. Schroeter J, Kimbell J, Walenga R, Babiskin A, Delvadia R. A CFD-PBPK model to simulate nasal absorption and systemic bioavailability of intranasal fluticasone propionate. *Journal of Aerosol Medicine and Pulmonary Drug Delivery*. 2017;30:13–14.

68. Stahlhofen W, Gebhart J, Heyder J. Biological variability of regional deposition of aerosol particles in the human respiratory tract. *American Industrial Hygiene Association Journal*. 1981;42(5):348–352.

69. Stahlhofen W, Gebhart J, Heyder J. Experimental determination of the regional deposition of aerosol particles in the human respiratory tract. *American Industrial Hygiene Association Journal*. 1980;41(6):385–398a.

70. Borgström L, Olsson B, Thorsson L. Degree of throat deposition can explain the variability in lung deposition of inhaled drugs. *Journal of Aerosol Medicine*. 2006;19(4):473–483.

71. Stapleton K-W, Guentsch E, Hoskinson M, Finlay W. On the suitability of k–ε turbulence modeling for aerosol deposition in the mouth and throat: A comparison with experiment. *Journal of Aerosol Science*. 2000;31(6):739–749.

72. Heenan A, Matida E, Pollard A, Finlay W. Experimental measurements and computational modeling of the flow field in an idealized human oropharynx. *Experiments in Fluids*. 2003;35(1):70–84.

73. Zhang Z, Kleinstreuer C. Low-Reynolds-number turbulent flows in locally constricted conduits: A comparison study. *AIAA Journal*. 2003;41(5):831–840.

74. Zhang Z, Kleinstreuer C, Kim C. Micro-particle transport and deposition in a human oral airway model. *Journal of Aerosol Science*. 2002;33(12):1635–1652.

75. Kleinstreuer C, Zhang Z. Laminar-to-turbulent fluid-particle flows in a human airway model. *International Journal of Multiphase Flow*. 2003;29(2):271–289.

76. Zhang Z, Kleinstreuer C. Airflow structures and nano-particle deposition in a human upper airway model. *Journal of Computational Physics*. 2004;198(1):178–210.

77. Matida EA, Finlay WH, Breuer M, Lange CF. Improving prediction of aerosol deposition in an idealized mouth using large-eddy simulation. *Journal of Aerosol Medicine*. 2006;19(3):290–300.

78. Xi J, Longest PW. Transport and deposition of micro-aerosols in realistic and simplified models of the oral airway. *Annals of Biomedical Engineering*. 2007;35(4):560–581.

79. Xi J, Longest PW. Effects of oral airway geometry characteristics on the diffusional deposition of inhaled nanoparticles. *Journal of Biomechanical Engineering*. 2008;130(1):011008.

80. Delvadia RR, Longest PW, Hindle M, Byron PR. In vitro tests for aerosol deposition. III: Effect of inhaler insertion angle on aerosol deposition. *Journal of Aerosol Medicine and Pulmonary Drug Delivery*. 2013;26(3):145–156.

81. Jayaraju S, Brouns M, Verbanck S, Lacor C. Fluid flow and particle deposition analysis in a realistic extrathoracic airway model using unstructured grids. *Journal of Aerosol Science*. 2007;38(5):494–508.

82. Sosnowski TR, Moskal A, Gradoń L. Dynamics of oropharyngeal aerosol transport and deposition with the realistic flow pattern. *Inhalation Toxicology*. 2006;18(10):773–780.

83. Sandeau J, Katz I, Fodil R, Louis B, Apiou-Sbirlea G, Caillibotte G et al. CFD simulation of particle deposition in a reconstructed human oral extrathoracic airway for air and helium–oxygen mixtures. *Journal of Aerosol Science*. 2010;41(3):281–294.

84. Gemci T, Shortall B, Allen G, Corcoran T, Chigier N. A CFD study of the throat during aerosol drug delivery using heliox and air. *Journal of Aerosol Science*. 2003;34(9):1175–1192.

85. Borgström L. On the use of dry powder inhalers in situations perceived as constrained. *Journal of Aerosol Medicine.* 2001;14(3):281–287.

86. Matida E, DeHaan W, Finlay W, Lange C. Simulation of particle deposition in an idealized mouth with different small diameter inlets. *Aerosol Science & Technology.* 2003;37(11):924–932.

87. DeHaan W, Finlay W. Predicting extrathoracic deposition from dry powder inhalers. *Journal of Aerosol Science.* 2004;35(3):309–331.

88. Longest PW, Hindle M, Choudhuri SD, Xi J. Comparison of ambient and spray aerosol deposition in a standard induction port and more realistic mouth–throat geometry. *Journal of Aerosol Science.* 2008;39(7):572–591.

89. Longest PW, Hindle M, Choudhuri SD. Effects of generation time on spray aerosol transport and deposition in models of the mouth–throat geometry. *Journal of Aerosol Medicine and Pulmonary Drug Delivery.* 2009;22(2):67–84.

90. Kleinstreuer C, Shi H, Zhang Z. Computational analyses of a pressurized metered dose inhaler and a new drug–aerosol targeting methodology. *Journal of Aerosol Medicine.* 2007;20(3):294–309.

91. Weibel ER. *Morphometry of the Human Lung.* Berlin, Germany: Springer; 1963.

92. Isaacs KK, Schlesinger R, Martonen TB. Three-dimensional computational fluid dynamics simulations of particle deposition in the tracheobronchial tree. *Journal of Aerosol Medicine.* 2006;19(3):344–352.

93. Zhang Z, Kleinstreuer C, Kim C. Flow structure and particle transport in a triple bifurcation airway model. *Journal of Fluids Engineering.* 2001;123(2):320–330.

94. Zhang Z, Kleinstreuer C. Effect of particle inlet distributions on deposition in a triple bifurcation lung airway model. *Journal of Aerosol Medicine.* 2001;14(1):13–29.

95. Comer J, Kleinstreuer C, Kim C. Flow structures and particle deposition patterns in double-bifurcation airway models. Part 2. Aerosol transport and deposition. *Journal of Fluid Mechanics.* 2001;435:55–80.

96. Comer J, Kleinstreuer C, Hyun S, Kim C. Aerosol transport and deposition in sequentially bifurcating airways. *Journal of Biomechanical Engineering.* 2000;122(2):152–158.

97. Comer J, Kleinstreuer C, Zhang Z. Flow structures and particle deposition patterns in double-bifurcation airway models. Part 1. Air flow fields. *Journal of Fluid Mechanics.* 2001;435:25–54.

98. Van Ertbruggen C, Hirsch C, Paiva M. Anatomically based three-dimensional model of airways to simulate flow and particle transport using computational fluid dynamics. *Journal of Applied Physiology.* 2005;98(3):970–980.

99. Nazridoust K, Asgharian B. Unsteady-state airflow and particle deposition in a three-generation human lung geometry. *Inhalation Toxicology.* 2008;20(6):595–610.

100. Spencer RM, Schroeter JD, Martonen TB. Computer simulations of lung airway structures using data-driven surface modeling techniques. *Computers in Biology and Medicine.* 2001;31(6):499–511. doi:10.1016/S0010-4825(01)00020-8.

101. Kitaoka H, Takaki R, Suki B. A three-dimensional model of the human airway tree. *Journal of Applied Physiology.* 1999;87(6):2207–2217.

102. Howatson Tawhai M, Pullan AJ, Hunter PJ. Generation of an anatomically based three-dimensional model of the conducting airways. *Annals of Biomedical Engineering.* 2000;28(7):793–802.

103. Horsfield K, Dart G, Olson DE, Filley GF, Cumming G. Models of the human bronchial tree. *Journal of Applied Physiology.* 1971;31(2):207–217. doi:10.1152/jappl.1971.31.2.207.

104. Gemci T, Ponyavin V, Chen Y, Chen H, Collins R. Computational model of airflow in upper 17 generations of human respiratory tract. *Journal of Biomechanics.* 2008;41(9):2047–2054. doi:10.1016/j.jbiomech.2007.12.019.

105. Tian G, Longest PW, Su G, Hindle M. Characterization of respiratory drug delivery with enhanced condensational growth using an individual path model of the entire tracheobronchial airways. *Annals of Biomedical Engineering.* 2011;39(3):1136–1153. doi:10.1007/s10439-010-0223-z.

106. Tian G, Longest P, Su G, Walenga R, Hindle M. Development of a stochastic individual path (SIP) model for predicting the tracheobronchial deposition of pharmaceutical aerosols: Effects of transient inhalation and sampling the airways. *Journal of Aerosol Science.* 2011;42(11):781–799.

107. Longest PW, Tian G, Walenga RL, Hindle M. Comparing MDI and DPI aerosol deposition using in vitro experiments and a new stochastic individual path (SIP) model of the conducting airways. *Pharmaceutical Research.* 2012;29(6):1670–1688. doi:10.1007/s11095-012-0691-y.

108. Lin CL, Tawhai MH, McLennan G, Hoffman EA. Characteristics of the turbulent laryngeal jet and its effect on airflow in the human intra-thoracic airways. *Respiratory Physiology & Neurobiology.* 2007;157(2–3):295–309. doi:10.1016/j.resp.2007.02.006.

109. Ley S, Mayer D, Brook B, Beek Ev, Heussel C, Rinck D et al. Radiological imaging as the basis for a simulation software of ventilation in the tracheo-bronchial tree. *European Radiology.* 2002;12(9):2218–2228.

110. Corley RA, Kabilan S, Kuprat AP, Carson JP, Minard KR, Jacob RE et al. Comparative computational modeling of airflows and vapor dosimetry in the

respiratory tracts of rat, monkey, and human. *Toxicological Sciences*. 2012;128(2):500–516. doi:10.1093/toxsci/kfs168.

111. Nowak N, Kakade PP, Annapragada AV. Computational fluid dynamics simulation of airflow and aerosol deposition in human lungs. *Annals of Biomedical Engineering*. 2003;31(4):374–390. doi:10.1114/1.1560632.

112. De Backer JW, Vos WG, Gorle CD, Germonpre P, Partoens B, Wuyts FL et al. Flow analyses in the lower airways: Patient-specific model and boundary conditions. *Medical Engineering & Physics*. 2008;30(7):872–879. doi:10.1016/j.medengphy.2007.11.002.

113. De Backer JW, Vos WG, Vinchurkar SC, Claes R, Drollmann A, Wulfrank D et al. Validation of computational fluid dynamics in CT-based airway models with SPECT/CT. *Radiology*. 2010;257(3):854–862. doi:10.1148/radiol.10100322.

114. Oakes JM, Marsden AL, Grandmont C, Darquenne C, Vignon-Clementel IE. Distribution of aerosolized particles in healthy and emphysematous rat lungs: Comparison between experimental and numerical studies. *Journal of Biomechanics*. 2015;48(6):1147–1157. doi:10.1016/j.jbiomech.2015.01.004.

115. Kuprat AP, Kabilan S, Carson JP, Corley RA, Einstein DR. A bidirectional coupling procedure applied to multiscale respiratory modeling. *Journal of Computational Physics*. 2013;244:148–167. doi:10.1016/j.jcp.2012.10.021.

116. Lin C, Tawhai M, McLennan G, Hoffman E. Computational fluid dynamics. *Engineering in Medicine and Biology Magazine, IEEE*. 2009;28(3):25–33.

117. Yin Y, Choi J, Hoffman EA, Tawhai MH, Lin CL. A multiscale MDCT image-based breathing lung model with time-varying regional ventilation. *Journal of Computational Physics*. 2013;244:168–192. doi:10.1016/j.jcp.2012.12.007.

118. Longest PW, Tian G, Khajeh-Hosseini-Dalasm N, Hindle M. Validating whole-airway CFD predictions of DPI aerosol deposition at multiple flow rates. *Journal of Aerosol Medicine and Pulmonary Drug Delivery*. 2016;29(6):461–481. doi:10.1089/jamp.2015.1281.

119. Walenga R, Longest P. Current inhalers deliver very small doses to the lower tracheobronchial airways: Assessment of healthy and constricted lungs. *Journal of Pharmaceutical Sciences*. 2016;105:147–159.

120. Khajeh-Hosseini-Dalasm N, Longest PW. Deposition of particles in the alveolar airways: Inhalation and breath-hold with pharmaceutical aerosols. *Journal of Aerosol Science*. 2015;79:15–30.

121. Kolanjiyil AV, Kleinstreuer C. Computational analysis of aerosol-dynamics in a human whole-lung airway model. *Journal of Aerosol Science*. 2017;114:301–316. doi:10.1016/j.jaerosci.2017.10.001.

122. Rudolf G, Kobrich R, Stahlhofen W. Modelling and algrebraic formulation of regional aerosol deposition in man. *Journal of Aerosol Science*. 1990;21:S403–S406.

123. Kim CS, Hu SC. Total respiratory tract deposition of fine micrometer-sized particles in healthy adults: Empirical equations for sex and breathing pattern. *Journal of Applied Physiology*. 2006;101(2):401–412. doi:10.1152/japplphysiol.00026.2006.

124. NCRP. *Deposition, Retention and Dosimetry of Inhaled Radioactive Substances*. Bethesda, MD: National Council on Radiation Protection and Measurements; 1997.

125. ICRP. Publication 66. Human respiratory tract model for radiological protection. *Annals of the ICRP*. 1994;24(1–3):1–482.

126. Yeh H-C, Schum G. Models of human lung airways and their application to inhaled particle deposition. *Bulletin of Mathematical Biology*. 1980;42(3):461–480.

127. Martonen TB. Mathematical-model for the selective deposition of inhaled pharmaceuticals. *Journal of Pharmaceutical Sciences*. 1993;82(12):1191–1199. doi:10.1002/jps.2600821202.

128. Koblinger L, Hofmann W. Analysis of human-lung morphometric data for stochastic aerosol deposition calculations. *Physics in Medicine and Biology*. 1985;30(6):541–556. doi:10.1088/0031-9155/30/6/004.

129. Asgharian B, Hofman W, Bergmann R. Particle deposition in a multiple-path model of the human lung. *Aerosol Science and Technology*. 2001;34(4):332–339. doi:10.1080/02786820151092478.

130. Miller FJ, Asgharian B, Schroeter JD, Price O. Improvements and additions to the multiple path particle dosimetry model. *Journal of Aerosol Science*. 2016;99:14–26. doi:10.1016/j.jaerosci.2016.01.018.

131. Asgharian B. A model of deposition of hygroscopic particles in the human lung. *Aerosol Science and Technology*. 2004;38(9):938–947. doi:10.1080/027868290511236.

132. Asgharian B, Price OT. Deposition of ultrafine (NANO) particles in the human lung. *Inhalation Toxicology*. 2007;19(13):1045–1054. doi:10.1080/08958370701626501.

133. Asgharian B, Price OT, Schroeter JD, Kimbell JS, Singal M. A lung dosimetry model of vapor uptake and tissue disposition. *Inhalation Toxicology*. 2012;24(3):182–193. doi:10.3109/08958378.2012.654857.

134. Lucey AD, King AJ, Tetlow G, Wang J, Armstrong JJ, Leigh MS et al. Measurement, reconstruction, and flow-field computation of the human pharynx with application to sleep apnea. *IEEE Transactions on Biomedical Engineering*. 2010;57(10):2535–2548.

135. Huang R, Rong Q. Respiration simulation of human upper airway for analysis of obstructive sleep apnea syndrome. In: Li K, Sun X, Jia L, Fei M, Irwin GW, editors. *Life System Modeling and Intelligent Computing*. Berlin, Germany: Springer-Verlag; 2010. pp. 588–596.

136. Kim S-H, Chung S-K, Na Y. Numerical investigation of flow-induced deformation along the human respiratory upper airway. *Journal of Mechanical Science and Technology*. 2015;29(12):5267–5272.

137. Wang Y, Wang J, Liu Y, Yu S, Sun X, Li S et al. Fluid–structure interaction modeling of upper airways before and after nasal surgery for obstructive sleep apnea. *International Journal for Numerical Methods in Biomedical Engineering*. 2012;28(5):528–546.

138. Rygg A, Hindle M, Longest PW. Absorption and clearance of pharmaceutical aerosols in the human nose: Effects of nasal spray suspension particle size and properties. *Pharmaceutical Research*. 2016;33(4):909–921.

139. Sukovic P. Cone beam computed tomography in craniofacial imaging. *Orthodontics & Craniofacial Research*. 2003;6(s1):31–36.

140. Chen W, Gillett E, Khoo MC, Davidson Ward SL, Nayak KS. Real-time multislice MRI during continuous positive airway pressure reveals upper airway response to pressure change. *Journal of Magnetic Resonance Imaging*. 2017;46(5):1400–1408.

141. Wu Z, Chen W, Nayak KS. Minimum field strength simulator for proton density weighted MRI. *PLoS One*. 2016;11(5):e0154711.

142. Visscher DO, Eijnatten M, Liberton NP, Wolff J, Hofman MB, Helder MN et al. MRI and additive manufacturing of nasal alar constructs for patient-specific reconstruction. *Scientific Reports*. 2017;7(1):10021.

143. Lazarow FB, Ahuja GS, Loy AC, Su E, Nguyen TD, Sharma GK et al. Intraoperative long range optical coherence tomography as a novel method of imaging the pediatric upper airway before and after adenotonsillectomy. *International Journal of Pediatric Otorhinolaryngology*. 2015;79(1):63–70.

144. Wijesundara K, Zdanski C, Kimbell J, Price H, Iftimia N, Oldenburg AL. Quantitative upper airway endoscopy with swept-source anatomical optical coherence tomography. *Biomedical Optics Express*. 2014;5(3):788–799.

145. Colletti AA, Amini R, Kaczka DW. Simulating ventilation distribution in heterogenous lung injury using a binary tree data structure. *Computers in Biology and Medicine*. 2011;41(10):936–945. doi:10.1016/j.compbiomed.2011.08.004.

146. Schroeter JD, Musante CJ, Hwang DM, Burton R, Guilmette R, Martonen TB. Hygroscopic growth and deposition of inhaled secondary cigarette smoke in human nasal pathways. *Aerosol Science and Technology*. 2001;34(1):137–143. doi:10.1080/027868201300082166.

147. Asgharian B, Price OT, Yurteri CU, Dickens C, McAughey J. Component-specific, cigarette particle deposition modeling in the human respiratory tract. *Inhalation Toxicology*. 2014;26(1):36–47. doi:10.3109/08958378.2013.851305.

148. Hindle M, Longest PW. Evaluation of enhanced condensational growth (ECG) for controlled respiratory drug delivery in a mouth-throat and upper tracheobronchial model. *Pharmaceutical Research*. 2010;27(9):1800–1811. doi:10.1007/s11095-010-0165-z.

149. Schroeter JD, Campbell J, Kimbell JS, Conolly RB, Clewell HJ, Andersen ME. Effects of endogenous formaldehyde in nasal tissues on inhaled formaldehyde dosimetry predictions in the rat, monkey, and human nasal passages. *Toxicological Sciences*. 2014;138(2):412–424. doi:10.1093/toxsci/kft333.

150. Weber B, Hochhaus G. A pharmacokinetic simulation tool for inhaled corticosteroids. *AAPS Journal*. 2013;15(1):159–171. doi:10.1208/s12248-012-9420-z.

151. Martin AR, Finlay WH. Model calculations of regional deposition and disposition for single doses of inhaled liposomal and dry powder ciprofloxacin. *Journal of Aerosol Medicine and Pulmonary Drug Delivery*. 2018;31(1):49–60. doi:10.1089/jamp.2017.1377.

4

Lung transporters and absorption mechanisms in the lungs

MOHAMMED ALI SELO, HASSAN H.A. AL-ALAK, AND CARSTEN EHRHARDT

Fate of inhaled matter	57		SLC22 subfamily	61
Mechanisms of absorption	58		Peptide transporters (PEPTs)/SLC15	62
Passive diffusion	58		Vesicle-mediated endocytosis/transcytosis	62
Transporter-mediated absorption and efflux	58		Uptake of particulate matters and macromolecules by immune cells	63
ABC transporters	59			
P-gp/ABCB1	60		Factors influencing the absorption process	63
Multidrug resistance-related proteins (MRP/ABCC)	60		Conclusion	64
BCRP/ABCG2	61		References	64
SLC transporters	61			

FATE OF INHALED MATTER

After an inhaled particle or aerosol droplet is deposited, the dissolved or suspended substance or particle has only two options to escape from the airspace: (1) it is absorbed across the epithelial barrier, or (2) it is removed via mucociliary clearance (see Chapter 2 for details of this process). In addition, the substance might be prone to extracellular pulmonary metabolism, and the resulting metabolites will share the fate explained above.

Particles deposited in the conducting airways are mainly removed through the mucociliary escalator into the trachea and are then swallowed into the gastrointestinal tract, and only a small percentage is absorbed into the blood or the lymphatic system (1). On the other hand, particles deposited in the alveolar region, where the epithelial barrier is much thinner, are either absorbed into the pulmonary circulation or phagocytosed by alveolar macrophages, and are then cleared either by the lymphatic system or transported into the ciliated airways and cleared via the mucociliary escalator to the larynx and subsequently swallowed (1,2). In summary, absorption from the airspace can occur in various compartments: (1) the lung interstitium, (2) the pulmonary circulation, (3) the bronchial circulation, and (4) the lymphatic system (Figure 4.1).

The lung interstitium is the connective tissue-rich supportive framework of the lung. It can be divided into three zones: the alveolar interstitium surrounding the pulmonary parenchyma, the axial interstitium surrounding the bronchovascular tree, and the peripheral interstitium adjacent to the pleura. In addition to connective tissue, the lung interstitium also contains smooth muscle, lymphatics, capillaries, and a variety of other cells and tissues.

The lung has two separate blood supplies: the pulmonary circulation and the bronchial circulation. The pulmonary arteries carry deoxygenated blood from the right ventricle to the lungs, where a dense network of pulmonary capillaries with very large surface area surrounds the alveoli. This is where removal of CO_2 and oxygenation of the blood takes place. After being oxygenated, the blood is returned to the left atrium through the pulmonary vein (3). The bronchial arteries, on the other hand, arise from the aorta and carry oxygenated blood to provide nutrients and oxygen to the conducting airways and lung interstitium and tissues. Only approximately one-third of the blood returns to the right atrium via the bronchial veins; the remaining blood drains into the left atrium through the pulmonary veins (4).

A network of lymphatic vessels drains the airways and the pulmonary parenchyma and terminates in the hilar and mediastinal lymph nodes (5). Anatomically, the pulmonary lymphatics can be divided into two sets: a surface pleural set of lymphatic vessels located in the connective tissue of the visceral pleura and a deep intrapulmonary network of lymphatic vessels that run on the pulmonary surface and the major conducting airways (6–8).

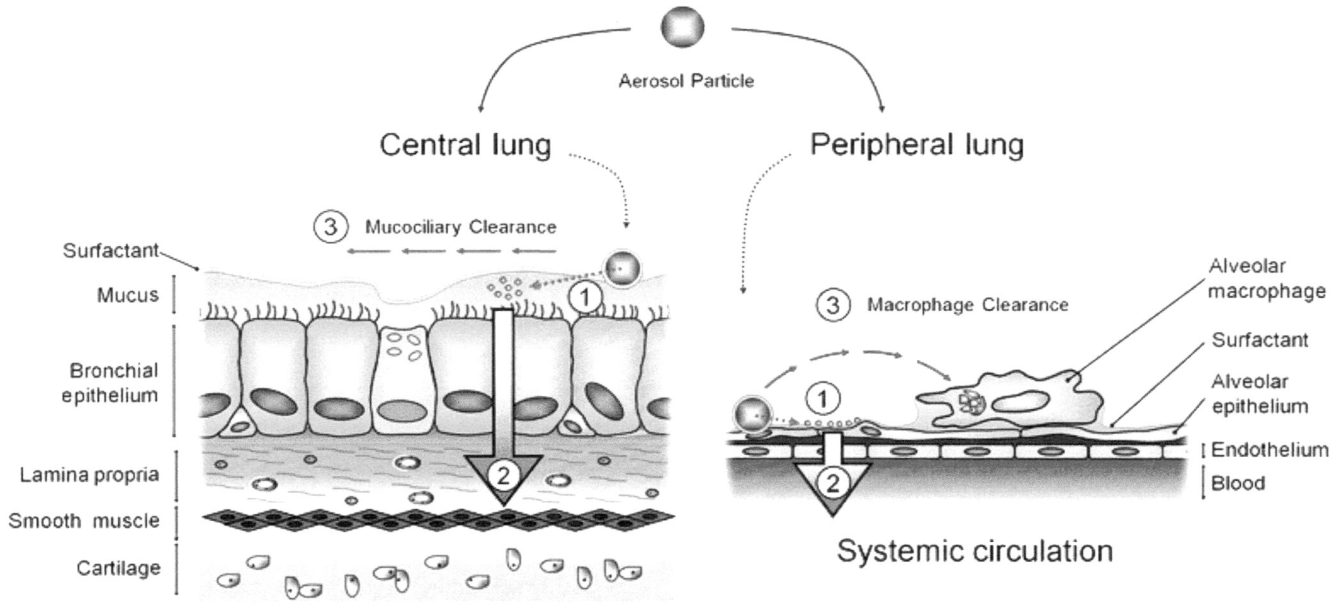

Figure 4.1 What happens to an aerosol particle after deposition in the lungs? **(1)** First contact with the lung lining fluid and dissolution of the active pharmaceutical ingredient (API), depending on the amount and composition of the locally available lining fluid and intrinsic properties of the API, and the carrier particle. **(2)** Absorption of the API across the pulmonary epithelium. This process is mainly controlled by the API physicochemical properties and physiological factors such as membrane transporters. **(3)** Clearance of the undissolved particle or drug. (Adapted from Ruge, C.A. et al., *Lancet Respir. Med.*, 1, 402–413, 2013.)

Pulmonary-delivered lipid-based nanoparticles have been suggested to be cleared predominantly by the pulmonary lymphatics, either after direct uptake through the pulmonary epithelium or following uptake by antigen-presenting cells. Thus, pulmonary delivered solid lipid nanoparticles (SLNs), nanostructured lipid carriers (NLCs), as well as liposomal formulations can potentially be used as drug carrier systems to specifically deliver vaccines and anticancer drugs into the pulmonary lymphatics and to visualize the pulmonary lymphatic network (5,7–16).

MECHANISMS OF ABSORPTION

Different absorption pathways have been described for pulmonary administered drugs and drug particles, including (1) passive diffusion (paracellular and transcellular), (2) transporter-mediated absorption and efflux (i.e., facilitated diffusion, primary active transport, secondary active transport), (3) vesicle-mediated endocytosis/transcytosis (mostly receptor-mediated), and (4) internalization into immune cells (i.e., macrophages or dendritic cells), followed by subsequent transepithelial translocation within the immune cell (Figure 4.2).

Passive diffusion

Passive diffusion of inhaled drugs along a concentration gradient from the airspace into the submucosa can occur through the epithelial cells (i.e., transcellular diffusion) or

via the intercellular junctions between the pulmonary epithelial cells (i.e., paracellular diffusion). Passive diffusion is dependent on physicochemical properties of the drug and the thickness of the air-blood barrier. Absorption of lipophilic compounds occurs generally through transcellular passive diffusion, whereas hydrophilic compounds diffuse mainly through the intercellular junctional pores (17,18). Within the molecular weight range of 100–1000 Da, pulmonary absorption is dependent mainly on the lipophilicity of the drug compound, with absorption half-life in the range of minutes for lipophilic molecules and hours for hydrophilic ones (19,20). Several mechanisms are implicated in the pulmonary uptake of macromolecules (i.e., peptides and proteins). However, the inverse relationship between the pulmonary absorption rate and the size of macromolecules with molecular weight range of 1–500 kDa indicates the uptake to be at least partially mediated by passive diffusion through the intercellular junction pores as smaller molecules diffuse faster than the large ones (17,21,22).

Transporter-mediated absorption and efflux

Transporters are membrane-bound proteins that facilitate the translocation of their substrates across biological membranes. They can be classified into passive and active transporters. Passive transporters, also known as facilitated transporters, allow diffusion of solutes (e.g., glucose, amino acids, and urea) across biological membranes down their concentration gradient without the need for metabolic energy. Active

Airways Lumen

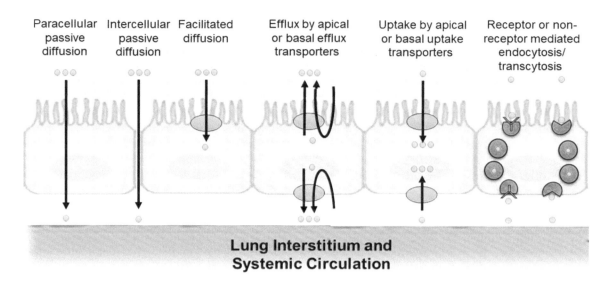

Figure 4.2 Endogenous and exogenous molecules passively diffuse down their concentration gradient either paracellularly or intracellularly or with the aid of membrane transporters (i.e., facilitated diffusion). Apically localized (e.g., P-gp, BCRP, MRP2) and basolaterally localized (e.g., MRP1, 3 and 5) efflux transporters extrude their substrates out of the cells to the airway lumen and to lung interstitium and systemic circulation, respectively. Uptake transporters, either apically (e.g., OCTN1 and PEPT2) or basolaterally localized, take up their substrates into epithelial cells. Therapeutic and endogenous macromolecules are often transported via receptor or non-receptor-mediated endocytosis/transcytosis into/across epithelial cells.

transporters, on the other hand, require energy to transport their substrates across cell membranes (often against a concentration gradient) and are further classified as primary or secondary active transporters according to the source of energy used. Primary active transporters use energy derived directly from the hydrolysis of adenosine triphosphate (ATP), whereas secondary active transporters use the energy derived from the movement of one molecule down its concentration gradient to power the uphill movement of another molecule against its concentration gradient (23,24).

The two-main superfamilies of membrane transporters are the ATP-binding cassette (ABC) family and the solute carrier (SLC) family. Transporters belonging to the ABC family are mainly involved in the efflux of their relevant substrates from the cells in an ATP dependent mechanism, whereas transporters belonging to the SLC family are mainly involved in the uptake of small molecules into cells (25). ABC transporters are considered primary active transporters; SLC transporters are predominantly facilitative or secondary active transporters (24,26,27).

The role that membrane transporters in the lung play in the absorption of inhaled drugs into the systemic circulation and in drug distribution into lung tissues is the topic of ongoing investigations. Evidence (mostly from *in vitro* studies) shows a potential influence of membrane transporters on the pharmacokinetic, pharmacodynamic, and the safety profiles of many

inhaled drugs (25,28). In addition, drug transporters in the lung may also mediate the uptake of drugs from the systemic circulation into lung tissue, resulting in increased pulmonary drug accumulation, which carries therapeutic benefits but also toxicological concerns (28). Furthermore, dysfunctions of pulmonary transporters may play a role in the pathogenesis and etiology of lung disorders, particularly chronic obstructive pulmonary disease (COPD) and asthma (25,29–31).

ABC transporters

The ABC family of transporters constitute a large superfamily of membrane proteins that are involved in the transport of a wide variety of substrates across biological membranes in an ATP-dependent mechanism. Many act as efflux transporters; i.e., they pump their substrates outside the cells. Thus, they play a crucial role in protecting against many endogenous and exogenous toxic compounds including xenobiotics (32,33).

Approximately 50 genes that are divided into eight subfamilies are encoding ABC transporters in humans (34,35). Among these, P-glycoprotein (P-gp), multidrug resistance-related protein 1–8 (MRP1–8), and breast cancer resistance protein (BCRP) are expressed in lung tissues at varying levels and are well known for their role in multidrug resistance (MDR).

P-gp/ABCB1

P-gp, also called multidrug resistance protein 1 (MDR1), a 170 kDa transporter was detected in apical membranes of bronchial and bronchiolar epithelial cells (36). Furthermore, it has been found to be expressed and be functionally active in apical membranes of rat and human alveolar type 1–like (AT1-like) epithelial cells but was absent in freshly isolated alveolar type 2 (AT2) cells. It is proposed to be involved in providing a barrier against xenobiotic transfer from alveolar airspace to pulmonary interstitium and systemic circulation (37,38). Similarly, P-gp was found to be functionally active in normal human bronchial epithelial cells (NHBECs) because the efflux P-gp substrate rhodamine 123 (Rh123) was sensitive to inhibition by the P-gp inhibitor, verapamil (39,40).

P-gp in lung tissue may influence the pharmacokinetics/pharmacodynamics of inhaled drugs and may lead to drug-drug interactions. For example, the co-administration of oral verapamil with either inhaled umeclidinium bromide alone or in combination with vilanterol, two P-gp substrates, in healthy volunteers, caused a 40% increase in both bronchodilators' area under the curve (AUC). However, the rise in the systemic concentration was of no clinical significance in terms of toxicity (41).

Many inhaled glucocorticoids are substrates and/or modulator of P-gp expression, and involvement of the glucocorticoid receptor in the regulation of P-gp expression has been reported (42,43). For example, many in vitro studies conducted on primary NHBEC, BEAS-2B, and A549 cell models have shown that fluticasone propionate, beclomethasone dipropionate, ciclesonide, and budesonide can increase P-gp expression, implicating a possible interaction with other inhaled drugs that are substrates of P-gp (44–46). Similarly, an in vivo study reported increased P-gp level by 140% after treatment of Male Sprague-Dawley rats with dexamethasone for 4 days (47).

Thus, a significant body of data shows the expression and functional activity of P-gp in the lung, where it transports its substrates out to the apical surface (37,48). However, several studies have also shown a negligible role for pulmonary P-gp on limiting the airway to blood absorption of its inhaled substrates. One example is an in vivo study conducted in rats that revealed a high bioavailability for the two P-gp substrates, talinolol and losartan, with 81% and 92%, respectively (49). Similarly, an ex vivo study performed in an isolated perfused rat lung (IPRL) model reported a high overall absorption for losartan. Despite having the physicochemical properties indicative of a high permeability drug, losartan displayed one of the slowest absorption half-lives ($t_{1/2}$ of 26 min) among the range of investigated drugs (49).

In addition, there is some evidence that P-gp in the lung also increases the pulmonary uptake of systemically administered drugs (25). For example, orally administered clarithromycin and to a lesser extent azithromycin were found to be accumulated in the epithelial lining fluid (ELF), the infection site of pathogens. After being taken up by pulmonary epithelial cells, they have been suggested to be actively effluxed to and retained in the airway lumen by the activity of P-gp, highlighting a beneficial role for treatment of lung infections (50,51).

Multidrug resistance-related proteins (MRP/ABCC)

Of the thirteen members of the MRP family, eight (i.e., MRP1–8) are involved in drug transport and are expressed in the plasma membranes of different cell types (28). MRP1, 3, and 5 are known to be localized mainly to basolateral membranes, whereas MRP2 and 4 are predominantly localized to apical membranes of the epithelial cells (33,36,52). Six of the MRP (i.e. MRP1, MRP3, MRP4, MRP5, MRP6, and MRP8) were detected by liquid chromatography–mass spectrometry/mass spectrometry (LC–MS/MS) in human whole lung tissue at varying levels with MRP1 having the highest abundance among all ABC transporters studied (53).

Apart from MRP1 (ABCC1), which is the best studied member of the subfamily in terms of activity and drug transport in the lung, few data on the pulmonary function of other MRP are available (25). The pulmonary activity of MRP1 has been determined by positron emission tomography (PET) imaging technique in vivo in mice (54).

The products of Phase II metabolism (i.e., glutathione, glucuronide, and sulphate conjugates) of xenobiotic organic anions are substrates of MRP1 (55–57). Thus, MRP1 is believed to have an important role in protecting lung tissues from oxidative stress and from the toxic insults of xenobiotics (57,58)

Many studies proposed an association between COPD and MRP1, which may have a protective role against damage induced by tobacco smoke. For example, a lower expression of MRP1 was found in bronchial epithelial cells and lung tissue of patients with COPD, in comparison with healthy nonsmoker volunteers, and the degree of decrement was associated with the severity of the disease (30). A reduction in MRP1 activity was also observed in 16HBE14o-bronchial epithelial cells, after incubation with cigarette smoke extract (CSE), as indicated by increased cellular retention of the MRP1 substrate, carboxyfluorescein (CF). Furthermore, inhibition of MRP1 by MK-571 resulted in increased CSE-induced toxicity, proposing a protective role for the transporter against the development of COPD (31). In addition, the two ABCC1 single-nucleotide polymorphisms (SNPs), rs4148382 and rs212093, were found to be associated with a higher and lower forced expiratory volume in 1 s (FEV1), respectively (59). However, another study revealed ABCC1 to be expressed highly at both the central and peripheral airways with no differences in the expression levels between healthy volunteers and patients with severe COPD (60).

In addition, many inhaled pharmaceuticals used for the treatment of COPD have been found to modulate MRP1 activity. For example, an in vitro study conducted on

16HBE14o-bronchial epithelial cells revealed budesonide, an inhaled corticosteroid, to inhibit MRP1-mediated CF transport, with the effect being compensated by the long-acting β_2-agonist formoterol, while ipratropium bromide and N-acetylcysteine (NAC) increased MRP1-mediated CF transport in a concentration dependant manner (61).

BCRP/*ABCG2*

BCRP belongs to the G subfamily of the human ABC super-family with an apparent molecular weight of 72 kDa. It was first cloned from a multidrug-resistant breast cancer cell line, hence the name (35,62). BCRP has a broad range of substrates of diverse physicochemical properties, including anticancer drugs, antiviral drugs, HMG-CoA reductase inhibitors, antibiotics, calcium-channel blockers, and flavonoids (63).

Generally, BCRP is localized to the apical membrane of epithelial cells and effluxes its substrates out to the apical surface, thus limiting the systemic exposure to many endogenous and exogenous toxic substrates (64,65). Moreover, an important role for BCRP has been suggested in detoxification of xenobiotics by extruding toxic metabolites, such as sulphate conjugates (66).

In human whole lung tissue and bronchial epithelial cells in primary culture, BCRP was detected by LC–MS/MS and found to have the second highest expression level among all ABC transporters. However, it was below the detection limits in alveolar and tracheal epithelial cells (53). Furthermore, using the same detection technique, it was found to have the highest expression level of all ABC transporters in many continuously growing cell lines of human lung origin, i.e., Calu-3, BEAS-2B, NCI-H292, NCI-H441, and A549 (67).

Despite being highly abundant, the pulmonary activity of BCRP is still poorly investigated. A recent *in vitro* study from our lab showed the protein to be expressed to the apical membranes of both NCI-H441 and AT1-like cells in primary culture, and it was functionally active in NCI-H441 but not in AT1-like monolayers. The study also revealed a higher abundance in freshly isolated AT2 cells than AT1-like cells (68). In addition to the cell membrane, BCRP was detected in cell nuclei of the primary alveolar epithelial cells, proposing a transcriptional role in distal lung epithelium (68,69).

Many inhaled drugs, such as ciprofloxacin, beclomethasone dipropionate, budesonide, ciclesonide, and mometasone furoate, have been shown to be substrates of BCRP (70,71). BCRP is also an important player in development of resistance to many chemotherapeutic agents such as doxorubicin, topotecan, and imatinib (72). BCRP mRNA in non-small-cell lung cancer (NSCLC) tissues was found to be expressed at sufficient levels, proposing a role in conferring resistance to chemotherapeutics, particularly after finding the activity of BCRB, as measured by topotecan efflux, to be very well correlated with the mRNA expression levels in many lung cancer cell lines such as NCI-H460, NCI-H441, and NCI-H1299 (73).

SLC transporters

SLC transporters are a superfamily of more than 300 membrane-bound proteins that facilitate the cellular uptake of a broad range of substrates, including nutrients and drugs. The *SLC22* and *SLC15* subfamilies are the best-studied SLC transporters in the lung and thus will be discussed in more detail below (25,27).

SLC22 subfamily

Organic cation transporters (i.e., OCT1-3) and the novel organic cation transporters (i.e., OCTN1 and 2) are members of the *SLC22* subfamily and are characterized by their ability to transport organic cations and the zwitterionic L-carnitine (28,74). OCT1, OCT2, and OCTN1 were detected by LC–MS/MS in human whole lung tissue as well as tracheal and bronchial cells in primary culture, while only OCT2 and OCTN1 were detected in alveolar cells. OCTN1 was found to have the highest expression level among all SLC transporters in the lung tissue and all those primary cells (53).

Using immunohistochemistry, OCTN1 and OCTN2 were shown to be expressed to the apical membranes of human tracheal and lung parenchymal epithelial cells (75). OCT1 and OCT2 were shown to be localized to the apical membrane of ciliated airway epithelial cells and OCT3 to the basolateral membrane of bronchial epithelial cells (29,76,77). Similarly, all organic cation transporters (i.e., OCT1, OCT2, OCT3, OCTN1, and OCTN2) were detected by Western blotting in human alveolar epithelial cells in primary culture (i.e., AT2 and AT1-like cells) and in NCI-H441 cells at similar levels, and the cell line was therefore suggested as a suitable *in vitro* model for transport studies of human distal lung epithelial barrier (78).

Physiological substrates of OCT/N include L-carnitine, which is mainly transported by OCTN2, antioxidants such as L-ergothioneine, the main substrate of OCTN1, hormones like prostaglandin E2 (PGE2), and neurotransmitters such as dopamine (25,79,80).

OCTs, particularly OCT3, has been suggested to mediate serotonin-induced acetylcholine (ACh) release, a potent physiological bronchoconstrictor, from the respiratory epithelium of mice, leading to airway constriction and thus implying a possible role for OCTs in asthma. This effect was found to be reversed by corticosteroids by inhibiting OCT3 localized in smooth muscle cells (29,81).

A great variety of pulmonary-administered drugs such as β_2-adrenergic agonists and anticholinergic bronchodilators are either cations or bases, and OCT/N may therefore play a role in their pulmonary absorption and distribution. OCT/N transporters have the highest impact on compounds with low passive permeability, and the transporter-mediated uptake is therefore expected to be the rate-limiting step in the transepithelial transport of such compounds (82).

Many *in vitro* an *ex vivo* studies suggest OCT/N-mediated active absorption of salbutamol, rather than passive diffusion, is the driving force for transport of the compound across airway epithelial cells. However, there are some contradictory data regarding the exact member being the main mediator of the active absorption process (75,83–85). One *in vitro* study compared alveolar (A549) and bronchial (16HBE14o- and Calu-3) epithelial cells and suggested a regional difference in the transport of organic cations across pulmonary epithelial cells, with the apically localized OCT2 to be predominantly involved in the alveolar epithelium and the basolaterally localized OCT3 having a role in both alveolar and bronchial epithelial cells (77). Likewise, the transport of salbutamol base and salbutamol sulphate across Calu-3 monolayers showed the involvement of OCT/N mediated transport. However, a contribution of passive diffusion in the uptake process was also shown (86). In contrast, another *in vitro* study investigated the uptake and transport of salbutamol across fully differentiated human bronchial epithelial cell (HBEC) monolayers found the transport to be mediated mainly by paracellular diffusion with the active transport having only a minor role (87).

Using primary human bronchial and vascular smooth muscle cells, corticosteroids such as budesonide and fluticasone were found to inhibit OCT3 mediated clearance of a cationic β_2-agonists (e.g., formoterol), but not a lipophilic one (e.g., salmeterol), from the bronchial smooth muscle cells, implying a beneficial effect for the use of a combination therapy of corticosteroids with cationic β_2-agonists in the treatment of asthma (88,89).

Another *in vitro* study conducted on BEAS-2B bronchial epithelial cells and an *in vivo* study conducted on mice revealed the uptake of the inhaled anti-muscarinic drugs, ipratropium, and tiotropium, to be mediated mainly by OCTN2/Octn2, with possible minor contribution of other OCT/N transporters (90,91). Similarly, a study investigating drug absorption and distribution in precision cut rat lung slices also suggested a transporter-mediated uptake of ipratropium and MPP$^+$ but not of tiotropium (92). In contrast, absorption of both L-carnitine and ipratropium across intact isolated and perfused rat lung epithelial barrier into the pulmonary circulation was shown to be mediated mainly by passive processes, with no evidence of OCT/N transporter involvement in the overall pulmonary absorption (93).

OCT2 together with OATP2B1 was also found to be involved in ciprofloxacin absorption, which has been approved by the Food and Drug Administration (FDA) as inhalation therapy for emergency treatment after anthrax exposure, as shown by uptake studies in Calu-3 cell monolayers (94,95).

Peptide transporters (PEPTs)/*SLC15*

The oligopeptide transporters PEPT1 and PEPT2 are proton-coupled transporters belonging to the *SLC15* subfamily (96,97). PEPTs can transport a wide range of substrates ranging from di- and tri-peptides to peptidomimetic drugs, such as angiotensin-converting enzyme inhibitors,

β-lactam antibiotics, antivirals, anti-neoplastics, and delta-aminolevulinic acid (98–101).

In the airways, PEPT2/Pept2 mRNA was detected at moderate to high levels in mammalian lung tissues and primary airways epithelial cells, respectively. PEPT1/Pept1, on the other hand, was either very weak or undetectable (102–106). Similarly, PEPT2 protein was detected by LC–MS/MS in human whole lung tissue and in the primary bronchial epithelial cells, while PEPT1 was under the detection limits (53). An *in vitro* study showed PEPT2 to be functionally active and to be mainly localized to the apical membrane of fully differentiated monolayers of human upper airway epithelial cells in primary culture (107). Likewise, PEPT2 protein was detected in human, rat, and mice tracheal, bronchial, and smaller airway epithelia, with stronger signal at the apical membrane, as well as endothelium of small vessels. PEPT2 immunostaining was also observed in the cytoplasm of type 2 pneumocytes and the *ex vivo* uptake studies of the fluorescent dipeptide, D-Ala-Lys-AMCA, conducted on isolated human and mouse lung specimens showed PEPT2 to be functionally active in the bronchial epithelium and AT2 but not AT1 pneumocyte (108,109).

PEPT2 was found to be functionally expressed in NCI-H441 cells, as indicated by the cefadroxil-sensitive glycylsarcosine uptake, and the cell line was therefore proposed as suitable *in vitro* model to study PEPT2 function in distal lung epithelium. In addition, the study revealed a cefadroxil sensitive apical to basal transport of cephalexin across NCI-H441 cell monolayers (110). A study conducted in primary rat alveolar macrophages and the NR8383 cell line revealed involvement of PEPT2-dependent uptake of s-nitrosothiols uptake, together with L-type amino-acid transporters, to the inhaled nitric oxide–mediated modulation of the immune responses in alveolar macrophages (111).

Vesicle-mediated endocytosis/transcytosis

Endocytosis is a form of active transport by which a molecule gains entry into the cell after being surrounded by an area of plasma membrane, which then buds off inside the cell forming a vesicle containing the ingested molecule. Transcytosis is a transcellular transport mechanism in which the internalized molecules are transported across the epithelial cells from one side to the opposite side. Among many endocytic pathways in mammalian cells, clathrin-dependent endocytosis and caveolar endocytosis are the most common and well-studied pathways. However, other pathways that use neither clathrin nor caveolae have been recognized (112).

Endocytosis/transcytosis is considered the main route for transport of therapeutic and endogenous macromolecules such as proteins and peptides across alveolar epithelial cells (22,113,114).

Clathrin-dependent and caveolar endocytosis are selective uptake mechanisms for specific macromolecules, as the substrate needs to binds to specific cell surface receptors concentrated in specialized regions of the plasma membrane (i.e., in caveolae or clathrin-coated pit) (115,116).

Many studies proposed involvement of transcytosis in the alveolar transport of albumin; for example, the transport of albumin across rat primary AT2 and AT-like cells was suggested to be through receptor-mediated transcytosis via caveolae-localized gp60 receptors (117–120). Another study conducted, also in rat primary alveolar cells, similarly suggested a transcytosis mediated uptake, but through the clathrin-mediated pathway (121). The pathway of uptake was similar in both AT2 and AT1-like cells, but with higher rate and activity in AT2 (i.e., approximately five to six times higher) than in AT1-like cells, implying an important role for AT2 cells in albumin clearance from the lung (121).

Similarly, transcytosis was found to be involved in the uptake of insulin across both primary rat AT2 and AT1-like cells, through both clathrin and caveolae-independent but dynamin-dependent and non-dynamin-dependent pathways, respectively (122).

Uptake of particulate matters and macromolecules by immune cells

Nanoparticles of 100 nm or less have been demonstrated to be rapidly transported, within a few minutes, from the lung into the systemic circulation, following intratracheal instillation into hamsters and aerosol inhalation in humans (123,124). The exact mechanisms involved in pulmonary nanoparticle transport remains poorly understood (123,124). However, phagocytosis by immune cells (i.e., alveolar macrophages and dendritic cells) and subsequent translocation into the pulmonary lymphatics has been suggested to play a role in the pulmonary uptake of insoluble particles and macromolecules (5,125). Alveolar macrophages, in addition to dendritic cells, are the predominant phagocytic cells in alveoli (126,127). For example, inhaled ultrafine silver particles deposited in rat lung parenchyma have been observed to be phagocytosed by alveolar macrophages, which were subsequently translocated into the pulmonary lymph nodes, suggesting a role for lymphatic drainage in translocation of nanoparticles from the lung into the systemic circulation (128). Moreover, an *in vivo* study conducted in mice showed the capacity of dendritic cells to take up the intratracheally instilled fluorescein isothiocyanate-conjugated macromolecules and subsequently migrate to thoracic lymph nodes, relying on their Ag-carrying properties (127).

FACTORS INFLUENCING THE ABSORPTION PROCESS

How a substance or particle is absorbed from the airspace depends on many different aspects. The morphology and cell physiology of the barrier obviously play an important role. Absorption processes across columnar bronchial epithelium are certainly different from absorption processes

across the extremely thin, squamous alveolar epithelium. Moreover, certain diseases might affect pulmonary absorption. For example, in smokers, the systemic availability of inhaled insulin has been shown to be significantly increased due to the higher rate and extent of absorption, which resulted in smoking becoming an exclusion criterion for the treatment with Exubera (129,130). In contrast, significantly lower absorption and metabolic effect of AIR-inhaled insulin has been reported in subjects with emphysema and chronic bronchitis compared with healthy subjects (131). Similarly, lower absorption of inhaled insulin has been reported in asthmatic patients compared to healthy subjects, with asthmatics requiring a higher dose of inhaled insulin to obtain similar glycaemic control (132,133).

Although there was a comparable pulmonary bioavailable fraction after oral olodaterol inhalation, a long acting β_2 agonist, between patients with asthma and COPD and healthy volunteers, the pulmonary absorption after olodaterol inhalation was slower in patients with COPD and asthma than in healthy individuals, resulting in longer pulmonary residence time and more beneficial lung targeting in patients when compared to healthy volunteers (134). It also has been demonstrated that the dose absorbed after nedocromil inhalation with a pressurized metered-dose inhaler (pMDI) in asthmatic patents was lower than in healthy volunteers, resulting in approximately 40% lower bioavailability in the patients (135). The pharmacokinetics of inhaled fluticasone propionate were significantly different in asthmatic patients and healthy volunteers, with more than 50% lower systemic availability with subsequent less hypothalamic–pituitary–adrenal suppression in patients with asthma than in healthy controls (136). On the other hand, there was no difference in the amount of drug deposited after inhalation of beclomethason dipropionate (BDP)/formoterol extra-fine hydrofluoroalkane (HFA) fixed combination between asthmatic and COPD patients and healthy subjects (137). Furthermore, lung diseases may influence the absorption of pulmonary-delivered drug indirectly by affecting the expression of drug transporters. For example, salbutamol transport was increased twofold when Calu-3 cell monolayers were treated with lipopolysaccharide (LPS) to induce an inflammatory reaction similar to that of asthmatic epithelium. This was attributed to an increased abundance of OCT1 by 20% and OCTN1 and OCTN2 protein levels by approximately 50% (138).

In addition, the properties of the drug substance (e.g., particle size, shape, charge, metabolic stability, transporter substrate, lipophilicity, molecular polar surface area [PSA], percentage polar surface area of the total molecular surface area [%PSA], and hydrogen bonding potential) are important factors governing which pathway will ultimately be dominant for the molecule's absorption from the airspace.

Lipophilic molecules permeate easily across cellular membranes, while hydrophilic molecules cross mainly through extracellular pathways, such as intercellular junctional pores or by active transport (139). The pulmonary epithelium was found to be highly permeable to compounds with high-molecular PSA and %PSA (140).

Although the molecular weight has a negligible effect on pulmonary absorption of compounds weighing less than 1000 Da, an inverse relationship exists between the alveolar absorption rate and the molecular weight of the larger molecules (17). For example, the serum level of 1-desamino-8-d-arginine vasopressin (DDAVP) (1.1 kDa) peaked at 1 h, compared with 16–24 h for bovine serum albumin (BSA) (67 kDa) after intratracheal instillation into rats (141).

The particle size greatly influences the site of deposition within the respiratory tract, with particles smaller than 3 µm being more likely to deposit in the deep lungs where the maximal absorption into the systemic circulation takes place. Larger particles of more than 5 µm are prone to removal by mucociliary clearance mechanism, whereas the majority of particles smaller than 1 µm are removed by exhalation without being deposited or conveying any therapeutic effect (142). Particles of smaller size have higher dissolution rates, and nanoparticle formulations of poorly soluble active pharmaceuticals such as fluticasone propionate are being assessed to enhance their solubility and pulmonary absorption (143,144). Furthermore, particle size influences the rate of phagocytosis by alveolar macrophages, which is probably the most significant clearance pathway of slowly dissolving particles from the deep lungs. Alveolar macrophages efficiently phagocytose particles with a diameter range of 0.5–5 µm, which is the optimal size range for alveolar deposition, resulting in significant reduction in the alveolar residence time and systemic bioavailability (144,145). Many approaches have been assessed to overcome this issue, such as the use of large porous particles which are too large for uptake by alveolar macrophages but with suitable aerodynamic properties for alveolar deposition (146). In addition, a drug particle's shape has a significant role in phagocytosis by alveolar macrophages and the shape can be engineered to overcome clearance of drug particles by alveolar macrophages; for example, wormlike particles with a high aspect ratio shape exhibit negligible uptake by alveolar macrophages (147).

CONCLUSION

Inhaled drug molecules deposited in the central airways are mainly cleared by mucocilliary clearance pathway, whereas those deposited in the alveoli are either cleared by alveolar macrophages or absorbed into the systemic circulation through various mechanisms. The rate, extent, and pathway of pulmonary absorption depend on many factors such as the physicochemical properties of the drug molecule as well as the diseases of the respiratory system. Among many absorption mechanisms, transporter-mediated uptake and efflux have the potential to affect inhaled drugs, and many studies, mainly *in vitro*, propose an important impact of membrane transporters on the absorption and distribution profiles of pulmonary-delivered drugs. However, the limited set of experiments in more complex systems, conducted mainly in rodent isolated and perfused lung models, shows negligible effect of membrane transporters on systemic absorption of inhaled drugs, while the role of transporters on pulmonary drug distribution is entirely unclear. Thus, more systems that allow for prediction of the human *in vivo* conditions need to be developed and more investigation needs to be conducted in such models to realistically assess the influence of drug transporters on the biopharmaceutics of inhaled drugs biopharmaceutics.

REFERENCES

1. Labiris, N. R. and M. B. Dolovich (2003). "Pulmonary drug delivery. Part I: Physiological factors affecting therapeutic effectiveness of aerosolized medications." *Br J Clin Pharmacol* **56**(6): 588–599.
2. Folkesson, H. G. et al. (1996). "Alveolar epithelial clearance of protein." *J Appl Physiol* **80**(5): 1431–1445.
3. Sharara, R. S. et al. (2017). "Introduction to the Anatomy and Physiology of Pulmonary Circulation." *Crit Care Nurs Q* **40**(3): 181–190.
4. Deffebach, M. E. et al. (1987). "The bronchial circulation. Small, but a vital attribute of the lung." *Am Rev Respir Dis* **135**(2): 463–481.
5. Videira, M. A. et al. (2002). "Lymphatic uptake of pulmonary delivered radiolabelled solid lipid nanoparticles." *J Drug Target* **10**(8): 607–613.
6. Rabaca Roque Botelho, M. F. et al. (2009). "Nanoradioliposomes molecularly modulated to study the lung deep lymphatic drainage." *Rev Port Pneumol* **15**(2): 261–293.
7. Pabst, R. and T. Tschernig (2010). "Bronchus-associated lymphoid tissue: An entry site for antigens for successful mucosal vaccinations?" *Am J Respir Cell Mol Biol* **43**(2): 137–141.
8. Botelho, M. F. et al. (2011). "[Visualization of deep lung lymphatic network using radioliposomes]." *Rev Port Pneumol* **17**(3): 124–130.
9. Beloqui, A. et al. (2016) "Nanostructured lipid carriers: Promising drug delivery systems for future clinics." *Nanomed Nanotechnol, Bio Med* **12**(1): 143–161.
10. Jain, R. K. (1994). "Barriers to drug delivery in solid tumors." *Sci Am* **271**(1): 58–65.
11. Harivardhan Reddy, L. et al. (2005). "Influence of administration route on tumor uptake and biodistribution of etoposide loaded solid lipid nanoparticles in Dalton's lymphoma tumor bearing mice." *J Control Release* **105**(3): 185–198.
12. Videira, M. A. et al. (2006). "Lymphatic uptake of lipid nanoparticles following endotracheal administration." *J Microencapsul* **23**(8): 855–862.
13. Cai, S. et al. (2011). "Lymphatic drug delivery using engineered liposomes and solid lipid nanoparticles." *Adv Drug Deliv Rev* **63**(10–11): 901–908.

14. Khan, A. A. et al. (2013). "Advanced drug delivery to the lymphatic system: Lipid-based nanoformulations." *Int J Nanomedicine* **8**: 2733–2744.

15. Weber, S. et al. (2014). "Solid lipid nanoparticles (SLN) and nanostructured lipid carriers (NLC) for pulmonary application: A review of the state of the art." *Eur J Pharm Biopharm* **86**(1): 7–22.

16. Trevaskis, N. L. et al. (2015). "From sewer to saviour – targeting the lymphatic system to promote drug exposure and activity." *Nat Rev Drug Discov* **14**(11): 781–803.

17. Effros, R. M. and G. R. Mason (1983). "Measurements of pulmonary epithelial permeability in vivo." *Am Rev Respir Dis* **127**(5 Pt 2): S59–S65.

18. Schneeberger, E. (1991). "Airway and alveolar epithelial cell junctions." In: Crystal, R. G et al. (eds) *The Lung*. Raven Press, New York, pp 205–214.

19. Schanker, L. S. and J. A. Hemberger (1983). "Relation between molecular weight and pulmonary absorption rate of lipid-insoluble compounds in neonatal and adult rats." *Biochem Pharmacol* **32**(17): 2599–2601.

20. Patton, J. S. et al. (2004). "The lungs as a portal of entry for systemic drug delivery." *Proc Am Thorac Soc* **1**(4): 338–344.

21. Kobayashi, S. et al. (1995). "Permeability of peptides and proteins in human cultured alveolar A549 cell monolayer." *Pharm Res* **12**(8): 1115–1119.

22. Patton, J. S. (1996). "Mechanisms of macromolecule absorption by the lungs." *Adv Drug Deliv Rev* **19**(1): 3–36.

23. Forrest, L. R. et al. (2011). "The structural basis of secondary active transport mechanisms." *Biochim Biophys Acta* **1807**(2): 167–188.

24. Hediger, M. A. et al. (2013). "The ABCs of membrane transporters in health and disease (SLC series): Introduction." *Mol Aspects Med* **34**(2–3): 95–107.

25. Nickel, S. et al. (2016). "Transport mechanisms at the pulmonary mucosa: Implications for drug delivery." *Expert Opin Drug Deliv* **13**(5): 667–690.

26. Sahoo, S. et al. (2014). "Membrane transporters in a human genome-scale metabolic knowledgebase and their implications for disease." *Front Physiol* **5**: 91.

27. Lin, L. et al. (2015). "SLC transporters as therapeutic targets: Emerging opportunities." *Nat Rev Drug Discov* **14**(8): 543–560.

28. Gumbleton, M. et al. (2011). "Spatial expression and functionality of drug transporters in the intact lung: Objectives for further research." *Adv Drug Deliv Rev* **63**(1–2): 110–118.

29. Lips, K. S. et al. (2005). "Polyspecific cation transporters mediate luminal release of acetylcholine from bronchial epithelium." *Am J Respir Cell Mol Biol* **33**(1): 79–88.

30. van der Deen, M. et al. (2006). "Diminished expression of multidrug resistance-associated protein 1 (MRP1) in bronchial epithelium of COPD patients." *Virchows Arch* **449**(6): 682–688.

31. van der Deen, M. et al. (2007). "Cigarette smoke extract affects functional activity of MRP1 in bronchial epithelial cells." *J Biochem Mol Toxicol* **21**(5): 243–251.

32. Choudhuri, S. and C. D. Klaassen (2006). "Structure, function, expression, genomic organization, and single nucleotide polymorphisms of human ABCB1 (MDR1), ABCC (MRP), and ABCG2 (BCRP) efflux transporters." *Int J Toxicol* **25**(4): 231–259.

33. Bosquillon, C. (2010). "Drug transporters in the lung– do they play a role in the biopharmaceutics of inhaled drugs?" *J Pharm Sci* **99**(5): 2240–2255.

34. Vasiliou, V. et al. (2009). "Human ATP-binding cassette (ABC) transporter family." *Hum Genomics* **3**(3): 281–290.

35. Jani, M. et al. (2014). "Structure and function of BCRP, a broad specificity transporter of xenobiotics and endobiotics." *Arch Toxicol* **88**(6): 1205–1248.

36. Scheffer, G. L. et al. (2002). "Multidrug resistance related molecules in human and murine lung." *J Clin Pathol* **55**(5): 332–339.

37. Campbell, L. et al. (2003). "Constitutive expression of p-glycoprotein in normal lung alveolar epithelium and functionality in primary alveolar epithelial cultures." *J Pharmacol Exp Ther* **304**(1): 441–452.

38. Endter, S. et al. (2007). "P-glycoprotein (MDR1) functional activity in human alveolar epithelial cell monolayers." *Cell Tissue Res* **328**(1): 77–84.

39. Lehmann, T. et al. (2001). "Expression of MRP1 and related transporters in human lung cells in culture." *Toxicology* **167**(1): 59–72.

40. Lin, H. et al. (2007). "Air-liquid interface (ALI) culture of human bronchial epithelial cell monolayers as an in vitro model for airway drug transport studies." *J Pharm Sci* **96**(2): 341–350.

41. Mehta, R. et al. (2013). "Effect of verapamil on systemic exposure and safety of umeclidinium and vilanterol: A randomized and open-label study." *Int J Chron Obstruct Pulmon Dis* **8**: 159–167.

42. Pavek, P. et al. (2007). "Examination of glucocorticoid receptor alpha-mediated transcriptional regulation of P-glycoprotein, CYP3A4, and CYP2C9 genes in placental trophoblast cell lines." *Placenta* **28**(10): 1004–1011.

43. Barnes, P. J. and I. M. Adcock (2009). "Glucocorticoid resistance in inflammatory diseases." *Lancet* **373**(9678): 1905–1917.

44. Kuzuya, Y. et al. (2004). "Induction of drug-metabolizing enzymes and transporters in human bronchial epithelial cells by beclomethasone dipropionate." *IUBMB Life* **56**(6): 355–359.

45. Crowe, A. and A. M. Tan (2012). "Oral and inhaled corticosteroids: Differences in P-glycoprotein (ABCB1) mediated efflux." *Toxicol Appl Pharmacol* **260**(3): 294–302.

46. Zerin, T. et al. (2012). "Protective effect of methylprednisolone on paraquat-induced A549 cell cytotoxicity via induction of efflux transporter, P-glycoprotein expression." *Toxicol Lett* **208**(2): 101–107.

47. Demeule, M. et al. (1999). "Dexamethasone modulation of multidrug transporters in normal tissues." *FEBS Lett* **442**(2–3): 208–214.

48. Ehrhardt, C. et al. (2003). "16HBE14o- human bronchial epithelial cell layers express P-glycoprotein, lung resistance-related protein, and caveolin-1." *Pharm Res* **20**(4): 545–551.

49. Tronde, A. et al. (2003). "Drug absorption from the isolated perfused rat lung–correlations with drug physicochemical properties and epithelial permeability." *J Drug Target* **11**(1): 61–74.

50. Togami, K. et al. (2011). "Distribution characteristics of clarithromycin and azithromycin, macrolide antimicrobial agents used for treatment of respiratory infections, in lung epithelial lining fluid and alveolar macrophages." *Biopharm Drug Dispos* **32**(7): 389–397.

51. Togami, K. et al. (2012). "Transport characteristics of clarithromycin, azithromycin and telithromycin, antibiotics applied for treatment of respiratory infections, in Calu-3 cell monolayers as model lung epithelial cells." *Pharmazie* **67**(5): 389–393.

52. Toyoda, Y. et al. (2008). "MRP class of human ATP binding cassette (ABC) transporters: Historical background and new research directions." *Xenobiotica* **38**(7–8): 833–862.

53. Sakamoto, A. et al. (2013). "Quantitative expression of human drug transporter proteins in lung tissues: Analysis of regional, gender, and interindividual differences by liquid chromatography-tandem mass spectrometry." *J Pharm Sci* **102**(9): 3395–3406.

54. Okamura, T. et al. (2013). "Imaging of activity of multidrug resistance-associated protein 1 in the lungs." *Am J Respir Cell Mol Biol* **49**(3): 335–340.

55. Manciu, L. et al. (2003). "Intermediate structural states involved in MRP1-mediated drug transport. Role of glutathione." *J Biol Chem* **278**(5): 3347–3356.

56. Deeley, R. G. and S. P. Cole (2006). "Substrate recognition and transport by multidrug resistance protein 1 (ABCC1)." *FEBS Lett* **580**(4): 1103–1111.

57. Cole, S. P. (2014). "Targeting multidrug resistance protein 1 (MRP1, ABCC1): Past, present, and future." *Annu Rev Pharmacol Toxicol* **54**: 95–117.

58. Wang, D. et al. (2014). "Allyl isothiocyanate increases MRP1 function and expression in a human bronchial epithelial cell line." *Oxid Med Cell Longev* **2014**. doi:10.1155/2014/547379.

59. Siedlinski, M. et al. (2009). "ABCC1 polymorphisms contribute to level and decline of lung function in two population-based cohorts." *Pharmacogenet Genom* **19**(9): 675–684.

60. Berg, T. et al. (2014). "Gene expression analysis of membrane transporters and drug-metabolizing enzymes in the lung of healthy and COPD subjects." *Pharmacol Res Perspect* **2**(4): e00054.

61. van der Deen, M. et al. (2008). "Effect of COPD treatments on MRP1-mediated transport in bronchial epithelial cells." *Int J Chron Obstruct Pulmon Dis* **3**(3): 469–475.

62. Mao, Q. and J. D. Unadkat (2015). "Role of the breast cancer resistance protein (BCRP/ABCG2) in drug transport–an update." *Aaps J* **17**(1): 65–82.

63. Robey, R. W. et al. (2009). "ABCG2: A perspective." *Adv Drug Deliv Rev* **61**(1): 3–13.

64. Takada, T. et al. (2005). "Characterization of polarized expression of point- or deletion-mutated human BCRP/ABCG2 in LLC-PK1 cells." *Pharm Res* **22**(3): 458–464.

65. Lee, C. A. et al. (2015). "Breast cancer resistance protein (ABCG2) in clinical pharmacokinetics and drug interactions: Practical recommendations for clinical victim and perpetrator drug–drug interaction study design." *Drug Metab Dispos* **43**(4): 490–509.

66. Suzuki, M. et al. (2003). "ABCG2 transports sulfated conjugates of steroids and xenobiotics." *J Biol Chem* **278**(25): 22644–22649.

67. Sakamoto, A. et al. (2015). "Drug transporter protein quantification of immortalized Human Lung cell lines derived from tracheobronchial epithelial cells (Calu-3 and BEAS2-B), bronchiolar-alveolar cells (NCI-H292 and NCI-H441), and alveolar type II-like cells (A549) by liquid chromatography-tandem mass spectrometry." *J Pharm Sci* **104**(9): 3029–3038.

68. Nickel, S. et al. (2017). "Expression and activity of breast cancer resistance protein (BCRP/ABCG2) in human distal lung epithelial cells in vitro." *Pharm Res* **34**: 2477–2487.

69. Liang, S. C. et al. (2015). "ABCG2 localizes to the nucleus and modulates CDH1 expression in lung cancer cells." *Neoplasia* **17**(3): 265–278.

70. Cooray, H. C. et al. (2006). "Modulation of p-glycoprotein and breast cancer resistance protein by some prescribed corticosteroids." *Eur J Pharmacol* **531**(1–3): 25–33.

71. Ando, T. et al. (2007). "Involvement of breast cancer resistance protein (ABCG2) in the biliary excretion mechanism of fluoroquinolones." *Drug Metab Dispos* **35**(10): 1873–1879.

72. Nakanishi, T. and D. D. Ross (2012). "Breast cancer resistance protein (BCRP/ABCG2): Its role in multidrug resistance and regulation of its gene expression." *Chin J Cancer* **31**(2): 73–99.

73. Kawabata, S. et al. (2003). "Expression and functional analyses of breast cancer resistance protein in lung cancer." *Clin Cancer Res* **9**(8): 3052–3057.

74. Koepsell, H. (2013). "The SLC22 family with transporters of organic cations, anions and zwitterions." *Mol Aspects Med* **34**(2–3): 413–435.

75. Horvath, G. et al. (2007). "Epithelial organic cation transporters ensure pH-dependent drug absorption in the airway." *Am J Respir Cell Mol Biol* **36**(1): 53–60.

76. Kummer, W. et al. (2008). "The epithelial cholinergic system of the airways." *Histochem Cell Biol* **130**(2): 219–234.

77. Salomon, J. J. et al. (2012). "Transport of the fluorescent organic cation 4-(4-(dimethylamino)styryl)-N-methylpyridinium iodide (ASP+) in human respiratory epithelial cells." *Eur J Pharm Biopharm* **81**(2): 351–359.

78. Salomon, J. J. et al. (2014). "The cell line NCI-H441 is a useful in vitro model for transport studies of human distal lung epithelial barrier." *Mol Pharm* **11**(3): 995–1006.

79. Grundemann, D. et al. (2005). "Discovery of the ergothioneine transporter." *Proc Natl Acad Sci U S A* **102**(14): 5256–5261.

80. Ingoglia, F. et al. (2016). "Functional activity of L-carnitine transporters in human airway epithelial cells." *Biochim Biophys Acta* **1858**(2): 210–219.

81. Kummer, W. et al. (2006). "Role of acetylcholine and polyspecific cation transporters in serotonin-induced bronchoconstriction in the mouse." *Respir Res* **7**: 65.

82. Shitara, Y. et al. (2006). "Transporters as a determinant of drug clearance and tissue distribution." *Eur J Pharm Sci* **27**(5): 425–446.

83. Ehrhardt, C. et al. (2005). "Salbutamol is actively absorbed across human bronchial epithelial cell layers." *Pulm Pharmacol Ther* **18**(3): 165–170.

84. Gnadt, M. et al. (2012). "Methacholine delays pulmonary absorption of inhaled beta(2)-agonists due to competition for organic cation/carnitine transporters." *Pulm Pharmacol Ther* **25**(1): 124–134.

85. Salomon, J. J. et al. (2015). "Beta-2 adrenergic agonists are substrates and inhibitors of human organic cation transporter 1." *Mol Pharm* **12**(8): 2633–2641.

86. Haghi, M. et al. (2012). "Deposition, diffusion and transport mechanism of dry powder microparticulate salbutamol, at the respiratory epithelia." *Mol Pharm* **9**(6): 1717–1726.

87. Unwalla, H. J. et al. (2012). "Albuterol modulates its own transepithelial flux via changes in paracellular permeability." *Am J Respir Cell Mol Biol* **46**(4): 551–558.

88. Horvath, G. et al. (2007). "The effect of corticosteroids on the disposal of long-acting beta2-agonists by airway smooth muscle cells." *J Allergy Clin Immunol* **120**(5): 1103–1109.

89. Horvath, G. et al. (2011). "Rapid nongenomic actions of inhaled corticosteroids on long-acting β(2)-agonist transport in the airway." *Pulm Pharmacol Ther* **24**(6): 654–659.

90. Nakamura, T. et al. (2010). "Transport of ipratropium, an anti-chronic obstructive pulmonary disease drug, is mediated by organic cation/carnitine transporters in human bronchial epithelial cells: Implications for carrier-mediated pulmonary absorption." *Mol Pharm* **7**(1): 187–195.

91. Nakanishi, T. et al. (2013). "In vivo evidence of organic cation transporter-mediated tracheal accumulation of the anticholinergic agent ipratropium in mice." *J Pharm Sci* **102**(9): 3373–3381.

92. Backstrom, E. et al. (2016). "Development of a novel lung slice methodology for profiling of inhaled compounds." *J Pharm Sci* **105**(2): 838–845.

93. Al-Jayyoussi, G. et al. (2015). "Absorption of ipratropium and l-carnitine into the pulmonary circulation of the ex-vivo rat lung is driven by passive processes rather than active uptake by OCT/OCTN transporters." *Int J Pharm* **496**(2): 834–841.

94. Meyerhoff, A. et al. (2004). "US food and drug administration approval of ciprofloxacin hydrochloride for management of postexposure inhalational anthrax." *Clin Infect Dis* **39**(3): 303–308.

95. Ong, H. X. et al. (2013). "Ciprofloxacin is actively transported across bronchial lung epithelial cells using a Calu-3 air interface cell model." *Antimicrob Agents Chemother* **57**(6): 2535–2540.

96. Daniel, H. and G. Kottra (2004). "The proton oligopeptide cotransporter family SLC15 in physiology and pharmacology." *Pflugers Arch* **447**(5): 610–618.

97. Smith, D. E. et al. (2013). "Proton-coupled oligopeptide transporter family SLC15: Physiological, pharmacological and pathological implications." *Mol Aspects Med* **34**(2–3): 323–336.

98. Saito, H. et al. (1995). "Cloning and characterization of a rat H+/peptide cotransporter mediating absorption of beta-lactam antibiotics in the intestine and kidney." *J Pharmacol Exp Ther* **275**(3): 1631–1637.

99. Yang, C. Y. et al. (1999). "Intestinal peptide transport systems and oral drug availability." *Pharm Res* **16**(9): 1331–1343.

100. Zhu, T. et al. (2000). "Differential recognition of ACE inhibitors in Xenopus laevis oocytes expressing rat PEPT1 and PEPT2." *Pharm Res* **17**(5): 526–532.

101. Groneberg, D. A. et al. (2004). "Molecular mechanisms of pulmonary peptidomimetic drug and peptide transport." *Am J Respir Cell Mol Biol* **30**(3): 251–260.

102. Saito, H. et al. (1996). "Molecular cloning and tissue distribution of rat peptide transporter PEPT2." *Biochim Biophys Acta* **1280**(2): 173–177.

103. Bleasby, K. et al. (2006). "Expression profiles of 50 xenobiotic transporter genes in humans and preclinical species: A resource for investigations into drug disposition." *Xenobiotica* **36**(10–11): 963–988.

104. Lu, H. and C. Klaassen (2006). "Tissue distribution and thyroid hormone regulation of Pept1 and Pept2 mRNA in rodents." *Peptides* **27**(4): 850–857.

105. Leclerc, J. et al. (2011). "Xenobiotic metabolism and disposition in human lung: Transcript profiling in non-tumoral and tumoral tissues." *Biochimie* **93**(6): 1012–1027.

106. Courcot, E. et al. (2012). "Xenobiotic metabolism and disposition in human lung cell models: Comparison with in vivo expression profiles." *Drug Metab Dispos* **40**(10): 1953–1965.

107. Bahadduri, P. M. et al. (2005). "Functional characterization of the peptide transporter PEPT2 in primary cultures of human upper airway epithelium." *Am J Respir Cell Mol Biol* **32**(4): 319–325.

108. Groneberg, D. A. et al. (2001). "Localization of the peptide transporter PEPT2 in the lung: Implications for pulmonary oligopeptide uptake." *Am J Pathol* **158**(2): 707–714.

109. Groneberg, D. et al. (2002). "Distribution and function of the peptide transporter PEPT2 in normal and cystic fibrosis human lung." *Thorax* **57**(1): 55–60.

110. Takano, M. et al. (2015). "Functional expression of PEPT2 in the human distal lung epithelial cell line NCI-H441." *Pharm Res* **32**(12): 3916–3926.

111. Brahmajothi, M. V. et al. (2013). "S-nitrosothiol transport via PEPT2 mediates biological effects of nitric oxide gas exposure in macrophages." *Am J Respir Cell Mol Biol* **48**(2): 230–239.

112. Kirkham, M. and R. G. Parton (2005). "Clathrin-independent endocytosis: New insights into caveolae and non-caveolar lipid raft carriers." *Biochim Biophys Acta* **1745**(3): 273–286.

113. Gumbleton, M. et al. (2003). "Targeting caveolae for vesicular drug transport." *J Control Release* **87**(1–3): 139–151.

114. Kim, K. J. and A. B. Malik (2003). "Protein transport across the lung epithelial barrier." *Am J Physiol Lung Cell Mol Physiol* **284**(2): L247–L259.

115. Sowa, G. (2012). "Caveolae, caveolins, cavins, and endothelial cell function: New insights." *Front Physiol* **2**: 120.

116. Ibrahim, M. and L. Garcia-Contreras (2013). "Mechanisms of absorption and elimination of drugs administered by inhalation." *Ther Deliv* **4**(8): 1027–1045.

117. Schnitzer, J. E. et al. (1988). "Albumin interacts specifically with a 60-kDa microvascular endothelial glycoprotein." *Proc Natl Acad Sci U S A* **85**(18): 6773–6777.

118. Matsukawa, Y. et al. (2000). "Rates of protein transport across rat alveolar epithelial cell monolayers." *J Drug Target* **7**(5): 335–342.

119. John, T. A. et al. (2001). "Evidence for the role of alveolar epithelial gp60 in active transalveolar albumin transport in the rat lung." *J Physiol* **533**(Pt 2): 547–559.

120. Kim, K. J. et al. (2003). "Absorption of intact albumin across rat alveolar epithelial cell monolayers." *Am J Physiol Lung Cell Mol Physiol* **284**(3): L458–L465.

121. Ikehata, M. et al. (2008). "Comparison of albumin uptake in rat alveolar type II and type I-like epithelial cells in primary culture." *Pharm Res* **25**(4): 913–922.

122. Ikehata, M. et al. (2009). "Mechanism of insulin uptake in rat alveolar type II and type I-like epithelial cells." *Biol Pharm Bull* **32**(10): 1765–1769.

123. Nemmar, A. et al. (2001). "Passage of intratracheally instilled ultrafine particles from the lung into the systemic circulation in hamster." *Am J Respir Crit Care Med* **164**(9): 1665–1668.

124. Nemmar, A. et al. (2002). "Passage of inhaled particles into the blood circulation in humans." *Circulation* **105**(4): 411–414.

125. Blank, F. et al. (2013). "Size-dependent uptake of particles by pulmonary antigen-presenting cell populations and trafficking to regional lymph nodes." *Am J Respir Cell Mol Biol* **49**(1): 67–77.

126. Stone, K. C. et al. (1992). "Allometric relationships of cell numbers and size in the mammalian lung." *Am J Respir Cell Mol Biol* **6**(2): 235–243.

127. Vermaelen, K. Y. et al. (2001). "Specific migratory dendritic cells rapidly transport antigen from the airways to the thoracic lymph nodes." *J Exp Med* **193**(1): 51–60.

128. Takenaka, S. et al. (2001). "Pulmonary and systemic distribution of inhaled ultrafine silver particles in rats." *Environ Health Perspect* **109**(Suppl 4): 547–551.

129. Himmelmann, A. et al. (2003). "The impact of smoking on inhaled insulin." *Diabetes Care* **26**(3): 677–682.

130. Becker, R. H. et al. (2006). "The effect of smoking cessation and subsequent resumption on absorption of inhaled insulin." *Diabetes Care* **29**(2): 277–282.

131. Rave, K. et al. (2007). "AIR inhaled insulin in subjects with chronic obstructive pulmonary disease: Pharmacokinetics, glucodynamics, safety, and tolerability." *Diabetes Care* **30**(7): 1777–1782.

132. Henry, R. R. et al. (2003). "Inhaled insulin using the AERx Insulin Diabetes Management System in healthy and asthmatic subjects." *Diabetes Care* **26**(3): 764–769.

133. Mudaliar, S. and R. R. Henry (2007). "Inhaled insulin in patients with asthma and chronic obstructive pulmonary disease." *Diabetes Technol Ther* **9**(Suppl 1): S83–S92.

134. Borghardt, J. M. et al. (2016). "Model-based evaluation of pulmonary pharmacokinetics in asthmatic and COPD patients after oral olodaterol inhalation." *Br J Clin Pharmacol* **82**(3): 739–753.

135. Neale, M. G. et al. (1987). "The pharmacokinetics of nedocromil sodium, a new drug for the treatment of reversible obstructive airways disease, in human volunteers and patients with reversible obstructive airways disease." *Br J Clin Pharmacol* **24**(4): 493–501.

136. Brutsche, M. H. et al. (2000). "Comparison of pharmacokinetics and systemic effects of inhaled fluticasone propionate in patients with asthma and healthy volunteers: A randomised crossover study." *Lancet* **356**(9229): 556–561.

137. De Backer, W. et al. (2010). "Lung deposition of BDP/formoterol HFA pMDI in healthy volunteers, asthmatic, and COPD patients." *J Aerosol Med Pulm Drug Deliv* **23**(3): 137–148.

138. Mukherjee, M. et al. (2017). "Enhanced expression of Organic Cation Transporters in bronchial epithelial cell layers following insults associated with asthma – Impact on salbutamol transport." *Eur J Pharm Sci* **106**: 62–70.

139. Summers, Q. A. (1991). "Inhaled drugs and the lung." *Clin Exp Allergy* **21**(3): 259–268.

140. Tronde, A. et al. (2003). "Pulmonary absorption rate and bioavailability of drugs in vivo in rats: Structure-absorption relationships and physicochemical profiling of inhaled drugs." *J Pharm Sci* **92**(6): 1216–1233.

141. Folkesson, H. G. et al. (1990). "Permeability of the respiratory tract to different-sized macromolecules after intratracheal instillation in young and adult rats." *Acta Physiol Scand* **139**(2): 347–354.

142. Carvalho, T. C. et al. (2011). "Influence of particle size on regional lung deposition–what evidence is there?" *Int J Pharm* **406**(1–2): 1–10.

143. Yang, J. Z. et al. (2008). "Fluticasone and budesonide nanosuspensions for pulmonary delivery: Preparation, characterization, and pharmacokinetic studies." *J Pharm Sci* **97**(11): 4869–4878.

144. Ruge, C. A. et al. (2013). "Pulmonary drug delivery: From generating aerosols to overcoming biological barriers-therapeutic possibilities and technological challenges." *Lancet Respir Med* **1**(5): 402–413.

145. Geiser, M. (2010). "Update on macrophage clearance of inhaled micro- and nanoparticles." *J Aerosol Med Pulm Drug Deliv* **23**(4): 207–217.

146. Edwards, D. A. et al. (1998). "Recent advances in pulmonary drug delivery using large, porous inhaled particles." *J Appl Physiol* **85**(2): 379–385.

147. Champion, J. A. and S. Mitragotri (2009). "Shape induced inhibition of phagocytosis of polymer particles." *Pharm Res* **26**(1): 244–249.

5

Bioavailability of inhaled compounds

LUCILA GARCIA-CONTRERAS

Introduction	71
Bioavailability	72
Definition of bioavailability	72
Factors that affect the bioavailability of inhaled compounds	74
Physicochemical properties of the compound	75
Formulation and delivery devices	77
Site of deposition	78
Clearance mechanisms	78
Drug release and dissolution	79
Permeability	80
Mechanisms of drug absorption	81

Methods to determine bioavailability of inhaled compounds	83
Selection of the subject	83
Dose calculation	85
Biological samples	87
Pharmacokinetic parameters to determine bioavailability	88
Pharmacodynamic parameters to determine bioavailability	89
Case studies of the bioavailability and bioequivalency of inhaled products	90
References	100

INTRODUCTION

Therapeutic aerosols have been used for many years to treat lung diseases such as asthma and chronic obstructive pulmonary diseases (COPD) and to alleviate and correct the pulmonary signs and symptoms of cystic fibrosis (CF) (1). The use of the pulmonary route of administration was considered in the 1990s to deliver compounds for systemic effects (2,3), and tuberculosis (4), while aerosolized chemotherapy was proposed for the treatment of lung cancer in the late 2000s (5). Given the large number of compounds delivered as therapeutic aerosols to treat this wide variety of diseases, it is not surprising that their physicochemical characteristics are diverse, encompassing a wide range of molecular weights, solubility, lipophilicity, and permeability. Although the disposition (absorption, distribution, and excretion) of these therapeutic compounds is influenced by their physicochemical properties, other factors strongly determine their disposition and consequently their bioavailability when delivered to the lungs as aerosols. These are depicted in Figure 5.1 and include the formulation, delivery device, site of deposition, disease state, clearance mechanisms, the desired site of drug action, and drug availability at the desired site of action.

Throughout the years, aerosols of therapeutic compounds have been generated from liquid or solid formulations employing nebulizers, metered-dose inhalers (MDIs), and dry powder inhalers (DPIs). The complexity of these

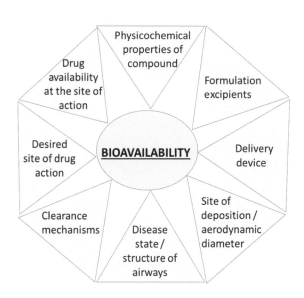

Figure 5.1 The different factors that affect the bioavailability of therapeutic compounds delivered as aerosols to the lungs.

formulations has increased over the years, with dry powder formulations affording the use of a wider variety of excipients and methods of preparation, ranging from physical mixtures of micronized drug and lactose to sophisticated particle engineering approaches. The efficiency of aerosol delivery depends on the device, the aerodynamic diameter and size distribution of the aerosol, as well as the site of deposition in the airways. In turn, the site of aerosol deposition is influenced by the extent to which the disease state of the patient has modified the original airway structure, whereas drug residence time and action are contingent on the clearance mechanisms in that region of the lungs. The effects of these factors on drug bioavailability will be discussed in this chapter as well as the methods employed to determine bioavailability and bioequivalence as outlined by the United States Food and Drug Administration (U.S. FDA).

BIOAVAILABILITY

Definition of bioavailability

Inhalation of therapeutic compounds to treat local diseases has the benefit of achieving high local concentrations and results in a rapid onset of drug actions. Administration of therapeutic compounds by inhalation has the additional benefit of increasing the bioavailability of drugs with low oral bioavailability, which allows the use of a smaller dose and the reduction of systemic side effects. Traditional pharmacokinetics books define *bioavailability* simply as "the rate and extent of drug absorption" (6), whereas others specify

that the rate and extent of drug absorption is into systemic circulation (7) because, particularly for oral administration, the fraction of the dose reaching systemic circulation is frequently correlated with drug action. However, this traditional definition of bioavailability cannot be extended to all drugs administered by the pulmonary route, as the site of drug action depends on the particular drug. The US FDA published a broader definition of *bioavailability* in their Guidance for Industry (Bioavailability and Bioequivalence Studies for Orally Administered Drug Products—General Considerations) based on Chapter 320.1 of the Code of Federal Regulations (CFR § 320.1):

The rate and extent to which the active ingredient or active moiety is absorbed from a drug product and becomes available at the site of action. For drug products that are not intended to be absorbed into the bloodstream, bioavailability may be assessed by measurements intended to reflect the rate and extent to which the active ingredient or active moiety becomes available at the site of action.

This definition is more suitable for drugs administered by the pulmonary route as long as the *site of action* can be defined for each particular drug. Table 5.1 lists the most

Table 5.1 Common diseases of the lungs, the drug classes used to treat them and their desired site of action

Disease	Characteristics	Drug classes used in treatment	Desired site of action
Asthma	• Airway inflammation and episodic, reversible bronchospasms causing shortness of breath, cough, chest tightness, and rapid respiration	Bronchodilators: • β-adrenoceptor agonists • Muscarinic antagonists (Anticholinergics) • Methyl-xanthines • Leukotriene antagonists Anti-inflammatory drugs: • Corticosteroids • Mast cell stabilizers	• Bronchi • Bronchioles
Bronchiectasis	• Occurs when the walls of the airways (bronchi) thicken as a result of chronic inflammation and/or infection and results in mucus accumulating	Antibiotics: tobramycin, gentamicin, colistin Anti-inflammatory drugs Bronchodilators	• Bronchi
Cancer	• Small cell lung cancer: Usually seen in cells near the bronchi • Adenocarcinoma: Most prevalent form of cancer and usually arises in the cells lining the alveoli. • Squamous cell carcinoma: Tumors appear in the flat cells that line the inside of the airways, usually near the bronchi • Large cell carcinoma: Can begin in any part of the lung and often grows and spreads quickly	Chemotherapeutic agents: Selected depending of the type of cancer, the localization and the stage. Examples of inhaled chemotherapeutic agents include, cetuximab, cisplatin, doxorubicin, gemcitabine, and paclitaxel	• Bronchi • Alveoli

(Continued)

Table 5.1 (*Continued*) Common diseases of the lungs, the drug classes used to treat them and their desired site of action

Disease	Characteristics	Drug classes used in treatment	Desired site of action

Chronic obstructive pulmonary disease (COPD)	• Airflow limitation that is less reversible than in asthma and has a progressive course
	• Bronchioles lose their shape and become clogged with mucus (bronchitis) and walls of alveoli are destroyed, forming fewer larger alveoli (emphysema)
		Bronchodilators:
		  • β-adrenoceptor agonists
		  • Muscarinic antagonists (Anticholinergics)
		  • Methyl-xanthines
		  • Leukotriene antagonists
		Anti-inflammatory drugs:
		  • Corticosteroids
		  • Mast cell stabilizers
			• Bronchi
			• Alveoli

Cystic fibrosis	• Abnormal airway secretions • Abnormal rheology of airway secretions • Opportunistic bacterial infections • Bronchoconstriction • Chronic inflammation	Mucolytics Amiloride, ATP, UTP Antibiotics Bronchodilators Anti-inflammatory drugs Gene therapy	• Bronchi • Bronchioles
Fungal infections	• Inhalation of fungi that are not effective cleared by the patient • Patients with weakened immune systems are more likely to develop more severe forms of the infection	*Anti-fungal drugs:* Examples: Itraconazole, fluconazole, voriconazole, amphotericin B	• Alveoli
NTM: Non-tuberculosis mycobacteria	• Caused by patient inhaling environmental NTM • If not cleared will infect the patient	*Antibiotics:* Effective treatment requires 2–3 drugs that are selected depending on the infecting NTM species, their drug susceptibility and extent of the infection	• Alveoli
Pneumonia	• Infection caused by bacteria, viruses, and fungi • The infection can quickly spread through the bloodstream and invade the entire body	*Antimicrobials*, depending on the causative agent and the severity of the disease; for bacterial pneumonia, macrolides can be used	• Alveoli
Pulmonary hypertension	• High blood pressure that affects arteries in the lungs and in the heart • Caused by blood vessels that become narrowed blocked or destroyed	*Prostacyclins:* Epoprostenol, iloprost and treprostinil Inhaled nitric oxide (INO)	• Alveoli
Transplant rejection	• Small airways of the transplanted lung, or graft, begin scarring and slowly become completely scarred and close up • Chronic rejection (also called bronchiolitis obliterans, BO) is characterized by a narrowing and disintegration of the small bronchioles	There is no cure BO, but therapies that may stop or reverse its course may include macrolide antibiotics, corticosteroids and immunosuppressant drugs such as cyclosporine A	• Bronchioles
Tuberculosis	• Caused by patient inhaling Mycobacterium tuberculosis • If not cleared will infect the patient	*Antibiotics:* Examples: Isoniazid, rifampicin, pyrazinamide, capreomycin, clofazimine	• Alveoli

Sources: Compiled from Trevor, A.J. et al., *Katzung & Trevor's pharmacology: Examination & board review*, 10th ed., *Lange Medical Books*, New York, McGraw-Hill, 2012; Crystal, R.G. et al., Eds. *The Lung Scientific Foundations*, Philadelphia, PA, Lippincott-Raven Publishers, 1997.

prevalent diseases of the lungs, the drug classes used to treat them, and their desired site of action.

According to the US FDA definition, the site of action for compounds intended to treat asthma and the symptoms of cystic fibrosis are the bronchi and bronchioles, whereas the site of action to treat fungal infections and pulmonary hypertension is the alveoli. For most of these compounds it is extremely difficult to measure the rate and the extent to which they become available at the site of action using drug concentrations. Thus, the second part of the definition applies for these compounds, which is to adapt measurements that can quantify indirectly these parameters.

On the other hand, the pulmonary route has been considered to deliver other compounds for systemic action, including insulin, leuprolide acetate, and salmon calcitonin, among several others. For these compounds, the traditional definition of bioavailability can be applied because the concentration of these compounds in serum or plasma is a good measure of their absorption and availability at the site of action.

The determination of bioavailability becomes even more complicated when the site of action is in both the lung tissue and other organs in the body, such as the proposed treatment of tuberculosis using inhaled therapies. For this purpose, the drug must be available in therapeutic concentration locally in the lung tissue and systemically so that it can reach other organs. It is practically impossible to achieve both without significant toxicities, and therefore it is no surprise that there are no commercially available products with this indication. Figure 5.2 illustrates the site of action for drugs that have

been considered for pulmonary delivery and that are commercially available or remain in the early stages of development.

Factors that affect the bioavailability of inhaled compounds

Bioavailability is traditionally calculated as the ratio of the extent of drug absorbed from an extravascular route of administration, either parenteral, oral, vaginal, rectal, or pulmonary, as measured by the area under the drug concentration versus time curve ($AUC_{0\to\infty}$), divided by the AUC after intravenous (IV) administration and corrected by their respective dose (6):

$$F = \frac{AUC_{0\to\infty} extravascular}{AUC_{0\to\infty} IV} \times \frac{Dose_{IV}}{Dose_{extravascular}} \tag{5.1}$$

Unlike any other extravascular route of administration, the absorption (into lung tissue or systemic circulation) of therapeutic compounds delivered by the pulmonary route is influenced by the formulation, the delivery device and anatomical factors, including the site of deposition, mechanisms of clearance, and permeability of the compound, as illustrated in Figure 5.3. The type of formulation is influenced by the physicochemical properties of the compound and the intended therapeutic dose. The efficiency of delivery of the selected formulation depends on the formulation and device, which in conjunction with the manner in which the patient inhales will dictate the site of aerosol deposition.

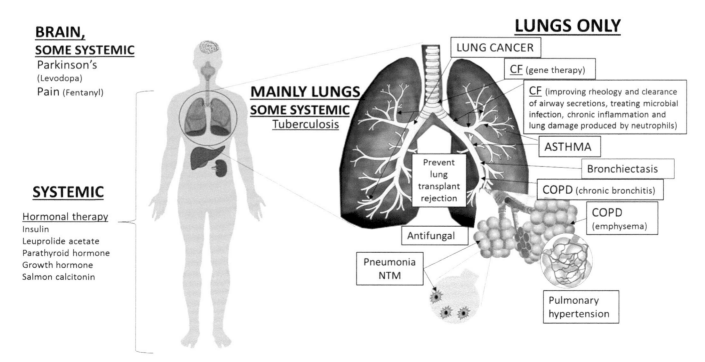

Figure 5.2 The required site of action where inhaled compounds must be available in therapeutic concentrations for an effective treatment.

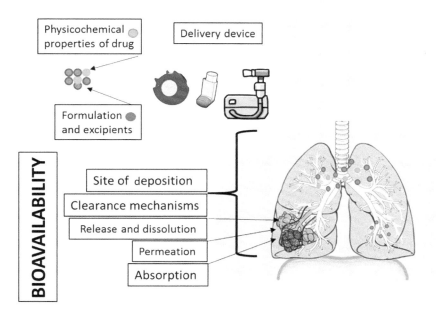

Figure 5.3 Anatomical considerations for the bioavailability of drugs delivered by the pulmonary route.

The site of deposition will determine the clearance mechanisms to which the aerosol would be subject, which sequentially will influence the fraction of the dose that would be available for absorption. In turn, drug absorption will be influenced by the permeability of the compound and, if the formulation is solid or is still encapsulated in the carrier, the release and dissolution of the compound will also limit the extent of its absorption. These factors will be discussed in this section.

PHYSICOCHEMICAL PROPERTIES OF THE COMPOUND

Besides the size of the intended dose, one of the factors that determines if a compound would be best formulated as liquid or solid for pulmonary delivery is its apparent solubility in the liquid media, which could be aqueous for nebulizers or liquified propellant for MDIs. The aqueous solubility of the compound plays a much smaller role in its dissolution in the lung environment because of the presence of a mucus layer in the airways and of surfactant in the alveolar region (10).

The physicochemical parameter that most influences the permeation of the drug into lung tissue is the partition coefficient (Log P), which is defined as the log of the ratio of the equilibrium concentrations of a dissolved substance in a two-phase system consisting of two largely immiscible solvents, most commonly 1-octanol and water (11), as follows:

$$P_{o/w} = \frac{Conc_{1-octanol}}{Conc_{1-octanol}} \qquad (5.2)$$

Here, $P_{o/w}$ is octanol-water partition coefficient, $Conc_{water}$ is concentration of solute in water and $Conc_{1-octanol}$ is concentration of solute in 1-octanol.

Lipinski et al. proposed the "rule of five" to predict the permeability and absorption of compounds through biological membranes, based on the molecular weight, Log P, number of groups in the molecule that can donate H^+ to hydrogen bonds, and the number of groups that can accept atoms to form hydrogen bonds (12). More specifically, drug absorption from the airways into lung tissue has been hypothesized to be influenced by the molecular weight of the compound. In a comprehensive review of the anatomy of the lung as it pertains to the mechanisms of drug absorption, Patton hypothesized that absorption of small compounds (<40 kDa) may be favored by paracellular mechanisms, whereas larger compounds may be better absorbed by transcytosis (13).

Table 5.2 lists the physicochemical properties for the main classes of therapeutic compounds that are commercially available or that have been administered by the pulmonary route to laboratory animals or humans in a preclinical or clinical setting.

Most of the commercially available compounds formulated specifically for inhalation follow the Lipinski rule of five in terms of molecular weight and LogP, including anticholinergic compounds, corticosteroids, muscarinic agonists, and β-2 agonists. However, other commercially available compounds such as insulin, leuprolide acetate, and growth hormone have molecular weights significantly higher than the 500 g/moL proposed by Lipinski. Since these compounds are intended for systemic action, their aerosol deposition is usually intended to target the alveolar region, where its large surface area (approximately 75 m²) offers high capacity for solute exchange due to the ultra-thin alveolar epithelium and excellent vascularization (3,17,18). In contrast, the other compounds that have been used off label in clinical settings or in preclinical studies do not follow the Lipinski rule of

Table 5.2 Physicochemical properties of the compounds that have been delivered by the pulmonary route

Class	Compound	Molecular weight (g/moL)*	Log P	Aqueous solubility (mg/mL)*
Antibiotic	Amikacin sulfate(C)	683.68	−7.4	185
	Carbenicillin(C)	378.4	1.13	0.39
	Ceftazidime(C)	546.58	−1.2	0.00573
	Ciprofloxacin(C)	331.35	0.28	30
	Clarithromycin(C)	747.95	3.16	0.33 mg/L
	Colistin(M)	1155.45	−2.4	564
	Colistimethate(M)	1634.87	−1.2	4.17
	Doxycycline(C)	444.43	−0.72	0.63
	Gentamicin(C)	477.6	−3.1	100
	Tobramycin(M)	467.52	−5.8	94
	Vancomycin(C)	1449.25	1.11	0.225
Anticancer	Cetuximab(P)	145,781.60	n.r	soluble
	Cisplatin(P)	298.04	0.041	2.5
	Doxorubicin(P)	543.52	1.27	soluble
	Fluorouracil(P)	130.08	−0.58	5.86
	Gemcitabine(P)	263.2	−1.4	soluble
	Paclitaxel(P)	853.91	3.2	insoluble
	Vitamin A(P)	286.45	5.68	0.671 mg/L
Anticholinergic	Ipratropium bromide(M)	412.37	0.21	freely soluble
	Tiotropium bromide(M)	472.42	−2.2	25
Antifungal	Amphotericin B(C)	924.08	−0.66	0.0819
	Itraconazole(C)	705.64	5.66	insoluble
	Voriconazole(C)	349.31	1.65	0.0978
Anti-tuberculosis	Capreomycin(P)	668.71	−9.69	soluble
	Clofazimine(P)	473.4	7.6	0.225 mg/L
	Ethionamide(P)	166.24	0.5	practically insoluble
	Isoniazid(P)	137.14	−0.7	140
	Levofloxacin(P)	361.37	2.1	insoluble
	Pretomanid(P)	359.26	2.8	0.0117
	Para-aminosalycilic acid(P)	153.14	1.01	1.69
	Pyrazinamide(P)	123.11	−1.88	150
	Rifabutin(P)	847.01	4.1	0.19
	Rifampicin(P)	822.14	4	1.4
	Rifapentin(P)	877.03	5.29	0.0213
β-2 agonist	Formoterol fumarate(M)	344.41	2.2	slightly soluble
	Indacaterol maleate(M)	508.571	3.3	0.00798
	Salmeterol xinafoate(M)	603.76	4.2	0.06
	Vilanterol(M)	486.43	3.39	0.00118
Corticosteroid	Beclomethasone dipropionate(M)	521.04	1.3	49.39
	Budesonide(M)	430.53	2.8	insoluble
	Ciclesonide(M)	540.7	4.08	0.00157
	Fluticasone propionate(M)	500.57	3.4	0.51 mg/L
	Flunisolide(M)	434.5	2.2	0.0374
	Mometasone furoate(M)	521.43	2.1	practically insoluble
	Triamcinolone acetonide(M)	394.43	0.84	0.847

(Continued)

Table 5.2 (*Continued*) Physicochemical properties of the compounds that have been delivered by the pulmonary route

Class	Compound	Molecular weight (g/moL)*	Log P	Aqueous solubility (mg/mL)*
Muscarinic antagonist	Aclidinium bromide[M]	564.55	3.4	hardly soluble
	Nedocromil sodium[M]	371.34	2.22	0.145
	Revefenacine[M]	597.76	4.24	0.00721
	Umeclidinium[M]	508.49	2.88	1.94e–05
Other	Estradiol[P]	272.38	4.01	3.6 mg/L
	Fentanyl[P]	336.47	4.05	0.2
	Growth hormone[M]	22,124 Da	n.r.	40
	Insulin (human)[M]	5808 Da	n.r.	soluble
	Leuprolide acetate[M]	1269.47	0.798	Slightly soluble
	Midazolam[C]	325.78	3.89	0.024
	Parathyroid hormone (human)[M]	9424.62	n.r.	0.40
	Salmon calcitonin[M]	2890.256	−3.89	1.0

Sources: Compiled from Ibrahim, M. and L. Garcia-Contreras, *Ther. Deliv.*, 4, 1027–1045, 2013; Ibrahim, M. and L. García-Contreras, Preclinical pharmacokinetics of antitubercular drugs, in *Delivery Systems for Tuberculosis Prevention and Treatment.*, A.J. Hickey, Editor 2016, John Wiley & Sons, West Sussex, UK, 131–155; Canadian-Institutes-of-Health-Research, Alberta Innovates Health-Solutions, and The-metabolomics-innovation-centre, *DrugBank database*, 2018.

* = otherwise indicated; [M] = a compound that has been marketed as a formulation for inhalation; [C] = a drug product intended for parenteral administration that has been used in clinical settings; [P] = a drug product or chemical compound used in pre-clinical studies.

five in terms of molecular weight, (123–145,782 g/moL) and LogP (−7.4–7.6), but these may not be a limitation for their commercial development as noted for compounds such as insulin and growth hormone.

Tronde et al. looked at two slightly different physico chemical properties to predict the absorption of 34 inhaled drugs in the market that they termed "first dimension or $t[1]$" and a "second dimension or $t[2]$" (19). The $t[1]$ was related to size (including molecular volume; surface area [polar/nonpolar]; hydrogen bonding donors/acceptors; electronic parameters, including charge and dipoles; and topological parameters, including molecular weight, atom/bond/ring counts, and connectivities), and $t[2]$ was related to lipophilicity (including LogD and LogP). They concluded that the absorption rate correlated better with the molecular polar surface area and the hydrogen bonding potential. However, this conclusion may be viewed with caution because the compounds that they studied mainly included beta 2-agonists and corticosteroids, with a few anesthetics (19).

FORMULATION AND DELIVERY DEVICES

Therapeutic compounds have been administered for decades as aerosols generated from liquid or dry powder formulations, using nebulizers, MDIs, and DPIs. In addition to the intended size of the dose and the physicochemical characteristics of the therapeutic compound, the selection of the formulation–delivery system combination is driven by other factors such as the age of the target population and issues related to the device, the extent to which the disease

of these patients affects their breathing pattern, the length of treatment, as well as econometric evaluations and regulatory issues (20).

It was generally believed that a more efficient delivery and control of the deposition site could be achieved with DPIs, but this hypothesis was proven to be incorrect by Rau et al., who compared the distribution of drugs from the aerosol devices most commonly used (21). They compared the fractions of the dose deposited in the oropharyngeal region and in the lungs, the fraction exhaled, and the fraction remaining in the different devices from different studies. They concluded that the fraction of the dose deposited in the lungs with these devices was about 10%–15%, but that the oropharyngeal deposition and the fractions exhaled and remaining in the device differed significantly among the devices. While the efficiency of drug delivered as measured by deposition in the lung may be the same, it is important to note that the nominal dose in each device is different, with nominal doses in the nebulizer being 10 to 12 times larger than those in MDIs and DPIs. Zainudin et al. also reported that all three devices may be equivalent to deliver salbutamol, as the lung deposition was very similar (9.1%–11.2%) with the three devices (22). However, the corresponding change in FEV1 was significantly higher (35.6%) after delivery with the MDI compared to that after delivery of the same dose with the DPI (25.2%) or the nebulizer (25.8%), suggesting that the percentage of the dose deposited in the lung by itself is not a good indicator of the bioavailability of a therapeutic compound.

SITE OF DEPOSITION

The site of deposition for aerosols generated from liquids or dry powders is determined by particle shape, size and distribution, hygroscopicity, static charge, anatomy of the airways, and breathing patterns (23). From these, the factors that most influence bioavailability are particle shape, size and distribution, anatomy of the airways, breathing frequency, and tidal volume.

In general, the size of therapeutic aerosols generated from commercial inhalers ranges from 0.1 to 60 μm and are polydisperse, with geometric standard deviation (GSD) between 1.5 and 3 μm, which results in their deposition in different regions of the lungs. Aerosols with sizes greater than 5 μm usually deposit by inertial impaction in the upper airways, whereas aerosols in sizes smaller than 5 μm deposit by sedimentation in the peripheral airways (24). Studies have established that the narrower the size distribution, the better the therapeutic effect. Zanen et al. demonstrated that smaller doses (8 μg) of ipratropium bromide delivered as monodisperse aerosols (2.8 μm) generated by a spinning disk can elicit similar effects to larger doses (40 μg) of this compound delivered as polydisperse aerosols with a commercial MDI (25,26). They also demonstrated that using the smaller dose (160 μg) of a monodisperse fenoterol aerosol produced the same therapeutic effect and reduced the adverse effects observed after inhalation of a larger dose (800 μg) delivered with a commercial MDI (27).

The deposition of aerosol droplets/particles in lungs is heavily influenced by the branching of the airways in the respiratory tree. Each bifurcation, directional change, and reduction in the diameter of the lumen of the airways as well as an increase in the airway generation number also increases the probability of aerosol deposition by inertial impaction (28). For most aerosols, the greatest, abrupt directional change occurs when the air moves from the pharynx and larynx into the trachea and bronchi, where the air velocity is maximum upon the first inhalation of the aerosol (23). Thus, the manner in which a patient inhales can influence the site of aerosol deposition and the deposited dose. In general, the patient is instructed to take a deep breath while inhaling the medication and hold her or his breath for a few seconds to enhance the deposition of the aerosol by sedimentation in the alveolar region (24). Consequently, a deep, fast breath may enhance the bioavailability of medications whose site of action is the larger airways, whereas a deep breath and holding the breath for a few seconds may enhance the bioavailability of drugs whose site of action is in the alveoli, or of medications intended for systemic action. However, modification or control of the breathing mode is not possible in obligated-nose-breathers, including infants or animal models such as rodents, and this also limits the dose of aerosol that they can inhale (29). Moreover, it is important to note that the cut-off diameter of aerosols that can be inhaled by humans is also significantly different from that of rodents. For example, while the cut-off diameter for particles inhaled through the nose of humans is about 10 μm, for small rodents like the rat is about 1 μm (30).

The disease type and stage also influence the architecture of the airways and in turn the aerosol deposition. Cystic fibrosis is perhaps the most studied disease because the type and amount of secretions modifies the diameter and humidity in the airways of these patients. The effect of the decrease in airway diameter on the deposition of inhaled aerosols has been studied by Martonen using a mathematical model and validated using *in vivo* data (31). In this model, when the obstruction in the airways increased and the diameter of the airways decreased by 5%–40%, aerosol deposition increased in a monotonic manner because the deposition by inertial impaction was favored and was directly proportional to the velocity of particles or droplets going through the airways (31).

CLEARANCE MECHANISMS

After deposition, clearance of aerosols droplets/particles is one of the biggest determinants of the bioavailability of inhaled drugs. Depending on the site or sites of the respiratory tract where the aerosol deposited, the droplets/particles may be cleared from the lungs by mechanical clearance, mucociliary clearance, uptake by alveolar macrophages, or degradation by enzymes (14), the latter being more relevant for protein/peptide type of drugs.

Aerosol droplets/particles of about 10 μm (MMAD) are usually deposited in the larger airways and cleared mechanically by sneezing or coughing, with aerosol droplets of this size also having the probability of being swallowed. If aerosol droplets/particles are deposited in the tracheobronchial region, they may be removed by mucociliary clearance within 24 h of aerosol administration to healthy subjects (32). Disease states such as cystic fibrosis can impair the mucociliary clearance mechanism in these patients due to their dehydrated mucus secretions, as reported by Boucher (33,34) and Corcoran (35).

In the smaller airways and the alveolar region, uptake by alveolar macrophages has a more significant effect on the bioavailability of inhaled drugs because it can sequester the drug into the lymph nodes and thus prevent its effect at the site of action (36). However, it should be noted that there are significant differences in the extent of particle uptake by alveolar macrophages between humans and other species: it has been reported that alveolar macrophages from rodent lungs uptake insoluble particles to a larger extent than human lungs (37). The residence time of aerosol particles and the solubility or the drug or carrier also influence the extent of macrophage uptake: the longer that the particle remains in the alveolar region, the higher the probability that it would be engulfed by alveolar macrophages. This factor has been one of the main limitations to achieving controlled release of drugs by the pulmonary route, but clever approaches such as formulation of compounds in "large porous particles" have addressed this limitation. These particles have geometric diameters of 10 μm or more but have mass densities of less than 0.4 g/mL, which allows them to behave aerodynamically, like particles of 1–3 μm for efficient alveolar deposition (38). This formulation strategy was used to provide sustained release of albuterol sulfate in the lungs of guinea pigs for up to 24 h (39) and to increase the bioavailability of estradiol in rats from 38% to 86% (40).

Although the presence of metabolic enzymes in the lung is less abundant than in other organs such as the intestine and liver, isoforms of the CYP450 family, such as CYP2S and CYP2F, as well as esterases and peptidases have been found in different regions of the lungs (41,42). The presence of these enzymes in the lungs has not been reported to influence significantly the bioavailability of inhaled drugs until now, but an increase in their expression has been reported to occur in patients that smoke (43). The efficacy of inhaled corticosteroids such as fluticasone propionate is reported to be reduced in patients with mild asthma who smoke (44).

DRUG RELEASE AND DISSOLUTION

Drugs in aerosols generated from solutions do not require release or dissolution, but if the aerosol is generated from a suspension of a drug alone or a dry powder consisting of a blend of micronized drug and carrier, the drug would have to be dissolved to some extent to be absorbed or to exert its pharmacological action. Furthermore, if the drug was formulated by particle engineering approaches using excipients or encapsulated into a polymeric matrix, then the drug would have to be released from the matrix or dissolved at the same time as the excipient, as in the case of sugars. Given the limited amount of fluid available for dissolution in the different regions of the lung (3,13), it is very likely that the dissolution of the compound would also limit the extent of its absorption.

Until a few years ago, the dissolution of dry powders for inhalation was not required or even performed in most cases, but after it was discovered that the dissolution of compounds in the lung environment may affect their effect or absorption, research groups were using this determination to predict, indirectly, the performance of their formulation in the lungs. Since there was no official dissolution apparatus to evaluate the dissolution of dry powders for inhalation or guidelines in the British, European, or United States Pharmacopeia (USP) on how to perform this determination, the experimental setup was widely variable. In some cases, adaptation of the current USP dissolution apparatuses were used, whereas others employed custom-made devices. Likewise, the volume and type of dissolution media varied, ranging from a few milliliters to the 900 mL specified by the USP, and from water and saline to simulated lung fluid with different compositions. For example, although the actual pulmonary surfactant contains dipalmitoyl-phosphatidyl-choline (DPPC), sodium dodecyl sulfate (SDS) or tween 80 were used interchangeably with DPPC in these earlier dissolution studies. Regardless of the type of surfactant used, the concentration used in the dissolution media varied among these studies and was reported to significantly influence the rate and extent of drug dissolution (45,46).

One of the first publications reporting a method to study the dissolution of powders for inhalation was that of Pham and Wiedmann (47), who collected aerosol particles of budesonide in a liquid impinger filled with saturated solutions of budesonide either in water or in 0.01% (SDS). The dissolution of budesonide was evaluated by placing a diluted aliquot of the solution from the impinger in scintillation vials that were oscillated on a shaking water bath and then taking samples at predetermined points. Another pioneer study by Davies and Feddah employed a flow-through cell as a dissolution apparatus to pump liquid through the cell that retained fluticasone propionate powder in order to maintain sink conditions (45). They reported an increase from 20% to 80% in the dissolution rate of fluticasone propionate in simulated lung fluid (SLF) after the addition of 0.02% DPPC. Son et al. were the first to use a USP apparatus to evaluate the dissolution of inhalable powders (46). To better mimic the in vivo situation, they used the New Generation Impactor (NGI) to aerodynamically separate hydrocortisone dry powders from stages 2, 3, 5, and 6. They held each powder fraction in a membrane cassette that was placed at the bottom of the standard USP method 5 (paddle over disc) containing 100 mL of SLF and stirred at 50 rpm. Even though this experimental setup separated and collected the respirable fraction of the powder in a more physiologic manner, the dissolution volume was at least three times larger than the volume of dissolution available in the alveolar region (3,13). This was resolved by Wang et al. using the Franz diffusion cell to sandwich a membrane containing the powder collected from stage 4 of the NGI between the donor and receiving compartments (48). They filled the receiving compartment with 23 mL of dissolution media so that the liquid would have a positive meniscus to wet and subsequently dissolve the dry powder in the sandwiched membrane, thus more closely resembling the dissolution of an inhaled dry powder in vivo. One of the conditions that the Son et al. (46) and Wang et al. (48) dissolution setups lack is the assurance of the existence of sink conditions (defined as one-third the concentration of the maximum solubility [Cs] of the drug) during the test, which is present in the dissolution setup described by Davies and Feddah (45). The dissolution apparatus reported by Ibrahim et al. addressed these limitation using the Franz diffusion cell in the same manner as Wang et al. (48), but they added 1 mL of the SLF in the donor compartment of the cell to facilitate drug dissolution and used a pump in the same manner as Davies and Feddah (45) to maintain sink conditions during the test (49).

In order to develop guidelines to establish the bioequivalency of inhaled generic drug products, in 2013, the US FDA provided support for a small number of projects to develop clinically relevant methods to evaluate the dissolution of orally inhaled drug products. Among these, the group at Virginia Commonwealth University (VCU) proposed a setup based on their previous work in which they used the Andersen Cascade Impactor (ACI) to collect the 2.1–3.3 or 4.7–5.8 μm aerosol fraction into a filter membrane (50). Unlike earlier studies that used the Franz diffusion cell, they used the Transwell® system containing 1.4 mL of PBS pH 7.4 in the acceptor compartment and placed the filter membrane with the collected powder onto the donor compartment, adding 0.04 mL of PBS or distilled deionized water to initiate the dissolution process. A second project awarded to the University of Florida also employed the ACI or NGI to collect the aerosolized powder and the Transwell system to test the dissolution, but the authors also studied the influence of adding a surfactant in the dissolution media and/or a stirrer in the acceptor compartment (51). This group evaluated the applicability of their novel dissolution method in the capability to predict the systemic disposition of three inhaled corticosteroids (ICSs) using two semimechanistic pharmacokinetic simulation approaches (52). They developed two multicompartmental models, which assumed that the ICS solubility and dissolution rate would control their absorption rate, but they differed from each other in the way that the dissolution and absorption rate constant were estimated. In approach 1, they first identified a dissolution media that would mimic, in vitro, the manner in which the compound was absorbed in the lung tissue, whereas in approach 2, they determined if the kinetics of pulmonary absorption could be derived from their in vitro dissolution tests in the Transwell system. They concluded that approach 1 was only useful to predict the systemic disposition of ICSs, while the input parameters for the pulmonary absorption rate constant that were estimated from dissolution experiments in approach 2 predicted better the pharmacokinetic profiles of ICSs reported in the literature (52). A third project at the University of Bath developed a proprietary aerosol dose collection system for the dissolution testing called The UniDose apparatus (53). This novel aerosol collection system deposits the whole lung dose directly onto a high surface area filter membrane under laminar flow and low impaction velocity. These filters can be placed in different dissolution setups such as Franz diffusion cell and the USP IV and V apparatuses. This aerosol collection system, used in conjunction with advanced techniques such as morphology-directed Raman spectroscopy and validated in silico mechanistic modeling, may increase the robustness and the discriminatory capacity of dissolution methods that could establish the bioequivalence of inhaled generic drug products.

In a privately funded study, Gerde et al. employed the Precise Inhale® exposure system to collect the inhalable fraction of aerosolized budesonide or fluticasone propionate powders onto a glass cover slip and evaluated their dissolution in a novel device called DissolvIt® (54). This system is composed of a dissolution chamber, a precision-controlled peristaltic pump, and an inverted microscope with a high resolution camera that was developed to evaluate the dissolution of respirable powders in an environment that simulates the lung epithelium. A feature that is present in the DissolvIt system and absent in the three dissolution systems described above is the presence of a mucus simulant and a polycarbonate membrane that mimics the basal membrane of the airway mucosa and separates the diffusion barrier of the mucus simulant from the "simulated blood" streaming on the other side of the membrane (54).

PERMEABILITY

Once the drug is in solution at the desired site of action, it is not certain that it would be absorbed because it still has to cross several anatomical barriers that differ in cell composition and thickness in the different regions of the lungs. For example, drugs deposited in the bronchi would have to cross the mucus layer and relatively thick epithelium that is composed mainly of ciliated, goblet, brush, and basal cells. It is estimated that the anatomical barrier that a drug needs to cross in the bronchi is about 66 μm, from the surface of the mucus (including cilia) to the blood vessels (55). In the terminal bronchioles, the barriers that a drug must cross in order to be absorbed are the lining fluid and epithelium, which is composed mainly of Clara cells. This pathway is about 13 μm, including mucus in the surface (13). In contrast, the alveolar epithelium is quite thin (0.5 –1.0 μm), and is composed mainly of the extremely broad and thin Type I cell and the small and compact Type II cell (13,55). Last, the drug must either cross through the cell or by the tight junctions (TJs), which is a complex structure of multiple proteins that connect the cells in the epithelium with each other (56).

The permeability of inhaled drugs has been studied in cell cultures using different cell lines, including the human bronchial cell lines 16HBE14o-, Calu-3 and BEAS-2B; alveolar cell lines L-2, A549, H441, MLE-15; and alveolar epithelial cells in primary culture (57). The Calu-3 and 16HBE14o- cell lines are most often used because they are readily available and well characterized, and they express features of the airway epithelium and several transport and metabolic systems relevant to drug absorption (58). Among the first published studies, Mathias et al. determined that the permeability of compounds was directly correlated to their lipophilicity and inversely correlated to their molecular weight (MW) (59). Their observations in the Calu-3 cell line correlated well with those in primary cultured rabbit tracheal epithelial cells and with the absorption of these compounds in vivo, after pulmonary administration to rats. The correlation of lipophilicity and permeability was also observed by Forbes et al. in the 16HBE14o- cell line, but the permeability of this cell line to hydrophilic compounds was significantly greater than that observed in alveolar cell cultures, which may be due to the lower resistance reported for the 16HBE14o- cell line (60). These early studies were performed with relatively small MW compounds, but the growing interest in developing a formulation for inhaled insulin fueled the evaluation of the permeability of protein/peptide compounds.

The first study evaluating the permeability of a series of peptides and proteins across alveolar epithelial cells in primary culture was published by Bur et al. in 2006 (61). Unlike small MW compounds, the permeability of the studied peptides and proteins did not depend on their size, with the growth hormone (MW = 22,125 Da) exhibiting a larger permeability (P_{app} = 8.33×10^{-7} cm/s) compared to that of insulin (MW = 5800 Da; P_{app} = 0.77×10^{-7} cm/s) or transferrin (MW = 76,500 Da; P_{app} = 0.88×10^{-7} cm/s). These results confirmed the hypothesis published by Patton a decade earlier, stating that molecules greater than 40 kDa traverse the epithelium via transcellular pathways (13). Therefore, it is no surprise that the bioavailability of macromolecules after pulmonary administration is higher than that after administration by any other nonparenteral route of delivery (62).

Most of these early studies that elucidated the correlation of the physicochemical properties of compounds with their permeability employed model compounds such as dextrans, mannitol (a low permeability marker), and propranolol (a high permeability marker). However, a smaller number of these studies report the actual permeability of therapeutic compounds clinically used to treat lung diseases. The permeability of anti-asthmatic compounds such as budesonide, salbutamol, and cromolyn has been reported in Caco-2, Calu-3, hAEpC, and 16HBE14o- cell lines (10,57), even though they are not required to be absorbed to exert their pharmacological activity. Fewer studies report the permeability of compounds that may require absorption into tissue or systemic circulation, including insulin and growth hormone in hAEpC (61) and a few antibiotics such as azithromycin, ciprofloxacin, doxycycline, moxifloxacin, rifampicin, and tobramycin in Calu-3 cells (63).

Other factors that could decrease the bioavailability of inhaled compounds due to a decrease in the permeability through the anatomical barriers may be the distortion or transformation of the mucus or epithelial barrier, which can be caused by disease states such as CF. In these patients, the mucus lining layer can be a substantial barrier to drugs having to reach the epithelium, especially when there is infection and inflammation. In addition, the hydration state of mucus may affect the ability of the drug to permeate through the mucus barrier as there is an inverse relationship between the molecular weight of the drug and its diffusion through mucus (64).

MECHANISMS OF DRUG ABSORPTION

The seminal review published by Schanker (65), of mostly qualitative pulmonary absorption studies performed up until 1978, ushered in a series of more quantitative studies that form the basis of the so-called inhalation biopharmaceutics field, which encompasses all the factors that influence drug absorption and bioavailability discussed in the previous sections (66). Notably, this review and other pivotal studies published by Effros and Mason (67), Brown et al. (68), and Schanker et al. (69), reported *in vivo* many of the findings recently confirmed in more controlled studies performed in cell cultures and perfused lung models. Most of these studies used model compounds that were absorbed by passive diffusion and showed the dependence of absorption on the lipophilicity and molecular weight of the compound. Schanker was the first to suggest in 1978 the possibility of transport-mediated absorption in the lungs (65), and although the active transport of sodium and proteins was described in lung epithelia in the 1980s (70–72), it was not until the late 1990s that the first drug transporters were identified in lung cell lines (73). Based on these studies, the mechanisms that have been postulated for drug absorption in the lungs are passive diffusion either through intracellular TJs (paracellular transport) or through pores in the membrane, vesicular transport, transporter mediated and drainage to the lymphatics (14). These are illustrated in Figure 5.4.

Intracellular tight junctions are the "kissing points" that bring the adjacent cells within a few nanometers of each other. Due to the changing cell composition in the different regions of the respiratory tract, the lung epithelium exhibits different forms and types of TJ with variable degree of tightness, as measured by their transepithelial electrical resistance (TEER) value. Sporty et al. reported that the apical-to-basal TEER value of the airway epithelium decreases from the trachea to a minimum in the distal airways before returning to a high value in the alveoli (74). Under this criteria, the bioavailability of drugs that are absorbed through the TJs could be increased if the aerosol is deposited mainly in the distal airways right before the alveoli. This has been reported to be the case

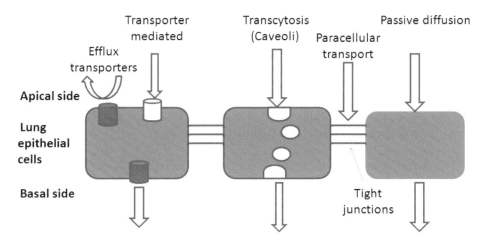

Figure 5.4 Mechanisms that have been postulated for drug absorption in the lungs. (Modified from Ibrahim, M. and Garcia-Contreras, L., *Ther. Deliv.*, 4, 1027–1045, 2013.)

for small hydrophilic molecules and small peptides such as insulin (62). Besides the TJs, drugs can be absorbed through "pores" on the basement membrane that are transiently formed due to cell death (13).

Drugs may also be absorbed through the cell membrane lipid bilayers of the lung epithelium by passive diffusion driven by a concentration gradient. The existence of this mechanism is supported by a rapid nonsaturable membrane permeability observed for several drugs but especially the hydrophobic drugs (75). Another mechanism of drug absorption across cell layers occurs when the drug is directly transported through the cell cytoplasm through membrane vesicles called caveoli (76). This mechanism of absorption is thought to be size-dependent and has been reported for albumin, insulin, and low-density lipoproteins (58). Despite the identification of transporter molecules in lung cells in the late 1990s, it was not until 2005 that Ehrhardt et al. reported that albuterol was absorbed by a transporter molecule in the 16HBE14o- human bronchial epithelial cell line (77). Since then, transporters belonging to the solute carrier transporters superfamily (SLC) and ATP binding cassette transporters (ABC) have been identified in the human lung (58) and are listed in Table 5.3 with their possible substrates.

The SLC family of transporters has been actively studied in the past two decades because a large number of anti-asthmatic compounds, particularly the beta-2-adrenergic agonists, antimuscarinics, and several ICSs are substrates for the transporters in this family, including the organic cation transporters OCT1-3 and OCTN2.

Only a few compounds have been delivered experimentally by the pulmonary route that are confirmed substrates for the ABC family of transporters, but it is anticipated that more research will be performed in this area as new entities are developed into commercial products. Particularly for compounds that may be substrates to efflux transporters, such as Pgp, BCRP, and the MRP1–3 transporters, this would be crucial as it would have determinant effects on the bioavailability and therapeutic efficacy of these compounds. *In vitro* studies performed by Stigliani et al. in bronchial epithelial cells suggested that the absorption of azithromycin, doxycycline, moxifloxacin, rifampicin, and tobramycin may be transport-mediated (63). In particular, if moxifloxacin and tobramycin are subject to efflux transporters, their use should be closely monitored to avoid the emergence of drug-resistant bacteria, which will decrease the therapeutic options for patients infected with mycobacteria (*M. tuberculosis or M. bovis*) or *Pseudomonas aeruginosa*.

Table 5.3 Transporters identified in human lungs and their location within the lung and substrates

Transporter	Cells where expressed and their location in the lung	Possible substrates
SLC Family		
OCT1	• Bronchial ciliated cells • Airway smooth muscle cells	Salbutamol Beclomethasone dipropionate Budesonide Formoterol Pentamidine Salmeterol xinafoate Para-amino-salicylic acid
OCT2	• Bronchial ciliated cells • Basal cells	Beclomethasone dipropionate Budesonide Fluticasone propionate Ipratropium bromide Levofloxacin Pentamidine Tiotropium bromide Para-amino-salicylic acid
OCT3	• Bronchial basal cells • Bronchial intermediate cells • Bronchial epithelial ciliated cells • Pulmonary blood vessels • Airway smooth muscle cells	Salbutamol Budesonide Ciprofloxacin Fluticasone propionate Formoterol Pentamidine Salmeterol xinafoate
OCTN2	• Airway epithelial cells	Ciprofloxacin Formoterol Ipratropium bromide Tiotropium bromide

(*Continued*)

Table 5.3 (*Continued*) Transporters identified in human lungs and their location within the lung and substrates

Transporter	Cells where expressed and their location in the lung	Possible substrates
ABC Family		
P-gp	• Bronchial epithelial cells • Alveolar macrophages • Alveolar epithelium • Serous cells of bronchial mucosa • Bronchial capillaries	Rifampicin Clarithromycin Itraconazole
MRP1	• Bronchi/bronchiolar epithelium • Alveolar macrophages • Bronchial ciliated epithelial cells • Mucus secreting cells of bronchial mucosa • Basal cells of bronchial mucosa	Doxorubicin Pacitaxel
MRP2	• Primary bronchial and epithelial cells	Cisplatin Clarithromycin
BCRP	• Bronchial epithelial cells and seromucinous glands • Small endothelial capillaries of the lung • Alveolar pneumocytes	Cisplatin

Sources: Compiled from Ibrahim, M. and L. Garcia-Contreras, *Ther. Deliv.*, 4, 1027–1045, 2013; Ehrhardt, C. et al., *J. Pharm. Sci.*, 106, 2234–2244, 2017; Gumbleton, M. et al., *Adv. Drug Deliv. Rev.*, 63, 110–118. 2011; van der Deen, M. et al., *Respir. Res.*, 20, 59, 2005; Miyama, T. et al., *Antimicrob. Agents Chemother.*, 42, 1738–1744, 1998; Parvez, M.M. et al., *Antimicrob. Agents Chemother.*, 61, 2017; Peters, J. et al., *Drug Metab. Dispos.*, 40, 522–528, 2012.

Methods to determine bioavailability of inhaled compounds

The traditional procedure to determine the bioavailability of a compound is to first administer the compound systemically (usually a solution intravenously) and then by the route of interest (usually extravascular), preferentially in the same subject, with an interval between administrations of one day to one week (84). Bioavailability is then calculated as the ratio of the total area under the drug concentration in plasma (or serum) versus time curve (AUC) after extravascular administration divided by the AUC after IV administration, corrected by the dose using Equation 5.1 (6), described in "Factors that affect the bioavailability of inhaled compounds" of this chapter.

The design of a study to calculate the bioavailability of an inhaled compound includes the selection of (1) the subject, either an animal model, healthy volunteer, or patient; (2) the dose, formulation, and device; (3) the type of biological samples and the time points at which they will be collected; and (4) the method to calculate the AUC and other relevant pharmacokinetic parameters. These factors will be discussed in the following sections.

SELECTION OF THE SUBJECT

Considering all factors that affect bioavailability, the best study design to calculate the bioavailability of inhaled compounds should be the patient population for which the treatment is intended. A study like this would have the advantages of directly benefitting the patients, measuring drug levels in the disease state to account for changes in the structure of the airways, giving a better assessment of the therapeutic efficacy of the drug, and avoiding the ethical dilemma of administering potentially harmful drugs to healthy volunteers. However, there are a number of drawbacks if the bioavailability determination is performed in patients. For example, depending on the disease state and stage, the health of the patient may be further compromised if stringent conditions such as fasting are required, and thus a rigorous medical examination should be performed before the subject is enrolled in the study. In addition, some studies require a drug washout period of at least 10 biological half-lives between drug administrations, which may also pose a danger for patients. Therefore, it is generally preferred to perform initial bioavailability studies in healthy volunteers and subsequently evaluate the bioavailability in patients, but the difference in drug disposition between these two populations should be thoroughly documented. For instance, healthy volunteers are considered more discriminative to evaluate the bioavailability of anticholinergic compounds than asthmatic patients because the bronchoconstriction in the airways of patients may cause greater lung deposition in the central airways (85). In contrast, the bioavailability of an inhaled antibiotic may be higher in healthy volunteers than in CF patients because of the presence of the thick mucus that reduces the airway diameter; limits drug permeation; and can inactivate some polycationic antibiotics, such as aminoglycosides, from inactivation by polyanionic components present in sputum, such as mucins or DNA (86).

A limitation of performing bioavailability studies in healthy volunteers and/or patients is the type and number of samples that can be collected throughout the study to determine drug concentrations at the relevant site of action. For example, it is impossible to determine concentrations of anti-asthmatic drugs in the airways of patients over a period of time, but it may be possible to measure the concentration of an antibiotic in the sputum of patients with CF to evaluate the bioavailability of the antibiotic in their airways. The simplest case would be to determine the bioavailability of a compound intended for systemic action such as the inhaled growth hormone because its concentration can be easily measured in plasma and it is relatively easy to collect blood samples over a period of time.

An attractive alternative is the use of animal models because, besides blood and plasma, they allow the collection of other biological samples, such as lung fluids and tissues. This task is simpler if small laboratory animals including mice, rats, and guinea pigs are employed, but the anatomical and physiological differences between these species and humans should be considered because they influence the size of the dose that can be inhaled, its deposition, and its clearance mechanisms. In contrast, larger animal models such as rabbits, dogs, and nonhuman primates are likely to inhale therapeutic aerosol to a larger extent, but the type and amount of biological samples that can be collected from these models over a period of time would be limited.

The main factors that determine the aerosol doses that each animal model can inhale by passive inhalation are the route of breathing, breathing frequency, and tidal volume. Small laboratory animals are obligated nose breathers, and the aerosol dose that they can inhale is first limited by the cut-off diameter of particles that can be inhaled through their nose, which is between 1 and 3 μm, in mice and guinea pigs, respectively (30). In contrast, dogs, nonhuman primates, and humans can breathe by their nose and mouth, which increases the amount of aerosol that they can inhale. The differences in breathing frequency and tidal volumes in the different animal models compared to that of humans are illustrated in Figure 5.5. The tidal volume is shown in the form of a cloud to illustrate the volume of aerosol that each model can inhale in one breath, as an estimation of the possible dose of aerosol that can be achieved by passive inhalation in the different species.

After the aerosol has been inhaled by the animal, the fraction deposited in each region will be influenced by the size and distribution of the aerosol as well as the airway branching and diameter of the airways. The anatomical features of the lungs in the different animal models have been described by Sakagami (88), Fernandes (89), Cryan et al. (29), and Guillon (90). The review published by Cryan et al. (29) gives a detailed description of the comparative airway structure of small and large animal models, including the type of airway branching and major bifurcations, as well as the dimension of their tracheas. Figure 5.6 illustrates some of these differences.

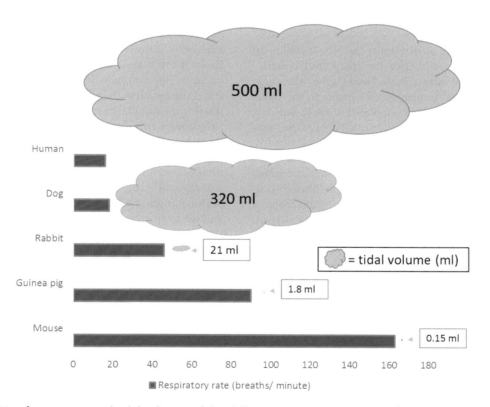

Figure 5.5 Breathing frequencies and tidal volumes of the different animal models compared to those of a 70 kg adult. (Scheme was drawn with data from Cryan, S.A. et al., *Adv. Drug Deliv. Rev.*, 59, 1133–1151, 2007; García-Contreras, L. In vivo models for controlled release pulmonary drug delivery, in *Controlled Pulmonary Drug Delivery*, H.D. Smyth and A.J. Hickey, Editors, Springer Science and Business Media, LLC, New York, 443–474, 2011.)

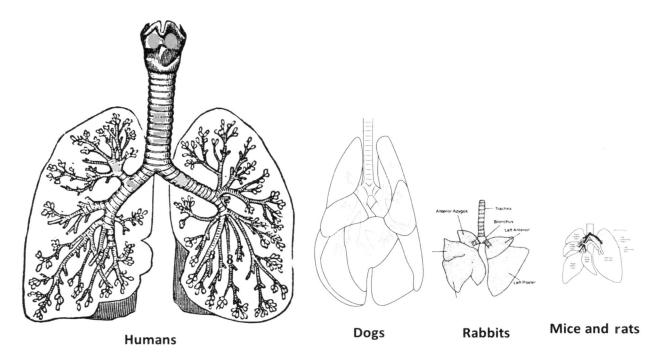

Figure 5.6 Schematic illustration of the size of the lungs in each species, the number of lobes, and the branching of the airways. (Compiled from Cook, M.J., *The Anatomy of the Laboratory Mouse*, 1965; FCIT, F.C.F. I.T. *Human lungs*, 2018; Pokusay, A. *Lungs of the Dog Vector Illustration*, Medical veterinary illustrations, 2018; Samiksha, S., *Respiratory System: Useful notes on Respiratory System of Different Animals*, http://www.yourarticlelibrary.com/respiration/respiratory-system-useful-notes-on-respiratory-system-of-different-animals/23265, 2018.)

In general, human lungs are oval and more symmetrical, reflecting the relatively symmetrical airway branching scheme at all airway generations in humans compared with the long tapering monopodial airways with small lateral branches characteristic of all the other species (95). The lungs among the different species also differ in terms of the number of lobes. In humans, the left human lung is divided into two lobes and the right lung is divided into three lobes, whereas the right lungs from laboratory mammals, including nonhuman primates, are divided into four lobes. In contrast, the left lungs from mice and rats are not divided, but those from larger mammals such as guinea pigs and rabbits are divided (96).

Differences in the type and number of cell in the lungs of the different species and the characteristics of the pulmonary vasculature are described elsewhere (87), but they should be considered when extrapolating the rate and extent of absorption of a therapeutic compound with respect to humans.

DOSE CALCULATION

Studies designed to determine the bioavailability of inhaled compounds ideally should administer the aerosolized medication using the same formulation (wet or dry aerosol, drug concentration, and excipients) and device (DPI, MDI, or nebulizer) that would be routinely used by the patient. The aerosol should be preferably administered to awake, ambulatory patients as a bolus (DPI, MDI) or by continuous passive inhalation (nebulizer) during the period of time that would achieve the desired dose. The dose delivered per

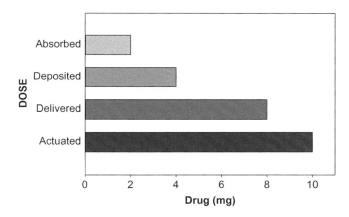

Figure 5.7 Schematic illustration of the relative size of the doses that could be used in the calculation of bioavailability of inhaled compounds.

actuation by DPIs or MDIs and the time that the patient should passively inhale from a nebulized solution should have been optimized prior to use *in vivo* so that the dose is precisely known when it is used to calculate the bioavailability. According to the FDA definition, the type of "dose" that should be used in the bioavailability calculation using Equation 5.1, described in the 'Factors that affect the bioavailability of inhaled compounds' section should match the amount of drug that would be available at the intended site of drug action. This is illustrated in Figure 5.7.

For example, if a dry powder aerosol is formulated into a DPI to deliver a 10 mg dose and the efficiency of delivery with that particular DPI is 80%, the actual "dose delivered" is 8 mg. Subsequently, if the respirable fraction is 50%, it is likely that the "deposited dose" in the airways would be about 4 mg. This would be the dose that should be used to calculate the bioavailability of compounds whose site of action is in the airways, including compounds to treat asthma, bronchiectasis, and the signs and symptoms of CF (Table 1, Figure 5.2). However, if a compound is intended for systemic action (insulin and growth hormone), then the "absorbed dose" should be used in the calculation of bioavailability, which is assumed to be 50% of the deposited dose, i.e., 2 mg, in the example illustrated in Figure 5.7.

The procedure of aerosol administration and dose calculation is much more complex when animal models are employed in bioavailability studies because the device to be used in patients cannot be used in the same manner in laboratory animals. The process is further complicated due to the differences in the route of breathing, breathing frequency, and tidal volume of the different animal models, which can significantly influence the dose delivered to the animal. Moreover, anatomical differences in airway branching and number of airway generations would also influence the actual aerosol dose deposited in their airways. Both of these differences can affect the bioavailability of drugs intended for local action in the airways, such as anti-asthmatic drugs, and also the absorbed dose that will affect the bioavailability of drugs intended for systemic delivery. Consequently, it is imperative that the "dose" employed in the calculation of bioavailability matches the amount of drug that would be available at the site of drug action.

In order to have an accurate estimation of the dose and to circumvent oropharyngeal deposition, researchers have employed direct administration methods to deliver the aerosolized compound to animals using intratracheal tubes or the Penn century devices, the Dry Powder Insufflator™, or the MicroSprayer®. However, aerosol delivery to conscious animals by passive inhalation is considered to resemble more closely the inhaled therapy in humans, and the dose delivered can be determined fairly accurately using the equation recommended by the Association of Inhalation Toxicologists (97):

$$DD = \frac{C \times RMV \times D (\times IF)}{BW} \qquad (5.3)$$

where DD is the delivered dose (mg/Kg), C is the concentration of drug in the aerosol (mg/L), RMV is the respiratory minute volume of the animal (L/min), D is the duration of exposure (min), BW is the bodyweight of the animal (Kg), and IF is the proportion by weight of particles that are inhalable by the test species (respirable fraction). The RMV can be calculated using Equation 5.4:

$$RMV = 0.608 \times BW^{0.852} \qquad (5.4)$$

where RMV and BW should be expressed in L/min and Kg, respectively.

Although it can be argued that the method of aerosol administration resembles more the "bolus" aerosol doses delivered with DPIs and MDIs, aerosol scientists can claim that the devices used for direct administration do not produce a "true" aerosol. This statement could be debated if the aerosol was generated from dry powders using the Penn Century Dry Powder Insufflator, but since the company went out of business there is no other company that can currently fill the gap in producing such a device. Other considerations before selecting one of these two methods of aerosol administration to animals include the amount of drug or formulation available for the study, the size of the dose, and the number of doses to be evaluated. These are compared for both methods in Table 5.4.

Direct aerosol administration methods are particularly useful when the amount of drug or formulation is limited, but depending on the size and distribution of the aerosol generated, the site of deposition may be altered because the aerosol is "forced" into the lungs of animals (87). Also, direct administration may work for daily dosing regimens if animals can tolerate the daily sedation and intubation, such as mice, but this method may not be suitable for sensitive species such as guinea pigs.

Although aerosol administration by passive inhalation using nebulizers for liquid aerosols or the sonic sifter and dry powder generators such as the Wright dust feed require large amounts of material (100 mg), newer devices such as the fluidized-bed aerosol generator (TSI Inc.), or the PreciseInhale

Table 5.4 Characteristics to be considered when selecting a method of aerosol administration to laboratory animals

Direct administration	Passive inhalation
Dose accurately measured	Dose estimated
Circumvents oropharyngeal deposition	Deposition depends on nose cut-off diameter
Highly efficient (small or large doses)	Low efficiency (large quantities needed)
Performed under light sedation or anesthesia	Performed in conscious animals
Multiple or consecutive doses may not be possible	Appropriate for multiple doses
Smaller inter-subject variability	Large inter-subject variability

Sources: Cryan, S.A. et al., *Adv. Drug Deliv. Rev.*, 59, 1133–1151, 2007; García-Contreras, L., In vivo models for controlled release pulmonary drug delivery, in *Controlled Pulmonary Drug Delivery*, H.D. Smyth and A.J. Hickey, Editors, Springer Science and Business Media, LLC, New York, 443–474, 2011.

system require only tenths of grams. While the fluidized-bed aerosol generator was developed for inhalation toxicology studies, the PreciseInhale system was specifically designed for use with pharmaceutical aerosols and requires 50 mg or less to perform a full PK study (98). In addition, this system has the capability of measuring the aerosol concentration and breathing pattern in real time, which allows modification of the aerosol characteristics to be used in different species that may have different nose cut-off diameters.

In passive inhalation studies, the aerosol can be administered to animals in whole-body chambers, head only and nose only. The whole-body inhalation chambers have the advantage of delivering aerosol to unrestrained animals, but the disadvantage is that the aerosolized drug may be absorbed by other routes including oral and percutaneous, which would overestimate the bioavailability of the studied compound. Therefore, head-only and nose-only inhalation chambers are preferred for PK and bioavailability studies because they reduce the probability of drug exposure by other routes, but they have the disadvantage that animals experience distress due to the restraint in the ports of the chamber.

One of the most important considerations in selecting the mode of aerosol administration for bioavailability studies is the size of the dose that can be achieved in an animal model. In general, direct administration can deliver large doses, and the whole dose can be administered as a bolus, but passive inhalation methods require a period of exposure and a rigorous control of the formulation, drug concentration, and the aerosol-generating device. For instance, direct administration of 5 mg and 10 mg of capreomycin microparticles by insufflation to guinea pigs required a few minutes and achieved plasma concentrations that were three to six time higher than the minimum inhibitory concentration (MIC) of the drug, respectively. The capreomycin plasma concentration was maintained above MIC for 3 and 4.5 h for the 5 and 10 mg doses, respectively (Figure 5.8). In contrast, administration of a nominal dose of 10 mg of these particles by passive inhalation required loading the dosing chamber with 100 mg of these microparticles and exposing the guinea pigs for 1 hour. It achieved capreomycin plasma concentrations that were two times higher than the MIC, and these concentrations were maintained above MIC for 2.5 h.

BIOLOGICAL SAMPLES

The type and number of the biological samples that should be collected in bioavailability studies with inhaled drugs depend on the particular drug and the intended site of action. Depending on the subjects employed in a study, blood, bronchoalveolar lavage (BAL) fluid, tissues, and urine may be collected to determine drug concentrations. BAL is usually performed to measure the fraction of the inhaled dose that remains unabsorbed. The collected BAL fluid contains lung cells, soluble proteins, lipids, and other chemical constituents from the epithelial surface of the lung. Determination of drug concentration in the cellular fraction and the supernatant of BAL can reveal if the drug or aerosol particles were engulfed by alveolar macrophages, which may reduce the

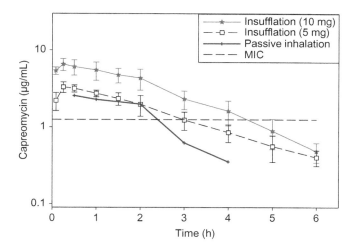

Figure 5.8 Capreomycin plasma concentration versus time curves after pulmonary administration of microparticles by insufflation or passive inhalation to guinea pigs in a nose only inhalation chamber. (Modified from Garcia-Contreras, L. et al., *Antimicrob Agents Chemother.*, 51, 2830–2836, 2007.)

bioavailability of an inhaled compound. It is also recommended that the concentration of urea in the BAL are measured to assess the magnitude of the dilution that may have occurred by the addition of saline solution employed in the BAL procedure (100). Determination of drug concentrations in tissue will help in determining the fraction of the dose absorbed, particularly for drugs intended to be absorbed for local action, such as antibiotics, antifungal agents, and anticancer drugs (Tables 5.1 and 5.2), but they may also provide information on drug metabolism in lung tissue that affects the bioavailability of drugs intended for systemic action such as insulin (101).

None of the studies in patients or healthy volunteers to evaluate the bioavailability of compounds used to treat asthma and COPD (Table 5.1) use biological samples to determine their availability at the airways, the main site of drug action. This is not surprising because it would be impossible to determine concentrations of these drugs in the airways of patients over a period of time. A few studies measure drug concentration in plasma, but the great majority employ indirect measurements of the acute pharmacodynamic effect of these compounds, such as pulmonary function, to evaluate their bioavailability. These studies will be discussed in the "Pharmacodynamic parameters to determine bioavailability" section.

Ideally, studies to evaluate the bioavailability of antibiotics, such as those used to treat the opportunistic infections in CF patients, would measure drug concentration in sputum because the site of effect is the bacterial biofilm on the airways of these patients. Other studies measure the concentration of antibiotic in plasma to evaluate the concentration of drug absorbed as marker of efficacy, but determination of antibiotic concentration in both fluids would give the best knowledge of its disposition. A single study was found to measure the concentration of laninamivir octanoate, a compound to treat influenza, in the BAL fluid of healthy male volunteers (102). This procedure is rarely performed in humans because of the high risk it represents.

Bioavailability studies performed in animals allow the collection of several biological samples, including blood, BAL, tissues and urine. For drugs intended for local action, collection of BAL and lung tissue would give the best estimation of drug concentrations at the site of action, whereas for bioavailability studies of drugs intended for systemic action, such as insulin or antibiotics to treat tuberculosis (Table 5.2), blood, BAL and tissues (lungs and other relevant tissues) should be collected. A limitation for this approach is that BAL and tissue collection are terminal in small laboratory animals; thus, a large number of subjects would be required. However, a recent study performed in horses to determine the concentration of salbutamol after pulmonary administration employed a novel technique that allows the sampling of the epithelial lining fluid throughout the study in the live animal (103). A tube was inserted into the nose of the horse all the way until the trachea, with cotton swabs attached at the end of the tube. Microdialysis is another semi-invasive sampling technique that has been used to study the disposition of drugs in the lungs (104). It involves the implantation of microdialysis probes with a semipermeable membrane into the tissue that is continuously perfused with a physiological solution at a very slow flow rate followed by gentle aspiration of the solution, which is analyzed for drug concentration by LC-MS (90). However, this sampling method may be limited to studies using water-soluble compounds because it is likely that compounds that are poorly soluble in water may not be dissolved in the physiological solution.

The number and frequency of samples collected in a determined study should be selected based on the half-life of the compound for all bioavailability studies. In general, it is suggested that samples should be collected for 4–5 half-lives of the compound, but it is recommended that the sampling time be extended at least twice for inhaled compounds if the half-life of the compound considered was determined after parenteral administration of the compound. A sufficient number of biological samples must be collected so that the terminal (elimination) phase of the PK profile contains at least 4–5 time points. Samples should be collected more frequently at the initial time points and around the time of maximum plasma concentration to accurately calculate the absorption rate constant.

PHARMACOKINETIC PARAMETERS TO DETERMINE BIOAVAILABILITY

The bioavailability of an inhaled compound is determined using the AUC after administration of the inhaled compound having as reference the AUC after its IV administration to determine absolute bioavailability, as shown in Equation 5.1, or after administration by another parenteral or oral route to determine relative bioavailability (6). In these studies is also important to determine the peak drug concentration (C_{max}) in the biological sample of interest as well as the time of peak concentration (T_{max}). Quantitatively,

the ratio of AUCs measures the extent of drug bioavailability, whereas the T_{max} measures of the rate of drug absorption, and the relationship of AUC:C_{max} measures both the rate of absorption and the extent of bioavailability.

The simplest method to determine the AUC after pulmonary delivery is by the linear trapezoidal rule, which involves the description of a given plasma concentration versus time curve by a function that represents the curve as a series of straight lines. This allows the AUC to be divided into a series of trapezoids (Figure 5.9). The area of each trapezoid can be calculated using two concentrations and two time points, and the sum of all areas of all the trapezoids is an estimate of the AUC of the particular drug (6).

The thinner the trapezoid, i.e., the more time points and concentrations, the more accurate is the calculated AUC because the trapezoidal rule tends to underestimate the area during the ascending part of the curve and overestimate the area during the descending phase, assuming that the elimination is first-order (84).

The noncompartmental analysis (NCA) method involves the mathematical integration of the different areas delineated by the trapezoidal rule using different algorithms (84). The easiest way to calculate the pharmacokinetic (PK) parameters to characterize the disposition of a drug after pulmonary administration is using NCA methods because it does not require the assumption of a specific compartmental model. The PK parameters that can be calculated by NCA are the elimination rate constant (K_e), half-life ($t_{1/2}$), clearance (CL), volume of distribution (V_d), mean residence time (MRT), and AUC. C_{max} and T_{max} can be determined directly from the plasma concentration versus time profiles. If a more detailed PK characterization is required using compartmental analysis, the initial estimates of PK parameters that are necessary can be obtained by NCA. A number of computer programs are available for PK analysis, but Phoenix WinNonlin, NONMEM, and MATLAB have been more commonly used in preclinical PK studies of inhaled drugs (98,105–107).

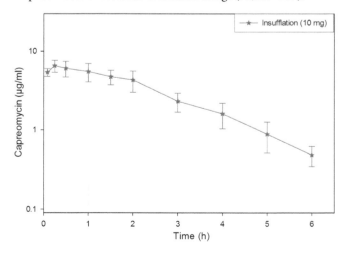

Figure 5.9 Application of the linear trapezoidal rule to estimate the area under the plasma concentration versus time curve after pulmonary administration of capreomycin microparticles by insufflation.

One of the limitations of the NCA is that the rate of drug absorption cannot be calculated by these methods, but MRT can be used to calculate a similar parameter, the mean absorption time (MAT), which can be calculated using Equation 5.5:

$$MAT = MRT_{(pulmonary)} - MRT_{IV} \qquad (5.5)$$

Alternatively, the rate of drug absorption, K_a, can be calculated from the plasma concentration versus time data using the method of residuals, the Wagner-Nelson or the Loo-Riegelman methods, or by compartment modeling (6,84). Compartmental modeling proposes that the body consists of different interconnecting compartments, each of these having a different volume of distribution and variable drug concentrations that are in equilibrium with each other. Different compartmental models can be evaluated and the best model is selected based on visual comparison of the observed versus predicted values, and by the goodness-of-fit criteria including the Akaike Criteria and the weighted sum of squares residuals (6,84).

Besides AUC and bioavailability, it is really important to calculate the rate of drug absorption for inhaled compounds which site of action is the lung tissue such as antibiotics or systemic action such as insulin because one of the causes of low drug bioavailability may be a slow rate of absorption. It is also very important to have the PK parameters after IV administration of the drug available because any significant differences between PK parameters (K_e, CL, $t_{1/2}$) of a drug after IV and pulmonary administration may reveal the existence of specific kinetic phenomena such as flip-flop kinetics. Typically, K_a is much higher than K_e because, in general, the absorption of a drug is faster than the elimination process, but for drugs exhibiting flip-flop kinetics, the situation is "flipped" and the K_a is smaller than K_e due to a slow rate of absorption. The best evidence for flip-flop kinetics is when the $t_{1/2}$ of a drug administered by the pulmonary route is longer than the $t_{1/2}$ after IV administration irrespective of the dose (108). The occurrence of flip-flop kinetics after pulmonary administration is particularly observed for compounds that are formulated for controlled release or for drugs that have poor water solubility such as rifampicin and ethionamide (105,107). The $t_{1/2}$ after pulmonary administration of rifampicin microparticles was almost two times longer than when it was administered IV as solution, and the bioavailability of rifampicin after pulmonary administration was slightly higher (87%) than that after oral administration (59%) (107). Likewise, the $t_{1/2}$ after pulmonary administration of ethionamide microparticles was almost two times longer than when it was administered IV as solution, but notably the bioavailability of ethionamide after pulmonary administration was significantly higher (85%) than that after oral administration (17%) (105). These studies highlight the advantage of delivering compounds with poor water solubility by the pulmonary route to enhance their bioavailability.

PHARMACODYNAMIC PARAMETERS TO DETERMINE BIOAVAILABILITY

Early studies to determine the efficacy of inhaled anti-asthmatic compounds employed lung deposition data as a surrogate for clinical response (109), but their use has decreased over the years with the advent of more sensitive parameters that can detect the drug accurately over time. Drugs can be radio-labeled (^{14}C, ^{3}H, and $^{99m}T_c$), and the detection method depends on the characteristic properties of the compound that is quantified (half-life, energy, and dose). Detection methods often used in animal studies include gamma scintigraphy, single photon emission computed tomography (SPECT), and positron emission tomography (PET). These techniques have been employed to quantify the deposition of radio-labeled drugs and particles delivered by the pulmonary route to small animals such as mice and rats (110–112) and large animals such as dogs and baboons (113–117). In general, PET images are considered to be more accurate to quantify *in vivo* the regional distribution by deposition of the drug in the large airway versus small airways (118).

The second part of the FDA definition of bioavailability states that "*For drug products that are not intended to be absorbed into the bloodstream, bioavailability may be assessed by measurements intended to reflect the rate and extent to which the active ingredient or active moiety becomes available at the site of action.*" This applies to compounds such as those intended to treat asthma and COPD and whose concentrations cannot be measured at the site of action. In these cases, it is acceptable to measure their acute pharmacodynamic (PD) effect or another reliable surrogate that indicates their availability at the site of action. This requires demonstration of a dose-related response, and the measurement of the pharmacodynamic effect should be frequent enough to enable estimation of the total AUC for a time period of at least three times the half-life of the drug (7). The bioavailability is then determined by characterization of an acute dose-response curve or acute pharmacodynamic (PD) effect–time curve, as shown in Figure 5.10. The PD effects that can be determined from such a curve are (1) total area under the acute PD effect–time curve, (2) peak PD effect, (3) time for peak PD effect, (4) minimum effective concentration (MEC) or minimum inhibitory concentration (MIC) for antimicrobials, (5) maximum safe concentration (MSC), (6) duration of action, (7) onset of action, and (8) intensity of action.

Table 5.5 lists some of the pharmacodynamic measurements that have been employed to quantify the availability of inhaled drugs at their site of action. Therapy with inhaled steroids has been found to cause suppression of the overnight urinary cortisol:creatinine ratio, and thus it has been considered to be a sensitive surrogate of relative lung dose delivered. Fluticasone proprionate (FP) has almost null oral bioavailability because is completely destroyed by hepatic first metabolism (119); thus, any FP detected in systemic circulation indicates solely lung absorption, which is correlated with the dose delivered by inhalation. For that reason, the systemic bioavailability of FP has been correlated with the suppression of the overnight urinary cortisol:creatinine ratio (120).

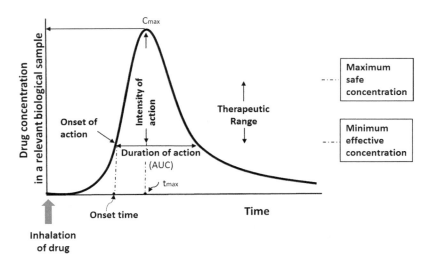

Figure 5.10 Acute dose-response curve or acute pharmacodynamic effect—Time curve.

Table 5.5 PD parameters employed to quantify the disposition and bioavailability of inhaled drugs

Parameter	Drug	References
Suppression of the overnight urinary cortisol:creatinine ratio	Fluticasone proprionate	(120,123)
Changes in the potassium serum concentration	Salmeterol	(120,123)
Forced expiratory volume in one second (FEV1)	Revefenacin	(124)
	Ipratropium bromide	(124)
Drug concentration in urine	Salbutamol	(125)
Drug concentration in plasma, AUC, C_{max}	Fluticasone proprionate	(126)
	Fluticasone proprionate and salmeterol	(127)
	Tiotropium bromide	(128)
	Beclomethasone diproprionate	(129)
	Fluticasone proprionate and salmeterol	(130)

Likewise, Salmeterol is also highly inactivated by first pass hepatic metabolism (121), and it has been observed that upon inhalation, the maximum plasma concentration of this compound is correlated with a significant decrease of the potassium concentration in serum (122). Thus, it has been used as surrogate marker for salmeterol bioavailability (120,123).

The forced expiratory volume in one second (FEV1) is the maximal amount of air that a person can forcefully exhale in one second, and it is normally expressed as a percentage of normal (131). In asthmatic patients, FEV1 is measured frequently to evaluate the degree of obstruction caused by the asthma (132); thus, it has been used to evaluate the bioavailability of compounds such as revefenacin and ipratropium bromide. On the other hand, a few studies have correlated the concentration of salbutamol in urine with the inhaled dose (133,134). Furthermore, it has been shown that the amount of salbutamol determined in the urine collected cumulatively for 24 h after inhalation of salbutamol correlates with the total dose that the patient has inhaled (125).

In the last decade, newer analytical instruments have enabled determination of minute concentrations of drugs in biological matrices. Thus, researchers have opted for measuring drug concentrations in plasma and calculating the bioavailability of inhaled compounds in systemic circulation to avoid some inter-subject variabilities such as asthma severity, baseline pulmonary function, race/ethnicity, pharmacogenetic influences, and duration of asthma (135). Similar to other PD parameters discussed above, however, this method is suitable only for drugs that have null oral bioavailability to make certain that the drug measured in systemic circulation has been absorbed only from lungs. The bioavailability of compounds such as fluticasone proprionate, salmeterol, tiotropium bromide, and beclomethasone diproprionate have been evaluated in this manner.

CASE STUDIES OF THE BIOAVAILABILITY AND BIOEQUIVALENCY OF INHALED PRODUCTS

Most of the studies reporting the bioavailability of inhaled compounds for local action in the airways, where absorption is not needed, either investigate new compounds (136), new formulations for existing compounds (137), and the performance of two devices for the same formulation (130), or they compare the use of accessories such as chambers and masks (120,126,127). All of these compounds are indicated for the treatment of asthma and COPD. For example, it has been reported that the size of the dose of a drug inhaled from a valved holding chamber (VHC) after delivery from an MDI depends on several factors, including the characteristics of the VHC used (size, shape, plastic versus antistatic composition, and dead-space volume), the drug formulation (drug, propellant, and excipient), and patient characteristics (tidal volume, calm versus crying, and facemask seal) (126). Examples of these studies are presented in Table 5.6.

Similarly, studies reporting the bioavailability of inhaled compounds for local action in the lungs, either in the airways, such as for compounds to treat opportunistic infections in CF patients, or where absorption into the tissue may be required, such as for pneumonia or influenza, investigate either new compounds (102,142) or new formulations for existing compounds (143–145). Most of these compounds and formulations are not commercially available. Examples of these studies are presented in Table 5.7.

Only a handful of studies report the bioavailability of newer formulations of inhaled antibiotics that are commercially available, such as tobramycin. Two of the most complete studies reporting the pharmacokinetics (PK) of inhaled tobramycin in serum and sputum to determine bioavailability were published by Geller et al. (148,149). In one study, they evaluated the PK and bioavailability of inhaled aerosols generated from liquid tobramycin formulated for inhalation (TOBI, Chiron Corporation) in patients from 69 CF centers. The concentration of tobramycin in the sputum of patients at 10 minutes after inhalation of the aerosol was 1237 µg/g, and the concentration of tobramycin in serum was 0.95 µg/mL one hour after inhalation of the aerosol. The bioavailability of inhaled tobramycin calculated from the serum data with IV administration as referenced was 11.7%. Most important, 95% of the patients achieved tobramycin concentration in the sputum that was more than 25 times higher than the minimum inhibitory concentration (MIC) of the antibiotic (149). A later study evaluated the PK and safety of escalating doses of inhaled tobramycin powder and compared them to that after nebulized tobramycin (148). The PK parameters obtained from this study are summarized in Table 5.8.

As expected, the tobramycin AUC and C_{max} were significantly higher in sputum than in serum, and they increased proportionally with the dose in serum but not in sputum (148). This may be due to limitations in the dissolution of the tobramycin powder with the higher dose of powder.

A few studies have measured the concentrations of antibiotics such as tobramycin in plasma mainly as a measure of possible systemic toxicity. For instance, Miller et al. determined the presence of tobramycin in concentrations ≥ 0.5 µg/mL in children younger than 18 years of age receiving tobramycin for more than 6.5 years and correlated it with acute kidney injury (150). They noted a clinically significant decrease in kidney function in children that had detectable concentrations of tobramycin and thus suggested that monitoring was required in that patient population.

For several decades, the pulmonary route has been considered as an attractive one for delivering compounds for systemic action because the alveolar region of the lungs offers a large surface area, thin epithelium, and rich blood supply that can enable rapid drug absorption and suitable systemic bioavailability (3,13,62). Although Exhubera® was the first inhaled insulin product commercialized (151), it was not the first inhalable compound intended for systemic action that showed reasonable bioavailability in humans. In 1990, Adjei et al. reported a bioavailability of 35%–45% when corrected for the respirable fraction of the leuprolide acetate aerosol generated by a MDI (152). Since then, a number of compounds intended for systemic action have been formulated for inhalation. Examples are presented in Table 5.9.

The determination of bioavailabilty in the last 10 years has had the newer objective of establishing the bioequivalence of generic inhalable compounds with the brand-name products that have been in the market for many years. Bioequivalence has been simply defined as "a pharmaceutical product that equals another in bioavailability and potency." Traditional clinical pharmacokinetic textbooks define it as follows: "The drug substance in two or more identical dosage form reaches the systemic circulation at the same rate and to the same extent" (7), but the official definition was published in the Code of Federal Regulations (CFR) 320.1 as:

The absence of significance difference in the rate and extent to which the active ingredient or active moiety in pharmaceutical equivalent or pharmaceutical alternative becomes available at the site of drug action when administered at the same molar dose under similar conditions in an appropriately designed study.

Under the FDA criteria, two products are bioequivalent if the bioavailabilities (both rate and extent of absorption) after administration in the same molar dose are similar to such a degree that their effects can be expected to be the same (158). Thus, generic drug manufacturers must demonstrate that a drug is bioequivalent to a reference drug product, which in this case is a commercially available product that has been approved for the specific indication that the generic is intended. In order of FDA preference, methods used to determine bioequivalence are (158): (1) pharmacokinetic studies, (2) pharmacodynamic studies, (3) comparative clinical trials, and (4) *in vitro* studies. Accordingly, most studies use pharmacodynamic parameters such as AUC and C_{max} to evaluate the bioequivalence of two products, some use both pharmacokinetic and pharmacodynamic parameters, and a few also evaluate the *in vitro* characteristics of the aerosol. Examples of bioequivalence studies are presented in Table 5.10.

Most of these bioequivalence studies are performed in healthy volunteers instead of patients having the disease of interest. The reason is that healthy volunteers are considered more discriminative than patients because the extent of bronchoconstriction is different in the patient population and it would influence the site of deposition. This carries the risk that two inhaled products may appear to be more

Table 5.6 Examples of bioavailability studies of inhaled compounds intended for local action in the airways, without the need of absorption

Drug/formulation	Device	Objective of the study	Subjects	Measurement	Outcomes	References
A2D5423 (a non-steroidal glucocorticoid)	Dosimetric nebulizer Spira Electra 2, vibrating mesh nebulizer I-neb AAD	Compare the absorption PK of A2D5453 after inhalation from different devices	Healthy (n = 6) and asthmatic (n = 7) male adults	Plasma concentration	Pulmonary bioavailability found as 27% for I-neb 30% for Turbohaler 46% for DPI and 35%–49% for Spira	(138)
Budesonide (BUD) nanocrystal-loaded hyaluronic acid microparticles (MPs)	Insufflator (Penn Century)	Evaluation of pulmonary retention and PK of BUD-loaded MPs to prolong the PK effect without compromising dissolution rate of BUD	Rats	Plasma concentration	Prolonged T_{max} and increased bioavailability but not higher than Pulmicort®	(137)
Salmeterol and FP	Easyhaler® and Diskus®	Demonstrate no inferiority in total systemic exposure and bioequivalence in lung deposition	Healthy volunteers n = 65	Delivered doses, FPF, systemic exposure assessed as surrogate for safety using C_{max}, AUC, lung deposition surrogate for efficacy	Bioequivalence calculated from statistics and C_{max} and AUC were analyzed	(130)
Fluticasone propionate (FP), pMDI	pMDI and babyhaler® (AeroChamber Plus®, Facemask VHC	Determine the bioavailability of FP in lung	Children ages 1–4 n = 17	Blood collection/AUC Population mean AUC	Clinically significant differences observed in pulmonary bioavailability with devices	(126)
Salmeterol and FP	pMDI Mini-spacer and Trudell Aerochamber	Compare the systemic exposure of FP and SAL after delivery with Mini-spacer or Aerochamer	Healthy volunteers n = 21	Plasma concentration, AUC_{0-24}, C_{max}	Mini-spacer use is not recommended with pMDI	(139)

(Continued)

Table 5.6 (Continued) Examples of bioavailability studies of inhaled compounds intended for local action in the airways, without the need of absorption

Drug/formulation	Device	Objective of the study	Subjects	Measurement	Outcomes	References
Umeclidinium and Vilanterol	Ellipta DPI	Evaluation of PK for umeclidinium and vilanterol	COPD Patients n = 1635	Plasma concentration	Body weight, age significantly covariate on umeclidinium and vilanterol CL/F	(140)
Revefenacin	PARI LC Plus	Evaluate PD, PK and safety of single and multiple dose administration in patients with moderate COPD	COPD patients n = 32	Change from baseline in FEV_1, AUC FEV_{1-t} and FEV_1, AUC_{0-24} post-administration	RAPID, onset and sustained duration of action; Low plasma concentration after inhalation due to extra-sensitivity of drug converting to major metabolite	(124)
FP and Salmeterol	Aerochamber Plus (AP), Volumatic Spacers (VM), Synchro-Breathe Device (SB), Evohaler pMDI (EH)	Compare in vivo pulmonary bioavailability	Healthy volunteers n = 10	Adrenal suppression and early fall in serum potassium (K) and overnight urinary cortisol/creatinine (OUCC)	Significant suppression of OUCC and K occurred from baseline with the SB, AP and VM, but not with the EH devices	(120)
Umeclidinium and Vilanterol	Ellipta DPI	Effect of umeclidinium and vilanterol on the QT interval corrected using QTcF correction	Healthy non-smokers n = 103	QT interval, cardiac parameters, PK, PD and safety, C_{max}, AUC	No change was observed in QT after use of umeclidinium/ vilanterol or umeclidium alone	(141)

Table 5.7 Examples of bioavailability studies of inhaled compounds intended for local action in the lungs, either in the airways or where absorption into the tissue may be required

Drug/formulation	Device	Disease	Objective of the study	Subjects	Measurement	Outcomes	References
D, L-lysine acetylsalicylate. glycine (LASAG)	Directed-flow nose-only exposure system	Influenza	Determination of antiviral properties of LASAG and comparison with acetyl salicylic acid	C57BL/6 Female mice	Blood, lung tissue collection	Total bioavailability of LASAG was 14% in plasma and more than 100% in lung and protected 50% of mice from death.	(142)
Laninamivir octanoate (LO)	PARI LC Sprint	Influenza	Evaluation of the PK of laninamivir after single nebulized administration of LO to identify a safe and effective nebulizer regimen for those who have difficulties with DPIs	Healthy male volunteers n = 64 (Japanese)	Blood and BAL collection	Nebulized LO lasted in the lungs for 7 days after administration. LO found as long-acting neuraminidase inhibitor. Accumulation of LO in AMs and BAL was observed.	(102)
Itraconazole (ITZ)-based dry powder or/with phospholipid	Insufflator	Invasive and chronic pulmonary aspergillosis	Evaluation of the influence of different powders prepared by spray drying a crystalline suspension (F1), a solution of ITZ alone (F2), and a suspension of ITZ and phospholipids (F3)	Outbred ICR male mice	Concentrations of ITZ with respect to MIC; blood and tissue collection	The apparent solubility of ITZ was enhanced in F2 and F3 resulting in faster absorption for F3, but AUC was larger from F2 due to faster excretion of F3.	(143)
Levofloxacin (LEV) as a solution, chitosan microparticles (MP) or PLGA MP	Micro-sprayer, insufflator	CF	Evaluation of LEV PK in plasma, tissue, epithelial lining fluid (ELF), after delivery of the three formulations by the IV or pulmonary routes	Male Sprague-Dawley rats) n = 80	Blood collection, BAL	The bioavailability of LEV was 98%, 71% and 92% from the solution, chitosan MP and PLGA MP, respectively. LEV concentration in ELF was sustained for 72 h after delivery of PLGA MP.	(144)
Liposomal amikacin for inhalation	PARI LC Star nebulizer	Pulmonary non-tuberculosis mycobacterial infections	Evaluation of pulmonary deposition, elimination, and effect on macrophage functions	CDIGS female rats n = 180	Deposition; blood, serum, tissue and BAL collection	Equal dose dependent deposition across all lungs, lobes and regions.	(145)

(Continued)

Table 5.7 (*Continued*) Examples of bioavailability studies of inhaled compounds intended for local action in the lungs, either in the airways or where absorption into the tissue may be required

Drug/formulation	Device	Disease	Objective of the study	Subjects	Measurement	Outcomes	References
						Diffusion and extracellular co-localization followed by uptake and gradual amikacin elimination. Amikacin concentration was detectable for 28 in lungs of the rats treated for 27 days. Amikacin was found in AMs and BAL.	
Colistin, DPI or IV	Insufflator or IV	CF	Investigation the PK of colistin as DPI form in healthy rats after pulmonary administration	Male Sprague-Dawley rats	Blood collection, BALF	Systemic absorption and bioavailability of DPI Colistin was higher than administration with nebulizer. Improved patients' life expectancy.	(146)
Tobramycin (TOBI)	LC Plus Nebulizer	CF	Investigation of the PK of TOBI in pediatric patients below 7 years of age	CF patients (6 months to 7 years of age) n = 145	Blood collection	Bioavailability of the drug increased linearly with age from 48% in patients of 6 months, to 97% in patients of 7 years of age. However, efficacy was similar in all groups regardless of differences in bioavailability.	(147)

Table 5.8 PK parameters after aerosol administration of TIP and TIS to CF patients to determine bioavailability

Dose (mg)	Formulation	AUC_{0-12} (µg × h/mL)		C_{max} (µg/mL)	
		Serum	Sputum	Serum	Sputum
28 = (2 × 14)	Dry powder	1.3 ± 0.6	261 ± 168	0.33 ± 0.09	258 ± 194
56 = (2 × 28)	Dry powder	2.5 ± 1.2	652 ± 421	0.5 ± 0.21	574 ± 527
84 = (3 × 28)	Dry powder	3.5 ± 1.3	1340 ± 1320	0.70 ± 0.33	1092 ± 1052
112 = (4 × 28)	Dry powder	4.6 ± 2.0	1307 ± 978	1.02 ± 0.53	1048 ± 1080
300	Liquid	4.8 ± 2.5	974 ± 1143	1.04 ± 0.58	737 ± 1028

Source: Adapted from Geller, D.E. et al., *Pediatr. Pulmonol,* 42, 307–313, 2007.

Table 5.9 Examples of bioavailability studies of inhaled compounds intended for systemic action that require absorption

Drug/formulation	Device	Disease	Objective of the study	Subjects	Measurement	Outcomes	References
Leuprolide Acetate (LA)	50 μL metering valve with micron-4 actuator	Hormonally sensitive diseases	Evaluation of *in vivo* absorbance kinetics, preclinical safety of aerosol formulation of LA	Beagle dog n = 8	Blood and tissue collection	Linear dose-plasma AUC relationship between 1.5 mg and 9 mg of LA per day. No changes in bioavailability after multiple dosing.	(153)
Exubera, Afrezza (insulin)	Exubera Inhaler, Afrezza inhaler	Diabetes	Comparison between Exubera and Afrezza products	Healthy volunteers for Exubera, n = 17 Patients with type 2 diabetes for Afrezza	Blood collection	Insulin T_{max} and peak effect were shorter (15 min and 53 min, respectively) after inhalation of Afrezza compared to Exubera (78 min and 120 min, respectively). The duration of action was longer for Exubera (360 min) than for Afrezza (180 min). Compared with insulin SC, the apparent bioavailability was higher for Afrezza (30%) compared to Exubera (11%).	(154)
Fentanyl	SmartMist breath-actuated metered-dose inhaler	Acute pain	Comparison of the PK of fentanyl between pulmonary and IV administration	Healthy volunteers n = 15	Blood collection	Similar profiles were observed for drug concentration vs time after pulmonary and IV administration. T_{max} after pulmonary administration was longer (9 min) than that after IV administration (4 min).	(155)

(Continued)

Table 5.9 (Continued) Examples of bioavailability studies of inhaled compounds intended for systemic action that require absorption

Drug/formulation	Device	Disease	Objective of the study	Subjects	Measurement	Outcomes	References
Fentanyl	Nebulizer, IV	Acute pain	Comparison of the PK of fentanyl between pulmonary and IV administration	Healthy volunteers n = 45	Blood collection	Bioavailability of nebulized fentanyl was 96.8%. T_{max} of fentanyl after nebulization was 20.5 min and 31.5 min after IV administration.	(155)
Morphine	Nebulizer, IM	Acute pain	Comparison of bioavailability of morphine between pulmonary and IM administration	Patients undergoing abdominal surgery n = 7	Blood collection	The apparent bioavailability of inhaled morphine was between 8.9% and 34.6% with respect to IM administration.	(155)
Technosphere Insulin (TI, 12 U), Regular Human Insulin (RHI, 15 U)	Gen2 Inhaler, IV	Diabetes	Determination of PK of TI vs RHI	Healthy volunteers n = 32	Blood collection	T_{max} and C_{max} of TI were 15 min and 190 mIU/mL compared to >60 min and 50 mIU/mL for RHI.	(151)
Technosphere Insulin (TI, 8 U), Insulin lispro (8 U)	Gen2 Inhaler, SQ	Diabetes	Determination of PK of TI vs RHI	Patients with type 1 diabetes n = 12	Blood collection	T_{max} and C_{max} of TI were 8 min and 51 mIU/ml compared to 50 min and 34 mIU/ml for insulin lispro.	(151)
Technosphere Insulin (TI, 8 U)	Gen2 Inhaler, MedTone Inhaler	Diabetes	Determination of PK profiles of TI with two different inhalers	Healthy volunteers n = 46	Blood collection	Inhalation of TI from the Gen2 inhaler resulted in an AUC_{0-120} = 4294 min.µU/mL and C_{max} = 105 µU/mL, whereas with the Medtone inhaler AUC_{0-120} = 4060 min.µU/mL and C_{max} = 97 µU/mL.	(151)

(Continued)

Table 5.9 (*Continued*) Examples of bioavailability studies of inhaled compounds intended for systemic action that require absorption

Drug/ formulation	Device	Disease	Objective of the study	Subjects	Measurement	Outcomes	References
Oxytocin	Modified air inlet Rotahaler, (50, 200, 400, and 600 µg), IM (17 µg)	Postpartum hemorrhage	Evaluation of the PK of inhalable oxytocin and comparison of the results to IM administration	Healthy female volunteers n = 15	Blood collection	PK profiles after the inhaled and IM oxytocin were similar. C_{max} was 15.3, 103.03, 255.95 and 365.42 pg/mL for the 50, 200, 400 and 600 µg, respectively, for the inhaled doses, compared to C_{max} = 189.96 pg/mL after IM. AUC was 9.16, 65.02, 153.83 and 224.34 pg.h/mL, respectively, for the inhaled doses and 119.83 pg.h/mL for the IM dose.	(156)
Technosphere Insulin (TI) (Afrezza)	Afrezza inhaler	Diabetes	Generate a dose-response model to compare the effects of TI and regular human insulin (RHI) on the induced glucose infusion rate (GIR) in heathy volunteers	Healthy volunteers n = 31	Blood collection	The PK-GIR model generated was capable to simulate GIR for a time window of up to 20 h and for higher doses. A subsequent dose–response model was then generated from the simulated GIR profiles. This second model provided for TI a dose of half maximum effect (ED_{50}) that is 5-fold higher than for RHI. This ratio could be used as conversion factor for equivalent doses of RHI and TI.	(157)

Table 5.10 Examples of bioequivalence (BE) studies of inhaled compounds in humans

Compound	Reference product	Test product	Subjects	Parameters measured to determine BE	Was BE declared?	References
Salmeterol and fluticasone proprionate (FP) combination product (SFC 50/250)	Multidose DPI (Diskus)	Capsule-based DPI (Rotahaler)	Asthma and COPD patients	• MMAD, GSD, fine particle mass, emitted dose • Plasma AUC, C_{max} • Serum cortisol	No	(123)
Salmeterol and FP (SFC 50/100, SFC 50/250)	Multidose DPI (Diskus)	Capsule-based DPI (Rotahaler)	Healthy volunteers	• Plasma AUC, C_{max} • Adverse events	Yes for SFC 50/250 No for SFC 50/100	(159)
Tiotropium bromide	Spiriva HandiHaler	Monodose capsule DPI	Healthy volunteers	• Plasma AUC, C_{max} • Tolerability and safety profile	Yes	(128)
Beclomethasone dipropionate (160, 320 µg)	Metered dose inhaler	Breath-actuated inhaler	Healthy volunteers	• Plasma AUC, C_{max}	Yes for the 320 µg dose	(129)
Salmeterol and FP	Seretide Diskus DPI	Easyhaler DPI	Healthy volunteers	• Plasma AUC, C_{max}	Yes	(130)

similar than they actually are (128). For this reason, the use of healthy volunteers instead of patients is supported by the European Medicines Agency (EMA) guidance on bioequivalence (160).

There have not been any bioequivalence studies based on clinical trials or *in vitro* data performed for inhalable products that have been published to this date. In fact, the *in vitro* measurements alone have been reported to lack predictive power (123), but there has been a research effort to develop a biopharmaceutics classification system (BCS) similar to that developed in the 1990s for oral dosage forms for immediate drug release. A group of scientists in the pharmaceutical inhalation field gathered to evaluate if such classification would be possible, and the results of these meeting were later reported (161). The authors concluded that, if such a classification system were developed, it may be useful for formulators and discovery chemists, but not suitable for regulatory purposes.

Based on the official FDA definitions for bioavailability and bioequivalence, as well as the studies discussed for the different compounds formulated for inhalation described in this chapter, it is unlikely that such system can be developed for all inhalable compounds. The BCS was established around the properties of solubility and permeability of a compound and three theoretical numbers (absorption, dose, and dissolution) (162), but these properties and numbers do not have the same relevance in the lung environment. The intrinsic solubility of the compound is less important in the lung environment than in the GI tract for bioavailability due to the presence of surfactant in the epithelial lining fluid and longer residence time. As shown for compounds with poor water solubility (105,107), permeability or absorption are not required for anti-asthmatic compounds to exert their therapeutic effect, and there is a huge range of doses indicated for these compounds (from micrograms for anti-asthmatic compounds to hundreds of milligrams for antibiotics). However, it may be plausible to have different types of BCS classifications for inhalable compounds if the system is based on either the range of doses or the intended site of action for the inhaled compound.

REFERENCES

1. García-Contreras, L. and A.J. Hickey, Aerosol treatment of cystic fibrosis. *Crit Rev Ther Drug Carrier Syst* 2003. **20**(5): p. 317–356.
2. Patton, J.S., J. Bukar, and S. Nagarajan, Inhaled insulin. *Adv Drug Deliv Rev* 1999. **35**: p. 235–247.
3. Patton, J.S., C.S. Fishburn, and J.G. Weers, The lungs as a portal of entry for systemic drug delivery. *Proc Am Thorac Soc* 2004. **1**(4): p. 338–344.
4. Muttil, P., C. Wang, and A.J. Hickey, Inhaled drug delivery for tuberculosis therapy. *Pharm Res* 2009. **26**(11): p. 2401–2416.
5. Gagnadoux, F. et al., Aerosolized chemotherapy. *J Aerosol Med Pulm Drug Deliv* 2008. **21**(1): p. 61–70.
6. Gibaldi, M. and D. Perrier, *Pharmacokinetics*. 1982, New York: Marcel Dekker.
7. Rowland, M. and T.N. Tozer, *Clinical Pharmacokinetics and Pharmacodynamics: Concepts and Applications*. 2011, Baltimore, MD: Wolters Kluwer| Lippincott Williams & Wilkins.
8. Trevor, A.J. et al., *Katzung & Trevor's pharmacology: Examination & board review*. 10th ed. *Lange Medical Books* 2012, New York: McGraw-Hill.
9. Crystal, R.G. et al., Eds. *The Lung. Scientific Foundations*. 1997, Philadelphia, PA: Lippincott-Raven Publishers.
10. Eixarch, H. et al., Drug delivery to the lung: Permeability and physicochemical characteristics of drugs as the basis for a pulmonary biopharmaceutical classification system (pBCS). *J Epithel Biol Pharmacol* 2010 **3**: p. 1–14.
11. OECD, *Test No. 107: Partition Coefficient (n-octanol/water): Shake Flask Method*. Paris, France: OECD Publishing.
12. Lipinski, C.A. et al., Experimental and computational approaches to estimate solubility and permeability in drug discovery and development settings. *Adv Drug Deliv Rev* 2001. **46**(1–3): p. 3–26.
13. Patton, J.S., Mechanisms of macromolecule absorption by the lungs. *Adv Drug Deliv Rev* 1996. **19**(1): p. 3–36.
14. Ibrahim, M. and L. Garcia-Contreras, Mechanisms of absorption and elimination of drugs administered by inhalation. *Ther Deliv* 2013. **4**(8): p. 1027–1045.
15. Ibrahim, M. and L. García-Contreras, preclinical pharmacokinetics of antitubercular drugs, in *Delivery Systems for Tuberculosis Prevention and Treatment.*, A.J. Hickey, Editor 2016, John Wiley & Sons: West Sussex, UK, p. 131–155.
16. Canadian-Institutes-of-Health-Research, Alberta Innovates Health-Solutions, and The-metabolomics-innovation-centre. *DrugBank Database*. 2018 March 13–21, 2018.
17. Agu, R.U. et al., The lung as a route for systemic delivery of therapeutic proteins and peptides. *Resp Res* 2001. **2**(4): p. 198.
18. Sanjar, S. and J. Matthews, Treating systemic diseases via the lung. *J Aerosol Med* 2001. 14 Suppl 1: p. S51–S518.
19. Tronde, A. et al., Pulmonary absorption rate and bioavailability of drugs in vivo in rats: Structure-absorption relationships and physicochemical profiling of inhaled drugs. *J Pharm Sci* 2003. **92**(6): p. 1216–1233.
20. Garcia-Contreras, L. and H.D. Smyth, Dry powder and liquid spray systems for inhaled delivery of peptides and proteins. *Am J Drug Deliv* 2005. **3**(1): p. 29–45.
21. Rau, J.L., The inhalation of drugs: Advantages and problems. *Respir Care* 2005. **50**(3): p. 367–382.

22. Zainudin, B.M. et al., Comparison of bronchodilator responses and deposition patterns of salbutamol inhaled from a pressurised metered dose inhaler, as a dry powder, and as a nebulised solution. *Thorax* 1990. **45**(6): p. 469–473.

23. Gonda, I., Targeting by deposition, in *Pharmaceutical Inhalation Aerosol Technology*, A.J. Hickey, Editor 1992, Marcel Dekker: New York. p. 61–82.

24. Verma, R., M. Ibrahim, and L. Garcia-Contreras, Lung anatomy and physiology and their implications for pulmonary drug delivery, in *Pulmonary Drug Delivery: Advances and Challenges*, A. Nokhodchi and G. Martin, Editors. 2015 John Wiley Publishers: Oxford UK.

25. Zanen, P., L.T. Go, and J.-W.J. Lammers, The optimal particle size for parasympatholytic aerosols in mild asthmatics. *Int J Pharm* 1995. **114**(1): p. 111–115.

26. Zanen, P., L.T. Go, and J.-W.J. Lammers, The efficacy of a low-dose, monodisperse parasympatholytic aerosol compared with a standard aerosol from a metered-dose inhaler. *Eur J Clin Pharmacol* 1998. **54**(1): p. 27–30.

27. Zanen, P. and J.-W.J. Lammers, Reducing adverse effects of inhaled fenoterol through optimization of the aerosol formulation. *J Aerosol Med* 1999. **12**(4): p. 241–247.

28. Newman, S.P., Aerosol deposition considerations in inhalation therapy. *Chest* 1985. **88**(2 Suppl): p. 152S–160S.

29. Cryan, S.A., N. Sivadas, and L. Garcia-Contreras, In vivo animal models for drug delivery across the lung mucosal barrier. *Adv Drug Deliv Rev* 2007. **59**(11): p. 1133–1151.

30. Yeh, H.C. and G.M. Schum, Models of human lung airways and their application to inhaled particle deposition. *Bull Math Biol* 1980. **42**(3): p. 461–480.

31. Martonen, T.B., I. Katz, and W. Cress, Aerosol deposition as a function of airway disease: Cystic fibrosis. *Pharm Res* 1995. **12**(1): p. 96–102.

32. Oberdorster, G., Pulmonary deposition, clearance and effects of inhaled soluble and insoluble cadmium compounds. *IARC Sci Publ* 1992(118): p. 189–204.

33. Boucher, R.C., Cystic fibrosis: A disease of vulnerability to airway surface dehydration. *Trends Mol Med* 2007. **13**(6): p. 231–240.

34. Boucher, R.C., Airway surface dehydration in cystic fibrosis: Pathogenesis and therapy. *Annu Rev Med* 2007. **58**: p. 157–170.

35. Corcoran, T.E. et al., Absorptive clearance of DTPA as an aerosol-based biomarker in the cystic fibrosis airway. *Eur Respir J* 2010. **35**(4): p. 781–786.

36. Lombry, C. et al., Alveolar macrophages are a primary barrier to pulmonary absorption of macromolecules. *Am J Physiol Lung Cell Mol Physiol* 2004. **286**(5): p. L1002–L1008.

37. Kreyling, W. and G. Ferron, Macrophage mediated particle transport from the lungs. *J Aerosol Med Pulm Drug Deliv* 1990. **3**: p. 285.

38. Edwards, D.A. et al., Large porous particles for pulmonary drug delivery. *Science* 1997. **276**(5320): p. 1868–1871.

39. Ben-Jebria, A. et al., Large porous particles for sustained protection from carbachol-induced bronchoconstriction in guinea pigs. *Pharm Res* 1999. **16**(4): p. 555–561.

40. Wang, J., A. Ben-Jebria, and D.A. Edwards, Inhalation of estradiol for sustained systemic delivery. *J Aerosol Med* 1999. **12**(1): p. 27–36.

41. Pacifici, G.M. et al., Tissue distribution of drug-metabolizing enzymes in humans. *Xenobiotica* 1988. **18**(7): p. 849–56.

42. Somers, G.I. et al., A comparison of the expression and metabolizing activities of phase I and II enzymes in freshly isolated human lung parenchymal cells and cryopreserved human hepatocytes. *Drug Metab Dispos* 2007. **35**(10): p. 1797–805.

43. Kroon, L.A., Drug interactions with smoking. *Am J Health Syst Pharm* 2007. **64**(18): p. 1917–1921.

44. Chalmers, G.W. et al., Influence of cigarette smoking on inhaled corticosteroid treatment in mild asthma. *Thorax* 2002. **57**(3): p. 226–230.

45. Davies, N.M. and M.R. Feddah, A novel method for assessing dissolution of aerosol inhaler products. *Int J Pharm* 2003. **255**(1–2): p. 175–187.

46. Son, Y.J. and J.T. McConville, Development of a standardized dissolution test method for inhaled pharmaceutical formulations. *Int J Pharm* 2009. **382**(1–2): p. 15–22.

47. Pham, S. and T.S. Wiedmann, Note: Dissolution of aerosol particles of budesonide in Survanta, a model lung surfactant. *J Pharm Sci* 2001. **90**(1): p. 98–104.

48. Wang, W. et al., Effects of surface composition on the aerosolisation and dissolution of inhaled antibiotic combination powders consisting of colistin and rifampicin. *AAPS J* 2016. **18**(2): p. 372–384.

49. Ibrahim, M., M.K. Hatipoglu, and L. Garcia-Contreras, SHetA2 dry powder aerosols for tuberculosis: Formulation, design, and optimization using quality by design. *Mol Pharm* 2018. **15**(1): p. 300–313.

50. Arora, D. et al., In vitro aqueous fluid-capacity-limited dissolution testing of respirable aerosol drug particles generated from inhaler products. *Pharm Res* 2010. **27**(5): p. 786–795.

51. Rohrschneider, M. et al., Evaluation of the transwell system for characterization of dissolution behavior of inhalation drugs: Effects of membrane and surfactant. *Mol Pharm* 2015. **12**(8): p. 2618–2624.

52. Bhagwat, S. et al., Predicting pulmonary pharmacokinetics from in vitro properties of dry powder inhalers. *Pharm Res* 2017. **34**(12): p. 2541–2556.

53. Price, R. et al., Demonstrating Q3 structural equivalence of dry powder inhaler blends: New analytical concepts and techniques, in Respiratory Drug

Delivery 2018, R.N. Dalby et al., Editors. 2018, *Davis Healthcare International Publishing*, LCC.: River Grove, IL. p. 265–276.

54. Gerde, P. et al., Dissolvlt: An in vitro method for simulating the dissolution and absorption of inhaled dry powder drugs in the lungs. *Assay Drug Dev Technol* 2017. **15**(2): p. 77–88.

55. Lubman, R.L., K.J. Kim, and E.D. Crandall, Alveolar epithelial barrier properties, in *The Lung: Scientific Foundations*, R.G. Crystal et al., Editors. 1997, Lippincott-Raven, Publishers: Philadelphia, PA. p. 585–602.

56. Schneeberger, E.E. and R.D. Lynch, Structure, function and regulation of cellular tight junctions. *Am J Physiol* 1992. **262**: p. L647–L661.

57. Forbes, B. and C. Ehrhardt, Human respiratory epithelial cell culture for drug delivery applications. *Eur J Pharm Biopharm* 2005. **60**(2): p. 193–205.

58. Bosquillon, C., Drug transporters in the lung—Do they play a role in the biopharmaceutics of inhaled drugs? *J Pharm Sci* 2010. **99**(5): p. 2240–55.

59. Mathias, N.R. et al., Permeability characterisitcs of calu-3 human bronchial epithelial cells: In vitro-in vivo correlation to predict lung absorption in rats. *J Drug Target* 2002. **10**(1): p. 31–40.

60. Forbes, B. et al., The human bronchial epithelial cell line 16HBE14o- as a model system of the airways for studying drug transport. *Int J Pharm* 2003. **257**(1–2): p. 161–7.

61. Bur, M. et al., Assessment of transport rates of proteins and peptides across primary human alveolar epithelial cell monolayers. *Eur J Pharm Sci* 2006. **28**(3): p. 196–203.

62. Patton, J.S. and P.R. Byron, Inhaling medicines: Delivering drugs to the body through the lungs. *Nat Rev Drug Discov* 2007. **6**(1): p. 67–74.

63. Stigliani, M. et al., Antibiotic transport across bronchial cells: Effects of molecular weight, LogP and apparent permeability. *Eur J Pharm Sci* 2016. **83**: p. 45–51.

64. Rubin, B.K., Experimental macromolecular aerosol therapy. *Respir Care* 2000. **45**(6): p. 684–694.

65. Schanker, L.S., Drug absorption from the lung. *Biochem Pharmacol* 1978. **27**(4): p. 381–385.

66. Ehrhardt, C., Inhalation biopharmaceutics: Progress towards comprehending the fate of inhaled medicines. *Pharm Res* 2017. **34**(12): p. 2451–2453.

67. Effros, R.M. and G.R. Mason, Measurements of pulmonary epithelial permeability in vivo. *Am Rev Respir Dis* 1983. **127**(5 Pt. 2): p. S59–S65.

68. Brown, R.A., Jr. and L.S. Schanker, Absorption of aerosolized drugs from the rat lung. *Drug Metab Dispos* 1983. **11**(4): p. 355–360.

69. Schanker, L.S., E.W. Mitchell, and R.A. Brown, Jr., Species comparison of drug absorption from the lung after aerosol inhalation or intratracheal injection. *Drug Metab Dispos* 1986. **14**(1): p. 79–88.

70. Berg, M.M. et al., Hydrophilic solute transport across rat alveolar epithelium. *J Appl Physiol* 1989. **66**: p. 2320–2327.

71. Goodman, M.R. et al., Ultrastructural evidence of transport of secretory IgA across bronchial epithelium. *Am Rev Respir Dis* 1981. **123**: p. 115–119.

72. Kim, K.-J. and E.D. Crandall, Heteropore populations of bullfrog alveolar epithelium. *J Appl Physiol* 1983. **54**: p. 140–146.

73. Elbert, K.J. et al., Monolayers of human alveolar epithelial cells in primary culture for pulmonary absorption and transport studies. *Pharm Res* 1999. **16**(5): p. 601–608.

74. Sporty, J.L., L. Horalkova, and C. Ehrhardt, In vitro cell culture models for the assessment of pulmonary drug disposition. *Expert Opin Drug Met* 2008. **4**(4): p. 333–345.

75. Murata, M. et al., Carrier-mediated lung distribution of HSR-903, a new quinolone antibacterial agent. *J Pharmacol Exp Ther* 1999. **289**(1): p. 79–84.

76. Gumbleton, M. et al., Targeting caveolae for vesicular drug transport. *J Control Release* 2003. **87**(1–3): p. 139–151.

77. Ehrhardt, C. et al., Salbutamol is actively absorbed across human bronchial epithelial cell layers. *Pulm Pharmacol Ther* 2005. **18**(3): p. 165–170.

78. Ehrhardt, C. et al., Current progress toward a better understanding of drug disposition within the lungs: Summary proceedings of the first workshop on drug transporters in the lungs. *J Pharm Sci* 2017. **106**(9): p. 2234–2244.

79. Gumbleton, M. et al., Spatial expression and functionality of drug transporters in the intact lung: Objectives for further research. *Adv Drug Deliv Rev* 2011. **63**(1–2): p. 110–118.

80. van der Deen, M. et al., ATP-binding cassette (ABC) transporters in normal and pathological lung. *Respir Res* 2005. **20**(6): p. 59.

81. Miyama, T. et al., P-glycoprotein-mediated transport of itraconazole across the blood-brain barrier. *Antimicrob Agents Chemother* 1998. **42**(7): p. 1738–1744.

82. Parvez, M.M. et al., Evaluation of para-Aminosalicylic acid as a substrate of multiple solute carrier uptake transporters and possible drug interactions with nonsteroidal anti-inflammatory drugs in vitro. *Antimicrob Agents Chemother* 2017. **61**(5).

83. Peters, J. et al., Clarithromycin is absorbed by an intestinal uptake mechanism that is sensitive to major inhibition by rifampicin: Results of a short-term drug interaction study in foals. *Drug Metab Dispos* 2012. **40**(3): p. 522–528.

84. Gabrielsson, J. and D. Weiner, *PK/PD Data Analysis: Concepts and Applications*. 3rd ed 2000, Stockholm, Sweden: Swedish Pharmaceutical Press.

85. Garcia-Arieta, A., A European perspective on orally inhaled products: In vitro requirements for a biowaiver. *J Aerosol Med Pulm Drug Deliv* 2014. **27**(6): p. 419–429.

86. Döring, G. et al., Treatment of lung infection in patients with cystic fibrosis: Current and future strategies. *J Cyst Fibros* 2012. **11**(6): p. 461–479.

87. García-Contreras, L., In vivo models for controlled release pulmonary drug delivery, in *Controlled Pulmonary Drug Delivery*, H.D. Smyth and A.J. Hickey, Editors. 2011, Springer Science and Business Media, LLC: New York, p. 443–474.

88. Sakagami, M., In vivo, in vitro and ex vivo models to assess pulmonary absorption and disposition of inhaled therapeutics for systemic delivery. *Adv Drug Deliv Rev* 2006. 58: p. 1030–1060.

89. Fernandes, C.A. and R. Vanbever, Preclinical models for pulmonary drug delivery. *Expert Opin Drug Deliv* 2009. **6**(11): p. 1231–1245.

90. Guillon, A. et al., Insights on animal models to investigate inhalation therapy: Relevance for biotherapeutics. *Int J Pharm* 2018. **536**(1): p. 116–126.

91. Cook, M.J. *The Anatomy of the Laboratory Mouse*. 1965, London, UK: Academic Press. p. 51–53.

92. FCIT, Florida Center for Instructional Technology. Human lungs. The Florida Center for Instructional Technology, College of Education, University of South Florida. https://etc.usf.edu/clipart/. Accessed May 15, 2018.

93. Pokusay, A. *Lungs of the Dog Vector Illustration*. Medical veterinary illustrations. 2018 [Publisher: 123RF, LLC Chicago, IL. https://www.123rf.com/ photo 46796442. cited 2018 May 15, 2018].

94. Samiksha, S. *Respiratory System: Useful Notes on Respiratory System of Different Animals*. http://www.yourarticlelibrary.com/respiration/respiratory-system-useful-notes-on-respiratory-system-of-different-animals/23265 2018 [cited 2018 May 15, 2018].

95. Phalen, R.F. and M.J. Oldham, Airway structures: Tracheobronchial airway structure as revealed by casting techniques. *Am Rev Respir Dis* 1983. **128**(2): p. s1–s4.

96. Tyler, W.S., Small Airways and Terminal Units: Comparative Subgross Anatomy of Lungs. *Am Rev Respir Dis* 1983. **128**(2): p. s32–s36.

97. Alexander, D.J. et al., Association of inhalation toxicologists (AIT) working party recommendation for standard delivered dose calculation and expression in non-Clinical aerosol inhalation toxicology studies with pharmaceuticals. *Inhal Toxicol* 2008. **20**(13): p. 1179–1189.

98. Fioni, A. et al., Investigation of lung pharmacokinetic of the novel PDE4 Inhibitor CHF6001 in preclinical models: Evaluation of the preciselnhale technology. *J Aerosol Med Pulm Drug Deliv* 2018. **31**(1): p. 61–70.

99. Garcia-Contreras, L. et al., Inhaled large porous particles of capreomycin for treatment of tuberculosis in a guinea pig model. *Antimicrob Agents Chemother* 2007. **51**(8): p. 2830–2836.

100. Kipnis, E., Using urea as an endogenous marker of bronchoalveolar lavage dilution. *Crit Care Med* 2005. **33**(9): p. 2153.

101. Hsu, M.C.-P. and J.P.F. Bai, Investigation into the presence of insulin-degrading enzyme in culture type II alveolar cells and the effects of enzyme inhibitors on pulmonary bioavailability of insulin in rats. *J Pharm Pharmacol* 1998. **50**: p. 507–514.

102. Toyama, K., H. Furuie, and H. Ishizuka, Intrapulmonary pharmacokinetics of laninamivir, a neuraminidase inhibitor, after a single nebulized administration of laninamivir octanoate in healthy Japanese subjects. *Antimicrob Agents Chemother* 2018. **62**(1).

103. Jacobson, G.A. et al., Bronchopulmonary pharmacokinetics of (R)-salbutamol and (S)-salbutamol enantiomers in pulmonary epithelial lining fluid and lung tissue of horses. *Br J Clin Pharmacol* 2017. **83**(7): p. 1436–1445.

104. de la Pena, A., P. Liu, and H. Derendorf, Microdialysis in peripheral tissues. *Adv Drug Deliv Rev* 2000. **45**(2–3): p. 189–216.

105. Garcia-Contreras, L. et al., Pharmacokinetics of ethionamide delivered in spray-dried microparticles to the lungs of guinea pigs. *J Pharm Sci* 2017. **106**(1): p. 331–337.

106. Garcia-Contreras, L. et al., Evaluation of novel particles as pulmonary delivery systems for insulin in rats. *AAPS PharmSci* 2003. **5**(2): p. E9.

107. Garcia Contreras, L. et al., Pharmacokinetics of inhaled rifampicin porous particles for tuberculosis treatment: Insight into rifampicin absorption from the lungs of guinea pigs. *Mol Pharm* 2015. **12**(8): p. 2642–2650.

108. Yanez, J.A. et al., Flip-flop pharmacokinetics--delivering a reversal of disposition: Challenges and opportunities during drug development. *Ther Deliv* 2011. **2**(5): p. 643–672.

109. Newman, S.P. and I.R. Wilding, Gamma scintigraphy: In vivo technique for assessing the equivalence of inhaled products. *Int. J. Pharm* 1998. **170** p. 1–9.

110. Batrakova, E.V. et al., Effects of pluronic and doxorubicin on drug uptake, cellular metabolism, apoptosis and tumor inhibition in animal models of MDR cancers. *J Control Release* 2010. **143**(3): p. 290–301.

111. Gagnadoux, F. et al., Safety of pulmonary administration of gemcitabine in rats. *J Aerosol Med* 2005. **18**(2): p. 198–206.

112. Richter, T. et al., Effects of posture on regional pulmonary blood flow in rats as measured by PET. *J Appl Physiol* 2010. **108**(2): p. 422–429.

113. Deshpande, D.S. et al., Gamma scintigraphic evaluation of a miniaturized AERx pulmonary delivery system for aerosol delivery to anesthetized animals using a positive pressure ventilation system. *J Aerosol Med* 2005. **18**(1): p. 34–44.

114. Gagnadoux, F. et al., Gemcitabine aerosol: In vitro antitumor activity and deposition imaging for preclinical safety assessment in baboons. *Cancer Chemother Pharmacol* 2006. **58**(2): p. 237–244.

115. Khanna, C. et al., Nebulized interleukin 2 liposomes: Aerosol characteristics and biodistribution. *J Pharm Pharmacol* 1997. **49**(10): p. 960–971.

116. Kreyling, W.G. et al., Anatomic localization of 24– and 96–h particle retention in canine airways. *J Appl Physiol* 1999. **87**(1): p. 269–284.

117. Young, B.C. et al., Toxic pneumonitis caused by inhalation of hydrocarbon waterproofing spray in two dogs. *J Am Vet Med Assoc* 2007. **23**(1): p. 74–78.

118. Dolovich, M.B., Measuring total and regional lung deposition using inhaled radiotracers. *J Aerosol Med* 2001. **14** (Suppl 1): p. S35–S44.

119. Thorsson, L. et al., Pharmacokinetics and systemic effects of inhaled fluticasone propionate in healthy subjects. *Br J Clin Pharmacol* 1997. **43**(2): p. 155–161.

120. Nair, A. et al., Comparative lung bioavailability of fluticasone/salmeterol via a breath-actuated spacer and conventional plastic spacers. *Eur J Clin Pharmacol* 2011. **67**(4): p. 355–363.

121. Bennett, J.A., T.W. Harrison, and A.E. Tattersfield, The contribution of the swallowed fraction of an inhaled dose of salmeterol to it systemic effects. *Eur Respir J* 1999. **13**(2): p. 445–448.

122. Kempsford, R. et al., Comparison of the systemic pharmacodynamic effects and pharmacokinetics of salmeterol delivered by CFC propellant and non-CFC propellant metered dose inhalers in healthy subjects. *Respir Med* 2005. 99 Suppl A: p. S11–S119.

123. Daley-Yates, P.T. et al., Pharmacokinetics and pharmacodynamics of fluticasone propionate and salmeterol delivered as a combination dry powder from a capsule-based inhaler and a multidose inhaler in asthma and COPD patients. *J Aerosol Med Pulm Drug Deliv* 2014. **27**(4): p. 279–289.

124. Quinn, D. et al., Pharmacodynamics, pharmacokinetics and safety of revefenacin (TD-4208), a long-acting muscarinic antagonist, in patients with chronic obstructive pulmonary disease (COPD): Results of two randomized, double-blind, phase 2 studies. *Pulm Pharmacol Ther* 2018. **48**: p. 71–79.

125. Moustafa, I.O.F. et al., Lung deposition and systemic bioavailability of different aerosol devices with and without humidification in mechanically ventilated patients. *Heart Lung* 2017. **46**(6): p. 464–467.

126. Blake, K. et al., Bioavailability of inhaled fluticasone propionate via chambers/masks in young children. *Eur Respir J* 2012. **39**(1): p. 97–103.

127. Mehta, R. et al., Systemic exposures of fluticasone propionate and salmeterol following inhalation via metered dose inhaler with the mini spacer compared with the aerochamber plus spacer. *J Aerosol Med Pulm Drug Deliv* 2016. **29**(4): p. 386–92.

128. Algorta, J. et al., Pharmacokinetic bioequivalence of two inhaled tiotropium bromide formulations in healthy volunteers. *Clin Drug Investig* 2016. **36**(9): p. 753–762.

129. Small, C.J. and M. Gillespie, Pharmacokinetics of beclomethasone dipropionate delivered by breath-actuated inhaler and metered-dose inhaler in healthy subjects. *J Aerosol Med Pulm Drug Deliv* 2017. **31**(3): p. 182–190.

130. Kirjavainen, M. et al., Pharmacokinetics of salmeterol and fluticasone propionate delivered in combination via easyhaler and diskus dry powder inhalers in healthy subjects. *J Aerosol Med Pulm Drug Deliv* 2018. **31**(5): p. 290–297.

131. Brown, L.K., Static lung volumes: Functional residual capacity, residual volume and total lung capacity, in *Pulmonary Function Tests in Clinical and Occupational Lung Disease*, A.L. Miller, Editor 1986, Grune and Stratton: Orlando, FL. p. 77–114.

132. Sheldon, R.L., Pulmonary function testing, in *Clinical Assessment in Respiratory Care*, R.L. Wilkins et al., Editors. 2000, Mosby: St. Louis, MO. p. 144–155.

133. Hussein, R.R.S. et al., In vitro/in vivo correlation and modeling of emitted dose and lung deposition of inhaled salbutamol from metered dose inhalers with different types of spacers in noninvasively ventilated patients. *Pharm Dev Technol* 2017. **22**(7): p. 871–880.

134. Rabea, H. et al., Modelling of in-vitro and in-vivo performance of aerosol emitted from different vibrating mesh nebulisers in non-invasive ventilation circuit. *Eur J Pharm Sci* 2017. **97**: p. 182–191.

135. Blake, K. et al., Population pharmacodynamic model of bronchodilator response to inhaled albuterol in children and adults with asthma. *Chest* 2008. **134**(5): p. 981–989.

136. Melin, J. et al., Pharmacokinetics of the inhaled selective glucocorticoid receptor modulator AZD5423 following inhalation using different devices. *Aaps j* 2017. **19**(3): p. 865–874.

137. Liu, T. et al., Budesonide nanocrystal-loaded hyaluronic acid microparticles for inhalation: In vitro and in vivo evaluation. *Carbohydr Polym* 2018. **181**: p. 1143–1152.

138. Melin, J. et al., Pharmacokinetics of the inhaled selective glucocorticoid receptor modulator AZD5423 following inhalation using different devices. *The AAPS J* 2017. **19** (3): p. 865–874.

139. Mehta, R. et al., Systemic exposures of fluticasone propionate and salmeterol following inhalation via metered dose inhaler with the mini spacer compared with the aerochamber plus spacer. *J Aerosol Med Pulm Drug Deliv* 2016. **29**(4): p. 386–392.

140. Goyal, N. et al., Population pharmacokinetics of inhaled umeclidinium and vilanterol in patients with chronic obstructive pulmonary disease. *Clin Pharmacokinet* 2014. **53**(7): p. 637–648.

141. Kelleher, D. et al., A randomized, placebo- and moxifloxacin-controlled thorough QT study of umeclidinium monotherapy and umeclidinium/vilanterol combination in healthy subjects. *Pulm Pharmacol Ther* 2014. **29**(1): p. 49–57.

142. Droebner, K. et al., Pharmacodynamics, pharmacokinetics, and antiviral activity of BAY 81–8781, a Novel NF-kappaB inhibiting anti-influenza drug. *Front Microbiol* 2017. **8**: p. 2130.

143. Duret, C. et al., Pharmacokinetic evaluation in mice of amorphous itraconazole-based dry powder formulations for inhalation with high bioavailability and extended lung retention. *Eur J Pharm Biopharm* 2014. **86**(1): p. 46–54.

144. Gaspar, M.C. et al., Pulmonary pharmacokinetics of levofloxacin in rats after aerosolization of immediate-release chitosan or sustained-release PLGA microspheres. *Eur J Pharm Sci* 2016. **93**: p. 184–191.

145. Malinin, V. et al., Pulmonary deposition and elimination of liposomal amikacin for inhalation and effect on macrophage function after administration in rats. *Antimicrob Agents Chemother* 2016. **60**(11): p. 6540–6549.

146. Lin, Y.W. et al., Pulmonary pharmacokinetics of colistin following administration of dry powder aerosols in rats. *Antimicrob Agents Chemother* 2017. **61**(11).

147. Wang, X. et al., Population pharmacokinetics of tobramycin inhalation solution in pediatric patients with cystic fibrosis. *J Pharm Sci* 2017. **106**(11): p. 3402–3409.

148. Geller, D.E. et al., Novel tobramycin inhalation powder in cystic fibrosis subjects: Pharmacokinetics and safety. *Pediatr Pulmonol* 2007. **42**(4): p. 307–313.

149. Geller, D.E. et al., Pharmacokinetics and bioavailability of aerosolized tobramycin in cystic fibrosis. *Chest* 2002. **122**(1): p. 219–226.

150. Miller, J.L. et al., Detectable concentrations of inhaled tobramycin in critically Ill children without cystic fibrosis: Should routine monitoring be recommended? *Pediatr Crit Care Med* 2017. **18**(12): p. e615–e620.

151. Heinemann, L. et al., Pharmacokinetic and pharmacodynamic properties of a novel inhaled insulin. *J Diabetes Sci Technol* 2017. **11**(1): p. 148–156.

152. Adjei, A. and J. Garren, Pulmonary delivery of peptide drugs: Effect of particle size on bioavailability of leuprolide acetate in healthy male volunteers. *Pharm Res* 1990. **7**(6): p. 565–569.

153. Adjei, A. et al., Pulmonary bioavailability of leuprolide acetate following multiple dosing to beagle dogs: Some pharmacokinetics and preclinical issues. *Int. J. Pharm* 1994. **104**: p. 57–66.

154. Al-Tabakha, M.M., Future prospect of insulin inhalation for diabetic patients: The case of afrezza versus exubera. *J Control Release* 2015. **215**: p. 25–38.

155. Thompson, J.P. and D.F. Thompson, Nebulized fentanyl in acute pain: A systematic review. *Ann Pharmacother* 2016. **50**(10): p. 882–891.

156. Fernando, D. et al., Safety, Tolerability and pharmacokinetics of single doses of oxytocin administered via an inhaled route in healthy females: Randomized, single-blind, phase 1 study. *EBioMedicine* 2017. **22**: p. 249–255.

157. Ruppel, D. et al., A population dose-response model for inhaled technosphere insulin administered to healthy subjects. *CPT Pharmacometrics Syst Pharmacol* 2017. **6**(6): p. 365–372.

158. FDA, United States Food and Drug Administration, *Guidance for Industry: Bioequivalence Studies with Pharmacokinetic Endpoints for Drugs Submitted Under an ANDA* U.S. Department of Health and Human Services, Editor 2013, Food and Drug Administration; Center for Drug Evaluation and Research (CDER) Silver Spring, MD.

159. Mehta, R. et al., Pharmacokinetics of fluticasone propionate and salmeterol delivered as a combination dry powder via a capsule-based inhaler and a multi-dose inhaler. *Pulm Pharmacol Ther* 2014. **29**(1): pp. 66–73.

160. CHMP, Committee for Medicinal Products for Human Use, *Guideline on the Investigation of Bioequivalence*, E.M. Agency, Editor 2010, European Medicines Agency: London, UK.

161. Hastedt, J. et al., Scope and relevance of a pulmonary biopharmaceutical classification system AAPS/FDA/USP workshop march 16th–17th, 2015 in Baltimore, MD. *AAPS Open* 2017. **2**(1): p. doi 10.1186/s41120-015-0002-x.

162. Amidon, G.L. et al., A theoretical basis for a biopharmaceutic drug classification: The correlation of in vitro drug product dissolution and in vivo bioavailability. *Pharm Res* 1995. **12**(3): p. 413–420.

6

3D models as tools for inhaled drug development

SALLY-ANN CRYAN, JENNIFER LORIGAN, AND CIAN O'LEARY

Introduction	107
Current preclinical models used in the development of drugs for inhalation and their limitations	107
In vitro cell culture models and ex vivo models	108
Animal models	109
Three-dimensional culture platforms for respiratory drug development	110
Scaffold biomaterial-based platforms	111
Spheroid-based platforms	112

Microfluidic-based platforms	112
Three-dimensional culture models of respiratory disease	114
Chronic obstructive pulmonary disease	114
Cystic fibrosis	115
Other diseases	115
Opportunities and challenges for 3D models for the translation of inhaled drug therapies	115
References	116

INTRODUCTION

Respiratory drug delivery and development have been slowed by a lack of anatomically and physiologically relevant in vitro models of the respiratory tract. The human respiratory tract contains 50 different cell types along its hierarchical structure in the conducting (the tracheobronchial and bronchiolar regions) and the respiratory (alveolar region) zones. Within the tracheobronchial region alone, a pseudostratified epithelial layer composed of three main cell types—ciliated epithelial cells, goblet cells, and basal cells—is supported by the extracellular matrix (ECM) of pulmonary interstitium and cartilage in a macroscopically and microscopically specific three-dimensional (3D) arrangement. Equally, the alveolar region is a complex mix of cell types and ECM. In contrast, common in vitro models often consist of two-dimensional (2D) monolayers of a single epithelial cell line cultured on a semipermeable polyester membrane at an air-liquid interface (ALI). These models often fail to capture the key multicellular, disease-specific ECM composition and/or mechanical stretch associated with respiration to fully represent the in vivo organization of the healthy or diseased human lungs that thereby limits their utility during drug development. Animal models have been the most prominent tools used to provide pharmacokinetic and pharmacodynamic information that is not attainable with in vitro models. There is an increasing awareness, however, that the interspecies structural and physiological differences between animal models and human lungs can limit their predictive capacity. Inadequate data obtained from the use of current in vitro models can increase the risk of drug candidate/formulation failure in in vivo preclinical or clinical studies due to poor in vitro–in vivo correlation (IVIVC), culminating in great expense and time lost that delay the development process of new medicines. In addition, the ethical drive to reduce dependence on animal testing for drug research purposes means that there are both sound scientific and ethical reasons to improve the in vitro cell models available to the respiratory medicine research community. The need for improved models therefore is driven by (1) the desire for reduction, refinement, and replacement of animal models in research; and (2) the need to establish improved IVIVCs for inhalation toxicology to provide more complete and/ or ineffective preclinical assessment.

CURRENT PRECLINICAL MODELS USED IN THE DEVELOPMENT OF DRUGS FOR INHALATION AND THEIR LIMITATIONS

Current preclinical models for respiratory drug discovery and development consist of a range of in vitro, ex vivo, and in vivo approaches that aim to obtain valuable data on aspects of drug deposition, absorption, efficacy, and toxicity (1). Traditionally, in vitro cell culture models grow cells on tissue culture plastic or polymer membrane cell inserts as a single layer of cells (2D culture) (2). These models are an invaluable tool in many areas of biomedical science, including the initial stages of drug discovery where fundamental pharmacological and toxicological endpoints are being investigated and can often enable high-throughput screening of potential drug candidates. Animal models are currently an essential preclinical step in assessing the safety and efficacy of new drugs or formulations. The utilization of an *in vivo* model addresses the issues of oversimplification inherent in 2D models. Although each model has its own advantages and disadvantages, an examination of their major limitations assists in highlighting key problems that need to be addressed and identifying how advanced 3D respiratory culture models could address some of these unmet needs.

In vitro cell culture models and *ex vivo* models

Respiratory *in vitro* cell culture models include a range of immortalized cell lines and primary respiratory cells utilized for mechanistic, drug transport, and toxicity studies. Ideally, a cell culture model should offer a less resource-intensive and more high-throughput method for drug development than an *in vivo* alternative, while at the same time faithfully representing *in vivo* behavior. However, developing a model that meets all of these criteria poses a significant technical challenge.

The most basic form of 2D culture model involves culture of a single cell type. The European Collection of Authenticated Cell Cultures (ECACC) and the American Type Culture Collection (ATCC) contain thousands of cell lines representative of a range of tissue types and genetic disorders (3,4). An advantage of cell lines in basic research is that, unlike patient- or animal-derived primary cells, the production of steadily proliferating and phenotypically stable cells is standardized, which in turn facilitates consistency in assay design and a subsequent improvement in comparison between respiratory drug candidates (2). They are also more readily available than donor primary cells, facilitating larger sample sizes and a greater range of test groups. Therefore, cell lines are an important tool in testing a new or repurposed drug, in assessing how cells respond to a new system, or in answering basic biological questions of cell function or disease states.

Respiratory cell lines have been predominantly derived from either lung carcinoma or from virally transformed epithelial cells (Table 6.1). For the respiratory epithelium, bronchial cells are a popular candidate, based on their propensity for tight junction formation (5) and the secretion of an apical mucous layer, similar to *in vivo* secretions (6). The bronchial cell line 16HBE14o-, for example, has been shown

Table 6.1 Prominent epithelial cell sources for respiratory cell culture models

Cell type	Features	Studies
Bronchial cell lines		
16HBE14o-	Transformed bronchial cell line Tight junction formation Limited ciliation and mucus secretion	(5,7,8,13,14)
BEAS-2B	Transformed bronchial cell line Cytochrome P450 metabolic activity Lack tight junctions, ciliation, and mucus secretion	(15,16)
Calu-3	Derived from adenocarcinoma of the lung Tight junction formation and mucus secretion Limited ciliation	(9,17–19)
Bronchiolar cell lines		
NCI-H441	Derived from adenocarcinoma of the lung Tight junction formation post-dexamethasone stimulation Limited ciliation	(11,12,20)
Alveolar cell lines		
A549	Derived from adenocarcinoma of the lung Surfactant secretion Potential for tight junction formation	(21–23)
Primary cells		
NHBE cells	Obtained from tracheobronchial tissue Tight junction formation, mucus secretion, and ciliation Donor variability and limited passage number	(24,25)
MatTek EpiAirway® Epithelix MucilAir® Epithelix SmallAir®	Specialized primary cell culture models Tight junction formation, mucus secretion, and ciliation Long lifespan Expensive	(26–28)

to form physiologically comparable tight junctions, making it an important tool for the investigation of drug transport (7,8), while Calu-3 cells, capable of mucin–production, are valuable in assessing drug transport and inflammatory responses (9,10). As the alveolar region represents both an attractive candidate site for aerosolized drug absorption and is the target site for a number of respiratory diseases, alveolar cell models have also been developed (11,12).

However, the properties that make cell lines such valuable tools also limit their utility. The immortalized nature of cell lines means that they can be grown more rapidly and used for greater periods than can patient-derived primary cells, but they may not replicate the behavior and responses of native tissue (6,29). Two-dimensional monoculture cell line models display limited recapitulation of full *in vivo* conditions, without the mechanical influences, global and local metabolism, and reciprocal relationships with other cell types that are present *in vivo*; as a result, 2D cell line models may not be reliable predictors of *in vivo* response or absorption (30).

As a result of these limitations, efforts have increased to optimize the use of primary respiratory cells that can display the organotypic characteristics of the *in vivo* epithelium. This also facilitates direct comparison of healthy and diseased cell types, without the confounding effects of immortalization. However, inter-donor variability poses an issue, creating the need for large sample sizes to promote accuracy, their availability and cost, and the requirement for complex culture conditions and the rapid de-differentiation of primary cells *in vitro* also pose ongoing challenges to their application in drug development.

Many *in vitro* respiratory models of both cell lines and primary cells are cultured on cell insert systems that can facilitate the growth of epithelial cells at an air-liquid interface (ALI), better mimicking the lung environment (26,31), and ALI culture has been found to induce cell polarization, differentiation, and mucus production (6,18,32). These cell insert cultures are sometimes referred to as 3D cultures and can support co-culture of different cell types on opposite sides of a membrane. In modeling the respiratory tract, epithelial cells can be co-cultured with other cells from the relevant region, for example, immune cells, providing a better mimic of the *in vivo* environment (5,11,18,23) and can potentially provide improved physiological responses over monoculture systems in response to aerosolized particles (32). However, the cell insert membranes between the cells, generally composed of polycarbonate (PC) and polyethylene terephthalate (PET), although permeable, prevent formation of an integrated interface and prohibit full cellular cross-talk. Furthermore, while some regions of the respiratory epithelium constitute a monolayer, a single cell-type monolayer does not reflect the *in vivo* situation, limiting the physiological accuracy of results. Although these cell insert models are a valuable tool for drug transport studies (6), their simplicity means that they are not a reliable tool for investigating toxicity in depth because they lack a native immune response (32,33).

The development of innovative methods for creating/harnessing effective human tissue models and excised human tissue models such as the lung slice model and the *ex vivo* lung perfusion model (EVLP) could improve predictive assessment of drug compounds and materials in humans (34,35). Excised human tissue models have obvious advantages, including the presence of multiple airway cell types arranged in the required spatial pattern within an appropriate respiratory tract ECM structure, better mimicking the natural environment to improve cell proliferation and differentiation. A number of agencies are actively cataloging these alternative animal-free methods for *in vitro* assessment (34). The major limitation for models, of course, is the limit in availability of human tissue/lungs, which makes these models difficult to scale up for drug development purposes.

Animal models

Animal models have been the most prominent biological tools used to provide pharmacokinetic and pharmacodynamic information for respiratory drug development to date. Promising drugs are usually investigated through a series of animal models of increasing physiological similarity to humans. Rodents are typically used in the first phase of animal studies, and indeed a wide range of imaging and molecular technologies can be used for mouse, rat, and guinea pig models (36,37). However, small animals can present issues as a result of their size. There is a limitation to the volumes of blood, urine, and tissue which can be extracted for pharmacokinetic analyses. The anatomy and physiology of small animals also presents difficulties in terms of dose administration. To address more complex questions, larger animals, such as dogs, sheep, and nonhuman primates have also been used in testing aerosolized drugs. However, while it is argued that such animals constitute a more physiologically relevant mimic of humans, larger animals also present difficulties in drug development. Logistical constraints such as housing and handling, as well as ethical concerns, limit the number of large animals which can be used in a given study (38). Larger animal studies, therefore, often lack the statistical power of small animal studies.

While animal models can provide pharmacokinetic and pharmacodynamic information that might not be currently attainable with *in vitro* models, some animal species used in preclinical testing are not always suitable for human respiratory drug research because of interspecies structural and physiological differences. Branching divisions within the respiratory tract and the relative position of the right and left main bronchi are not equivalent between humans and common animal models; as a result, the assessment of drug disposition in animals can inaccurately reflect that in humans and have consequences for reliable estimation of tracheobronchial and alveolar drug/material exposure (36,39). Early-stage screening methods in small animals such as endotracheal delivery may produce artificial toxicological and pharmacological effects, while simultaneously bypassing the upper airway (40–42). Nose-only exposure chambers (43,44) and the whole-body exposure chambers (45) can provide more information about the effect the drug may have more broadly on airway tissues post-inhalation.

Immunological differences between species are perhaps of even more significance. Novel treatments for asthma that showed promise in animal studies, for example, have failed when brought forward to clinical trials. For example, extreme systemic inflammatory responses occurred in human volunteers to novel agents when they were originally safe in animals, in the tragic case of the phase I trial of TGN1412. This discordance between inflammatory pathways and the immune system between rodents and humans is clearly evident in the lack of a model that efficiently demonstrates the respiratory pathophysiology of respiratory diseases such as asthma and cystic fibrosis. The shortcomings in these models are reflected in the attrition rate of candidate drugs proposed for clinical use, with only 7.5% of investigational new drugs obtaining approval after Phase III clinical trials (46). It is clear that there is an unmet need for improved tools for the clinical and commercial translation of inhaled medicines. The need for improved models therefore is driven by (1) the desire for reduction, refinement, and replacement of animal models in research; and (2) the need to establish improved IVIVCs for inhalation toxicology to provide more complete and/or effective preclinical assessment.

THREE-DIMENSIONAL CULTURE PLATFORMS FOR RESPIRATORY DRUG DEVELOPMENT

Three-dimensional models in which cells can grow in multiple directions are well-poised to fill the current gap between *in vitro* 2D work and *in vivo* work. They overcome several of the shortcomings presented by 2D models, while delaying and potentially reducing the use of animal models until a more advanced stage of the project. Cells in a 3D system can signal and influence each other in a more physiologically realistic way than cells growing in monoculture. Among other shortcomings, cells cultured on polymeric inserts lack an extracellular matrix; this oversimplification may affect the rate of drug uptake (47,48). Cells cultured on polymeric inserts also

show phenotypic alterations, with proliferation rates, protein expression, and differentiation varying between different compositions of natural and synthetic polymers (31,49–51). Furthermore, in 3D platforms, different cell types can be grown on different components of a system, mimicking cellular stratification *in vivo*. Different microenvironments can be created to reflect the requirements of different cell types and to promote a more physiologically relevant response. Mechanical stimuli can also be introduced if appropriate. These amendments could provide more physiologically accurate data about novel compounds and drug formulations before progressing to *in vivo* testing (26).

Three-dimensional models may also address some of the issues encountered in animal testing. They represent a more gradual transition from the 2D environment to an animal model and can support the use of human cells that may provide more detailed information about the inflammatory response and localized reactions to the candidate drug and drug formulations before moving into more complex, less controlled systems *in vivo*.

Although 3D models do not represent a perfect solution to all current issues with respiratory models, they show great potential as a tool to refine drug and drug formulation studies in an environment more complex than 2D culture systems, and they are potentially more reflective of the human response than animal models. Such a tool would reduce the cost and time investment associated with candidate drug investigations and enable drug formulation and the delivery process to be better refined at an earlier stage of development than is currently possible.

The three main types of 3D culture platforms under current investigation for inhaled drug development are scaffold biomaterial-based systems, spheroid culture systems, and microfluidic chip systems (Figure 6.1). Scaffold systems and microfluidic lung-on-a-chip platforms have been the subject of much interest because of the opportunities to alter the composition of the polymeric substrate for cell culture in conjunction with ALI culture (52,53), while spheroids have garnered interest as models of disease (54). In the following sections, the principal characteristics of each platform will be outlined, with reference to appropriate examples.

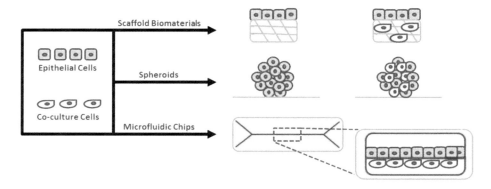

Figure 6.1 3D culture platforms for respiratory drug development. Epithelial cells are cultured with or without other cells in co-culture such as fibroblasts or endothelial cells on polymeric scaffold biomaterial substrates, as spheroid cell aggregates, or in microfluidic chip systems with fluid-flow chambers.

Scaffold biomaterial-based platforms

Scaffold biomaterials are traditionally the main platform for 3D respiratory culture models. The biomaterials employed are typically composed of natural polymeric materials (e.g., collagen), donor extracellular matrix (decellularized [DC] tissue), synthetic polymeric materials (e.g., poly-ε-caprolactone [PCL]), and composites of synthetic and natural materials (55). Although hydrogel-based platforms surged in popularity in the early twenty-first century, porous polymeric scaffolds were among the first 3D airway models (56,57). Today, multiple varieties of hydrogels, porous polymeric scaffolds, and DC tissue are evident in the literature. In tandem with these models, a plethora of tissue-engineering fabrication techniques that can reproducibly control parameters such as porosity and mechanical rigidity have been employed to facilitate control of cellular infiltration, differentiation, and behavior (58,59). This is of particular note for respiratory modeling, as varying the properties of the scaffold can facilitate modeling of the distinct anatomical regions of the lungs.

Hydrogels have historically been the most commonly investigated biomaterial for tracheobronchial modeling. Hydrogels are two- or multicomponent systems consisting of a network of polymer chains and water that fills the space between macromolecules in a state of dynamic equilibrium (60). Models of the tracheobronchial respiratory tract consist of epithelial cells cultured on a cell-free gel substrate or as a set gel suspension containing fibroblasts and other submucosal cells. Alveolar hydrogel platforms utilize the surrounding pliable matrix of the gel environment to permit the growth of alveolar buds embedded within them that express markers of type I and type II alveolar epithelial cells (61–63). This property of gel matrices has been reported as early as the 1980s with the use of Matrigel®, a reconstituted, sarcoma-derived basement membrane, to produce spherical clusters of fetal rabbit type II alveolar epithelial cells around a central lumen (64).

While hydrogel systems are a dynamic environment with random polymer assembly and arrangement following gelation, DC tissue, by contrast, provides a biomaterial scaffold with an organ-specific architecture that has already been structured by natural morphogenic processes during fetal development and is used following the removal of the antigenic components of the donor tissue (65). In this manner, the *in vivo* tissue structure, relevant natural polymer composition, and embedded growth factors for seeded cells are already tailored for efficient 3D respiratory cell culture. Although DC tissue such as whole lung has been envisaged as a possible alternative for lung transplantation and tissue regeneration in the future (66), the challenges related to the vast quantities of multiple cell types and standardization of tissue quality, storage, and DC methods make this implausible at present (67–71). On the other hand, reseeded DC lungs hold promise as a sophisticated *in vitro* drug development platform that could provide information on drug deposition fate in the lungs following pulmonary administration (72) and analysis of systemic absorption, given that the vascular and airway systems remain intact and independent of each other in the DC organ (73). Additionally, the use of DC tissue slices provides the opportunity for high-throughput screening with the use of a single human or animal donor organ (74).

Porous scaffolds exhibit many similarities to DC tissue matrices but differ in that they can provide more scope for customization of composition and structure. These biomaterials are sponge-like in architecture, where the struts of the pores can provide a framework on which physiological structures such as alveoli can grow (75). Unlike hydrogels and DC tissue, the ability to tailor pore size and interconnectivity in porous scaffolds can provide customizable space for development into the luminal airway and for neovascularization (76–78). Porous polymeric scaffolds also represent an improvement to the *in vitro* representation of the tissue architecture and composition of the tracheobronchial region, creating fibrous structures more similar to tracheobronchial architecture than those produced by hydrogels. In order to recapitulate such architecture, however, porous scaffold models must have a basement membrane analog incorporated into its structure for epithelial monolayer culture at the ALI; this has been achieved through the development of multilayered scaffolds with dense or nanoporous regions that these cells cannot migrate through (53,79,80). The model described by O'Leary et al., for example, consists of a thin 2D film fused to a porous 3D sub-layer for Calu-3 cells that are cultured at an ALI with 3D fibroblast culture in the submucosa (Figure 6.2) (53). Such systems can provide organotypic tissue reconstruction for drug mechanistic, transport, and toxicological studies without the need for a supply of donors or complex tissue preparation.

Scaffold-based biomaterials utilize a variety of natural and synthetic polymers as building blocks for hydrogel and porous platforms. As collagen is a major structural tissue component in the human body (81), it has been particularly popular as a hydrogel constituent. The culture of primary tracheobronchial epithelial cells at the ALI on a type I collagen gel has consistently provided an organotypic pseudostratified epithelium (82–85). The expression of the mucus biomarker MUC5AC, for example (86), is increased when respiratory cells are cultured on collagen-coated substrates (31), verifying its value as a natural substrate. Additionally, epithelial cells grown on collagen-based hydrogels and porous scaffolds show improved tight junction formation, cilia development, and extracellular matrix secretion over 2D models (53,87,88). Matrigel has been utilized for alveolar hydrogel acini formation, as previously mentioned; more refined substrates, such as Gelfoam® (a purified gelatin product) (78); highly porous, lyophilized collagen-glycosaminoglycan scaffolds (76); and a composite of polyglycolic acid (PGA) mesh and Pluronic F127 (PF127) gel (77) have also shown promise for alveolar modeling applications. Other natural polymers and composites that have shown promise for 3D respiratory culture models include chitosan (89), fibrin (90), and hyaluronan (91–93). Overall, natural substrates for scaffold biomaterial platforms have prevailed, although synthetic polymers are of interest to bolster these substrates and increase mechanical integrity during the cell culture period for the assessment of inhaled drug products.

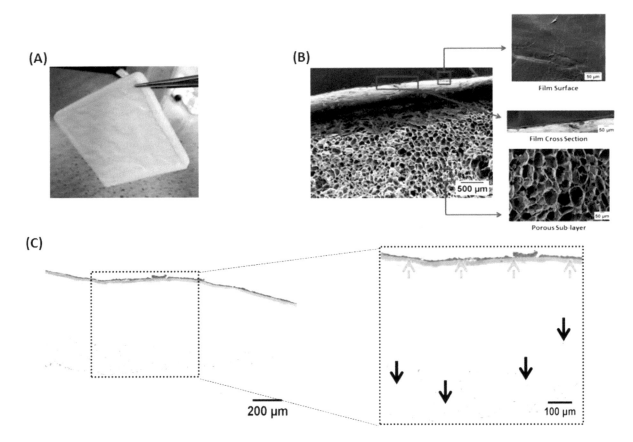

Figure 6.2 Bilayered collagen-hyaluronate scaffolds as a scaffold-based respiratory cell culture platform. (A) A representative macroscopic image of the porous polymeric scaffold. (B) A representative image of scaffold ultrastructure, consisting of a dense film layer and connected porous sub-layer. (C) Respiratory epithelial (blue arrows) and fibroblast (black arrows) co-culture on the scaffold platform. (Adapted from O'Leary, C., et al., *Biomaterials*, 85, 111–127, 2016. With permission from Elsevier [53].)

Spheroid-based platforms

The use of 3D cellular spheroids has gained particular popularity over the last decade. Spheroids are self-assembled aggregates of single or multiple cell types that exhibit 3D shape and extensive cell-cell connections beyond that in 2D culture, with resultant phenotypic features and toxicity responses undetected in conventional culture (94). Originally developed as a means of investigating hypoxia, vascularization, and drug infiltration within tumors (95,96), they have shown promise as models for drug investigation beyond cancer research, as they provide a more accurate recapitulation of *in vivo* extracellular matrices, cytoskeletal arrangement, and cell-cell interactions than 2D cultures (97,98). Methods for producing spheroids include the hanging drop method, use of nonadherent surfaces, micropatterned surfaces, suspension culture, and microfluidic systems (99–103). More recent assembly procedures have been developed for large-scale automated, standardized production of spheroids (98), making them attractive as an intermediate model between 2D cultures and *in vivo* studies for the investigation of novel drugs and drug formulations.

The application of spheroid platforms for respiratory drug discovery and toxicology has not been as extensively investigated as scaffold-based systems; validation studies primarily exist for other applications such as cancer and liver metabolism (104,105). Nevertheless, lung spheroid studies have provided encouraging results. They have been shown to retain characteristics of pseudostratified respiratory epithelia, including ciliation and mucus production (106,107), representing an improvement over 2D culture models. For instance, a recent study by Tan and colleagues combined adult human primary bronchial epithelial cells, lung fibroblasts, and lung microvascular endothelial cells together in multicellular aggregates that were able to recapitulate features of both the tracheobronchial and alveolar respiratory regions (Figure 6.3) (54). With respect to toxicological applications, lung spheroid platforms have been used to assess the safety of reagents employed for EVLP (108), indicating their feasibility as *in vitro* tools for toxicity testing of novel respiratory drugs and formulations.

Microfluidic-based platforms

In the past few years, research into the organ-on-a-chip microfluidic platform technology has significantly

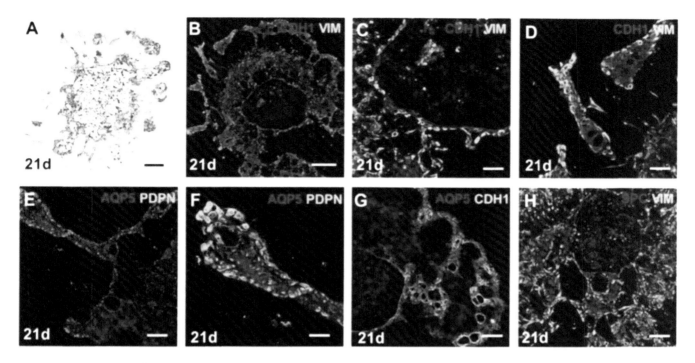

Figure 6.3 Expression of distal lung epithelial lineage markers in airway organoids. **(A)** H&E staining of airway organoid section. **(B–D)** Co-staining of E-cadherin (red) and vimentin (green) reveals diverse architecture of epithelial and mesenchymal compartments within airway organoids at day 21 *in vitro* with low- and high-power imaging. **(E–G)** Type I alveolar epithelial cell markers aquaporin 5 (red) and podoplanin (green) were seen throughout the airway organoids with low- and high-power magnification, as well as with E-cadherin (green) in the airway organoids. **(H)** The type II alveolar epithelial cell surfactant protein C (red) co-staining with Vimentin (green) the airway organoids was also detected. (Adapted from Tan, Q., et al., *Biomaterials*, 113, 118–132, 2017. With permission from Elsevier [54].)

expanded. Novel microfluidic approaches have led to the creation of lung-on-a-chip technology to model the bronchoalveolar region. Chip platforms are microengineered biomimetic systems that represent key functional units of living human organs. They often consist of transparent 3D polymeric microchannels lined by living human cells and replicate three important aspects of intact organs: the 3D microarchitecture defined by the spatial distribution of multiple tissue types; functional tissue–tissue interfaces; and complex organ-specific mechanical and biochemical microenvironments, as reviewed in (109). As such, these systems are more integrated than the 2D models because they provide more detailed information about inflammatory responses and drug uptake (110,111).

The lung-on-a-chip technology is typified by the seminal paper from Huh and colleagues in 2010 (112). Within the chip, two closely apposed microchannels were separated by a thin (10 μm), porous, flexible membrane made of poly(dimethylsiloxane) (PDMS) that was coated with fibronectin or collagen. Human alveolar epithelial cells and human pulmonary microvascular endothelial cells were cultured on opposite sides of this membrane, and an ALI was introduced once cells had reached confluence (Figure 6.4). Mechanical stretch was built into the design to mimic the tidal expansion and collapse of alveoli during breathing; these factors were found to influence cell responses and permeability. Subsequent studies have developed a tracheobronchial version of this platform in addition to the pioneering alveolar-capillary model (113). This co-culture microfluidic model has incorporated similar cells to that seen in scaffold-based and spheroid-based platforms, i.e., epithelial, endothelial, and fibroblast cells, with confirmation of mucociliary differentiation and barrier formation. It might therefore be possible to tailor the lung-on-a-chip to recapitulate different regions of the airway using the lung-on-a-chip approach for novel drug and drug formulation investigation. Indeed, the potential of these 3D culture platforms has been acknowledged to the extent that in April 2017, the Food and Drug Administration (FDA) has committed to invest in this technology to develop tools for drug, food, and cosmetic evaluation.

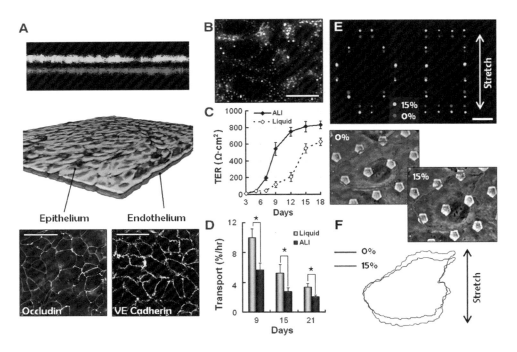

Figure 6.4 On-chip formation and mechanical stretching of an alveolar-capillary interface. (A) Long-term microfluidic coculture produces a tissue-tissue interface consisting of a single layer of the alveolar epithelium (epithelium, stained with CellTracker Green) closely apposed to a monolayer of the microvascular endothelium (endothelium, stained with CellTracker Red), both of which express intercellular junctional structures stained with antibodies to occludin or VE-cadherin, separated by a flexible ECM-coated PDMS membrane. Scale bar, 50 μm. (B) Surfactant production by the alveolar epithelium during air-liquid interface culture in our device detected by cellular uptake of the fluorescent dye quinacrine that labels lamellar bodies (white dots). Scale bar, 25 μm. (C) Air-liquid interface (ALI) culture leads to a greater increase in transbilayer electrical resistance (TER) and produces tighter alveolar-capillary barriers with higher TER (>800 Ω·cm²), as compared with the tissue layers formed under submerged liquid culture conditions. (D) Alveolar barrier permeability measured by quantitating the rate of fluorescent albumin transport is significantly reduced in ALI cultures compared with liquid cultures (*P < 0.001). Data in (C) and (D) represent the mean ± SEM from three separate experiments. (E) Membrane stretching–induced mechanical strain visualized by the displacements of individual fluorescent quantum dots that were immobilized on the membrane in hexagonal and rectangular patterns before (red) and after (green) stretching. Scale bar, 100 μm. (F) Membrane stretching exerts tension on the cells and causes them to distort in the direction of the applied force, as illustrated by the overlaid outlines of a single cell before (blue) and after (red) application of 15% strain. The pentagons in the micrographs represent microfabricated pores in the membrane. Endothelial cells were used for visualization of cell stretching. (Adapted from Huh, D. et al., *Science*, 328, 1662–1668, 2010. Reprinted with permission from AAAS [112].)

THREE-DIMENSIONAL CULTURE MODELS OF RESPIRATORY DISEASE

A key role for 3D culture models in the evolution of drug development is to provide physiologically representative models of disease for effective drug candidate screening at an early stage in the discovery and development process. For respiratory disease, incurable conditions such as asthma, chronic obstructive pulmonary disease (COPD), cystic fibrosis (CF), and idiopathic pulmonary fibrosis (IPF) contribute significantly to an enormous clinical and socioeconomic burden but lack effective preclinical models. COPD, in particular, has been identified as the fourth leading cause of mortality worldwide (114). Survival rates for CF decrease steadily beyond forty years, primarily as a result of death from respiratory causes in 68% of cases (115,116), while for patients diagnosed with IPF, the median survival is approximately 2.5–3.5 years post-diagnosis (117). Additionally, tracheal, bronchial, and other

lung cancers are predicted to become the sixth leading cause of mortality by 2030 (118). This section will outline some of the pertinent lung diseases for which 3D culture platforms can improve the translation of novel therapies into the clinic.

Chronic obstructive pulmonary disease

Chronic obstructive pulmonary disease (COPD) is an umbrella term for several airway diseases that are defined by the presence of chronic airflow limitation that is not fully reversible by clinical intervention (119). The two broad clinical phenotypes for COPD include chronic bronchitis and emphysema, of which research into the latter seeks to prevent alveolar destruction and loss of gas exchange in the lungs as a result of tissue remodeling (120). Therefore, 3D models are well positioned to offer a platform to investigate the structural aspects of the disease.

DC tissue platforms can provide such a structural model of emphysematous lungs. Wagner and colleagues, for example, directly compared healthy and diseased lungs to investigate the effects of different ECM components on cell viability (67). Although proteomic analysis of the tissues revealed no significant differences in composition, respiratory cells seeded onto diseased lungs appeared less adherent than on the healthy counterpart and only lasted around 7 days in culture, which led to the hypothesis that the microarchitectural arrangement of the tissue was influencing cell activity. Microfluidic chips are now being investigated to model COPD in a more high-throughput model for analysis of COPD exacerbations and inflammation (111), paving the way for screening of novel inhalable treatments to reduce the burden of mortality.

Cystic fibrosis

Cystic fibrosis (CF) is an autosomal recessive disorder that causes a defective cystic fibrosis transmembrane conductance regulator (CFTR) ion transporter in the body (121). This seemingly simple mutation results in a slew of clinical complications, including recurrent chest infection, malabsorption, and infertility. Within the respiratory tract, tracheobronchial epithelial cells secrete a thicker mucus barrier that is more tenacious in nature, potentially hindering drug diffusion (122), as well as providing a colonization site for bacteria and chronic inflammatory responses in the lungs (123). Accordingly, 3D disease models seek to incorporate these pathological features, as well as to address the issue that CF currently lacks an efficient preclinical animal model (124).

Spheroid models have shown promise as 3D disease models of CF, with the 3D structures cultured in media or in combination with Matrigel to emulate the disease features (125). Recent research indicates that spheroids can be used to induce other CF patient cells apart from bronchial brushings to express pathophysiological features to create a model. Indeed, one model has been developed to investigate CFTR function in primary human nasal spheroids (106), and other studies have highlighted drug development opportunities with rectal epithelial cells (126,127). These models can also incorporate the submucosal fibrotic aspect of the disease (128).

Other diseases

Other respiratory diseases of interest for 3D cell culture platforms include asthma and IPF. Like CF, asthma research suffers from a lack of effective animal models (129). As a chronic inflammatory disorder with unresponsive subsets of patients and a pathology that is still not fully understood, sophisticated in vitro models are required to fully delineate the mechanistic pathways of the condition. Hydrogels have shown promise in this regard, where 3D co-cultures of bronchial epithelial cells and fibroblasts have been combined with T-cells from healthy and asthmatic donors to better understand the relevant inflammatory processes (130,131). Spheroid assays have also been employed to examine the angiogenic properties of asthmatic airway smooth muscle cells (132). Spheroids have also been used to assess antifibrotic drugs for IPF (133) and hydrogels for the effects of matrix stiffness on IPF activity (134). Overall, the use of these 3D platforms for disease modeling reinforces

their core advantage over conventional in vitro cell models: the capacity to create a tool that accurately reflects the complex microenvironment of the diseased lung tissue, the additional barriers to efficacious drug delivery that the disease can bring, and the associated cell behaviors that can be targeted for the development of novel inhalable therapies.

OPPORTUNITIES AND CHALLENGES FOR 3D MODELS FOR THE TRANSLATION OF INHALED DRUG THERAPIES

As outlined above, advanced 3D cell culture systems can offer a number of advantages over conventional in vitro cell models for respiratory drug development, particularly in terms of their capacity to more accurately reflect the complex microenvironment of the diseased lung tissue; however, key to their becoming effective tools in inhaled drug development will be developing appropriate culture conditions, aerosol exposure systems, and valid analytical methods for endpoint readout.

Of course, as is the case with every preclinical model, each 3D culture platforms have their associated limitations that challenge their widespread implementation and need to be considered. The principal limitation of hydrogels is their high water content. In general, hydrogels have the inherently weakest mechanical properties of all 3D culture platforms and as a result extended ex vivo culture periods and combinations with synthetic polymers are employed to reduce scaffold collapse (60). Although DC tissue is mechanically stronger, differences are seen in structural integrity and ECM composition among the three most popular protocols (135). Beyond the more obvious challenge that this biomaterial scaffold platform requires a steady supply of donor tissue from animals or humans, tissue heterogeneity due to long-term storage is another caveat that must be taken into account (136). Porous polymeric scaffolds have the potential to overcome the limitations of the other scaffold systems, leaving scale-up and the high cost of manufacture as the primary challenges for their application to respiratory drug development. Spheroids, on the other hand, are theoretically more amenable for cheaper high-throughput studies once the method of 3D culture has been standardized, but their lack of an extracellular matrix component can remove a key contributor to cell behavior and resultant drug responses. Spheroids have not yet been used to assess drug uptake or penetration to the same degree as scaffold biomaterial platforms. Microfluidic chip platforms undoubtedly have the greatest translational potential at present for incorporation into the drug development process; once the technology becomes more widespread and the internal polymeric membrane is replaced with extracellular matrix components to fully facilitate 3D co-culture, this system will truly provide an in vitro iteration of the in vivo respiratory tract for drug and inhalable formulation development.

The method of cell exposure to aerosols has long been an area of research interest. In standard cell line studies, exposure is often achieved by adding the drug/formulation to the medium of a submerged culture. As mentioned previously, it is well established now in the field that culturing of airway cells at an ALI is a better recapitulation of the lung environment and can induce cell polarization, differentiation, and mucus production (6,18,32). Therefore, when establishing and validating models for respiratory drug delivery, being able to culture airway cells at an ALI to enhance differentiation and provide an appropriate environment for aerosol exposure studies would appear advantageous. Scaffold systems and microfluidic lung-on-a-chip platforms for cell culture (Figure 6.1) are particularly well suited to ALI culture (53,54); however, creation of an ALI with spheroid systems presents a significant technical challenge (55). A range of different scaffold systems have been used to successfully culture epithelial cells at an ALI, including type I collagen gels (83–86) and porous scaffolds (54). In the lung-on-a-chip studies, an ALI was successfully introduced once the epithelial and endothelial cells had reached confluence on the membrane (113).

Direct addition of drugs/formulations onto cell cultures via pipetting fails to represent the deposition patterns associated with aerosol exposure. In order to better represent the deposition patterns onto cells from aerosol delivery of drugs/formulations, a range of aerosol exposure systems have been developed, including commercially available systems such as CULTEX® and VITROCELL®. The air-liquid interface exposure (ALICE) system supports exposure of cell cultures to nebulized systems (137) while the Pharmaceutical Deposition Device on Cell Culture (PADDOCC) system was designed for dry powder inhaler formulations (138). If the overarching goal of 3D models application in respiratory drug development is to better recapitulate the *in vivo* environment, then it is critical that appropriate aerosol exposure systems are employed.

To date, spheroids have not been used primarily to study drug uptake or formulation transport, but their integration with high content analysis (HCA) systems could enable spheroids to be applied more in drug development as well as discovery. HCA is a tool that can provide quantitative multiparametric fluorescence-based data from cell populations. As a method, HCA has been used widely in drug discovery and toxicology research, but there is a growing appreciation that it can be used as an innovative tool in drug delivery research including respiratory drug delivery (139). While work on using spheroid cultures in HCA screening is in its infancy, its potential in both fundamental and applied respiratory research is vast.

Overall, the development of innovative methods for creating 3D human cell-based models and culture systems could improve predictive assessment for the field of inhalation toxicology (140) and inhalable therapeutics (34). In addition, these more advanced models can assist at a scientific level in better understanding the respiratory cell responses to drugs/drug formulations at a cellular/tissue level. Key to the application of these models is determining if they are suitable to provide information relevant to the endpoint being studied, for example, toxicity/safety, immune response, efficacy, local drug action, cell uptake/interaction, drug transport across the respiratory epithelium, and so on, and are representative of the appropriate target site, for example, alveolar versus bronchial (34).

In vitro cell-based methods are at present primarily used for scientific screening purposes and to support *in vivo* animal data in regulatory dossier submissions. Key to the

incorporation of more advanced 3D models into standardized scientific and industrial development programmes and further to their acceptance by the regulatory agencies will be robust validation of their reproducibility, sensitivity, availability and predictive abilities. Many of the novel 3D models emerging are still early in this validation process, and focus must in the first instance be on standardizing the methods; key after that is selection of an appropriate model against which to validate. There are agencies now which support this kind of validation work, for example, the European Union Reference Laboratory for Alternatives to animal testing (EURL-ECVAM). For human cell-based 3D models, validation against the current gold-standard animal model might not be most relevant, while *ex vivo* models, for example, EVLP model or lung slices, can perhaps offer better tools to compare drug/formulation effects.

There is no question that a new era of advanced 3D human cell models is rapidly emerging. These models will not necessarily completely replace well-established and robust 2D models that have been shown to provide useful information for certain endpoints in the past, but they can undoubtedly provide an extra toolkit for advanced preclinical screening prior to *in vivo* testing and better respiratory disease models for drug discovery. In addition, technological advances in the aerosol exposure systems and high-throughput screening methods (and indeed combining these two) will undoubtedly enable and support their more widespread introduction into academic and industry research laboratories. Their meaningful utility as valid alternatives or supplements to animal testing will be heavily dependent on matching the appropriate models to the relevant endpoints being assessed. What is important now is to build on the exciting work outlined herein to validate and challenge the models for their predictive abilities.

REFERENCES

1. Nahar K, Gupta N, Gauvin R, Absar S, Patel B, Gupta V, Khademhosseini A, Ahsan F. In vitro, in vivo and ex vivo models for studying particle deposition and drug absorption of inhaled pharmaceuticals. *European Journal of Pharmaceutical Sciences: Official Journal of the European Federation for Pharmaceutical Sciences*. 2013;49(5):805–818. doi:10.1016/j.ejps.2013.06.004.
2. Bérubé K, Aufderheide M, Breheny D, Clothier R, Combes R, Duffin R, Forbes B et al. In vitro models of inhalation toxicity and disease. The report of a FRAME workshop. *Alternatives to Laboratory Animals*. 2009;37(1):89–141.
3. European Collection of Authenticated Cell Cultures. "About ECACC" [cited 2017 21st August]; Retrieved from: https://www.phe-culturecollections.org.uk/collections/ecacc.aspx.
4. American Type Culture Collection. "Who We Are" [cited 2017 21st August]; Retrieved from: https://www.lgcstandards-atcc.org/en/About/About_ATCC/Who_We_Are.aspx.
5. Pohl C, Hermanns MI, Uboldi C, Bock M, Fuchs S, Dei-Anang J, Mayer E et al. Barrier functions and

paracellular integrity in human cell culture models of the proximal respiratory unit. *European Journal of Pharmaceutics and Biopharmaceutics: Official Journal of Arbeitsgemeinschaft fur Pharmazeutische Verfahrenstechnik eV*. 2009;72(2):339–349. doi:10.1016/j.ejpb.2008.07.012.

6. Forbes B, Ehrhardt C. Human respiratory epithelial cell culture for drug delivery applications. *European Journal of Pharmaceutics and Biopharmaceutics: Official Journal of Arbeitsgemeinschaft fur Pharmazeutische Verfahrenstechnik eV*. 2005;60(2):193–205. doi:10.1016/j.ejpb.2005.02.010.

7. Ehrhardt C, Kneuer C, Fiegel J, Hanes J, Schaefer UF, Kim KJ, Lehr CM. Influence of apical fluid volume on the development of functional intercellular junctions in the human epithelial cell line 16HBE14o-: Implications for the use of this cell line as an in vitro model for bronchial drug absorption studies. *Cell and Tissue Research*. 2002;308(3):391–400. doi:10.1007/s00441-002-0548-5.

8. Forbes B, Shah A, Martin GP, Lansley AB. The human bronchial epithelial cell line 16HBE14o- as a model system of the airways for studying drug transport. *International Journal of Pharmaceutics*. 2003;257(1–2):161–167.

9. Foster KA, Avery ML, Yazdanian M, Audus KL. Characterization of the Calu-3 cell line as a tool to screen pulmonary drug delivery. *International Journal of Pharmaceutics*. 2000;208(1–2):1–11.

10. Harcourt JL, Haynes LM. Establishing a liquid-covered culture of polarized human airway epithelial Calu-3 cells to study host cell response to respiratory pathogens in vitro. *Journal of Visualized Experiments*. 2013(72). doi:10.3791/50157.

11. Hermanns MI, Unger RE, Kehe K, Peters K, Kirkpatrick CJ. Lung epithelial cell lines in coculture with human pulmonary microvascular endothelial cells: Development of an alveolo-capillary barrier in vitro. *Laboratory Investigation; A Journal of Technical Methods and Pathology*. 2004;84(6):736–752. doi:10.1038/labinvest.3700081.

12. Kasper J, Hermanns MI, Bantz C, Utech S, Koshkina O, Maskos M, Brochhausen C et al. Flotillin-involved uptake of silica nanoparticles and responses of an alveolar-capillary barrier in vitro. *European Journal of Pharmaceutics and Biopharmaceutics: Official Journal of Arbeitsgemeinschaft fur Pharmazeutische Verfahrenstechnik eV*. 2013;84(2):275–287. doi:10.1016/j.ejpb.2012.10.011.

13. Cozens AL, Yezzi MJ, Kunzelmann K, Ohrui T, Chin L, Eng K, Finkbeiner WE et al. CFTR expression and chloride secretion in polarized immortal human bronchial epithelial cells. *American Journal of Respiratory Cell and Molecular Biology*. 1994;10(1):38–47.

14. Manford F, Tronde A, Jeppsson AB, Patel N, Johansson F, Forbes B. Drug permeability in 16HBE14o- airway cell layers correlates with absorption from the isolated

perfused rat lung. *European Journal of Pharmaceutical Sciences: Official Journal of the European Federation for Pharmaceutical Sciences*. 2005;26(5):414–420. doi:10.1016/j.ejps.2005.07.010.

15. Reddel RR, Ke Y, Gerwin BI, McMenamin MG, Lechner JF, Su RT, Brash DE et al. Transformation of human bronchial epithelial cells by infection with SV40 or adenovirus-12 SV40 hybrid virus, or transfection via strontium phosphate coprecipitation with a plasmid containing SV40 early region genes. *Cancer Research*. 1988;48(7):1904–1909.

16. Molloy EL, Adams A, Moore JB, Masterson JC, Madrigal-Estebas L, Mahon BP, O'Dea S. BMP4 induces an epithelial-mesenchymal transition-like response in adult airway epithelial cells. *Growth Factors (Chur, Switzerland)*. 2008;26(1):12–22. doi:10.1080/08977190801987166.

17. Fogh J, Fogh JM, Orfeo T. One hundred and twenty-seven cultured human tumor cell lines producing tumors in nude mice. *Journal of the National Cancer Institute*. 1977;59(1):221–226.

18. Grainger CI, Greenwell LL, Lockley DJ, Martin GP, Forbes B. Culture of Calu-3 cells at the air interface provides a representative model of the airway epithelial barrier. *Pharmaceutical Research*. 2006;23(7):1482–1490. doi:10.1007/s11095-006-0255-0.

19. Stentebjerg-Andersen A, Notlevsen IV, Brodin B, Nielsen CU. Calu-3 cells grown under AIC and LCC conditions: Implications for dipeptide uptake and transepithelial transport of substances. *European Journal of Pharmaceutics and Biopharmaceutics*. 2011;78(1):19–26. doi:10.1016/j.ejpb.2010.12.030.

20. Gazdar AF, Linnoila RI, Kurita Y, Oie HK, Mulshine JL, Clark JC, Whitsett JA. Peripheral airway cell differentiation in human lung cancer cell lines. *Cancer Research*. 1990;50(17):5481–5487.

21. Giard DJ, Aaronson SA, Todaro GJ, Arnstein P, Kersey JH, Dosik H, Parks WP. In vitro cultivation of human tumors: Establishment of cell lines derived from a series of solid tumors. *Journal of the National Cancer Institute*. 1973;51(5):1417–1423.

22. Lieber M, Smith B, Szakal A, Nelson-Rees W, Todaro G. A continuous tumor-cell line from a human lung carcinoma with properties of type II alveolar epithelial cells. *International Journal of Cancer*. 1976;17(1):62–70.

23. Rothen-Rutishauser BM, Kiama SG, Gehr P. A three-dimensional cellular model of the human respiratory tract to study the interaction with particles. *American Journal of Respiratory Cell and Molecular Biology*. 2005;32(4):281–289. doi:10.1165/rcmb.2004-0187OC.

24. Gray TE, Guzman K, Davis CW, Abdullah LH, Nettesheim P. Mucociliary differentiation of serially passaged normal human tracheobronchial epithelial cells. *American Journal of Respiratory Cell and Molecular Biology*. 1996;14(1):104–112. doi:10.1165/ajrcmb.14.1.8534481.

25. Fulcher ML, Gabriel S, Burns K, Yankaskas J, Randell S. Well-differentiated human airway epithelial cell

cultures. In: Picot J, ed. *Human Cell Culture Protocols*. Humana Press, New York; 2005. p. 183–206.

26. Bérubé K, Pitt A, Hayden P, Prytherch Z, Job C. Filter-well technology for advanced three-dimensional cell culture: Perspectives for respiratory research. *Alternatives to Laboratory Animals*. 2010;38(Suppl 1):49–65.

27. Reus AA, Maas WJ, Jansen HT, Constant S, Staal YC, van Triel JJ, Kuper CF. Feasibility of a 3D human airway epithelial model to study respiratory absorption. *Toxicology in Vitro: An International Journal Published in Association with BIBRA*. 2014;28(2):258–264. doi:10.1016/j.tiv.2013.10.025.

28. Huang S, Boda B, Vernaz J, Ferreira E, Wiszniewski L, Constant S. Establishment and characterization of an in vitro human small airway model (SmallAir). *European Journal of Pharmaceutics and Biopharmaceutics: Official Journal of Arbeitsgemeinschaft fur Pharmazeutische Verfahrenstechnik eV*. 2017;118:68–72. doi:10.1016/j.ejpb.2016.12.006.

29. Maqsood MI, Matin MM, Bahrami AR, Ghasroldasht MM. Immortality of cell lines: Challenges and advantages of establishment. *Cell Biology International*. 2013;37(10):1038–1045. doi:10.1002/cbin.10137.

30. Birgersdotter A, Sandberg R, Ernberg I. Gene expression perturbation in vitro–a growing case for three-dimensional (3D) culture systems. *Seminars in Cancer Biology*. 2005;15(5):405–412. doi:10.1016/j.semcancer.2005.06.009.

31. Davenport EA, Nettesheim P. Regulation of mucociliary differentiation of rat tracheal epithelial cells by type I collagen gel substratum. *American Journal of Respiratory Cell and Molecular Biology*. 1996;14(1):19–26. doi:10.1165/ajrcmb.14.1.8534482.

32. Klein SG, Hennen J, Serchi T, Blömeke B, Gutleb AC. Potential of coculture in vitro models to study inflammatory and sensitizing effects of particles on the lung. *Toxicology in Vitro: An International Journal Published in Association with BIBRA*. 2011;25(8):1516–1534. doi:10.1016/j.tiv.2011.09.006.

33. Bérubé K, Prytherch Z, Job C, Hughes T. Human primary bronchial lung cell constructs: The new respiratory models. *Toxicology*. 2010;278(3):311–318. doi:10.1016/j.tox.2010.04.004.

34. Hittinger M, Schneider-Daum N, Lehr CM. Review. Cell and tissue-based in vitro models for improving the development of oral inhalation drug products. *European Journal of Pharmaceutics and Biopharmaceutics*. 2017;118:73–78. doi:10.1016/j.ejpb.2017.02.019.

35. Frank JA, Briot R, Lee JW, Ishizaka A, Uchida T, Matthay MA. Physiological and biochemical markers of alveolar epithelial barrier dysfunction in perfused human lungs. *American Journal of Physiology. Lung Cellular and Molecular Physiology*. 2007;293(1):L52–L59.

36. Cryan SA, Sivadas N, Garcia-Contreras L. In vivo animal models for drug delivery across the lung mucosal barrier. *Advanced Drug Delivery Reviews*. 2007;59(11):1133–1151. doi:10.1016/j.addr.2007.08.023.

37. Zosky GR, Sly PD. Animal models of asthma. *Clinical and Experimental Allergy: Journal of the British Society for Allergy and Clinical Immunology*. 2007;37(7):973–988. doi:10.1111/j.1365-2222.2007.02740.x.

38. Tardif SD, Coleman K, Hobbs TR, Lutz C. IACUC review of nonhuman primate research. *ILAR Journal/National Research Council, Institute of Laboratory Animal Resources*. 2013;54(2):234–245. doi:10.1093/ilar/ilt040.

39. Wolff RK, Dorato MA. Toxicologic testing of inhaled pharmaceutical aerosols. *Critical Reviews in Toxicology*. 1993;23(4):343–369. doi:10.3109/10408449309104076.

40. Wolff RK. Toxicology studies for inhaled and nasal delivery. *Molecular Pharmaceutics*. 2015;12(8):2688–2696. doi:10.1021/acs.molpharmaceut.5b00146.

41. Scherließ R, Mönckedieck M, Young K, Trows S, Buske S, Hook S. First in vivo evaluation of particulate nasal dry powder vaccine formulations containing ovalbumin in mice. *International Journal of Pharmaceutics*. 2015;479(2):408–415. doi:10.1016/j.ijpharm.2015.01.015.

42. Ghasemian E, Vatanara A, Rouini MR, Rouholamini Najafabadi A, Gilani K, Lavasani H, Mohajel N. Inhaled sildenafil nanocomposites: Lung accumulation and pulmonary pharmacokinetics. *Pharmaceutical Development and Technology*. 2016;21(8):961–971. doi:10.3109/10837450.2015.1086369.

43. Cannon WC, Blanton EF, McDonald KE. The flow-past chamber: An improved nose-only exposure system for rodents. *American Industrial Hygiene Association Journal*. 1983;44(12):923–928. doi:10.1080/15298668391405959.

44. March TH, Cossey PY, Esparza DC, Dix KJ, McDonald JD, Bowen LE. Inhalation administration of all-trans-retinoic acid for treatment of elastase-induced pulmonary emphysema in Fischer 344 rats. *Experimental Lung Research*. 2004;30(5):383–404. doi:10.1080/01902140490463142.

45. Leberl M, Kratzer A, Taraseviciene-Stewart L. Tobacco smoke induced COPD/emphysema in the animal model-are we all on the same page? *Frontiers in Physiology*. 2013;4:91. doi:10.3389/fphys.2013.00091.

46. Ledford H. Translational research: 4 ways to fix the clinical trial. *Nature*. 2011;477(7366):526–528. doi:10.1038/477526a.

47. Kirkpatrick CJ. Developing cellular systems in vitro to simulate regeneration. *Tissue Engineering Part A*. 2014;20(9–10):1355–1357. doi:10.1089/ten.tea.2014.0002.

48. Kirkpatrick CJ, Fuchs S, Unger RE. Co-culture systems for vascularization–learning from nature. *Advanced Drug Delivery Reviews*. 2011;63(4–5):291–299. doi:10.1016/j.addr.2011.01.009.

49. Kim SW, Park KC, Kim HJ, Cho KH, Chung JH, Kim KH, Eun HC et al. Effects of collagen IV and laminin on the reconstruction of human oral mucosa. *Journal of Biomedical Materials Research.* 2001;58(1):108–112.

50. Lin YM, Zhang A, Rippon HJ, Bismarck A, Bishop AE. Tissue engineering of lung: The effect of extracellular matrix on the differentiation of embryonic stem cells to pneumocytes. *Tissue Engineering Part A.* 2010;16(5):1515–1526. doi:10.1089/ten. TEA.2009.0232.

51. Sorkio A, Hongisto H, Kaarniranta K, Uusitalo H, Juuti-Uusitalo K, Skottman H. Structure and barrier properties of human embryonic stem cell-derived retinal pigment epithelial cells are affected by extracellular matrix protein coating. *Tissue Engineering Part A.* 2014;20(3–4):622–634. doi:10.1089/ten. TEA.2013.0049.

52. Huh DD. A human breathing lung-on-a-chip. *Annals of the American Thoracic Society.* 2015;12(Suppl 1): S42–S44. doi:10.1513/AnnalsATS.201410-442MG.

53. O'Leary C, Cavanagh B, Unger RE, Kirkpatrick CJ, O'Dea S, O'Brien FJ, Cryan S-A. The development of a tissue-engineered tracheobronchial epithelial model using a bilayered collagen-hyaluronate scaffold. *Biomaterials.* 2016;85:111–127. doi:10.1016/j. biomaterials.2016.01.065.

54. Tan Q, Choi KM, Sicard D, Tschumperlin DJ. Human airway organoid engineering as a step toward lung regeneration and disease modeling. *Biomaterials.* 2017;113:118–132. doi:10.1016/j.biomaterials.2016.10.046.

55. O'Leary C, Gilbert JL, O'Dea S, O'Brien FJ, Cryan SA. Respiratory tissue engineering: Current status and opportunities for the future. *Tissue Engineering Part B,Reviews.* 2015;21(4):323–344. doi:10.1089/ten. TEB.2014.0525.

56. Douglas WH, Moorman GW, Teel RW. The formation of histotypic structures from monodisperse fetal rat lung cells cultured on a three-dimensional substrate. *In Vitro.* 1976;12(5):373–381.

57. Douglas WH, Teel RW. An organotypic in vitro model system for studying pulmonary surfactant production by type II alveolar pneumonocytes. *The American Review of Respiratory Disease.* 1976;113(1):17–23.

58. Breuls RG, Jiya TU, Smit TH. Scaffold stiffness influences cell behavior: Opportunities for skeletal tissue engineering. *The Open Orthopaedics Journal.* 2008;2:103–109. doi:10.2174/1874325000802010103.

59. Shkumatov A, Thompson M, Choi KM, Sicard D, Baek K, Kim DH, Tschumperlin DJ et al. Matrix stiffness-modulated proliferation and secretory function of the airway smooth muscle cells. *American Journal of Physiology-Lung Cellular and Molecular Physiology.* 2015;308(11):L1125–L1135. doi:10.1152/ ajplung.00154.2014.

60. Ahmed EM. Hydrogel: Preparation, characterization, and applications: A review. *Journal of Advanced Research.* 2015;6(2):105–121. doi:10.1016/j. jare.2013.07.006.

61. Mondrinos MJ, Koutzaki S, Jiwanmall E, Li M, Dechadarevian JP, Lelkes PI, Finck CM. Engineering three-dimensional pulmonary tissue constructs. *Tissue Engineering.* 2006;12(4):717–728. doi:10.1089/ ten.2006.12.717.

62. Mondrinos MJ, Koutzaki S, Lelkes PI, Finck CM. A tissue-engineered model of fetal distal lung tissue. *American Journal of Physiology-Lung Cellular and Molecular Physiology.* 2007;293(3):L639–L650. doi:10.1152/ajplung.00403.2006.

63. Sugihara H, Toda S, Miyabara S, Fujiyama C, Yonemitsu N. Reconstruction of alveolus-like structure from alveolar type II epithelial cells in three-dimensional collagen gel matrix culture. *The American Journal of Pathology.* 1993;142(3):783–792.

64. Blau H, Guzowski DE, Siddiqi ZA, Scarpelli EM, Bienkowski RS. Fetal type 2 pneumocytes form alveolar-like structures and maintain long-term differentiation on extracellular matrix. *Journal of Cellular Physiology.* 1988;136(2):203–214. doi:10.1002/jcp.1041360202.

65. Crapo PM, Gilbert TW, Badylak SF. An overview of tissue and whole organ decellularization processes. *Biomaterials.* 2011;32(12):3233–3243. doi:10.1016/j. biomaterials.2011.01.057.

66. Nichols JE, Niles JA, Cortiella J. Production and utilization of acellular lung scaffolds in tissue engineering. *Journal of Cellular Biochemistry.* 2012;113(7):2185–2192. doi:10.1002/jcb.24112.

67. Wagner DE, Bonenfant NR, Parsons CS, Sokocevic D, Brooks EM, Borg ZD, Lathrop MJ et al. Comparative decellularization and recellularization of normal versus emphysematous human lungs. *Biomaterials.* 2014;35(10):3281–3297. doi:10.1016/j. biomaterials.2013.12.103.

68. Petersen TH, Calle EA, Colehour MB, Niklason LE. Matrix composition and mechanics of decellularized lung scaffolds. *Cells, Tissues, Organs.* 2012;195(3):222–231. doi:10.1159/000324896.

69. Wallis JM, Borg ZD, Daly AB, Deng B, Ballif BA, Allen GB, Jaworski DM, Weiss DJ. Comparative assessment of detergent-based protocols for mouse lung de-cellularization and re-cellularization. *Tissue Engineering Part C, Methods.* 2012;18(6):420–432. doi:10.1089/ten. TEC.2011.0567.

70. Bonenfant NR, Sokocevic D, Wagner DE, Borg ZD, Lathrop MJ, Lam YW, Deng B et al. The effects of storage and sterilization on de-cellularized and re-cellularized whole lung. *Biomaterials.* 2013;34(13):3231–3245. doi:10.1016/j. biomaterials.2013.01.031.

71. Sokocevic D, Bonenfant NR, Wagner DE, Borg ZD, Lathrop MJ, Lam YW, Deng B et al. The effect of age and emphysematous and fibrotic injury on the re-cellularization of de-cellularized lungs. *Biomaterials.* 2013;34(13):3256–3269. doi:10.1016/j. biomaterials.2013.01.028.

72. Carvalho TC, Peters JI, Williams RO, 3rd. Influence of particle size on regional lung deposition–What evidence is there? *International Journal of Pharmaceutics*. 2011;406(1–2):1–10. doi:10.1016/j.ijpharm.2010.12.040.

73. Bosquillon C, Madlova M, Patel N, Clear N, Forbes B. A comparison of drug transport in pulmonary absorption models: Isolated perfused rat lungs, respiratory epithelial cell lines and primary cell culture. *Pharmaceutical Research*. 2017. doi:10.1007/s11095-017-2251-y.

74. Wagner DE, Fenn SL, Bonenfant NR, Marks ER, Borg ZD, Saunders P, Oldinski RA, Weiss DJ. Design and synthesis of an artificial pulmonary pleura for high throughput studies in acellular human lungs. *Cellular and Molecular Bioengineering*. 2014;7(2):184–195. doi:10.1007/s12195-014-0323-1.

75. Partap S, Lyons F, O'Brien FJ. IV.1. Scaffolds & surfaces. *Studies in Health Technology and Informatics*. 2010;152:187–201.

76. Chen P, Marsilio E, Goldstein RH, Yannas IV, Spector M. Formation of lung alveolar-like structures in collagen-glycosaminoglycan scaffolds in vitro. *Tissue Engineering*. 2005;11(9–10):1436–1448. doi:10.1089/ten.2005.11.1436.

77. Cortiella J, Nichols JE, Kojima K, Bonassar LJ, Dargon P, Roy AK, Vacant MP, Niles JA, Vacanti CA. Tissue-engineered lung: An in vivo and in vitro comparison of polyglycolic acid and pluronic F-127 hydrogel/somatic lung progenitor cell constructs to support tissue growth. *Tissue Engineering*. 2006;12(5):1213–1225. doi:10.1089/ten.2006.12.1213.

78. Andrade CF, Wong AP, Waddell TK, Keshavjee S, Liu M. Cell-based tissue engineering for lung regeneration. *American Journal of Physiology-Lung Cellular and Molecular Physiology*. 2007;292(2):L510–L518. doi:10.1152/ajplung.00175.2006.

79. Harrington H, Cato P, Salazar F, Wilkinson M, Knox A, Haycock JW, Rose F, Aylott JW, Ghaemmaghami AM. Immunocompetent 3D model of human upper airway for disease modeling and in vitro drug evaluation. *Molecular Pharmaceutics*. 2014;11(7):2082–2091. doi:10.1021/mp5000295.

80. Bridge JC, Aylott JW, Brightling CE, Ghaemmaghami AM, Knox AJ, Lewis MP, Rose FR, Morris GE. Adapting the electrospinning process to provide three unique environments for a tri-layered in vitro model of the airway wall. *Journal of Visualized Experiments*. 2015(101):e52986. doi:10.3791/52986.

81. Friess W. Collagen–biomaterial for drug delivery. *European Journal of Pharmaceutics and Biopharmaceutics: Official Journal of Arbeitsgemeinschaft fur Pharmazeutische Verfahrenstechnik eV*. 1998;45(2):113–136.

82. Paquette JS, Tremblay P, Bernier V, Auger FA, Laviolette M, Germain L, Boutet M, Boulet LP, Goulet F. Production of tissue-engineered three-dimensional human bronchial models. *In Vitro Cellular & Developmental Biology Animal*. 2003;39(5–6):213–220. doi:10.1290/1543-706x(2003) 039<0213:potthb>2.0.co;2.

83. Vaughan MB, Ramirez RD, Wright WE, Minna JD, Shay JW. A three-dimensional model of differentiation of immortalized human bronchial epithelial cells. *Differentiation; Research in Biological Diversity*. 2006;74(4):141–148. doi:10.1111/j.1432-0436.2006.00069.x.

84. Wang Y, Wong LB, Mao H. Creation of a long-lifespan ciliated epithelial tissue structure using a 3D collagen scaffold. *Biomaterials*. 2010;31(5):848–853. doi:10.1016/j.biomaterials.2009.09.098.

85. Pageau SC, Sazonova OV, Wong JY, Soto AM, Sonnenschein C. The effect of stromal components on the modulation of the phenotype of human bronchial epithelial cells in 3D culture. *Biomaterials*. 2011;32(29):7169–7180. doi:10.1016/j.biomaterials.2011.06.017.

86. Ali MS, Pearson JP. Upper airway mucin gene expression: A review. *The Laryngoscope*. 2007;117(5):932–938. doi:10.1097/MLG.0b013e3180383651.

87. Choe MM, Sporn PH, Swartz MA. An in vitro airway wall model of remodeling. *American Journal of Physiology-Lung Cellular and Molecular Physiology*. 2003;285(2):L427–L433. doi:10.1152/ajplung.00005.2003.

88. Choe MM, Tomei AA, Swartz MA. Physiological 3D tissue model of the airway wall and mucosa. *Nature Protocols*. 2006;1(1):357–362. doi:10.1038/nprot.2006.54.

89. Risbud M, Endres M, Ringe J, Bhonde R, Sittinger M. Biocompatible hydrogel supports the growth of respiratory epithelial cells: Possibilities in tracheal tissue engineering. *Journal of Biomedical Materials Research*. 2001;56(1):120–127.

90. Cornelissen CG, Dietrich M, Kruger S, Spillner J, Schmitz-Rode T, Jockenhoevel S. Fibrin gel as alternative scaffold for respiratory tissue engineering. *Annals of Biomedical Engineering*. 2012;40(3):679–687. doi:10.1007/s10439-011-0437-8.

91. Huang TW, Chan YH, Cheng PW, Young YH, Lou PJ, Young TH. Increased mucociliary differentiation of human respiratory epithelial cells on hyaluronan-derivative membranes. *Acta Biomaterialia*. 2010;6(3):1191–1199. doi:10.1016/j.actbio.2009.08.031.

92. Huang TW, Cheng PW, Chan YH, Yeh TH, Young YH, Young TH. Regulation of ciliary differentiation of human respiratory epithelial cells by the receptor for hyaluronan-mediated motility on hyaluronan-based biomaterials. *Biomaterials*. 2010;31(26):6701–6709. doi:10.1016/j.biomaterials.2010.05.054.

93. Huang CJ, Chien YL, Ling TY, Cho HC, Yu J, Chang YC. The influence of collagen film nanostructure on pulmonary stem cells and collagen-stromal cell

interactions. *Biomaterials*. 2010;31(32):8271–8280. doi:10.1016/j.biomaterials.2010.07.038.

94. Hoffmann OI, Ilmberger C, Magosch S, Joka M, Jauch KW, Mayer B. Impact of the spheroid model complexity on drug response. *Journal of Biotechnology*. 2015;205:14–23. doi:10.1016/j.jbiotec.2015.02.029.

95. Nath S, Devi GR. Three-dimensional culture systems in cancer research: Focus on tumor spheroid model. *Pharmacology & Therapeutics*. 2016;163:94–108. doi:10.1016/j.pharmthera.2016.03.013.

96. Leek R, Grimes DR, Harris AL, McIntyre A. Methods: Using three-dimensional culture (Spheroids) as an in vitro model of tumour hypoxia. *Advance in Experimental Medicine and Biology*. 2016;899:167–196. doi:10.1007/978-3-319-26666-4_10.

97. Laschke MW, Menger MD. Spheroids as vascularization units: From angiogenesis research to tissue engineering applications. *Biotechnology Advances*. 2017;35(6):782–791. doi:10.1016/j.biotechadv.2017.07.002.

98. Laschke MW, Menger MD. Life is 3D: Boosting spheroid function for tissue engineering. *Trends Biotechnology*. 2017;35(2):133–144. doi:10.1016/j.tibtech.2016.08.004.

99. Kelm JM, Timmins NE, Brown CJ, Fussenegger M, Nielsen LK. Method for generation of homogeneous multicellular tumor spheroids applicable to a wide variety of cell types. *Biotechnology Bioengineering*. 2003;83(2):173–180. doi:10.1002/bit.10655.

100. Su G, Zhao Y, Wei J, Han J, Chen L, Xiao Z, Chen B, Dai J. The effect of forced growth of cells into 3D spheres using low attachment surfaces on the acquisition of stemness properties. *Biomaterials*. 2013;34(13):3215–3222. doi:10.1016/j.biomaterials.2013.01.044.

101. Wang W, Itaka K, Ohba S, Nishiyama N, Chung UI, Yamasaki Y, Kataoka K. 3D spheroid culture system on micropatterned substrates for improved differentiation efficiency of multipotent mesenchymal stem cells. *Biomaterials*. 2009;30(14):2705–2715. doi:10.1016/j.biomaterials.2009.01.030.

102. Carpenedo RL, Sargent CY, McDevitt TC. Rotary suspension culture enhances the efficiency, yield, and homogeneity of embryoid body differentiation. *Stem Cells*. 2007;25(9):2224–2234. doi:10.1634/stemcells.2006-0523.

103. Li XJ, Valadez AV, Zuo P, Nie Z. Microfluidic 3D cell culture: Potential application for tissue-based bioassays. *Bioanalysis*. 2012;4(12):1509–1525. doi:10.4155/bio.12.133.

104. Torisawa YS, Takagi A, Shiku H, Yasukawa T, Matsue T. A multicellular spheroid-based drug sensitivity test by scanning electrochemical microscopy. *Oncology Reports*. 2005;13(6):1107–1112.

105. Fey SJ, Wrzesinski K. Determination of drug toxicity using 3D spheroids constructed from an immortal human hepatocyte cell line. *Toxicological Sciences*. 2012;127(2):403–411. doi:10.1093/toxsci/kfs122.

106. Brewington JJ, Filbrandt ET, LaRosa FJ, Ostmann AJ, Strecker LM, Szczesniak RD, Clancy JP. Detection of CFTR function and modulation in primary human nasal cell spheroids. *Journal of Cystic Fibrosis*. 2017. doi:10.1016/j.jcf.2017.06.010.

107. Hild M, Jaffe AB. Production of 3-D airway organoids from primary human airway basal cells and their use in high-throughput screening. *Current Protocols in Stem Cell Biology*. 2016;37:IE.9.1–IE.9.15. doi:10.1002/cpsc.1.

108. Pagano F, Nocella C, Sciarretta S, Fianchini L, Siciliano C, Mangino G, Ibrahim M et al. Cytoprotective and antioxidant effects of steen solution on human lung spheroids and human endothelial cells. *American Journal of Transplantation*. 2017;17(7):1885–1894. doi:10.1111/ajt.14278.

109. Esch EW, Bahinski A, Huh D. Organs-on-chips at the frontiers of drug discovery. *Nature Reviews Drug Discovery*. 2015;14(4):248–260. doi:10.1038/nrd4539.

110. Nichols JE, Niles JA, Vega SP, Cortiella J. Novel in vitro respiratory models to study lung development, physiology, pathology and toxicology. *Stem Cell Research & Therapy*. 2013;4(Suppl 1):S7. doi:10.1186/scrt368.

111. Benam KH, Villenave R, Lucchesi C, Varone A, Hubeau C, Lee HH, Alves SE et al. Small airway-on-a-chip enables analysis of human lung inflammation and drug responses in vitro. *Nature Methods*. 2016;13(2):151–157. doi:10.1038/nmeth.3697.

112. Huh D, Matthews BD, Mammoto A, Montoya-Zavala M, Hsin HY, Ingber DE. Reconstituting organ-level lung functions on a chip. *Science (New York, NY)*. 2010;328(5986):1662–1668. doi:10.1126/science.1188302.

113. Sellgren KL, Butala EJ, Gilmour BP, Randell SH, Grego S. A biomimetic multicellular model of the airways using primary human cells. *Lab on a Chip*. 2014;14(17):3349–3358. doi:10.1039/c4lc00552j.

114. Global Strategy for the Diagnosis, Management and Prevention of COPD, Global Initiative for Chronic Obstructive Lung Disease (GOLD) 2015. Available from: http://www.goldcopd.org/. 2015.

115. Dodge JA, Lewis PA, Stanton M, Wilsher J. Cystic fibrosis mortality and survival in the UK: 1947–2003. *The European Respiratory Journal*. 2007;29(3):522–526. doi:10.1183/09031936.00099506.

116. Foundation CF. *Cystic Fibrosis Foundation Patient Registry: 2013 Annual Data Report to the Center Directors*. Bethesda, MD: 2014.

117. King TE, Jr., Pardo A, Selman M. Idiopathic pulmonary fibrosis. *Lancet (London, England)*. 2011;378(9807):1949–1961. doi:10.1016/s0140-6736(11)60052-4.

118. Mathers CD, Loncar D. Projections of global mortality and burden of disease from 2002 to 2030.

PLoS Medicine. 2006;3(11):e442. doi:10.1371/journal.pmed.0030442.

119. Vanfleteren LEGW, Spruit MA, Wouters EFM, Franssen FME. Management of chronic obstructive pulmonary disease beyond the lungs. The Lancet Respiratory Medicine. 2016;4(11):911–924. doi:10.1016/S2213-2600(16)00097-7.

120. Rabe KF, Watz H. Chronic obstructive pulmonary disease. The Lancet. 2017;389(10082):1931–1940. doi:10.1016/S0140-6736(17)31222-9.

121. Elborn JS. Cystic fibrosis. The Lancet. 2016;388(10059):2519–2531. doi:10.1016/S0140-6736(16)00576-6.

122. Stigliani M, Manniello MD, Zegarra-Moran O, Galietta L, Minicucci L, Casciaro R, Garofalo E et al. Rheological properties of cystic fibrosis bronchial secretion and in vitro drug permeation study: The effect of sodium bicarbonate. Journal of Aerosol Medicine and Pulmonary Drug Delivery. 2016;29(4):337–345. doi:10.1089/jamp.2015.1228.

123. Hartl D, Gaggar A, Bruscia E, Hector A, Marcos V, Jung A, Greene C et al. Innate immunity in cystic fibrosis lung disease. Journal of Cystic Fibrosis. 2012;11(5):363–382. doi:10.1016/j.jcf.2012.07.003.

124. O'Sullivan BP, Freedman SD. Cystic fibrosis. Lancet (London, England). 2009;373(9678):1891–1904. doi:10.1016/s0140-6736(09)60327-5.

125. Cholon DM, Gentzsch M. Recent progress in translational cystic fibrosis research using precision medicine strategies. Journal of Cystic Fibrosis. 2017. doi:10.1016/j.jcf.2017.09.005.

126. Graeber SY, Hug MJ, Sommerburg O, Hirtz S, Hentschel J, Heinzmann A, Dopfer C et al. Intestinal current measurements detect activation of mutant CFTR in patients with cystic fibrosis with the G551D mutation treated with ivacaftor. American Journal of Respiratory and Critical Care Medicine. 2015;192(10):1252–1255. doi:10.1164/rccm.201507-1271LE.

127. Dekkers JF, Berkers G, Kruisselbrink E, Vonk A, de Jonge HR, Janssens HM, Bronsveld I et al. Characterizing responses to CFTR-modulating drugs using rectal organoids derived from subjects with cystic fibrosis. Science Translational Medicine. 2016;8(344):344ra84. doi:10.1126/scitranslmed.aad8278.

128. Durieu I, Peyrol S, Gindre D, Bellon G, Durand DV, Pacheco Y. Subepithelial fibrosis and degradation of the bronchial extracellular matrix in cystic fibrosis. American Journal of Respiratory and Critical Care Medicine. 1998;158(2):580–588. doi:10.1164/ajrccm.158.2.9707126.

129. Holmes AM, Solari R, Holgate ST. Animal models of asthma: Value, limitations and opportunities for alternative approaches. Drug Discovery Today. 2011;16(15–16):659–670. doi:10.1016/j.drudis.2011.05.014.

130. Darveau ME, Jacques E, Rouabhia M, Hamid Q, Chakir J. Increased T-cell survival by structural bronchial cells derived from asthmatic subjects cultured in an engineered human mucosa. The Journal of Allergy and Clinical Immunology. 2008;121(3):692–699. doi:10.1016/j.jaci.2007.11.023.

131. Chakir J, Pagé N, Hamid Q, Laviolette M, Boulet LP, Rouabhia M. Bronchial mucosa produced by tissue engineering: A new tool to study cellular interactions in asthma. The Journal of Allergy and Clinical Immunology. 2001;107(1):36–40. doi:10.1067/mai.2001.111929.

132. Keglowich L, Roth M, Philippova M, Resink T, Tjin G, Oliver B, Lardinois D et al. Bronchial smooth muscle cells of asthmatics promote angiogenesis through elevated secretion of CXC-chemokines (ENA-78, GRO-alpha, and IL-8). PloS One. 2013;8(12):e81494. doi:10.1371/journal.pone.0081494.

133. Surolia R, Li FJ, Wang Z, Li H, Liu G, Zhou Y, Luckhardt T et al. 3D pulmospheres serve as a personalized and predictive multicellular model for assessment of antifibrotic drugs. JCI Insight. 2017;2(2):e91377. doi:10.1172/jci.insight.91377.

134. Marinkovic A, Liu F, Tschumperlin DJ. Matrices of physiologic stiffness potently inactivate idiopathic pulmonary fibrosis fibroblasts. American Journal of Respiratory Cell and Molecular Biology. 2013;48(4):422–430. doi:10.1165/rcmb.2012-0335OC.

135. Haykal S, Soleas JP, Salna M, Hofer SO, Waddell TK. Evaluation of the structural integrity and extracellular matrix components of tracheal allografts following cyclical decellularization techniques: Comparison of three protocols. Tissue Engineering Part C, Methods. 2012;18(8):614–623. doi:10.1089/ten.

136. Baiguera S, Del Gaudio C, Jaus MO, Polizzi L, Gonfiotti A, Comin CE, Bianco A et al. Long-term changes to in vitro preserved bioengineered human trachea and their implications for decellularized tissues. Biomaterials. 2012;33(14):3662–3672. doi:10.1016/j.biomaterials.2012.01.064.

137. Lenz AG, Karg E, Lentner B, Dittrich V, Brandenberger C, Rothen-Rutishauser B et al. A dose-controlled system for air-liquid interface cell exposure and application to zinc oxide nanoparticles. Part Fibre Toxicology. 2009;16(6):32. doi:PMID: 20015351.

138. Hein S, Bur M, Kolb T, Muellinger B, Schaefer UF, Lehr CM. The Pharmaceutical Aerosol Deposition Device on Cell Cultures (PADDOCC) in vitro system: Design and experimental protocol. Alternatives to Laboratory Animals. 2010;38(4):285–295. doi:PMID: 20822321.

139. Brayden DJ, Cryan SA, Dawson KA, O'Brien PJ, Simpson JC. High-content analysis for drug delivery and nanoparticle applications. Drug Discovery Today. 2015;20(8):942–957.

140. Hiemstra PS, Grootaers, G., van der Does, A.M., Krul, C.A.M., Kooter, I.M.. Human lung epithelial cell cultures for analysis of inhaled toxicants: Lessons learned and future directions. Toxicology in Vitro. 2017;47:137–146. doi:PMID: 29155131.

7

Overview of the delivery technologies for inhalation aerosols

DANIEL F. MORAGA-ESPINOZA, ASHLEE D. BRUNAUGH, SILVIA FERRATI, LARA A. HEERSEMA, MATTHEW J. HERPIN, PATRICIA P. MARTINS, HAIRUI ZHANG, AND HUGH D.C. SMYTH

Physical principles of aerosol generation	123	Pressurized metered-dose inhalers	127
Atomization and nebulization	123	Nebulizers	131
Particle redispersion	124	Metered liquid dose inhalers	133
Particle-particle interaction forces	124	Particle redispersion devices	134
Mechanisms of redispersion	125	Dry powder inhalers	134
Evaporation–condensation	126	Evaporation–condensation devices	136
Aerosol device technology	127	Conclusion	137
Atomization devices	127	References	137

PHYSICAL PRINCIPLES OF AEROSOL GENERATION

Atomization and nebulization

Atomization is a key process in many inhalation aerosol systems and is defined as "the formation of droplets within a gaseous medium." Within the pharmaceutical industry, a regulatory distinction has been made between atomizers and nebulizers. Atomization refers to the generation of an aerosol that is dispersed into the air before contacting a patient, whereas nebulization and nebulizers deliver the aerosol directly to the patient (1). The production of droplets with the appropriate physicochemical and aerodynamic characteristics is fundamental to the performance and success of inhalation therapy. The following section will address some of the fundamental mechanisms for droplet formation, as well as the underlying physics and fluid dynamics that govern their behavior.

The breakup of droplets for nebulization or atomization can occur as a combination of several interacting mechanisms and, depending on the available sources of force and energy, the mathematical solution would quickly become unsolvable. However, the general principle of balancing equilibrium forces remains and allows a systematic understanding of overall droplet formation.

The overall physics of droplet formation is governed by the balance of internal and external forces on the bulk liquid or on the surface of the droplet (2). Before we consider more advanced cases, let us consider the simplest form: static or hanging drop formation. The formation of a static or hanging drop is dependent on the balance between gravitational forces and the surface tension on the drop. The balancing of these forces is directly related to the diameter of the orifice releasing the droplet and the flow rate through the nozzle. Under low flow, these droplets grow larger with an increase in orifice size, but ultimately the surface tension of the droplet is the predominant force that holds it intact as it begins to grow. As the droplet grows, the gravitational forces are increased to a point where they exceed the surface tension, and a droplet is thus formed and detaches itself from the orifice. Upon increasing the fluid velocity, laminar flow can be established. Within this laminar or Rayleigh flow regime, as flow increases, filaments begin to form within the jet due to local instabilities and primary droplets begin to form (3). Beyond this region (at higher jet velocities), a turbulent jet exists which further destabilizes the fluid and increases the droplet content of the spray (4). The mechanisms outlined above are for single fluid jets that are passing through a single nozzle. The mechanisms for droplet formation in common inhalation aerosol devices can be much more complex, as discussed below.

The same fundamental principles apply to the breakup of droplets in aerosols for inhalation therapy. However, depending on the configuration of the system, many more factors may come into play, thus rendering the mechanism of droplet formation much more complex. Primary droplet or liquid deformation can occur by several different mechanisms such as shear from high fluid flow (i.e., pressure differentials), localized turbulence, extrusion through micropumps, and even electrically induced ultrasonic waves (5). These mechanisms can produce primary droplets that are subject to further disintegration into secondary droplets, evaporation resulting in smaller droplet size, or coalescence/coagulation resulting in a larger droplet size. In many cases, a combination of these events can occur.

Due to the complexity of these phenomena, an index value, the Weber (We) number, is used to assess the probability of droplet breakup. The We number takes into account the density of air (ρ_a), the relative velocity of the droplet in an air stream (U), the diameter of the droplet (D), and the surface tension of the droplet (s). The mathematical relationship of these variables can be seen in Equation 7.1. The We number quantifies the ratio of the aerodynamic forces and the surface tension forces. The larger the We number, the greater the probability of droplet breakup. When these two forces are equal in magnitude, we have a condition known as the critical Weber number (We_{crit}). The We_{crit} is defined in Equation 2, where C_D is the coefficient of drag (0.45 for turbulent conditions). This number essentially represents the point where droplets disintegrate (6).

$$We = \frac{\rho_a U_R^2 D}{\sigma} \qquad (7.1)$$

$$We_{crit} = \frac{8}{C_D} \qquad (7.2)$$

In addition to the fundamental mechanisms, several physical and chemical properties of the system have a significant impact on the resulting aerosol formation. Within a fixed system, one of the largest factors that affect the formation of aerosols is the size and configuration of the nozzle system. Some of these systems include two-fluid gas/liquid nozzles, with internal mixing or postnozzle mixing. Others have natural feed or aspiration via the Venturi effect and have a baffle or impinger to assist in droplet breakup and to coalesce larger droplets to prevent their escape from the device.

Finally, factors associated with the characteristics of the liquids play a role in the formation of aerosols. With certain types of devices, such as plain air-jet nebulizers, the mean droplet is roughly inversely proportional to the relative velocity difference between the air/liquid interface and the original liquid jet diameter, but the density, viscosity, and surface tension all play a role (7,8). Density establishes the mass flow rate through the nozzle. However, in most aqueous systems, the differences in density from liquid to liquid can be quite small. The surface tension is a key component in the We number, as previously discussed, and represents the critical force that needs to be overcome to generate new droplets. In general, the minimum energy required for atomization is equal to the surface tension multiplied by the increase in liquid surface area. An important physicochemical property for liquids is viscosity. The viscosity of the liquid plays a large role in determining the Reynolds number of the fluid flow and thus alters the development of natural instabilities in the jet. This effectively slows the process of droplet disintegration and ultimately increases the droplet size (9). The relationship between viscosity and fluid flow through nozzles is highly dependent on the nature and geometry of the nozzle system. An in-depth description is beyond the scope of this chapter, but in general an increase in viscosity increases droplet size. This may be explained by the energy input being diverted into establishing fluid flow and thus being taken away from energy that can be utilized for the breakup of droplets and ultimately leads to a coarser aerosol. Therefore, when evaluating or considering atomization or nebulization systems, it important to account for the specific device atomization mechanism and the physicochemical properties of the drug product formulations.

Particle redispersion

The delivery of powders for pulmonary applications requires the redispersion of particle agglomerates into the air stream into primary particles. Therefore, the delivery efficiency of active pharmaceutical ingredients (APIs) is governed by the balance between the attractive forces holding the powder together and the external force applied to the agglomerates, generated during patient's inspiration through the device or from the device itself. Understanding these forces is necessary to control the formation and dispersion of agglomerates for optimum powder aerosol performance. A review of the basic interparticle forces, the factors affecting them, and the forces acting during redispersion is presented here. The mechanisms of dispersion in different inhaler devices will be further discussed in the section called "Particle re-dispersion devices."

PARTICLE-PARTICLE INTERACTION FORCES

Pharmaceutical powders for pulmonary delivery generally consist of fine drug particles (micronized API) mixed with excipient(s), such as the carrier lactose. When particle size is reduced to less than 10 μm, particle-particle interaction forces are stronger than gravity and their contribution to the overall system becomes significant, leading to potential challenges with agglomeration and deagglomeration (10–12).

Particle-particle attraction can be broadly classified as either adhesion or cohesion (10). *Adhesion* usually refers to the attraction of particles of two different chemical composition, while *cohesion* refers to the attraction of two particles of the same chemical nature. Although these forces are much weaker than covalent bonding, their range extends over greater distances, and thus they are called long-range forces (10). These interparticle interactions are the result of multiple concurrently acting forces, which include molecular interactions, electrostatic interactions, capillary forces, and mechanical interlocking (6,10–12). Uncharged particles can interact with each other through molecular interactions. Even overall neutral particles can possess temporary local concentrations of charge due to instantaneous different electronic configurations. This leads to the formation of permanent or transient dipoles, which can induce complementary dipoles in neighboring particles. Consequently, polarizable neutral charge molecules can attract each other through molecular interactions called London–van der Waals dispersion forces that exerts an influence over a range of approximately 10 nm, rapidly decreasing with increasing distance between the two particles (6,10). In a normal environment with low relative humidity, van der Waals forces are the main contributor to the cohesive/adhesive forces between two particles.

The van der Waals force between two macroscopic particles was calculated by Hamaker assuming the additivity property of the London–van der Waals forces. He integrated pair-wise all possible individual molecular interactions in a macroscopic, spherical solid body, obtaining the following equation (6,12):

$$F = \frac{A}{12r^2} \star \left(\frac{d_1 d_2}{d_1 + d_2} \right) \tag{7.3}$$

where A is the Hamaker constant (which depends on the materials involved), d_1 and d_2 are the diameters of the two spherical particles, and r is the separation distance between the two particles. Similarly, the adhesion of a sphere to a plane surface composed of different molecules can be calculated as:

$$F = \frac{\sqrt{A_{11} A_{22}}}{6r^2} d_1 \tag{7.4}$$

where A_{11} and A_{22} are the Hamaker constants for the fine particle and the plane surface, respectively; d_1 is the diameter of the particle; and r is the separation distance between the particle and the plane surface (10).

Contact, sliding, and friction between particles during powder processing, handling, and delivery can generate an electrical charge on insulating particles' surfaces (13). The term *triboelectrification* is often used to describe this process of charging. The electrostatic interaction force between charged particles can be described by Coulomb's law, in which the attractive (or repulsive) force is proportional to the charge of the particles and rapidly decreases with a separation distance between the two particles (6,12). Depending on the formulation and the device, the extent of this force can vary.

Liquid bridges originate when a material adsorbs water vapor onto its surface. This leads to an attractive force between particles or between a particle and the device surface due to the surface tension of adsorbed liquid films present at the contact point (capillary adhesion forces) (6,12). At low relative humidity, liquid bridges usually do not contribute significantly to the particle interactions. For hydrophilic particles, however, such forces are potentially prevalent over the other forces if the relative humidity is raised above 65% (10,12,14,15).

It is important to note that the equations that describe van der Waals forces, electrostatic interaction forces, and capillary adhesion forces have been determined for ideal spherical particles made of a hard material. The irregular shape of particles possessing asperities and imperfections, potential surface deformation, and heterogeneous chemical composition can lead to changes in the separation distance and contact area between the particles, leading to deviations from the theory. In particular, for powder blends containing particles with high surface roughness, mechanical interlocking can occur (e.g., entrapment of small particles in the asperities of larger carrier particles), which increase the overall adhesion forces (10,11). Several mathematical approaches have been explored to incorporate these parameters into the interparticle forces calculations, such as Johnson-Kendhal-Robert (JKR) theory (16), Derjaguin method (17), Maugis method (18), and the model derived by Rabinovich (19,20). However, these methods are complicated and are not easily applicable to experimental data.

In addition to particle morphology, other factors that affect particle-particle interactions include size distribution, polydispersity, physicochemical properties (such as the mechanical and electrical properties and hygroscopicity) (21), crystal form (11) (such as crystallinity and polymorphism), and external environmental conditions (such as relative humidity, temperature, and processing conditions). A summary of these main factors and their effects is reported in Table 7.1.

MECHANISMS OF REDISPERSION

For a powder to be emitted from a dry powder inhaler (DPI) device during inhalation, it needs to be fluidized, entrained in the air stream, and then emitted. During this process, the powder must deagglomerate. Deagglomeration has an inverse relationship with interparticle strength (41); cohesive forces must be overcome by dispersion forces for this process to be successful (11,12). The forces involved in powder dispersion can be broadly categorized into aerodynamic forces (shear, drag, and lift) and inertial forces (impaction, vibration, and centrifugal) (12).

During inhalation, airflow creates shear on the powder, which leads to lift and drag forces that are responsible for the fluidization and entrainment of the powder in the airflow. These forces are proportional to the square of the particle's diameter, which results in a greater effect on larger particles. This has been suggested as one of the reasons carrier particles have been traditionally used in DPIs as excipients to facilitate powder flow and delivery of fine API particles, which are adhered to the carrier surface. Once in the air stream, turbulence can create tumbling and rolling, thus facilitating the release of the APIs from the carrier.

Table 7.1 Factors related to powder redispersion

Factor	Force affected	Mechanism	Reference
Particles size	van der Waals	For size <10 μm, van der Waals are dominant over gravitational forces. Potential interlocking mechanism.	(11,22)
Size distribution and polydispersity	van der Waals	Increase packing and number of contacts between particles.	(11,23–25)
Shape	van der Waals and electrostatic forces	Effect the contact area between particles.	(11,26–29)
Surface texture	van der Waals	Surface asperities affect inter-particles distance. Potential interlocking.	(30–33)
Surface deformation	van der Waals	Can increase the adhesion force by increasing the contact area.	(30,34)
Surface energy	van der Waals, electrostatic forces, and liquid bridge/capillary forces	Affects forces at multiple levels specific for each type of material.	(35,36)
Hygroscopicity	Liquid bridge/capillary forces	Affects adsorption and/or absorption of water vapor onto particles.	(11)
Porosity	Liquid bridge/capillary forces	Porous particles have higher specific surface area which makes them more sensitive to humidity than coarser particles.	(37)
Environment relative humidity	Liquid bridge/capillary forces and electrostatic forces	Increased relative humidity results in increased rate and magnitude of water vapor adsorption onto solid particle surfaces. At low humidity, electrostatic forces are mainly important.	(14,15,37–39)
Physicochemical properties of particles and contacting surfaces	Electrostatic forces	Particles charge will depend upon their relative electron-donor or -acceptor properties as well as the material of the surfaces they come in contact with.	(40)
Crystal types	Electrostatic forces	Charge distribution and surface energy will depend on the crystallinity of the solid.	(11)
Processing conditions	van der Waals, electrostatic forces, and liquid bridge/capillary forces	Affects forces at multiple levels, e.g., increasing deformation, changing crystallinity, exposure to humidity.	(10)

The torque generated by turbulence can also lead to sudden acceleration, which creates centrifugal forces on the API particles (8,12,42). If the acceleration is directly opposite to the cohesive/adhesive force ($F_{inter-part}$), detachment can occur when:

$$ma > F_{inter-part} \quad (7.5)$$

where m is the mass of the particle and a is the acceleration (8). Due to the complexity of the process, computational models have been developed to calculate the separation torque for drug particles from carrier particle (43) and map powder cohesive strength distribution (44) in order to predict deagglomeration and powder performance (45).

Depending on the device, many particle-particle and particle-wall collisions can occur, and they further contribute to the dispersion of the powder (43). For a particle of mass m on the outside of an agglomerate, the force of detachment by impaction can be expressed as:

$$F = \frac{m\vartheta_0}{\Delta_t} \quad (7.6)$$

where ϑ_0 is the speed of impaction and is the collision time (8).

Finally, vibration of either carrier particle or of a film to which the powder is adhered, has also been used to disperse powders (43).

Each mechanism of deagglomeration occurs to a different extent in different types of inhalers. More detailed mechanisms related to different devices are provided in the section called "Aerosol device technology."

Evaporation–condensation

The first step in aerosol generation for devices governed by evaporation–condensation is the process of evaporation. Evaporation occurs when a liquid is heated, increasing the net loss of liquid from the surface to vapor, which means that the rate of molecules leaving the surface of a liquid is higher than the rate of molecules arriving at that surface or condensing (46–48).

The second step is condensation. In a supersaturated vapor system, as the temperature decreases, the partial vapor pressure increases above the saturated vapor pressure and condensation occurs (46,48). This temperature decrease may occur as the vapor moves away from the source of heat. Condensation can either occur by heterogeneous nucleation or homogeneous nucleation. Heterogeneous nucleation depends on the presence of condensation nuclei (such as small particles), while homogeneous nucleation (also known as self-nucleation) corresponds to the process of particle growth without the presence of condensation nuclei. Heterogeneous condensation generates more controlled monodisperse aerosols compared to homogeneous nucleation. Homogeneous nucleation requires higher supersaturation ratios than heterogeneous nucleation (46–48). Various factors influence the aerosol quality. For example, Leong (47) found an additional step can be included to improve monodispersity of the aerosol, by reheating and recondensing the droplets. Monodispersity could also be further improved by changing the geometry of the aerosol generator (e.g., the volume–to–surface area ratio of the container) (47,49).

Additional factors affecting droplet size include the excipients used in the formulation, the vapor concentration, and temperature. If the temperature is too high, it may degrade the drug; however, if the temperature is too low, insufficient vapor or aerosol will be formed. Therefore, these factors need to be considered when developing an aerosol by evaporation–condensation mechanisms. A solution to the avoidance of degradation due to high temperature could be the incorporation of low-volatile materials, as demonstrated by Hickey and Smyth (47,50).

AEROSOL DEVICE TECHNOLOGY

Atomization devices

PRESSURIZED METERED-DOSE INHALERS

Pressurized metered-dose inhalers (pMDIs) are handheld devices used in the treatment of lung diseases such as asthma and chronic obstructive pulmonary disease (COPD). Their first appearance in the market (1956, Medihaler Iso, Riker Laboratories, Inc) was revolutionary, considering the device size, ease of use, large number of doses (approximately 200 doses), and relatively low cost (51,52).

The technology behind pMDIs consists of an API either dissolved or dispersed in a high-pressure liquid propellant, which provides the energy to aerosolize the formulation. Upon actuation, a spray is delivered directly to the mouth of the patient, where a relatively high-velocity aerosol (30–60 m/s) is theoretically transported to the deep lung. The efficiency of these devices is significantly low (<50%) due to a significant amount of drug depositing in the oropharyngeal region by impaction

(53,54). The purpose of this section is to introduce the main components of pMDIs and their effect on the drug delivery efficiency.

Device components: Metered valves, actuators design, and nozzle

The basic components that make up the hardware of pMDI devices has remained generally the same for the past several decades. The three most important components of a pMDI device are the canister, the metering valve, and the actuator. The canister and the valve provide a sealed system that works as a reservoir for the liquefied high-pressure formulation. The metered chamber, located in the valve, controls the deliverable dose, typically between 25 and 100 µL, through a cyclic process of releasing the drug through the stem and loading the chamber after actuation (55,56). The actuator is an independent plastic platform that keeps the canister in position and provides support during actuation. The inner geometry of the actuator holds the expansion chamber, where the liquid propellant expands thanks to a recirculation region known as the sump. The plastic actuator provides the orifice through which formulation is emitted and the mouthpiece that interfaces with the patient (Figure 7.1).

Differences in the actuator have proven to have a significant impact on the final plume characteristics (Figure 7.2), and researchers in the past have shown great interest in understanding how the interaction between formulation and device affect the efficiency of the inhaler (57–60).

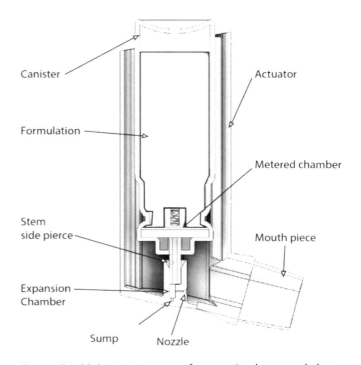

Figure 7.1 Main components of pressurized metered-dose inhalers.

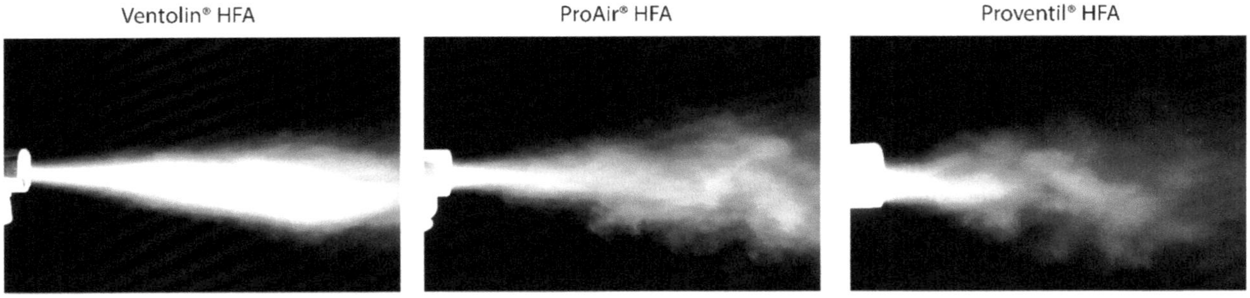

| Ventolin® HFA | ProAir® HFA | Proventil® HFA |

Figure 7.2 Composite image of pMDI plumes generated by three marketed albuterol sulfate-based formulations.

The formulation in pMDIs

The last 60 years have seen continuous developments in pressurized metered-dose inhaler (pMDI) formulations. The first products available on the market used chlorofluorocarbons (CFCs) as the liquid propellant to provide the energy for drug aerosolization and lung delivery. However, after years on the market, it was established that CFCs have serious environmental consequences and contributed to the depletion of the ozone layer. This led to a CFC phaseout process for almost two decades. After the global transition away from CFCs was endorsed by the Montreal Protocol revision in 1997, the last CFC-based pMDI product (Maxair Autohaler, Graceway Pharmaceuticals) was removed from the U.S. market in December 2013 (61). Consequently, an entire generation of pMDIs was reformulated using two new propellants known as hydrofluoroalkane (HFA134a and HFA227), which feature significantly lower ozone depletion effects than their CFC predecessors. The transition from pMDIs using CFCs to HFAs presented two significant complications. First, the solubility of previously used excipients was significantly lower in HFAs compared to CFCs, making it challenging to formulate CFC-free equivalent products (15,62,63). Second, banning these products had a significant economic impact on the public health policy of developing countries due to a reduction in the number of more affordable generic products. Therefore, the phaseout process was scheduled to be gradual, allowing the use of CFCs where required for a longer time period (64). On the other hand, reformulation using HFA propellants had some benefits. Some of the new formulations generated warmer and slower plumes, increasing the delivery efficiency and reducing oropharyngeal deposition (53,64,65).

Currently, pMDIs may be subject to a similar need for redesign after the Kigali amendment in the last Montreal Protocol revision (October 2016). This time, an international phase-down agreement for fluorinated gases was signed, wherein 197 countries agreed to cut the production and consumption of hydrofluorocarbons (HFCs) by more than 80% over the next 30 years (68). Therefore, HFCs such as HFA 134a and HFA 227, both used for orally inhaled and nasal drug products (OINDPs), may eventually be replaced by alternatives. At present, several candidates may exist. For example, HFA 152a has a global warming potential (GWP) ten times lower than HFA134a or 227 but a similar vapor pressure (Table 7.2), and it has preliminary data demonstrating formulation of pMDI solution and suspensions with comparable cascade impaction stage deposition profiles to HFA134a formulations (Figure 7.3) (69).

Excipients

Excipients approved for inhalation are scarce compared to other dosage forms, and in the case of pMDIs, the additional limitation of compatibility with propellants decreases the options further (62). Formulations usually

Table 7.2 Properties of current and potential alternative liquid propellants used in pMDIs

Propellant	Molecular weight	GWP[a]	Vapor pressure (psig) at 20°C	Boiling point (°C)	Density (g cm^{-3})
HFA 134a	102	1360	64.5	−26	1.21
HFA 227	170	3140	56	−16	1.39
HFA 152a	66.1	148	63	−25	0.908

Source: UNEP. Report of the refrigeration, air conditioning and heat pumps technical options committee, 2014. Available from: http://conf.montreal-protocol.org/meeting/mop/mop-27/presession/Background%20Documents%20are%20available%20in%20English%20only/RTOC-Assessment-Report-2014.pdf; Propellants, M.M., Zephex HFA Medical propellants. Mexichem, 2016, United Nations Environment Programme Report of the Technology and Economic Assessment Panel, Mexichem website, 2016.

[a] Global warming potential.

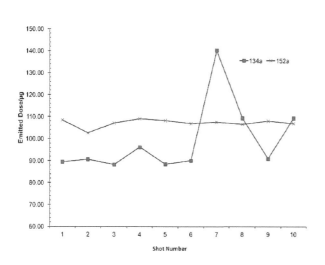

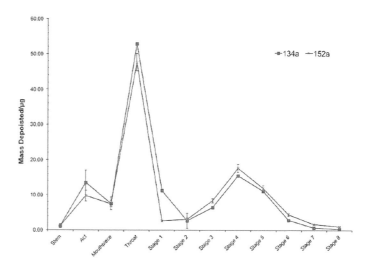

Figure 7.3 Emitted dose uniformity test and aerodynamic particle size distribution performance for Albuterol sulfate suspension formulation based on HFA152a. Formulations were bench filled. (From OINDPnews. Mexichem discusses potential for using HFA 152a as pMDI propellant 2016 [cited July 25, 2017]. Available from: http://www.oindpnews.com/2016/12/mexichem-discusses-potential-for-using-hfa-152a-as-pmdi-propellant/.)

include an API, a liquid propellant, and excipients, the function of which varies depending on whether the formulation is a solution or suspension.

The most commonly used excipients are cosolvents (e.g., ethanol). These solubilize the API or surfactant in the liquid propellant, and suspension stabilizers (e.g., oleic acid), working as dispersing agents. Other components such as valve lubricants (e.g., polyethylene glycol) are used if required, and other less common options such as antioxidants or buffering agents are used to increase stability.

The influence of these excipients on the aerosol performance has been investigated. In the case of the first generation of inhalers, by combining different proportions of CFCs, Clark determined that the velocity of the droplets in the aerosol was directly correlated to the vapor pressure of the mixture (70). Later, Dunbar and colleagues showed, using the same propellants and measurement method, that addition of surfactant and drug to CFC systems raises the droplet velocity (71). These were some of the first attempts on modulating the overall plume velocity of the pMDI by changing the components of the formulation; however, the limited solubility in the propellant was a limitation in this approach.

Studying the second generation of propellants (HFA 134a and HFA 227), Hoye, Gupta, and Myrdal investigated the variables involved in predicting the solubility of several organic solutes in HFA. The study also included the effect of the presence and absence of ethanol to build a predictive model for the solubility of new compounds in the liquid propellant (63,72). Unfortunately, even though some of the factors studied (melting point, logP, molar volume, entropy) shown some correlation, data did not allow an accurate prediction of the solubility in HFA.

For suspension formulations, the variation in dosing if the inhaler is not shaken before use, particle-particle interaction, potential clogging of the valve, and/or nozzle

blockage are the most common drawbacks (73,74). To overcome these issues, investigation of new excipients has increased. In some cases, these new excipients have successfully reached the market, as demonstrated by the recent incorporation of hollow porous microspheres (PulmoSpheres™) in Bevespi® (Pearl Therapeutics S.A). This new co-suspension delivery system enabled consistent aerosol performance of inhaled medication, ensuring a uniform dose of double or triple combination of drugs for the treatment of COPD. The technology relies on the incorporation of low-density phospholipid base microparticles into the suspension MDI, forming respirable agglomerates suitable for inhalation (75).

From actuation to aerosol formation

The aerosolization process in pMDIs is a complex, dynamic, and transient event that usually lasts no more than a few hundred milliseconds (76). Once actuated, a known volume of liquid propellant (20–100 μL) previously loaded into the metered valve is transferred to the expansion chamber through the valve stem. As soon as the valve opens, the propellant transfers from the canister to the expansion chamber and exits the actuator through the nozzle. During this process, the intermolecular attractive forces between liquid propellant molecules are overcome by the large pressure gradient, generating cavities filled with propellant vapor. This phenomenon, known as flashing or cavitation, occurs only at nucleation sites, naturally occurring small vapor pockets located in the irregular surfaces of suspended drug particles, and on the surface of the walls of the expansion chamber and actuator passage (4). These rapidly growing bubbles form and flash evaporation occurs. Versteeg et al. (77) confirmed the presence of bubble growth and the effect of the early cavitation process using a transparent actuator and

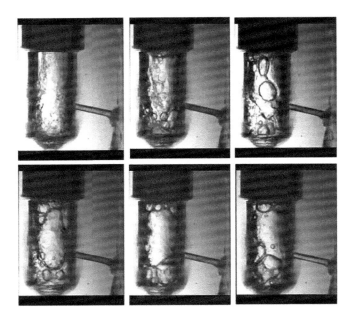

Figure 7.4 Internal view of an expansion chamber in a pMDI. (From Versteeg, H. et al. *J Phy Confer Ser.*, 45, 207–213, 2006.)

high-speed imaging (Figure 7.4). Their results described the presence of a two-phase (gas/liquid) mixture starting to flow from the metered valve, following an annular flow regime inside the expansion chamber. The mixtures presented a vapor core, flashing near the spray orifice exit and the sump (77).

After the formulation exits the expansion chamber through the nozzle orifice, two separate phases occur: (1) droplet formation (2) aerosol maturation (78). The first involves the atomization of the formulation in small droplets through disruption of the surface of the liquid propellant by shear, as described in the section called "Physical principles of aerosol generation." The second relates to the evaporation rate of the droplets in the aerosol, which depends on the content of volatile and semivolatile components such as the

hydrofluoroalkanes and ethanol. Prediction of droplet size, residual particle size, number of emitted droplets, and effect on drug delivery efficiency has been studied extensively in the past (58,79–81). In the case of solution formulations using nonvolatile components, the residual particle would be a matrix of drug and excipient, but if semivolatile and volatile excipients are used, this results in amorphous drug spheres (82). For suspensions, the result of the aerosol maturation is different since the formulation is not homogeneous and droplets generated may or may not contain the micronized drug. Because of this, the residual particle can vary in size depending on the number of suspended particles in the droplet (Figure 7.5) (79).

Dose counters and electronic monitoring devices

The inability to track the number of doses remaining in the canister has been an issue for many years because these inhalers can deliver several doses above the labeled claim, increasing the chances for the patient to receive sub-therapeutic doses. Moreover, the responsibility of dose tracking has been historically delegated to the patient, with one in every four patients finding their pMDIs empty during an asthma attack (83). In 2003, the United States Food and Drug Administration (FDA) developed a guidance for the industry to regulate the addition of an integrated dose counter in devices (71).

The use of electronic device technologies has grown exponentially in daily life during the last decade, and inhalation devices are also receiving attention. Electronic monitoring devices are gaining greater acceptance, and their claims to optimize the patient experience and compliance have attracted much attention. Devices like SmartTrack, CareTRx™, Doser, or Smartinhaler tracker offer valuable information about patient compliance and adherence (84), and have generated many publications over the last years (85–87). Regardless of the benefits claimed by the manufacturers, the acceptance of these new technologies has met with resistance. Experts reported that physician's concerns

QVAR® (solution)   Ventolin® (suspension)

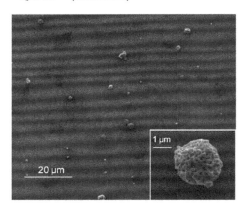 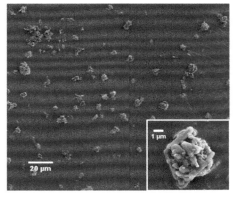

Figure 7.5 SEM images of residual particles from a solution (QVAR®) and a suspension formulation (Ventolin®). (From Grainger, C. et al. *Mol. Pharm.*, 9, 563–569, 2012.)

reside in the potential for increased burdens to the health-care system, liability, and clinical relevance of data. On the other hand, patients state that the use of these technologies should be intuitive and integrated into the device, but they have concerns about the utilization of the information, specifically in the case of retribution by insurance companies if their compliance is low (88).

NEBULIZERS

Nebulizers have been widely employed in liquid aerosol inhalation for the delivery of solutions and suspensions. As the development of nebulizer technologies advances, aerosol generation has progressed from manually compressing a hand-bulb to gas and electronic power systems (89). Lung deposition of drugs is determined by both aerosol characteristics (size, shape, density, and charge of droplets) and patient-dependent factors (airway anatomy, pathophysiology, respiratory pattern, etc.). Most research has focused on the improvement of aerosol properties to enhance lung deposition since different size ranges of particle possess different capacities to deposit in lung. Even though droplets generated by nebulizers often present heterogeneous size distribution, nebulizers have advantages such as high deposition in the lung, applicability to children, and the capability to aerosolize biomolecule-containing formulations compared to other delivery systems. Commercial nebulizers can be divided into three majora categories: jet nebulizers, ultrasonic nebulizers, and vibrating-mesh nebulizers (90).

Jet nebulizers

Jet nebulizers are powered by a compressed gas source. The general principle of jet nebulizers is that high-velocity gas flow leads to decreased pressure (Venturi effect) around the nozzle, which further draws the solution from the reservoir (Bernoulli effect) (Figure 7.6). As described in the section called "Physical principles of aerosol generation," droplet formation depends on the balance between internal and external forces. Here, the internal force is the surface tension of liquid bulk or droplet, and the external forces include shear generated by Venturi and Bernoulli effects as well as localized turbulence. The drug-containing solution can be broken up by the high-velocity compressed gas to form aerosol droplets. Most of the primary droplets have an impact on the baffle, to be further broken up or recycled into the reservoir since they are normally too large to be inhaled. As a result, part of the drug-containing liquid must experience several cycles to be inhaled by patients, which limits its application to the delivery of easily degradable drugs (91,92). Furthermore, droplet size is proportional to the square root of the liquid jet diameter. Jet nebulizers can be classified into four main categories based on their design: jet nebulizers with a reservoir tube, jet nebulizers with a collection bag, breath-enhanced nebulizers, and breath-actuated nebulizers.

Jet nebulizers with a reservoir tube

This type of jet nebulizer generates aerosol constantly during inspiration, expiration, and breath-hold. As a result, a significant portion of drug-containing aerosol can be exhaled to the environment. These nebulizers are generally considered to have low efficiency in drug delivery since only around 15% of aerosol can be inhaled (93). Although the requirement for a compressed gas source and variability between device design and operation introduces inconveniences in clinical operation, they are user-friendly and have good patient compliance (94). Sidestream Nebulizers™ and Micro Mist® are examples of this type of nebulizers available on the market.

Jet nebulizers with a collection bag

In this type of nebulizer, aerosol generated by compressed gas is temporarily stored in a collection bag. When patients

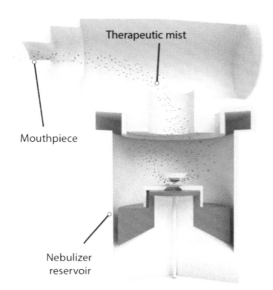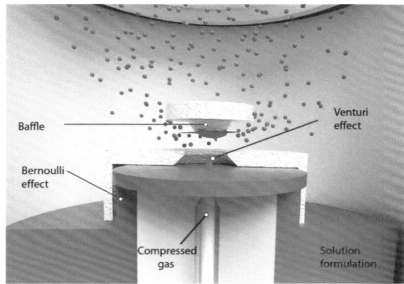

Figure 7.6 A schematic diagram showing the principle of conventional jet nebulizers.

inspire, the one-way valve between the bag and mouthpiece allows aerosol in the bag to be inhaled by the patient. When the patient exhales, the valve near the mouthpiece allows the aerosol to be released to the environment while the one-way valve is closed, which leads to the accumulation of the generated aerosol in the collection bag instead of being lost to the environment. Compared with jet nebulizers with a reservoir tube, this type of nebulizer generates aerosol with significantly smaller droplet sizes and provides less medication than jet nebulizers (95). The Circulaire® is an example of this type of nebulizer available on the market.

Breath-enhanced jet nebulizers

There are two one-way valves in this type of nebulizer: inspiratory valve and expiratory valve. Inspiratory valve is open during inhalation, and expiratory valve in the mouthpiece is open during the expiration process to prevent aerosol escaping into the environment. As a result, this design reduces the loss of aerosol and improves the delivery efficiency. Efficiency of breath-enhanced nebulizers is higher than for jet nebulizers with a reservoir tube. When comparing the drug output in vented and unvented nebulizers, vented nebulizers exhibited higher drug output as inspiratory flow increased, resulting in shorter nebulization times and a reduction in drug loss during the expiratory phase (96). PARI LC® Plus, NebuTech®, and SideStream Plus® are examples of this type of nebulizer available on the market.

Breath-actuated jet nebulizers

The design of this type of nebulizer allows devices to sense the respiratory pattern of patients and deliver aerosol only during the inhalation process. For example, AeroEclipse II® has a breath-actuated valve that can move up and down to trigger the delivery of drug aerosol. When patients exhale, the valve is closed, resulting in no generation or delivery of drug aerosol, which significantly decreases the loss of drug to the environment. In addition, both the breath-enhanced and breath-actuated nebulizers enhance efficiency of delivery of aerosol and reduce nebulization time compared with other jet nebulizers (97).

Ultrasonic nebulizers

The working mechanism underlying ultrasonic nebulizers is based on the power conversion from electrical signals to oscillatory mechanical movement through a piezoelectric transducer. High frequency, which can be as high as 20 kHz, enables the piezoelectric transducer to generate pressure disturbances propagating throughout the liquid. These pressure disturbances can further create liquid-air interfacial destabilization, which subsequently leads to bubble breakup and aerosol droplet formation (98) (Figure 7.7). Ultrasonic nebulizers can produce smaller droplets and a less heterodisperse aerosol than jet nebulizer systems (99).

Because of the high-energy input during the aerosol generation process, the local temperature can increase significantly, which potentially limits the use of this type of nebulizer for the delivery of macromolecules since they are more sensitive to thermal variation (100). In addition, ultrasonic nebulizers are not suitable for aerosolizing suspensions (101,102) and highly viscous solutions (101,103). However, lipid nanoparticles can be delivered to the lungs by using ultrasonic nebulizers without leading to the rupture or aggregation of lipid nanoparticles (104,105). Examples of this type of nebulizer include The MicroAir® Ultrasonic Model and MABISMist™ II.

Vibrating-mesh nebulizers

Vibrating-mesh nebulizers may apply micropump technology to force bulk liquid to pass through a mesh membrane, resulting in the formation of aerosol droplets. This type of nebulizer can be divided into two categories—passive vibrating-mesh and active vibrating-mesh systems—based on device design and mechanisms underlying aerosol generation. In the passive vibrating-mesh system, a piezo crystal connected to a transducer horn is powered by electricity and induces the vibration of the transducer horn, subsequently creating waves in the bulk liquid. As a result, the solution in the reservoir is forced to flow through the mesh membrane and disperse to form an aerosol (106). In contrast, the active vibrating-mesh system contains a mesh connected to a vibrating piezoelectric element. The vibration of the microperforated membrane forces liquid to pass through

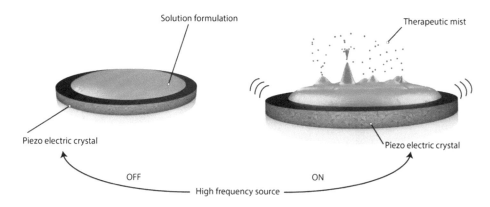

Figure 7.7 A schematic diagram showing the principle of aerosol formation in ultrasonic nebulizers.

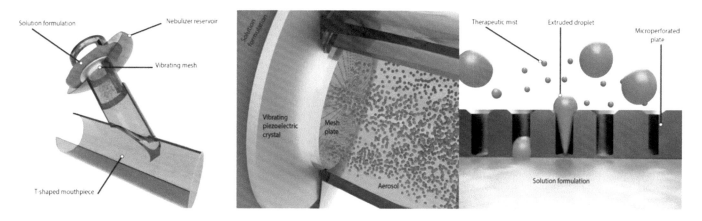

Figure 7.8 A schematic diagram showing the principle of an active vibrating-mesh system.

the mesh, which breaks up to create an aerosol (107) (Figure 7.8).

Overall, vibrating-mesh nebulizers cause minimal changes in temperature, low change in drug concentration, and have low residual volume. Use of the Aeroneb Pro® caused only a 5°C increase in temperature, while air-jet and ultrasonic nebulizers demonstrated considerable temperature change: approximately 10°C (108). This type of nebulizer has minimal residual volume of drug formulation following nebulization compared to jet-nebulizers and ultrasonic nebulizers (100). Notably, the performance of both types of vibrating-mesh nebulizers depends on the properties of drug formulations. A change in droplet size was observed as fluid viscosity increased, which also led to a prolonged nebulization time and decreased output rate. Ion concentration also affects the properties of aerosol. Liquid with a low ion concentration led to enhanced aerosol generation and reduced variability in droplet size and output (109). Omron MicroAir (passive) and Aeroneb Pro and Pari eFlow (active) are examples of this type of nebulizers.

METERED LIQUID DOSE INHALERS

Water-based metered liquid dose inhalers are a newer category of inhaler devices that generate aerosolized droplet mists using either electrical, mechanical, or kinetic energy (110,111). The development of these mist inhalers was driven by several factors, including (1) environmental effects of propellants, (2) patient-dependent drug deposition, (3) repeatable efficacy, and (4) portability and ease of maintenance (112). Aside from the methods mentioned previously in the overview of atomization and nebulization, liquids containing dissolved drug can be aerosolized by colliding liquid jets, mechanical extrusion, electrostatic charge, and vaporization. The Respimat® SoftMist™ Inhaler, developed by Boehringer Ingelheim, creates a spray by colliding two liquid jets. The Respimat SMI is mechanically driven and uses a spring rather than propellants to force the metered liquid dose through a two-channel nozzle. This produces two jets of liquid with narrow diameters that collide at a preset angle to generate the soft mist (110). The soft mist

inhaler may reduce patient-dependent drug deposition by increasing the fine particle fraction (approximately 65% to 80%) and particle size control, increasing plume duration (approximately 1.5 seconds) and decreasing mist velocity (89,110,113). In general, creating a spray using this method requires nozzles with orifices on the order of 10 μm in diameter (114). Additionally, the pressure needed to generate liquid jets can be hundreds of atmospheres, which may negatively affect the drug (114). The Respimat SoftMist™ Inhaler platform is currently available for five different formulations for the treatment of COPD and asthma (115–118).

Other methods for creating sprays are in various stages of development and adoption by the market. The AERx® platform, developed by Aradigm, creates a continuous, steady capillary microjet of atomized liquid (119). In versions of the AERx inhaler, the liquid formulation is contained in disposable bolus packages, each of which contains an aerosol nozzle with laser drilled holes (89). During atomization, the liquid dose is extruded through the laser drilled holes into an air channel that provides the necessary flow rate for droplet formation (120). The resulting droplets are controlled by the nozzle pore size and airflow rate. Aerosols generated by this device had 90% of droplets within the 2–3 μm diameter range (89). While the AERx Insulin Diabetes Management System (iDMS) reached phase III clinical trials, it has not been brought to the market (121). The AERx platform is also being tested for delivery of liposomal ciprofloxacin for bronchiectasis, cystic fibrosis, and biodefense applications (122). The Mystic Inhaler, which was under development by Battelle Memorial Institute, used electrostatic charging to atomize a bulk liquid to generate an electrohydrodynamic spray. For this type of device, an electric field of sufficient strength to charge ions in a liquid, overcome surface tension, and induce aerosolization is required (123,124). Electrostatic charging can be used to produce monodisperse and nonagglomerated particles in a range of sizes, as is needed for inhaled therapies (125). Liquids used in this type of device must have specific electrical and physical properties to be aerosolized by electrohydrodynamic spraying (124,125). Metered-dose liquid inhalers overcome some

Table 7.3 Aerosol mist inhalers currently available and under development

Manufacturer	Product	Disease indication	API
Boehringer Ingelheim	STIOLTO® Respimat	COPD	Tiotropium Bromide and Olodaterol
	SPIRIVA® Respimat	COPD	Tiotropium Bromide
	SPIRIVA® Respimat	Asthma	Tiotropium Bromide
	COMBIVENT® Respimat	COPD	Tiotropium Bromide and Albuterol
	STRIVERDI® Respimat	COPD	Olodaterol
Aradigm	AERx™ iDMS	Diabetes (Types I and II)	Insulin
	ARD-3150 Pulmaquin®	Bronchiectasis	Pulmaquin, Liposomal Ciprofloxacin
	ARD-3100 Lipoquin®	Cystic Fibrosis	Lipoquin, Liposomal Ciprofloxacin
Battelle Memorial Institute	Mystic	–	–
Pharmaero ApS	ADI	Lung Infections	Antibiotics

of the obstacles that current devices face, but aside from the Respimat system, they have yet to be commercialized (Table 7.3).

Particle redispersion devices

DRY POWDER INHALERS

DPIs are pulmonary delivery devices in which drug powder is aerosolized by energy supplied by the patient's inspiratory flow or the device itself. The delivery system consists of the device, the drug formulation, and the dose-metering system. Dose administration is breath actuated, thereby eliminating the need for coordination between patient inhalation and device actuation that is found with pMDIs. The first DPI, the Spinhaler®, became available in 1971 (126). The advent of the Montreal Protocol in 1987 further accelerated development of DPI technologies as an alternative to propellant-based systems (127), while still retaining the portability and rapid administration time of pMDIs. Other advantages of DPIs include the ability to deliver drugs that are unstable in aqueous environments, and the delivery of higher drug payloads, as exemplified by the commercialization of antibiotic dry powder delivery systems such as the TOBI® Podhaler (Tobramycin, 28 mg) (128).

However, DPIs are not without disadvantages. To be deposited in the lungs, drug particles must be less than 5 μm in aerodynamic diameter. This generally necessitates the use of micronization techniques to produce very small, geometrically sized particles. As discussed in the section called "Aerosol device technology," the increased surface area–to–mass ratio found in particles of this size range as well as the increased surface energy brought about by micronization processes results in highly cohesive particles (129). Particle redispersion is therefore one of the major challenges of powder delivery via DPI.

Many of the technological advancements made in DPI device and formulation design have been focused on improving the dispersibility of powders and predictably delivering drug to the lungs in a manner that is unconnected to the magnitude of airflow through the device. The actual dosage delivered to the lungs of the patient depends on properties of the drug formulation (powder flow, particle size, shape, and surface energy), device performance, aerosol generation, patient inhalation technique, and the patient's inspiratory flow rate (27).

Mechanisms of particle fluidization and redispersion from DPIs

While pMDIs tend to follow a standard device design with little deviation, DPIs are highly variable in design, with differences in dimensions, internal geometries, airflow velocity, and mechanisms of aerosol generation (130). Devices are often designed for a specific drug formulation. In general, dose delivery is achieved through fluidization of the powder bed, followed by entrainment in the air stream and then dose emission from the device. As the patient inhales, airflow moves over the static powder bed and particles are mobilized through gas-assist, capillary, and shear forces in the case of aerodynamic fluidization, or vibration and impaction forces in the case of mechanical fluidization (129). Fluidized powders are then deaggregated into primary particles by strong aerodynamic forces (turbulence and shear stress) and particle collisions within the inhaler. Successful deaggregation is crucial to device performance because it determines the particle size that entrained and delivered to the patient (11), which in turn affects where in the lungs the drug is deposited. Different methods of powder entrainment include gas-assisted, shear-force driven, capillary, and mechanical fluidization (129). The specific mechanisms of these processes are discussed further in the section called "Aerosol device technology."

Device-based methods to improve powder redispersion

The design of a DPI must accomplish several objectives, including predictable performance independent of patient lung function and inspiratory force, successful deagglomeration of drug particles, and low manufacturing costs (131).

To overcome the cohesive forces between particles, break up agglomerates, and aerosolize the drug powder, sufficient energy must be supplied through the device. DPIs are categorized as passive or active devices depending on the source of energy for aerosol dispersion. Passive DPIs depend on the inhalation force of the patient to provide the energy needed to disperse the drug powder. As the patient inhales, the airflow over the powder bed results in the creation of shear forces, which in turn leads to the lift and drag forces necessary for fluidization and entrainment. As a result, in passive devices, the strength of the patient's airflow can influence the degree of fluidization and entrainment and subsequently the amount of drug delivered to the lungs (132). If flow rate is too low, sufficient deagglomeration of the drug powder will not occur, while if the velocity of the airflow exiting the device is too high, excessive oropharyngeal deposition will occur and reduce overall device performance. Different passive devices have varying degrees of flow rate dependency (131). For each device, it is postulated that there is a critical point at which increasing inspiratory airflow does not result in increased deagglomeration or further improvements in performance (133). Identification of this point could be used to maximize device performance.

In contrast, active DPIs utilize an external energy source to generate powder dispersion rather than relying on the patient's inhalation efforts. Devices in development include those where powder fluidization is powered by electrical, pneumatic, or mechanical forces. Currently, there are no active DPIs on the market, though the previously marketed Exubera® (Pfizer) inhaler for insulin utilized a jet of compressed air to achieve powder dispersion (134).

Various design components are incorporated into DPIs to improve aerosolization efficiency. Typically, devices incorporate an airflow constriction downstream of the inlet to increase the velocity and energy of the flow stream when it encounters the drug powder bed, to enhance the shear forces necessary to ensure particle detachment (133). Design components intended to induce turbulent flow may be included to facilitate deagglomeration or detachment of drug from carrier particles. Turbulent flows consist of highly irregular and rapid fluctuations in velocity in both time and space. The presence of turbulence subjects drug agglomerates and particles to shear forces resulting from acceleration in different directions. At forces of sufficient magnitude, particles are detached from agglomerates or carrier particles. Methods for inducing turbulent airflow include the use of multiple air inlets, as well as tortuous pathways, baffles, and grids in the airflow.

Mechanical forces may also be incorporated into the device design to ensure powder deagglomeration. These may be mechanically driven, in the case of impellers, beads, and spring-driven hammers, or they may provide a method for impaction, as is the case of baffles, in which the entrained powder in the flow impacts the baffle and deagglomerates (135). Other deagglomeration methods utilized in patented active devices include the introduction of pneumatic forces to the powder bed or mechanical vibration through specifically arranged capsules, flutter films, and piezoelectric crystals (136).

A mesh or screen is typically included in DPI device design, often to prevent capsule fragments from being inhaled. The inclusion of a mesh can also affect the flow stream. For example, a mesh may suppress turbulence downstream by generating a spatially uniform airflow, or turbulence may be increased by the presence of a mesh in the flow stream through use of pores. The presence of the mesh can improve particle deagglomeration through the generation of turbulence or impaction forces; however, particles may remain trapped on the mesh, negating the overall effect.

Small variation in device design can greatly affect performance. For example, by utilizing computational fluid dynamics modeling of a modified Aerolizer® device, Coates and colleagues found that the degree of grid voidage is inversely related to aerosol performance (137,138), while inlet size influences the levels of turbulence and particle impaction velocities generated in the device (139).

Role of device resistance in powder redispersion

To deliver drug to the lungs of the patient, air must flow through the DPI device. Flow rate (Q) through the device is related to device resistance (R) and pressure drop (ΔP) across the device by the following equation:

$$\Delta P = QR \tag{7.7}$$

For a given pressure drop, a higher flow rate is achieved through a lower-resistance device. Likewise, a lower flow rate is expected to be produced through a high-resistance device. Device resistance is increased by constricting the flow of air through use of narrowing inlets (140). By narrowing the cross-sectional area of the flow stream, the linear velocity is increased and greater kinetic energy is carried by the flow stream. This leads to improvements in device performance with respect to dose delivery and aerodynamic particle size distribution. For passive DPIs, the aerosolization efficiency of the device is therefore related to the resistance of the device, and the performance of high resistance DPIs may often exceed that of low resistance DPIs. However, a potential concern with high-resistance devices is that certain patients may lack the lung function to generate a flow rate sufficient to disperse the aerosol through the high-resistance devices (133), though recent literature suggests this may not be the case for newer devices (141). In addition, the velocity of the flow must be reduced, or most of the particles will deposit in the mouth or back of the throat. This may be accomplished by widening the flow path through the mouthpiece, which reduces the axial velocity of the flow stream exiting the device. Baffles or curved paths can also be implemented to reduce flow velocity.

DPI formulations

Formulation-based methods can be used to reduce particle cohesiveness and improve dispersibility from DPIs. Powder flow is generally directly related to particle size, with larger particles (greater than 50 µm) exhibiting greater flow and fluidization potential (142). To overcome the poor powder flow and fluidization of micronized drug particles, various formulation strategies have been implemented, including spheronization to produce loose agglomerates of drug powder and the blending of large (50–200 μm) carrier particles with drug powder. Carrier-based or carrier-free formulations may also utilize flow control agents such as magnesium stearate, lecithin, or leucine to reduce particle surface energy and heterogeneity, and thereby improve flow and powder dispersion (134).

Carrier-based systems utilize a blend of micronized drug particles with larger excipient particles, typically lactose. The drug adheres to the lactose particles, which results in improved powder flow compared to the drug alone. Upon inhalation by the patient, the drug particles are separated from the carrier particles. This approach is especially useful for low-potency drugs, where the dose may be so low that it requires a diluent for uniform dose filling. The dispersion mechanism and the type of carrier best suited for the formulation are heavily intertwined (143). Most of the currently produced commercial inhalers rely on drag and lift forces in turbulent air streams, which require carrier particles with relatively smooth surfaces. However, dispersion via inertial separation forces are less dependent on carrier properties and may in fact perform better with carriers containing a high degree of rugosity (144). Attractive forces between the carrier and drug particle must not be so great that the dispersion forces generated by the inhaler do not result in detachment. If detachment does not occur, then the drug particle will not deposit in the respiratory region. Inclusion of fine powders (excipient particles < 10 μm) may be utilized to block highly energetic sites on the carrier particles to improve aerosol performance.

Agglomerate-based formulations can contain either pure drug or a mixture of drug and excipient(s). The large agglomerates provide improved powder flow. These agglomerates must be strong enough to withstand the manufacturing process but can be deagglomerated upon inhalation by the patient. An example of an agglomerate-based DPI is the Pulmicort Turbuhaler® (AstraZeneca) (145).

Few excipients have been approved for pulmonary administration by the FDA. Particle engineering of APIs and approved excipients has emerged to control morphology, size, and surface energy of particles to achieve desirable aerosolization performance and deagglomeration and to overcome the limited availability of excipients. For new high-dose formulations especially, particle engineering provides means to overcome particle cohesion and to achieve dispersion (146), as the doses required for efficacy may preclude the use of excipients. Spray drying, anti-solvent precipitation, and supercritical fluid technologies are widely used particle engineering methods, with several variables that can be adjusted to achieve the desired product (127). An example of a particle-engineering approach to improve powder flow and lung delivery is the use of porous particles. Though typically large in geometrical diameter, the low-density nature of these particles results in a small aerodynamic diameter. This allows for the improvement in particle flow without the need for carrier particles, and ensures peripheral lung deposition (127). Examples of porous particle technology include PulmoSphere® (147,148) and the AIR® pulmonary delivery system (149). It is important to note that, in addition to device design, the type of formulation approach utilized may also affect the flow rate dependency of the DPI performance. In general, spheronization results in a high flow rate dependency, lactose carrier blends have a medium flow rate dependency, and low-density porous particles have low flow rate dependency to achieve powder dispersion (150).

Dose-metering systems in DPIs

DPIs can be classified based on the dose-metering system utilized. Capsule-based metering systems are generally considered to be first-generation devices (see the example in Figure 7.9). More advanced multidose devices deliver the dose through a premetered blister or strip incorporated into the device design or by dispensing the dose from a powder reservoir housed in the device design. Factory-metered capsules, blisters, and strips generally offer better protection of the drug from the environment and dose dispensing may be less prone to variability. However, depending on the device design, the patient may need to reload the dosage unit system, which can be inconvenient and increase the number of technical maneuvers and chances for error in the dose administration. Device metered systems can potentially administer multiple doses without requiring reloading but may be prone to dose and dispensing variability. Protection of the drug powder from the environment (i.e., moisture) is also a concern.

Evaporation–condensation devices

The limitations present in other inhaler devices, such as challenging physicochemical properties of the drug, irreproducible dosing, lack of particle size uniformity, the

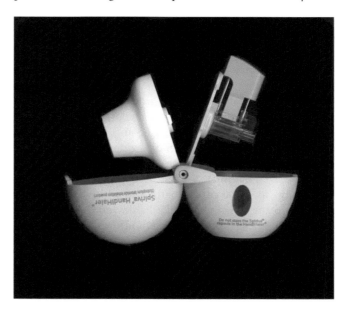

Figure 7.9 An example of a capsule-based DPI, the Spiriva Handihaler®.

difficulty of use, and targeting, have encouraged the development of delivery devices based on different mechanisms of aerosolization such as the ones characterized by evaporation-condensation technology.

Currently, only one FDA approved product is on the market: ADASUVE™ (utilizing the Staccato® technology), which is commercialized by Ferrer Therapeutic, Inc. Staccato ADASUVE was approved in 2012 by the FDA and in 2013 by EMA as a product containing loxepine for managing agitation in patients with schizophrenia and bipolar I disorder. The Staccato delivery device was developed by Alexza Pharmaceuticals. Ferrer Therapeutics, Inc., licensed and markets the ADASUVE product. This device is based on rapid vaporization by heating of a surface coated with a thin film of the drug. The device is breath-actuated and has a valve that controls airflow in order to achieve the desired particle size (151–153). Staccato produces an aerosol of small particle size (mass media aerodynamic diameter is in the 2 µm range for Loxapine), which is optimal for deep lung deposition and systemic delivery (154). This inhaler is handheld with single- or multi-dose capacity depending on the drug product (153). Besides ADASUVE, three more drug products are under development using the Staccato delivery device: AZ-003 (fentanyl) for oncologic pain; AZ-007 (zaleplon) for nocturnal awakening; and AZ-002 (alprazolam) for acute repetitive seizures, which is being developed by Engage Therapeutics and has recently raised $23 million to support its phase 2b clinical trials (155,156).

ARIA™ pulmonary delivery technology consists of a capillary tube that is heated in order to vaporize the liquid flowing inside it, which condenses when inhaled due to a decrease in temperature (50). This device was developed by Chrysalis Therapeutics, a division of Philip Morris, USA. More recently, Discovery Labs, now called Windtree Therapeutics, Inc., initiated a collaboration with Chrysalis to develop new drug delivery systems and transfer the technology to Windtree Therapeutics, Inc. (157–159). Aerosurf® is one of the products being developed by Windtree Therapeutics, and it is based on capillary technology for evaporation–condensation (158). Aerosurf just finished phase 2b clinical trials for the development of a noninvasive therapy using KL4 surfactants for the treatment of respiratory distress syndrome in premature infants (158).

Another drug delivery system based on rapid vaporization and the use of carriers with low vapor pressure (50). The device is composed of a heating filament, a surface coated with a carrier of low vapor pressure, and a therapeutic agent. In contrast with previous devices, the drug is not directly heated, which helps avoid drug degradation. Instead, a carrier of low vapor pressure is heated and vaporized, releasing the therapeutic agent afterward (50).

Recently, electronic cigarettes (e-cigarettes) have been considered for use in drug delivery (152). These devices are also based on evaporation-condensation technology. Briefly, electronic cigarettes are activated by an automatic flow sensor or a manual pushbutton which activates the heating element of the e-cigarette and vaporizes the solution inside. A wide variety of consumer devices are available with varying designs. Inhalation through the device introduces incoming air through inlet ports, over a heating element(s) and toward the mouthpiece. This airflow causes a drop in the temperature of the vapor, and condensation occurs to form liquid droplets that enter the respiratory tract (160).

CONCLUSION

Technology development for inhaled pharmaceutical products has evolved with our increased understanding of the mechanisms of aerosol formation and how devices interact with formulations. Although significant advances continue to be made, the search for the "ideal" inhaler remains a fascinating task for scientists in the field and ensures the continuous evolution of these important delivery systems.

REFERENCES

1. Medicinal Nonventilatory Nebulizer (Atomizer). 21 C.F.R. § 868.5640 (2017).
2. Klüsener O. The injection process in compressorless diesel engines. *VDI Z.* 1933;77(7):107–110.
3. Rayleigh L. On the instability of jets. *Proceedings of The London Mathematical Society.* 1878;1(1):4–13.
4. Hickey AJ. *Inhalation Aerosols: Physical and Biological Basis for Therapy.* Boca Raton, FL: CRC Press, 1996.
5. Qi A, Friend JR, Yeo LY, Morton DA, McIntosh MP, Spiccia L. Miniature inhalation therapy platform using surface acoustic wave microfluidic atomization. *Lab on a Chip.* 2009;9(15):2184–2193.
6. Hinds WC. *Aerosol Technology: Properties, Behavior, and Measurement of Airborne Particles.* New York: John Wiley & Sons, 2012.
7. McCallion ON, Taylor KM, Thomas M, Taylor AJ. Nebulization of fluids of different physicochemical properties with air-jet and ultrasonic nebulizers. *Pharmaceutical Research.* 1995;12(11):1682–1688.
8. Finlay WH. *The Mechanics of Inhaled Pharmaceutical Aerosols: An Introduction.* San Diego, CA: Academic Press, 2001.
9. Lefebvre AH, McDonell VG. *Atomization and Sprays.* Boca Raton, FL: CRC Press, 2017.
10. Zeng XM, Martin GP, Marriott C. *Particulate Interactions in Dry Powder Formulation for Inhalation.* Boca Raton, FL: CRC Press, 2003.
11. Dunber CA, Hickey AJ, Holzner P. Dispersion and characterization of pharmaceutical dry powder aerosols. *KONA Powder and Particle Journal.* 1998;16:7–45.
12. Donovan MJ, Gibbons A, Herpin MJ, Marek S, McGill SL, Smyth HD. Novel dry powder inhaler particle-dispersion systems. *Therapeutic Delivery.* 2011;2(10):1295–1311.

13. Feng JQ, Hays DA. Relative importance of electrostatic forces on powder particles. *Powder Technology*. 2003;135:65–75.

14. Lu X-Y, Chen L, Wu C-Y, Chan H-K, Freeman T. The Effects of Relative Humidity on the Flowability and Dispersion Performance of Lactose Mixtures. *Materials*. 2017;10(6):592.

15. Jashnani RN, Byron PR, Dalby RN. Testing of dry powder aerosol formulations in different environmental conditions. *International Journal of Pharmaceutics*. 1995;113(1):123–130.

16. Johnson K, Kendall K, Roberts A (eds). Surface energy and the contact of elastic solids. *Proceedings of the Royal Society of London A: Mathematical, Physical and Engineering Sciences*. 1971;324:301–313.

17. Derjaguin BV, Muller VM, Toporov YP. Effect of contact deformations on the adhesion of particles. *Journal of Colloid and Interface Science*. 1975;53(2):314–326.

18. Maugis D. Adhesion of spheres: The JKR-DMT transition using a Dugdale model. *Journal of Colloid and Interface Science*. 1992;150(1):243–269.

19. Rabinovich YI, Adler JJ, Ata A, Singh RK, Moudgil BM. Adhesion between nanoscale rough surfaces: I. Role of asperity geometry. *Journal of Colloid and Interface Science*. 2000;232(1):10–16.

20. Rabinovich YI, Adler JJ, Ata A, Singh RK, Moudgil BM. Adhesion between nanoscale rough surfaces: II. Measurement and comparison with theory. *Journal of Colloid and Interface Science*. 2000;232(1):17–24.

21. Peng T, Lin S, Niu B, Wang X, Huang Y, Zhang X, Li G, Pan X, Wu C. Influence of physical properties of carrier on the performance of dry powder inhalers. *Acta Pharmaceutica Sinica B*. 2016;6(4):308–318.

22. Mukherjee R, Gupta V, Naik S, Sarkar S, Sharma V, Peri P, Chaudhuri B. Effects of particle size on the triboelectrification phenomenon in pharmaceutical excipients: Experiments and multi-scale modeling. *Asian Journal of Pharmaceutical Sciences*. 2016;11(5):603–617.

23. Parteli EJ, Schmidt J, Blümel C, Wirth K-E, Peukert W, Pöschel T. Attractive particle interaction forces and packing density of fine glass powders. *Scientific Reports*. 2014;4:6227.

24. Dou X, Mao Y, Zhang Y. Effects of contact force model and size distribution on microsized granular packing. *Journal of Manufacturing Science and Engineering*. 2014;136(2):021003.

25. Safatov A, Yashin V, Kulkin S, Frolov V, Shishkin A, Buryak G. Variations in disperse composition of dry powders according to energy of their dispersion. *Powder Technology*. 1998;97(3):227–232.

26. Hassan MS, Lau RWM. Effect of particle shape on dry particle inhalation: Study of flowability, aerosolization, and deposition properties. *American Association Pharmaceutical Scientists*. 2009;10(4):1252.

27. Visser J. Van der Waals and other cohesive forces affecting powder fluidization. *Powder Technology*. 1989;58(1):1–10. doi:10.1016/0032-5910(89)80001-4.

28. Zeng XM, Martin GP, Marriott C, Pritchard J. The influence of carrier morphology on drug delivery by dry powder inhalers. *International Journal of Pharmaceutics*. 2000;200(1):93–106.

29. Murtomaa M, Mellin V, Harjunen P, Lankinen T, Laine E, Lehto V-P. Effect of particle morphology on the triboelectrification in dry powder inhalers. *International Journal of Pharmaceutics*. 2004;282(1):107–114.

30. Walton OR. Review of adhesion fundamentals for micron-scale particles. *KONA Powder and Particle Journal*. 2008;26:129–141.

31. Flament M-P, Leterme P, Gayot A. The influence of carrier roughness on adhesion, content uniformity and the in vitro deposition of terbutaline sulphate from dry powder inhalers. *International Journal of Pharmaceutics*. 2004;275(1):201–209.

32. Zou Y, Jayasuriya S, Manke CW, Mao G. Influence of nanoscale surface roughness on colloidal force measurements. *Langmuir*. 2015;31(38):10341–10350.

33. Rahimpour Y, Hamishehkar H. Lactose engineering for better performance in dry powder inhalers. *Advanced Pharmaceutical Bulletin*. 2012;2(2):183.

34. Rimai D, DeMejo L. Physical interactions affecting the adhesion of dry particles. *Annual Review of Materials Science*. 1996;26(1):21–41.

35. Cline D, Dalby R. Predicting the quality of powders for inhalation from surface energy and area. *Pharmaceutical Research*. 2002;19(9):1274–1277.

36. R Williams D. Particle engineering in pharmaceutical solids processing: Surface energy considerations. *Current Pharmaceutical Design*. 2015;21(19):2677–2694.

37. Fukuoka E, Kimura S, Yamazaki M, Tanaka T. Cohesion of particulate solids. VI. Improvement of apparatus and application to measurement of cohesiveness at various levels of humidity. *Chemical and Pharmaceutical Bulletin*. 1983;31(1):221–229.

38. Kwok PCL, Chan H-K. Effect of relative humidity on the electrostatic charge properties of dry powder inhaler aerosols. *Pharmaceutical Research*. 2008;25(2):277–288.

39. Rowley G, Mackin LA. The effect of moisture sorption on electrostatic charging of selected pharmaceutical excipient powders. *Powder Technology*. 2003;135:50–58.

40. Eilbeck J, Rowley G, Carter P, Fletcher E. Effect of materials of construction of pharmaceutical processing equipment and drug delivery devices on the triboelectrification of size-fractionated lactose. *Pharmacy and Pharmacology Communications*. 1999;5(7):429–433.

41. Adi S, Adi H, Chan H-K, Finlay WH, Tong Z, Yang R, Yu A. Agglomerate strength and dispersion of pharmaceutical powders. *Journal of Aerosol Science.* 2011;42(4):285–294.

42. Lee K, Suen K, Yianneskis M, Marriott C. Investigation of the aerodynamic characteristics of inhaler aerosols with an inhalation simulation machine. *International Journal of Pharmaceutics.* 1996;130(1):103–113.

43. Nichols S, Wynn E. New approaches to optimizing dispersion in dry powder inhalers-dispersion force mapping and adhesion measurements. *Respiratory Drug Delivery.* 2008;1:175–184.

44. Das SC, Behara SRB, Bulitta JB, Morton DA, Larson I, Stewart PJ. Powder strength distributions for understanding de-agglomeration of lactose powders. *Pharmaceutical Research.* 2012;29(10):2926–2935.

45. Tong Z, Yu A, Chan H-K, Yang R. Discrete Modelling of Powder Dispersion in Dry Powder Inhalers-A Brief Review. *Current Pharmaceutical Design.* 2015;21(27):3966–3973.

46. Hinds WC. Condensation and evaporation. 2012. In *Aerosol Technology Properties, Behavior, and Measurement of Airborne Particles* [*Internet*]. New York: John Wiley & Sons, 278–303. Available from: http://UTXA.eblib.com/patron/FullRecord. aspx?p=1120423.

47. Leong KH. Theoretical principles and devices used to generate aerosols for research. In: Hickey AJ, ed. *Pharmaceutical Inhalation Aerosol Technology.* Baco Raton, FL: CRC Press, 2003.

48. Kulkarni P, Baron PA, Willeke K. *Aerosol measurement: Principles, techniques, and applications.* 3rd ed. Hoboken, NJ: John Wiley & Sons; 2011, pp. xiv, 883.

49. Peters C, Altmann J. Monodisperse aerosol generation with rapid adjustable particle size for inhalation studies. *Journal of Aerosol Medicine.* 1993;6(4):307–315.

50. Hickey AJ, Smyth HDC. Coated filament for evaporation/condensation aerosol generation of therapeutic agents and methods for using. Google Patents; 2012.

51. Oversteegen L. Inhaled medicines: Product differentiation by device. *Innovation Pharmaceutical Technology.* 2008;28:62–65.

52. UNEP. Report of the technology and economic assessment panel. http://ozone.unep.org/en/assessment-panels/technology-and-economic-assessment-panel: United Nations Enviornment Programme TEAP; 2014.

53. Leach CL, Davidson PJ, Hasselquist BE, Boudreau RJ. Lung deposition of hydrofluoroalkane-134a beclomethasone is greater than that of chlorofluorocarbon fluticasone and chlorofluorocarbon beclomethasone: A cross-over study in healthy volunteers. *Chester.* 2002;122(2):510–516.

54. Dunbar C. Atomization mechanisms of the pressurized metered dose inhaler. *Particulate Science and Technology.* 1997;15(3–4):253–271.

55. Stein SW, Sheth P, Hodson PD, Myrdal PB. Advances in metered dose inhaler technology: Hardware development. *American Association Pharmaceutical Scientists.* 2014;15(2):326–338.

56. Smyth HDC, Hickey AJ. *Controlled Pulmonary Drug Delivery*: Springer, New York; 2011.

57. Smyth HDC, Hickey AJ, Brace G, Barbour T, Gallion J, Grove J. Spray pattern analysis for metered dose inhalers I: Orifice size, particle size, and droplet motion correlations. *Drug Development and Industrial Pharmacy.* 2006;32(9):1033–1041.

58. Stein SW, Myrdal PB. A theoretical and experimental analysis of formulation and device parameters affecting solution MDI size distributions. *Journal of Pharmaceutical Sciences.* 2004;93(8):2158–2175.

59. Brambilla G, Ganderton D, Garzia R, Lewis D, Meakin B, Ventura P. Modulation of aerosol clouds produced by pressurised inhalation aerosols. *International Journal of Pharmaceutics.* 1999;186(1):53–61.

60. Chen Y, Young PM, Murphy S, Fletcher DF, Long E, Lewis D, Church T, Traini D. High-speed laser image analysis of plume angles for pressurised metered dose inhalers: The effect of nozzle geometry. *American Association Pharmaceutical Scientists.* 2017;18(3):782–789.

61. (a) U.S.FDA. Phase-Out of CFC Metered-Dose Inhalers Containing flunisolide, triamcinolone, metaproterenol, pirbuterol, albuterol and ipratropium in combination, cromolyn, and nedocromil-Questions and Answers. https://www.fda.gov/Drugs/DrugSafety/InformationbyDrugClass/ucm208138.htm#3.WhenwilltheseCFCinhalersbegone. U.S. Food & Drug administration Press Announcements 2015. (b) Grainger C, Saunders M, Buttini F, Telford R, Merolla L, Martin G, Jones S, Forbes B. Critical characteristics for corticosteroid solution metered dose inhaler bioequivalence. Molecular Pharmaceutics. 2012;9(3):563–569.

62. Smith IJ. The challenge of reformulation. *Journal of Aerosol Medicine.* 1995;8(s1):S-19–S-27.

63. Hoye JA, Gupta A, Myrdal PB. Solubility of solid solutes in HFA—134a with a correlation to physicochemical properties. *Journal of Pharmaceutical Sciences.* 2008;97(1):198–208.

64. Leach CL. The CFC to HFA transition and its impact on pulmonary drug development. *Respiratory Care.* 2005;50(9):1201–1208.

65. Kempsford R, Handel M, Mehta R, De Silva M, Daley-Yates P. Comparison of the systemic pharmacodynamic effects and pharmacokinetics of salmeterol delivered by CFC propellant and non-CFC propellant metered dose inhalers in healthy subjects. *Respiratory Medicine.* 2005;99:S11–S9.

66. UNEP. Report of the refrigeration, air conditioning and heat pumps technical options committee 2014. Available from: http://conf.montreal-protocol.org/meeting/mop/mop-27/presession/Background%20Documents%20are%20available%20in%20English%20only/RTOC-Assessment-Report-2014.pdf.

67. (a) UNEP. Report of the refrigeration, air conditioning and Heat pumps. http://conf.montreal-protocol.org/meeting/mop/mop-27/presession/Background%20Documents%20are%20available%20in%20English%20only/RTOC-Assessment-Report-2014.pdf. Secretariat UsO; 2014. (b) Propellants MM. Zephex HFA Medical propellants. Mexichem; 2016. Source: United nations environment Programme Report of the technology and economic assessment panel 2016, Mexichem website.

68. EPA. Amendment to Address HFCs under the Montreal Protocol 2016. Available from: https://www.epa.gov/ozone-layer-protection/recent-international-developments-under-montreal-protocol.

69. OINDPnews. Mexichem discusses potential for using HFA 152a as pMDI propellant 2016 [cited 2017 25 July]. Available from: http://www.oindpnews.com/2016/12/mexichem-discusses-potential-for-using-hfa-152a-as-pmdi-propellant/.

70. Clark AR. *Metered Atomisation for Respiratory Drug Delivery*: Loughborough University; 1991.

71. Dunbar C, Watkins A, Miller J. An experimental investigation of the spray issued from a pMDI using laser diagnostic techniques. *Journal of Aerosol Medicine*. 1997;10(4):351–368.

72. Hoye JA, Myrdal PB. Measurement and correlation of solute solubility in HFA-134a/ethanol systems. *International Journal of Pharmaceutics*. 2008;362(1):184–188.

73. Sanchis J, Corrigan C, Levy ML, Viejo JL. Inhaler devices–from theory to practice. *Respiratory Medicine*. 2013;107(4):495–502.

74. Traini D, Young PM, Rogueda P, Price R. In vitro investigation of drug particulates interactions and aerosol performance of pressurised metered dose inhalers. *Pharmaceutical Research*. 2007;24(1):125–135.

75. Lechuga-Ballesteros D, Noga B, Vehring R, Cummings RH, Dwivedi SK. Novel cosuspension metered-dose inhalers for the combination therapy of chronic obstructive pulmonary disease and asthma. *Future Medicinal Chemistry*. 2011;3(13):1703–1718.

76. Gabrio BJ, Stein SW, Velasquez DJ. A new method to evaluate plume characteristics of hydrofluoroalkane and chlorofluorocarbon metered dose inhalers. *International Journal of Pharmaceutics*. 1999;186(1):3–12.

77. Versteeg H, Hargrave G, Kirby M (eds). Internal flow and near-orifice spray visualisations of a model pharmaceutical pressurised metered dose inhaler. *Journal of Physics: Conference Series*. 2006;45:207–213.

78. Stein SW, Myrdal PB. The relative influence of atomization and evaporation on metered dose inhaler drug delivery efficiency. *Aerosol Science and Technology*. 2006;40(5):335–347.

79. Stein SW, Sheth P, Myrdal PB. A model for predicting size distributions delivered from pMDIs with suspended drug. *International Journal of Pharmaceutics*. 2012;422(1):101–115.

80. Ganderton D, Lewis D, Davies R, Meakin B, Brambilla G, Church T. Modulite®: A means of designing the aerosols generated by pressurized metered dose inhalers. *Respiratory Medicine*. 2002;96:S3–S8.

81. Stein SW. Estimating the number of droplets and drug particles emitted from MDIs. *American Association Pharmaceutical Scientists*. 2008;9(1):112–115.

82. McKenzie L, Oliver M. Evaluation of the particle formation process after actuation of solution MDIs. *Journal of Aerosol Medicine*. 2000;13:59.

83. Sander N, Fusco-Walker SJ, Harder JM, Chipps BE. Dose counting and the use of pressurized metered-dose inhalers: Running on empty. *Annals of Allergy, Asthma & Immunology*. 2006;97(1):34–38.

84. Ingerski LM, Hente EA, Modi AC, Hommel KA. Electronic measurement of medication adherence in pediatric chronic illness: A review of measures. *The Journal of Pediatrics*. 2011;159(4):528.

85. Foster JM, Smith L, Usherwood T, Sawyer SM, Rand CS, Reddel HK. The reliability and patient acceptability of the SmartTrack device: A new electronic monitor and reminder device for metered dose inhalers. *Journal of Asthma*. 2012;49(6):657–662.

86. Wasserman RL, Sheth K, Lincourt WR, Locantore NW, Rosenzweig JC, Crim C, editors. Real-world assessment of a metered-dose inhaler with integrated dose counter. *Allergy and Asthma Proceedings*. OceanSide Publications, Inc., 2006.

87. Patel M, Pilcher J, Chan A, Perrin K, Black P, Beasley R. Six-month in vitro validation of a metered-dose inhaler electronic monitoring device: Implications for asthma clinical trial use. *Journal of Allergy and Clinical Immunology*. 2012;130(6):1420–1422.

88. George M. User perspectives on innovation in inhalers. Available from: http://ipacrs.org/news-events/events/2017-ipac-rs-isam-joint-workshop-new-frontiers-in-inhalation-technology. *International Society of Aerosol in Medicine*. 2017.

89. Watts AB, McConville JT, Williams RO, 3rd. Current therapies and technological advances in aqueous aerosol drug delivery. *Drug Development and Industrial Pharmacy*. 2008;34(9):913–922. doi:10.1080/03639040802144211.

90. Carvalho TC, Peters JI, Williams RO, 3rd. Influence of particle size on regional lung deposition–What evidence is there? *International Journal of Pharmaceutics*. 2011;406(1–2):1–10. doi:10.1016/j.ijpharm.2010.12.040.

91. Cipolla D, Gonda I, Chan HK. Liposomal formulations for inhalation. *Therapeutic Delivery.* 2013;4(8):1047–1072. doi:10.4155/tde.13.71.

92. Lelong N, Vecellio L, Sommer de Gelicourt Y, Tanguy C, Diot P, Junqua-Moullet A. Comparison of numerical simulations to experiments for atomization in a jet nebulizer. *PLoS One.* 2013;8(11):e78659. doi:10.1371/journal.pone.0078659.

93. Rau JL, Ari A, Restrepo RD. Performance comparison of nebulizer designs: Constant-output, breath-enhanced, and dosimetric. *Respiratory Care.* 2004;49(2):174–179.

94. Waldrep JC, Dhand R. Advanced nebulizer designs employing vibrating mesh/aperture plate technologies for aerosol generation. *Current Drug Delivery.* 2008;5(2):114–119.

95. Piper SD. In vitro comparison of the circulaire and AeroTee to a traditional nebulizer T-piece with corrugated tubing. *Respiratory Care.* 2000;45(3):313–319.

96. Coates AL, MacNeish CF, Lands LC, Meisner D, Kelemen S, Vadas EB. A comparison of the availability of tobramycin for inhalation from vented vs unvented nebulizers. *Chester.* 1998;113(4):951–956.

97. O'Callaghan C, Barry PW. The science of nebulised drug delivery. *Thorax.* 1997;52(Suppl 2):S31–S44.

98. Yeo LY, Friend JR, McIntosh MP, Meeusen EN, Morton DA. Ultrasonic nebulization platforms for pulmonary drug delivery. *Expert Opinion on Drug Delivery.* 2010;7(6):663–679. doi:10.1517/17425247.2010.485608.

99. Rajan R, Pandit AB. Correlations to predict droplet size in ultrasonic atomisation. *Ultrasonics.* 2001;39(4):235–255.

100. Arzhavitina A, Steckel H. Surface active drugs significantly alter the drug output rate from medical nebulizers. *International Journal of Pharmaceutics.* 2010;384(1–2):128–136. doi:10.1016/j.ijpharm.2009.10.012.

101. Nikander K, Turpeinen M, Wollmer P. The conventional ultrasonic nebulizer proved inefficient in nebulizing a suspension. *Journal of Aerosol Medicine.* 1999;12(2):47–53. doi:10.1089/jam.1999.12.47.

102. Najlah M, Parveen I, Alhnan MA, Ahmed W, Faheem A, Phoenix DA, Taylor KM, Elhissi A. The effects of suspension particle size on the performance of air-jet, ultrasonic and vibrating-mesh nebulisers. *International Journal of Pharmaceutics.* 2014;461(1–2):234–241. doi:10.1016/j.ijpharm.2013.11.022.

103. Mc Callion ONM, Patel MJ. Viscosity effects on nebulisation of aqueous solutions. *International Journal of Pharmaceutics.* 1996;130(2):245–249. doi:10.1016/0378-5173(95)04291-1.

104. Pardeike J, Weber S, Haber T, Wagner J, Zarfl HP, Plank H, Zimmer A. Development of an itraconazole-loaded nanostructured lipid carrier (NLC) formulation for pulmonary application. *International Journal of Pharmaceutics.* 2011;419(1–2):329–338. doi:10.1016/j.ijpharm.2011.07.040.

105. Videira MA, Botelho MF, Santos AC, Gouveia LF, de Lima JJ, Almeida AJ. Lymphatic uptake of pulmonary delivered radiolabelled solid lipid nanoparticles. *Journal of Drug Targeting.* 2002;10(8):607–613. doi:10.1080/1061186021000054933.

106. Elhissi A, Hidayat K, Phoenix DA, Mwesigwa E, Crean S, Ahmed W, Faheem A, Taylor KM. Air-jet and vibrating-mesh nebulization of niosomes generated using a particulate-based proniosome technology. *International Journal of Pharmaceutics.* 2013;444(1–2):193–199. doi:10.1016/j.ijpharm.2012.12.040.

107. Lass JS, Sant A, Knoch M. New advances in aerosolised drug delivery: Vibrating membrane nebuliser technology. *Expert Opinion on Drug Delivery.* 2006;3(5):693–702. doi:10.1517/17425247.3.5.693.

108. Beck-Broichsitter M, Kleimann P, Schmehl T, Betz T, Bakowsky U, Kissel T, Seeger W. Impact of lyoprotectants for the stabilization of biodegradable nanoparticles on the performance of air-jet, ultrasonic, and vibrating-mesh nebulizers. *European Journal of Pharmaceutics and Biopharmaceutics: Official Journal of Arbeitsgemeinschaft fur Pharmazeutische Verfahrenstechnik eV.* 2012;82(2):272–280. doi:10.1016/j.ejpb.2012.07.004.

109. Ghazanfari T, Elhissi AM, Ding Z, Taylor KM. The influence of fluid physicochemical properties on vibrating-mesh nebulization. *International Journal of Pharmaceutics.* 2007;339(1–2):103–111. doi:10.1016/j.ijpharm.2007.02.035.

110. Dalby R, Spallek M, Voshaar T. A review of the development of Respimat Soft Mist Inhaler. *International Journal of Pharmaceutics.* 2004;283(1–2):1–9. doi:10.1016/j.ijpharm.2004.06.018.

111. Nguyen TT, Irving CL, Cox KA, McRae DD, Nichols WA, inventors; Philip Morris USA Inc., assignee. *Aerosol Generating Devices and Methods for Generating Aerosols Suitable for Forming Propellant-Free Aerosols.* United States; 2006.

112. Wachtel H, Kattenbeck S, Dunne S, Disse B. The Respimat® Development Story: Patient-Centered Innovation. *Pulmonary Therapy.* 2017;3(1):19–30. doi:10.1007/s41030-017-0040-8.

113. Hess DR. Aerosol delivery devices in the treatment of asthma. *Respiratory Care.* 2008;53(6):699–725.

114. Finlay WH. Pharmaceutical aerosol sprays for drug delivery to the lungs. In: Ashgriz N, ed. *Handbook of Atomization and Sprays.* New York: Springer; 2011.

115. Prescribing Information STRIVERDI RESPIMAT Ridgefield, CT: Boehringer Ingelheim Pharmaceuticals, Inc.; 2016.

116. Prescribing Infromation STIOLTO RESPIMAT Ridgefield, CT: Boehringer Ingelheim Pharmaceuticals, Inc.; 2016.

117. Prescribing Infromation SPIRIVA RESPIMAT Ridgefield, CT: Boehringer Ingelheim Pharmaceuticals, Inc.; 2017.

118. Prescribing Infromation COMBIVENT RESPIMAT Ridgefield, CT: Boehringer Ingelheim Pharmaceuticals, Inc.; 2016.

119. Ganan-Calvo A, Ripoll AB, inventors; Aradigm Corporation, assignee. *Liquid Atomization Process*. United States; 2000.

120. Lloyd LJ, Lloyd PM, Rubsamen RM, Schuster JA, inventors; Aradigm Corporation, assignee. *Device and Method of Creating Aerosolized Mist of Respiratory Drug*. United States; 1999.

121. Stein SW, Thiel CG. The history of therapeutic aerosols: A chronological review. *Journal of Aerosol Medicine and Pulmonary Drug Delivery*. 2017;30(1):20–41. doi:10.1089/jamp.2016.1297.

122. Cipolla D, Blanchard J, Gonda I. Development of liposomal cirpofloxacin to treat lung infections. *Pharmaceutics*. 2016;8(6):31.

123. Sultan F, Ashgriz N, Guildenbecher DR, Sojka PE. Electrosprays. In: Ashgriz N, ed. *Handbook of Atomization and Sprays*. New York: Springer; 2011.

124. Trees GA, Fong JC, inventors; Ventaira Pharmaceuticals, Inc., assignee. *Dissociated Discharge EHD Sprayer with Electric Field Shield*. United States of America; 2008.

125. Chen D-R, Pui DYH. Electrospray and its medical applications. In: Marihnissen JCM, Gradon L, eds. *Nanoparticles in Medicine and Environment*. Dordrecht, the Netherlands: Springer, 2009.

126. Bell JH, Hartley PS, Cox JSG. Dry powder aerosols I: A new powder inhalation device. *Journal of Pharmaceutical Sciences*. 1971;60(10):1559–1564. doi:10.1002/jps.2600601028.

127. Hoppentocht M, Hagedoorn P, Frijlink HW, de Boer AH. Technological and practical challenges of dry powder inhalers and formulations. *Advanced Drug Delivery Reviews*. 2014;75:18–31. doi:10.1016/j.addr.2014.04.004.

128. VanDevanter DR, Geller DE. Tobramycin administered by the TOBI® Podhaler(®) for persons with cystic fibrosis: A review. *Medical Devices (Auckland, NZ)*. 2011;4:179–188. doi:10.2147/MDER.S16360.

129. Xu Z, Mansour HM, Hickey AJ. Particle interactions in dry powder inhaler unit processes: A review. *Journal of Adhesion Science and Technology*. 2011;25(4–5):451–482. doi:10.1163/016942410×525669.

130. Atkins PJ. Dry powder inhalers: An overview. *Respiratory Care*. 2012;50(10):1304.

131. Kopsch T, Murnane D, Symons D. Optimizing the entrainment geometry of a dry powder inhaler: Methodology and preliminary results. *Pharmaceutical Research*. 2016;33(11):2668–2679. doi:10.1007/s11095-016-1992-3.

132. Daniher DI, Zhu J. Dry powder platform for pulmonary drug delivery. *Particuology*. 2008;6(4):225–238. doi:10.1016/j.partic.2008.04.004.

133. Coates MS, Chan H-K, Fletcher DF, Raper JA. Influence of air flow on the performance of a dry powder inhaler using computational and experimental analyses. *Pharmaceutical Research*. 2005;22(9):1445–1453. doi:10.1007/s11095-005-6155-x.

134. Weers J, Clark A. The impact of inspiratory flow rate on drug delivery to the lungs with dry powder inhalers. *Pharmaceutical Research*. 2017;34(3):507–528.

135. White S, Bennett DB, Cheu S, Conley PW, Guzek DB, Gray S, Howard J et al. EXUBERA®: Pharmaceutical development of a novel product for pulmonary delivery of insulin. *Diabetes Technology & Therapeutics*. 2005;7(6):896–906. doi:10.1089/dia.2005.7.896.

136. Finlay WH. *The Mechanics of Inhaled Pharmaceutical Aerosols: An Introduction*. San Diego, CA: Academic Press, 2001.

137. Ashurst I, Malton A, Prime D, Sumby B. Latest advances in the development of dry powder inhalers. *Pharmaceutical Science & Technology Today*. 2000;3(7):246–256. doi:10.1016/S1461-5347(00)00275-3.

138. Longest PW, Son Y-J, Holbrook L, Hindle M. Aerodynamic factors responsible for the deaggregation of carrier-free drug powders to form micrometer and submicrometer aerosols. *Pharmaceutical Research*. 2013;30(6):1608–1627. doi:10.1007/s11095-013-1001-z.

139. Donovan MJ, Gibbons A, Herpin MJ, Marek S, McGill SL, Smyth HDC. Novel dry powder inhaler particle-dispersion systems. *Therapeutic Delivery*. 2011;2(10):1295.

140. Coates MS, Fletcher DF, Chan H-K, Raper JA. Effect of design on the performance of a dry powder inhaler using computational fluid dynamics. Part 1: Grid structure and mouthpiece length. *Journal of Pharmaceutical Sciences*. 2004;93(11):2863–2876. doi:10.1002/jps.20201.

141. Coates MS, Chan H-K, Fletcher DF, Raper JA. Effect of design on the performance of a dry powder inhaler using computational fluid dynamics. Part 2: Air inlet size. *Journal of Pharmaceutical Sciences*. 2006;95(6):1382–1392. doi:10.1002/jps.20603.

142. Laube BL, Janssens HM, de Jongh FHC, Devadason SG, Dhand R, Diot P, Everard ML et al. What the pulmonary specialist should know about the new inhalation therapies. *European Respiratory Journal*. 2011;37(6):1308.

143. Geldart D. Types of gas fluidization. *Powder Technology*. 1973;7(5):285–292. doi:10.1016/0032-5910(73)80037-3.

144. Begat P, Morton DAV, Shur J, Kippax P, Staniforth JN, Price R. The role of force control agents in high-dose dry powder inhaler formulations. *Journal of Pharmaceutical Sciences*. 2009;98(8):2770–2783. doi:10.1002/jps.21629.

145. Borgström L, Asking L, Thorsson L. Idealhalers or realhalers? A comparison of Diskus and Turbuhaler. *International Journal of Clinical Practice*. 2005;59(12):1488–1495. doi:10.1111/j.1368-5031.2005.00747.x.

146. Donovan MJ, Smyth HDC. Influence of size and surface roughness of large lactose carrier particles in dry powder inhaler formulations. *International Journal of Pharmaceutics*. 2010;402(1):1–9. doi:10.1016/j.ijpharm.2010.08.045.

147. Vehring R. Pharmaceutical particle engineering via spray drying. *Pharmaceutical Research*. 2008;25:999–1022. doi:10.1007/s11095-007-9475-1.

148. Chow AHL, Tong HHY, Chattopadhyay P, Shekunov BY. Particle engineering for pulmonary drug delivery. *Pharmaceutical Research*. 2007;24(3):411–437. doi:10.1007/s11095-006-9174-3.

149. Edwards DA, Hanes J, Caponetti G, Hrkach J, Ben-Jebria A, Eskew ML, Mintzes J et al. Large porous particles for pulmonary drug delivery. *Science*. 1997;276(5320):1868.

150. Weers J, Tarara T. The PulmoSphere™ platform for pulmonary drug delivery. *Therapeutic Delivery*. 2014;5(3):277–295. doi:10.4155/tde.14.3.

151. Healy AM, Amaro MI, Paluch KJ, Tajber L. Dry powders for oral inhalation free of lactose carrier particles. *Advanced Drug Delivery Reviews*. 2014;75:32–52. doi:10.1016/j.addr.2014.04.005.

152. Hickey AJ. Back to the future: Inhaled drug products. *Journal of Pharmaceutical Sciences*. 2013;102(4):1165–1172. doi:10.1002/jps.23465.

153. Alexza Pharmaceuticals. Staccato System 2017 [cited August 31, 2017]. Available from: http://www.alexza.com/staccato/staccato-overview.

154. Dinh K, Myers DJ, Glazer M, Shmidt T, Devereaux C, Simis K, Noymer PD et al. In vitro aerosol characterization of Staccato® loxapine. *International Journal of Pharmaceutics*. 2011;403(1):101–108.

155. Alexza Pharmaceuticals. Pipeline Overview 2017 [cited August 31, 2017]. Available from: http://www.alexza.com/alexza-pipeline/pipeline-overview.

156. Idrus AA. Engage Therapeutics bags $23M to trial epilepsy drug-device combo: Fierce Biotechnolog; 2017 [cited September 28, 2017]. Available from: http://www.fiercebiotech.com/medtech/engage-therapeutics-bags-23m-to-trial-epilepsy-drug-device-combo.

157. Nasdaq. Discovery Labs and Chrysalis Technologies Modify Collaboration for Future Development of Aerosolized Drug Device Products 2008. Available from: https://globenewswire.com/news-release/2008/04/02/375686/139358/en/Discovery-Labs-and-Chrysalis-Technologies-Modify-Collaboration-for-Future-Development-of-Aerosolized-Drug-Device-Products.html.

158. Windtree Therapeutics I. Windtree Announces Top-Line Results from AEROSURF® Phase 2b Clinical Trial for the Treatment of Respiratory Distress Syndrome (RDS) in Premature Infants: Windtree Therapeutics, Inc.; 2017 [cited August 31, 2017]. Available from: http://windtreetx.investorroom.com/2017-06-29-Windtree-Announces-Top-Line-Results-from-AEROSURF-R-Phase-2b-Clinical-Trial-for-the-Treatment-of-Respiratory-Distress-Syndrome-RDS-in-Premature-Infants.

159. Newswire CP. Discovery Labs Changes Name to Windtree Therapeutics, Inc. (NASDAQ: WINT) 2016 [cited August 31, 2017]. Available from: http://www.prnewswire.com/news-releases/discovery-labs-changes-name-to-windtree-therapeutics-inc-nasdaq-wint-300252562.html.

160. Ingebrethsen BJ, Cole SK, Alderman SL. Electronic cigarette aerosol particle size distribution measurements. *Inhalation Toxicology*. 2012;24(14):976–984. doi:10.3109/08958378.2012.744781.

PART II

Applications, Influence of Lung Disease Pathophysiology on Aerosol Deposition, Inhaler Device Technique in Respiratory Disease, and Clinical Outcomes in Drug Performance Assessment

8   Neonatal and pediatric inhalation drug delivery   147
    Ariel Berlinski
9   Asthma   161
    Omar S. Usmani
10 Drug delivery in pulmonary aspergillosis   167
    Sawittree Sahakijpijarn, Jay I. Peters, and Robert O. Williams, III
11 Lung cancer inhalation therapeutics   187
    Rajiv Dhand
12 Inhaled therapeutics in chronic obstructive pulmonary disease   215
    Tejas Sinha, Paul Dejulio, and Philip Diaz
13 Cystic fibrosis infection and biofilm busters   223
    Jennifer Fiegel and Sachin Gharse
14 Current and future CFTR therapeutics   239
    Marne C. Hagemeijer, Gimano D. Amatngalim, and Jeffrey M. Beekman
15 Innate and adaptive barrier properties of airway mucus   257
    Alison Schaefer and Samuel K. Lai
16 Nontuberculous mycobacteria   275
    M. Ghadiri, P.M. Young, and D. Traini
17 Inhalational therapies for non-cystic fibrosis bronchiectasis   291
    Ashvini Damodaran, Dustin R. Fraidenburg, and Israel Rubinstein
18 Pulmonary fibrosis   303
    Priya Muralidharan, Don Hayes, Jr., and Heidi M. Mansour
19 Therapeutics in pulmonary hypertension   313
    Maria F. Acosta, Don Hayes, Jr., Jeffrey R. Fineman, Jason X.-J. Yuan, Stephen M. Black, and Heidi M. Mansour

20 Overview of lung surfactant and respiratory distress syndrome 323
   Heidi M. Mansour, Debra Droopad, and Julie G. Ledford
21 Surfactant aerosol therapy for nRDS and ARDS 327
   Donovan B. Yeates
22 Fundamentals in nasal drug delivery 343
   Zachary Warnken, Yu Jin Kim, Heidi M. Mansour, Robert O. Williams, III, and Hugh D.C. Smyth
23 Inhaled therapeutics against TB: The promise of pulmonary treatment and prevention strategies in the clinic 361
   Dominique N. Price, Nitesh K. Kunda, Elliott K. Miller, and Pavan Muttil

Neonatal and pediatric inhalation drug delivery

ARIEL BERLINSKI

Introduction 147
Indications for inhalation therapy 147
    Neonatal population 147
    Pediatric population 148
Anatomical, physiological, and behavioral differences
between children and adults 148
Considerations for using different aerosol delivery
devices in children 148
    Nebulizers 148
    Pressurized metered-dose inhalers 149
    Soft mist inhalers 149
    Dry powder inhalers 149

Device selection 150
Delivery of inhalation therapies in patients receiving
respiratory support 150
    Transnasal aerosol delivery 150
    Aerosol delivery during noninvasive mechanical
    ventilation 151
    Aerosol delivery through tracheostomies 151
    Aerosol delivery during invasive mechanical
    ventilation 152
Unmet needs 154
Conclusion 154
References 154

INTRODUCTION

Inhalation therapy is used to treat many neonatal and pediatric respiratory conditions. As in adults, the inhaled route offers topical action, high *in situ* concentration, and the need for lower doses (1). Aerosol delivery in neonatal-pediatric patients is hindered by numerous factors. They have behavioral, anatomical, and physiological differences from adults. Patients receiving inhaled medications may or may not be receiving invasive or noninvasive ventilator support (noninvasive ventilation [NIV], continuous positive airway pressure [CPAP], bilevel ventilation, and heated high flow nasal cannula [HHFNC]). Inhaled treatments are given at home, at doctor offices, in emergency departments, and during hospitalization in pediatric wards and neonatal and pediatric intensive care units.

Our current understanding of aerosol delivery in the neonatal-pediatric population is based on *in vivo* (human and animal), *in vitro*, and *in silico* data (2). Due to ethical concerns with the administration of radiolabeled aerosols used in deposition studies, and the volume and frequency of blood extractions for pharmacokinetic and pharmacodynamics studies, human studies are limited (3). Animal models of neonatal size include rabbits, piglets, macaques, and lambs; pigs are the most commonly used

pediatric size model (4–8). *In vitro* models have evolved from very simple ones to three-dimensional printed anatomically correct models derived from computed tomography (CT)/magnetic resonance imaging (MRI) data (9). The latter have shown better correlation with *in vivo* studies (10). These new models are also used to investigate aerosol delivery using computational fluid dynamics techniques (9).

This chapter will focus on specific key aspects of neonatal-pediatric drug delivery for each type of device and delivery condition.

INDICATIONS FOR INHALATION THERAPY

Neonatal population

Inhaled medications given to neonates include bronchodilators (albuterol and ipratropium bromide) for relief of bronchoconstriction; corticosteroids for prevention of development of bronchopulmonary dysplasia; surfactant for replacement therapy in deficiency states, dornase alfa for atelectasis; antibiotics for intrapulmonary infections; and pulmonary vasodilators for primary pulmonary hypertension (11–17). All these medications are used off label except for surfactant, which is currently being tested in neonates receiving CPAP (18).

Pediatric population

Many pediatric conditions are treated with inhaled medications. Albuterol, ipratropium bromide, and inhaled corticosteroids are used for the treatment of asthma (19). Hypertonic saline is used in cystic fibrosis, and in bronchiolitis (20,21). Antibiotics are used in cystic fibrosis, in tracheostomized patients experiencing tracheitis, and in intubated patients suffering pneumonia (20,22). Dornase alfa is used in cystic fibrosis patients, but also off label for the treatment of atelectasis (20,23). Vasodilators are used in the treatment of pulmonary hypertension (17). Racemic epinephrine and budesonide are used in croup (24,25).

ANATOMICAL, PHYSIOLOGICAL, AND BEHAVIORAL DIFFERENCES BETWEEN CHILDREN AND ADULTS

Several anatomical differences between infants and young children, and adults explain the difference in intrapulmonary deposition between these populations (9,26). The tongue is relatively larger in the airway in children compared to adults. The pathway of aerosols to intrapulmonary deposition is hindered by the fact that in infants the larynx is situated much higher, and the epiglottis is closer to the palate. Another factor is that the pharynx and supraglottic tissues are less rigid and more prone to collapse during inspiration in infants and young children than in adults. The airway is funnel shaped and narrowest at the level of the cricoid cartilage. These anatomical differences partially explain why infants prefer to breathe through their nose (27). Due to the excellent filtration properties of the nose, intranasal inhalation results in a 50% decrease in intrapulmonary deposition when compared to an oral inhalation maneuver (28).

In addition to the anatomical differences, equipment used in the pediatric population generally has smaller internal diameters (IDs) such as endotracheal tubes (ETTs); tracheostomy tubes; nasal cannula prongs; and circuits used during invasive ventilation, NIV, CPAP, and HHFNC, than the adult ones.

Several physiological differences between infants and children, and adults explain in part why aerosol delivery to the pediatric population is less efficient. Infants have higher respiratory rates, shorter inspiratory times, lower inspiratory flows, and lower tidal volumes than adults (29,30).

Patient behavior hinders drug delivery in different ways across the age spectrum of the pediatric population. Different studies reported a four- to tenfold reduction in lung deposition when the patient cried (31,32). Facemasks are used in pediatric patients who could not cooperate with the inhalation maneuver (33). Many commercially available masks are made of hard material, thus they are more likely to upset the pediatric patient (34). During adolescence, adherence and contrivance may negatively impact the success of disease control (35).

CONSIDERATIONS FOR USING DIFFERENT AEROSOL DELIVERY DEVICES IN CHILDREN

Nebulizers

Infants younger than 6 months of age have an inspiratory flow that is typically lower than the nebulizer flow; thus, they receive undiluted aerosol (36). Particle size of the therapeutic aerosols play a significant role in aerosol deposition. A study in a group of infants with cystic fibrosis reported a greater than twofold intrapulmonary deposition of aerosols with smaller mass median aerodynamic aerosol (MMAD) (3.6 μm) and larger respirable fraction than aerosols with larger MMAD (7.7 μm) and lower respirable fraction (37). Another study reported a fourfold difference in intrapulmonary deposition of budesonide in toddlers when using aerosols with MMADs of 2.5 and 4.2 μm (38). Some authors question whether infants and toddlers would not require aerosols with a smaller MMAD to optimize drug delivery (39).

The choice of the right interface for the delivery of aerosolized medications cannot be minimized. The use of facemasks and mouthpieces rendered similar clinical responses (40,41). However, many children who, due to their cognitive abilities, are not able to properly use a mouthpiece use a facemask as their interface instead. The dead space of the mask does not seem to affect drug delivery during nebulization (42). The design of the facemask plays a role in delivery efficiency and in facial and ocular exposure (43,44). Facial and ocular exposure is responsible for some of the known side effects of inhaled medications (45,46). Facemasks with the aerosol stream aligned with the mouth/nostrils (front loaded) resulted in lower facial-ocular exposure and a higher amount of aerosol available for inhalation than masks that had an aerosol stream reaching the target at 90 degrees (bottom loaded) (43,44). This difference increased when a distance between the face and the mask was applied. Newer masks have been developed using three-dimensional scanning of children's faces (47). This mask has an aperture to thread a pacifier and help keep the mask seal during suckling, while the aerosol steam is directed to the nostrils. This mask showed similar lung deposition than a traditional bottom-loaded mask (48). Other interfaces that use the transnasal route were tested in an anatomically correct model of an infant and rendered similar lung deposition values to those previously reported in human studies (10). A facemask that is not tightly fitted also results in a significant decrease in lung deposition (10,49).

The use of a hood in infants has been reported to render similar lung deposition than aerosols given by nebulizer and mask (50). The same authors reported that clinical and physiological responses were at least as good for the hood than for the facemask (51,52). A study using computational fluid dynamic calculations estimated that head orientation during aerosol administration via hood affected the amount of facial deposition (53). Although the use of the hood appears to be an improvement in delivery method, the resulting facial, ocular, and high body surface exposure limits its clinical utilization.

The use of breath-actuated nebulizers in the pediatric population can be challenging because the devices require a minimum inspiratory flow to open the inspiratory valve. Some patients when well and even more while experiencing bronchoconstriction might not be able to reach the threshold flow. Therefore, practitioners need to verify that children can effectively use the device.

Some practitioners who are concerned with the risk of overdosing their young patient decrease the nebulizer's loading volume in half. This results in a more significant decrease in drug output because most jet nebulizers have high residual volumes (54). The two available options to reduce inhaled dose are either decreasing nebulization time, or decreasing loading dose but adding saline solution to restore the original loading volume.

Pressurized metered-dose inhalers

The portability of pressurized metered-dose inhalers (pMDIs) have made them a preferred method of aerosol administration in the pediatric population. Coordination of actuation of the pMDI with inhalation required for proper lung deposition is overcome by using a valved holding chamber (VHC) (55–56). Patients receiving inhaled medications with MDI and VHC can either use a mouthpiece or a mask, similar to nebulizer therapy. Whenever possible, a mouthpiece should be used instead of a facemask because the mouthpiece decreases facial and ocular deposition, and optimizes drug delivery. Many commercially available masks have dead-space volumes that are larger than a 6-month-old infant (34). The amount of dead-space volume inversely correlates with drug delivery (57). The mask seal is very important because minor facemask leaks have resulted in a decrease in drug delivery (58). It is not uncommon that, when delivering inhaled medications via pMDI and VHC to infants and young children, a delay occurs between either shaking and actuation, or actuation and inhalation. The former resulted in an increase in emitted dose of hydrofluoroalkane (HFA) fluticasone suspension on the actuation following the delay (59). The same was found for other HFA suspensions but not for solutions (60). Both studies were done at the beginning of the life of the canister; thus, the emitted dose is expected to be low toward the end of the life of the canister. A 10-second delay between actuation and inhalation resulted in a decrease in the HFA albuterol dose released from the VHC (61).

Spacers (valveless tubes) are also used in children who can coordinate actuation with inhalation and can perform a single slow maximal maneuver. Spacers have been shown to produce adequate lung deposition and bronchodilation in asthmatic children (62,63).

Drug delivery with pMDI and VHC is optimized when the infant is calm, since crying significantly decreased lung deposition (64). A study found that giving inhaled medications with pMDI and VHC while the children were asleep resulted in awakening and upsetting most of them (65). They also reported lower emitted dose and higher dose variability when a pMDI was given while asleep. Some small patients might not be able to open the inspiratory valve; thus, this needs to be verified by the practitioner (66).

Bronchodilator response was similar between children inhaling albuterol HFA with VHC while using tidal breathing and single slow maximal inhalation (67). However, when an HFA beclomethasone solution was used, the single slow inhalation with a breath hold resulted in higher intrapulmonary deposition than the tidal breathing maneuver (68). A breath-actuated HFA beclomethasone inhaler resulted in similar deposition than an HFA beclomethasone inhaler used with VHC and tidal breathing technique (68–69). Actuation of an HFA pMDI of fluticasone during coordinated and uncoordinated breathing maneuvers resulted in low variation when a nonelectrostatic VHC was used (70). The same study revealed that children 5–8 years old were capable of emptying the VHC in 3 breaths or less. In another study, 2- to 7-year-old children were able to empty VHCs in 2 to 3 breaths (71). They also reported that tidal breathing technique resulted in similar drug delivery than single slow inhalation technique. Some VHCs incorporated a whistle that is set to sound at high inspiratory flow. This feedback mechanism has two main drawbacks: (1) some children will try to produce the sound rather than avoid making the noise, and (2) the whistling threshold is different among different pMDIs (72).

Soft mist inhalers

Soft mist inhalers are propellant-free inhalation devices that use the energy of a spring to force liquids through a small nozzle (73). The aerosol plume of Respimat™ (Boeringher Ingelheim) is slower and lasts longer than pMDIs (74). Because of these characteristics and the deposition data, it is recommended that a VHC not be used (75). However, children younger than 5 years old have difficulty handling the device; thus, the use of a VHC is recommended (76). However, there is only one formulation approved in the United States for asthmatic children 12 years and older (tiotropium bromide) (77). Practitioners need to check that the child is able to coordinate actuation and inhalation, and inhale the mist for 1.5 seconds.

In a human study, the use of a soft mist inhaler with a VHC resulted in acceptable pulmonary deposition without waking up infants (78). In an *in vitro* study using a metallic VHC with facemask a soft mist inhaler, the results showed higher lung dose than a pMDI (79). The difference was greater at low tidal volumes (50 mL). Lung dose increased with tidal volume until the tidal volume reached the VHC's volume.

Dry powder inhalers

Currently available dry powder inhalers (DPIs) require the inspiratory flow to disaggregate the drug (1). An increase in inspiratory flow resulted in an increase in intrapulmonary deposition for most formulations (80). However, for some newly developed drugs, drug delivery did not increase when the threshold inspiratory flow was exceeded (81). Active DPIs are being developed and could potentially be used by pediatric patients in a similar fashion to a pMDI and VHC (82).

The two main challenges for pediatric patients are to be able to (1) follow all the steps required for inhalation of the DPI, and (2) generate enough inspiratory flow (82). Age alone cannot be used to determine patient's ability to properly use a device (83). Therefore, objective measurement of inspiratory flow at the device resistance is strongly recommended (84). Low-cost devices are currently available in the United State and European markets. In addition, many manufacturers provide training devices to help determine patient proficiency to use that specific device.

In summary, patient's proficiency and ability to use DPI devices need to be verified at the time of prescription and during follow-up visits. Newer, pediatric-friendly devices and formulations are needed.

Device selection

Several steps are necessary in selecting the appropriate device for a given neonatal-pediatric patient: (1) determine what formulation(s) is(are) available for a specific drug, (2) determine caregiver/patient's ability to use the specific device(s) containing the chosen formulations, (3) consider caregiver/patient's as well as physician's preferences if more than one formulation is available, and (4) consider cost. However, current practice in the United States and other countries shows that the second step of the process is to verify that the drug is part of a third-party payer formulary, and consider the cost of the drug.

Nebulizers and pMDIs with VHC can be used by all pediatric patients including those with impaired cognitive abilities and those receiving respiratory support. A mouthpiece should be used when possible to minimize facial and ocular exposure. DPIs can be used by older children but not by those with impaired cognitive abilities and those receiving respiratory support.

DELIVERY OF INHALATION THERAPIES IN PATIENTS RECEIVING RESPIRATORY SUPPORT

The use of respiratory support devices in pediatric patients inside and outside the intensive care unit has increased over the past few years. The number of pediatric patients receiving respiratory support has also increased due to improvements in technology and medical knowledge. Most of these patients also receive inhaled therapies (85,86). Some of these medications are given to treat chronic respiratory conditions, while others are given to treat the acute respiratory conditions. Some of the current challenges with aerosol delivery in these patients are due to unanswered questions: (1) How much drug does a specific patient need? (2) Does our understanding of particle size and intrapulmonary apply to aerosols delivered through artificial airways? (3) Do we want to

achieve very high deposition rates of specific products if a dose adjustment will not be done? (4) How do we implement new technologies into patient care?

Transnasal aerosol delivery

The use of HHFNC has become widespread over the past years, and newer systems allow the delivery of higher flows than before (87). While neonatal flows are generally low (< 2 L/min), pediatric flows are significantly higher (at least 6–8 L/min). This should be kept in mind when reviewing data from studies using this type of technology to deliver aerosols. Another limiting factor is the small ID of the nasal prongs.

Data on drug delivery through HHFNC in the pediatric population is limited and mostly based on *in vitro* studies and some animal data (88–92). A study using a nonanatomically correct model with a vibrating mesh nebulizer placed after the humidifier reported 18.6% and 25.4% drug delivery for the infant and pediatric cannula, respectively (88). Another study using a nonanatomically correct model and a vibrating mesh nebulizer placed before the humidifier reported 10.7% and 2% for flows of 3 and 6 L/min, respectively (89). The authors also reported that switching delivery gas from oxygen to 80:20 heliox did not improve drug delivery at low flow, but resulted in an increase in drug delivery of 2.8-fold for the highest flow. Another study compared aerosol delivery using a vibrating mesh nebulizer placed before the nasal cannula (90). The neonatal cannula size delivered 05%–0.6% with flows between 3 and 8 L/min, while the pediatric cannula delivered 0.1%–1.2% with flows between 3 and 10 L/min. The pediatric cannula delivered twice the amount of drug than the neonatal one at the lowest flow. The MMAD of the aerosols ranged between 0.49 and 1.38 μm. More recently, a study using an anatomically correct model of an infant reported drug delivery of 4.2%, 3.3%, and 0.5% with flows of 2, 4, and 8 L/min, respectively, while using a vibrating mesh placed before the humidifier (6). The jet nebulizer was placed before the humidifier, and on the face with and without nasal cannula and delivered 0.5%, 0.9%, and 1.7% of the loading dose, respectively. The MMAD ranged from 1.05 to 1.43 μm and from 1.07–2.62% for the vibrating mesh and jet nebulizer, respectively. The same study included a macaque model that showed five- to sevenfold and ten- to fifteenfold lower deposition than the *in vitro* study for the vibrating mesh and the jet nebulizer, respectively. Another study with an anatomically correct model of a preterm infant and using a vibrating mesh nebulizer placed before the cannula and before the humidifier reported a 1.3% and 0.9% drug delivery efficiency, respectively (91).

A study using a high-flow system but a facemask instead of a cannula reported that using a vibrating mesh nebulizer placed before the humidifier resulted in drug delivery of 6.4%, 4.2%, and 2.8% for 3, 6, and 12 L/min, respectively, when an infant breathing pattern was used (92). However, lung dose increased by 15%–38% with a pediatric breathing pattern. The MMAD ranged from 2.8 to 3.3 μm for flows ranging from 3 and 12 L/min.

In summary, studies clearly show that drug delivery with HHFNC systems is low (0.5%–1%), and this should be considered if poor clinical response is noted.

Aerosol delivery during noninvasive mechanical ventilation

Noninvasive ventilation is increasingly used in several clinical situations (93). It is used in acute care either to avoid invasive mechanical ventilation or after extubation. It is also used for chronic care, but most of these patients can be transiently removed support to receive inhalation therapy. This should be the preferred modality for these patients (85).

In a human study with children with cystic fibrosis, the administration of a radiolabeled aerosol coupled with pressure support resulted in 30% higher lung deposition without change in the distribution (94). However, studies in healthy volunteer adults and asthmatics experiencing exacerbation did not find difference in lung deposition between spontaneous and supported breathing (95,96).

Few *in vitro* studies have been reported on pediatric NIV and concomitant aerosol delivery (91,97–99). Figures 8.1 and 8.2 show schematics of drug delivery during NIV using single- and double-limb circuits (85). One study using an anatomically correct preterm infant model of CPAP reported drug delivery of 0.6%–0.7% and 0.8%–1.2% when a vibrating mesh

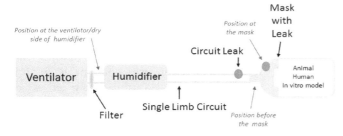

Figure 8.1 Schematic of drug delivery during NIV using a single-limb circuit. (Modified from Berlinski, A., Inhaled drug delivery for children on long-term mechanical ventilation, In Sterni, L.M. and Carroll, J.L., *Caring for the Ventilator Dependent Child, A Clinical Guide*, 1st edition, New York, Humana Press, 2016, pp. 217–239.)

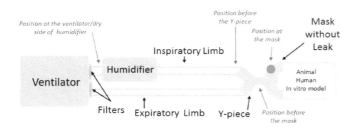

Figure 8.2 Schematics of drug delivery during NIV using double-limb circuit. (Modified from Berlinski, A., Inhaled drug delivery for children on long-term mechanical ventilation, In Sterni, L.M. and Carroll, J.L., *Caring for the Ventilator Dependent Child, A Clinical Guide*, 1st edition, New York, Humana Press, 2016, pp. 217–239.)

nebulizer was placed closer to the patient and on the dry side of the nebulizer, respectively (91). A study using an anatomically correct pediatric model of NIV with single-limb circuit reported drug delivery of 4%, 5%, and 11% placing a vibrating mesh nebulizer on the dry side of the humidifier, right before the mask and after the leak, and integrated into the mask, respectively (97). Another study using an anatomically correct pediatric model of NIV with single-limb circuit reported drug delivery of 16.6%, 4.7%, and 10% of a vibrating mesh nebulizer placed before the mask, at the ventilator, and incorporated to the mask, respectively (98). A jet nebulizer delivered 2.1% and 5.5% when placed at the ventilator and before the mask (after the circuit leak), respectively. A study using an anatomically correct pediatric model of NIV with a double-limb circuit reported drug delivery of 18%, 17.6%, 13.3%, and 10% when a vibrating mesh nebulizer was placed before the mask, before the Y-piece, at the ventilator, and incorporated into the mask, respectively (99). A jet nebulizer was tested at before the Y-piece and on the dry side of the humidifier and rendered 3.8% and 3.5% deposition, respectively. The use of higher ventilator setting did not improve drug delivery (99).

In summary, during pediatric NIV, placing the device before the mask, using a vibrating mesh nebulizer, and using a double-limb ventilator circuit improved drug delivery. Higher NIV settings did not improve drug delivery.

Aerosol delivery through tracheostomies

The number of neonatal-pediatric patients undergoing tracheostomy has increased over time in part due to improvements in medical technology and neonatal-pediatric critical care (100). Tracheostomized patients are prescribed inhaled medications including bronchodilators, corticosteroids, antibiotics, and others (101).

Tracheostomized patients may or may not receive respiratory support. Some of these patients can be transiently disconnected from the ventilator for the aerosol treatment. Those who cannot be disconnected are very few and should receive their medication inline. Pediatric data are limited and are mostly derived from *in vitro* studies (101,111).

A human study compared gentamicin delivery via different routes (102). They reported a 24- to 28-fold higher sputum concentration and blood levels with instillation than with aerosolization. An animal study using a neonatal model showed a 50% decrease in pulmonary deposition of a beclomethasone pMDI when assisted technique was used instead of a VHC (103). Few reports are available of modifications of devices to allow administration of inhaled medications to tracheostomized children (104,105).

In vitro studies have provided the greatest insight into the intricacies of drug delivery in pediatric patients with tracheostomy (106–111). Those studies evaluated the effects of type of device, type of interface, type of formulation, type of add-on devices, breathing pattern, ID of the tracheostomies, and use of different administration techniques on drug delivery through pediatric tracheostomies. One study compared several add-on devices used with pMDIs, several breathing patterns, tracheostomies of different IDs, and different administration techniques (106). The authors reported that a nonelectrostatic VHC was the most efficient device, that tidal volumes lower than the volume of the VHC delivered less drug, and that reducing ID below 4.5 mm decreased drug delivery. They also reported that assisted technique (use of resuscitation bag to augment tidal volume) was detrimental to drug delivery. Another study using a different model compared a jet nebulizer and two different nonelectrostatic VHCs using facial and tracheostomy delivery (107). The authors reported that equal nebulized doses delivered via tracheostomy resulted in higher lung doses than when delivered via oronasal route. However, results were variable for the pMDI with VHCs. They also found that decreasing the tracheostomy ID, and using assisted technique decreased lung delivery. The nebulizer delivered significantly higher doses than the pMDI. A follow-up study comparing a pMDI and a soft mist inhaler delivered via a metallic VHC was done using the same model (108). The authors reported that soft mist inhalers delivered more drug than the pMDI. They also reported that tracheostomy doses were higher than those achieved via oronasal route. Another study compared nebulization through tracheostomies in a pediatric model. The authors evaluated different nebulizers, breathing patterns, tracheostomy IDs, interfaces, and assisted technique (109). They reported that (1) a T-piece was more efficient than a tracheostomy mask, (2) a breath-enhanced nebulizer was equivalent to continuous output nebulizer with 15 cm extension tube using assisted technique, and (3) the use of assisted increased drug delivery both distally (beyond carina) and proximally (trachea). A study compared two nebulizers and a pMDI with spacer using two different administration techniques (110). They reported that (1) a vibrating mesh nebulizer delivered more drug than a jet nebulizer, and (2) an assisted technique did not change drug delivery. One study compared a DPI and a nebulizer delivering tobramycin and reported that three capsules were equivalent to standard nebulized dose (111).

Aerosols experience changes in their characteristics as they travel through a tracheostomy tube (107,109). A study using a tracheostomy with ID of 4.5 mm reported that the characteristics (MMAD/GSD/percentage of particles <5 μm) of albuterol aerosol generated by a pMDI with VHC changed from (2.14–2.15 μm/1.44–1.46/99%) to (1.65–1.74 μm/1.37–1.25/99%) (107). Another study reported the aerosol characteristics of nebulized albuterol generated by 4 different nebulizer setups. The authors found that characteristics of aerosols leaving a 3.5 mm ID tracheostomy were smaller in MMAD, but similar in GSD (1.68–1.93) and percentage of particles < 5 μm (99%–100%) than aerosols exiting a 5.5 mm ID tracheostomy. The difference in MMAD varied with nebulizer design being breath actuated, breath enhanced, and continuous output. The MMAD ranged from 1.20–1.43 μm and 1.38–1.77 μm for tracheostomies with IDs of 3.5 and 5.5 mm, respectively.

A recent report on aerosol delivery through tracheostomies made the following recommendations to improve drug delivery: (1) clean the tracheostomy tube before the aerosol treatment, (2) disconnect the heated trach collar before aerosol administration, (3) encourage when possible a breathing pattern characterized large and slow breaths, and (4) avoid the use of assisted techniques for pMDI but consider it for antibiotic treatment for intratracheal infections (112).

Aerosol delivery during invasive mechanical ventilation

Delivery of aerosols during invasive mechanical ventilation includes delivery through both tracheostomies and endotracheal tubes (85). Most patients receiving chronic mechanical ventilation can be disconnected from the ventilator for the duration of the inhaled treatment. Most patients receiving mechanical ventilation through endotracheal tubes for acute illnesses should receive inhaled treatments inline. Figure 8.3 shows a schematic of drug delivery during invasive mechanical ventilation using a double-limb circuit (85).

Although current knowledge about drug delivery to neonates receiving invasive mechanical ventilation is based on human, animal, and *in vitro* studies, most pediatric age data are based on *in vitro* studies (113–162). A survey of albuterol administration in intubated patients in neonatal intensive care units revealed great variation in practice (113). Different dosing, type of delivery device, and placement in the ventilator circuit were reported.

A study in intubated babies showed very low drug delivery and no difference between placement of the nebulizer at the endotracheal tube and in the inspiratory limb (60 cm before the tube) (114). There was no advantage to using submicronic aerosols despite a difference noted in the *in vitro* evaluation. Another study showed similar drug delivery of a pMDI with spacer placed before the endotracheal tube, and a nebulizer placed in the inspiratory limb (115). A study in intubated neonates with bronchopulmonary dysplasia reported marked variability in intrapulmonary deposition of both a pMDI with spacer and a jet nebulizer (116). Therapeutic response of albuterol administered via a nebulizer and pMDI with a spacer has been documented in intubated premature infants (117,118). Another study showed

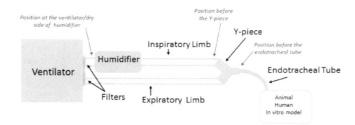

Figure 8.3 Schematic of drug delivery during invasive mechanical ventilation using a double-limb circuit. (Modified from Berlinski, A. Inhaled drug delivery for children on long-term mechanical ventilation, In Sterni, L.M. and Carroll, J.L., *Caring for the Ventilator Dependent Child, A Clinical Guide*, 1st edition, New York, Humana Press, 2016, pp. 217–239.)

that the use of an ultrasonic nebulizer resulted in better response than a pMDI with spacer or a jet nebulizer (119). A study in pediatric patients found similar serum concentrations and effects between a jet nebulizer placed in the inspiratory limb and a pMDI with spacer placed after the ventilator circuit (120).

Neonatal animal studies done in rabbits reported that (1) paralysis decreased drug delivery when compared to spontaneous breathing, (2) longer inspiratory times resulted in higher drug deposition, (3) a nebulizer producing submicronic aerosols increased lung deposition, and (4) an ultrasonic nebulizer delivered more drug than a pMDI with spacer (4,121–123). Neonatal animal studies with piglets reported that (1) lung injury severely decreased lung deposition of a pMDI given with spacer, and (2) a low-flow nebulizer placed in the inspiratory limb was able to deliver drug during high frequency ventilation (124,125). A neonatal animal model of macaques reported a 28-fold difference in lung deposition between a jet (05%) and a vibrating mesh nebulizer (126). Pediatric animal studies with pigs reported (1) an ultrasonic nebulizer and a vibrating mesh nebulizer provided similar lung deposition, (2) the use of an adapter for delivery of pMDI was very inefficient, and (3) vibrating mesh and ultrasonic nebulizers placed at the ventilator delivered significantly more drug than pMDI with VHC (8,127).

The use of inline therapy avoids breaking the integrity of the circuit-patient connection, thus minimizing the risk of ventilator associated pneumonia (128). Also, inline therapy avoids lung derecruitment that would occur in patients receiving support at high settings once the ventilator circuit is disconnected. The use of aerosol generators that add external flow to the system, such as jet nebulizers, require adjustment of the delivered tidal volume during and after the treatment to avoid overdistention and/or hypoventilation (129). Jet nebulizers are sometimes powered by the ventilator instead of using an external force and can show different performance according the selected ventilator model (130). Ultrasonic and vibrating mesh nebulizers do not require modification of the ventilator settings. Some ventilators allow the coordination of drug delivery with the inspiratory cycle (inspiratory, expiratory, and continuous), but results are inconclusive (131–133).

Neonatal in vitro models have been used to study the effect on drug delivery of several variables, such as formulation, type of device and placement, type of ventilator, ventilation modality, and endotracheal IDs (134–146). Nebulizers and pMDIs with spacers are used in neonatal circuits. Spacers are typically placed between the circuit and the endotracheal tube, and they are removed after its use. A pMDI HFA formulation delivered more drug than a CFC formulation of a corticosteroid but not of albuterol (134,135). A spacer was found to be 18 times more efficient than an adapter (136). The ventilation mode during conventional ventilation did affect drug delivery during albuterol nebulization (137). A nebulizer was reported to deliver more drug than a pMDI with spacer (138). Another study showed that

nebulizer flowrate significantly affected drug output (139). Placement of the nebulizer closer to the patient increased drug delivery in several studies (140–144). Vibrating mesh nebulizers were more efficient than jet nebulizers (140–141,143). Also, during high-frequency oscillatory ventilation, devices were more efficient when placed close to the patient, and a vibrating mesh nebulizer delivered larger amounts of drug than a jet nebulizer (142–144). A small volume adapter that allowed independent flow of aerosol and gas from the ventilator was reported to deliver more drug than a conventional adapter (145). The aerosol generated by jet and vibrating mesh nebulizers placed between the inspiratory limb and the Y-piece was similar to the aerosol released from the nebulizer alone (146). However, when the aerosol generators were moved to the dry side of the humidifier, the MMAD and delivered mass decreased, but the percentage of particle <5 µm increased (146). A study using computational fluid dynamics reported that 1 µm particles were not affected by inspiratory flows ranging from 3 to 5 L/min and endotracheal tubes with IDs ranging from 2.5 to 3.5 mm (147). However, as particle size, penetration decreased and the effect was greater at higher inspiratory flows. Optimization of connectors done with computational fluid dynamic tools resulted in significant increase in drug delivery (148). Also, delivery of aerosols at the beginning of the inhalation resulted in further improvement

Pediatric in vitro models have shaped current aerosol delivery practice during mechanical ventilation (149–162). Many variables were studied, such as type of device, type of ventilator, position in the ventilator circuit, effect of endotracheal tube ID, type of circuit, presence of bias flow, among others. Similarly to what has been reported for tracheostomy and for neonatal mechanical ventilation, smaller endotracheal tubes impaired drug delivery of aerosols generated by nebulizers and pMDI (149–152).

VHCs were more effective than adapters and spacers to deliver albuterol pMDI (152,154). Aerosol delivery was significantly increased with a pMDI and spacer when heliox was used in the circuit (155,156). Delivery of aerosol via pMDI was negligible during high-frequency ventilation (157). Drug delivery of pMDI was hindered by the presence of humidity in the circuit (151,152). Therefore, practitioners need to increase the dose to compensate for it because a delivery of dry gas would be harmful for the neonatal-pediatric patient.

Vibrating mesh and ultrasonic nebulizers delivered more drug than jet nebulizers during pediatric conventional mechanical ventilation (132,143,158–160). Placing vibrating mesh nebulizer on the dry side of the nebulizer resulted in higher drug output compared to placing it before the Y-piece (143,158–160). However, results for the jet showed either no difference or improvement in drug delivery when placing the nebulizer on the dry side of the ventilator (158–161). An intrapulmonary percussive ventilator delivered the same amount of drug as a jet nebulizer when placed before the Y-piece but less when placed at the ventilator (161). Increasing tidal volume did not improved drug delivery in a pediatric model of conventional mechanical ventilation (160,161). Bias flow negatively affected drug delivery during pediatric conventional mechanical ventilation (158). During pediatric high-frequency oscillatory ventilation, placing a vibrating mesh nebulizer close to the endotracheal tube increased drug delivery (142,143). Optimization of connectors and use of and excipient growth formulation at the first portion of the inhalation resulted in very high drug deposition.

In summary, optimal placement and choice of aerosol-generating devices depend on many variables that could be different in neonatal and pediatric patients. Although significant differences were reported in *in vitro* studies between different type of devices, it is not completely clear how that translates into clinical efficacy. Sometimes the device inefficiency can be overcome by increasing the loading dose (159). Highly efficient devices might require guidance for dose adjustment.

UNMET NEEDS

Pediatric and neonatal patients have historically used devices and formulations developed for adults. Surfactant replacement therapy is probably the only exception. Formulations and devices that match the unique anatomical, physiological, and behavioral characteristics of this population are desperately needed. Devices that can deliver maintenance and rescue medications are needed. Add-on devices with better facemask leak detectors, and inhaled volume and inspiratory flow detectors have the potential of improving drug delivery to this population.

CONCLUSION

Drug delivery to infants and children is a very challenging task due to their behavioral, physiological, and anatomical characteristics. In addition, these elements interact with equipment, drug formulations, and devices that have been primarily designed for adult use. The limited amount of human data with high reliance on recently improved models makes the decision of what device to use even more difficult than in adults. Although efficiency of delivery is important when comparing devices or formulations, it is deposition at the desired target that really matters. The cost of the drug and device, and time spent during the inhalation maneuver are also important. Devices and formulations designed for their use in the pediatric population are needed.

REFERENCES

1. Laube BL et al. What the pulmonary specialist should know about the new inhalation therapies. *Eur Respir J*. 2011;37(6):1308–1331.
2. Carrigy NB, Ruzycki CA, Golshahi L, Finlay WH. Pediatric in vitro and in silico models of deposition via oral and nasal inhalation. *J Aerosol Med Pulm Drug Deliv*. 2014;27(3):149–169.
3. Everard ML. Studies using radiolabelled aerosols in children. *Thorax*. 1994;49(12):1259–1266.
4. Fok TF, al-Essa M, Monkman S, Dolovich M, Girard L, Coates G, Kirpalani H. Delivery of metered dose inhaler aerosols to paralyzed and nonparalyzed rabbits. *Crit Care Med*. 1997;25(1):140–144.
5. Linner R, Perez-de-Sa V, Cunha-Goncalves D. Lung deposition of nebulized surfactant in newborn piglets. *Neonatology*. 2015;107(4):277–282.
6. Réminiac F, Vecellio L, Loughlin RM, Le Pennec D, Cabrera M, Vourc'h NH, Fink JB, Ehrmann S. Nasal high flow nebulization in infants and toddlers: An in vitro and in vivo scintigraphic study. *Pediatr Pulmonol*. 2017;52(3):337–344.
7. Hütten MC, Kuypers E, Ophelders DR, Nikiforou M, Jellema RK, Niemarkt HJ, Fuchs C, Tservistas M, Razetti R, Bianco F, Kramer BW. Nebulization of Poractant alfa via a vibrating membrane nebulizer in spontaneously breathing preterm lambs with binasal continuous positive pressure ventilation. *Pediatr Res*. 2015;78(6):664–669.
8. Berlinski A, Holt S, Thurman T, and Heulitt M. Albuterol delivery during mechanical ventilation in an ex-vivo porcine model. *J Aerosol Med Pulm Drug Deliv*. 2013;26(2):A-57.
9. Xi J, Si X, Zhou Y, Kim J, Berlinski A. Growth of nasal and laryngeal airways in children: Implications in breathing and inhaled aerosol dynamics. *Respir Care*. 2014;59(2):263–273.
10. El Taoum KK, Xi J, Kim J, Berlinski A. In Vitro Evaluation of Aerosols Delivered via the Nasal Route. *Respir Care*. 2015;60(7):1015–1025.
11. Armangil D, Yurdakök M, Korkmaz A, Yiğit S, Tekinalp G. Inhaled beta-2 agonist salbutamol for the treatment of transient tachypnea of the newborn. *J Pediatr*. 2011;159(3):398–403.e1.
12. Fayon M, Tayara N, Germain C, Choukroun ML, De La Roque ED, Chêne G, Breilh D, Marthan R, Demarquez JL. Efficacy and tolerance of high-dose inhaled ipratropium bromide vs. terbutaline in intubated premature human neonates. *Neonatology*. 2007;91(3):167–173.
13. Shah SS, Ohlsson A, Halliday HL, Shah VS. Inhaled versus systemic corticosteroids for preventing bronchopulmonary dysplasia in ventilated very low birth weight preterm neonates. *Cochrane Database Syst Rev*. 2017 Oct 17;10:CD002058.
14. Pillow JJ, Minocchieri S. Innovation in surfactant therapy II: Surfactant administration by aerosolization. *Neonatology*. 2012;101(4):337–344.
15. Scala M, Hoy D, Bautista M, Palafoutas JJ, Abubakar K. Pilot study of dornase alfa (Pulmozyme) therapy for acquired ventilator-associated infection in preterm infants. *Pediatr Pulmonol*. 2017;52(6):787–791.
16. Nakwan N, Lertpichaluk P, Chokephaibulkit K, Villani P, Regazzi M, Imberti R. Pulmonary and systemic pharmacokinetics of colistin following a

single dose of nebulized colistimethate in mechanically ventilated neonates. *Pediatr Infect Dis J.* 2015; 34(9):961–963.

17. Casa N, Costa Jr. E. Inhaled pulmonary vasodilators for persistent pulmonary hypertension of the newborn: Safety issues relating to drug administration and delivery devices. *Med Devices* 2016;9:45–51.

18. https://www.anzctr.org.au/Trial/Registration/TrialReview.aspx?id=373412&isReview=true. Accessed December 25, 2017.

19. Global Strategy for Asthma Management and Prevention. Updated 2017, www.ginasthma.org. Accessed December 25, 2017.

20. Agent P, Parrott H. Inhaled therapy in cystic fibrosis: Agents, devices and regimens. *Breathe (Sheff).* 2015; 11(2):110–118.

21. Heikkilä P, Renko M, Korppi M. Hypertonic saline inhalations in bronchiolitis-A cumulative meta-analysis. *Pediatr Pulmonol.* 2018;53(2):233–242.

22. Rusakow LS, Guarín M, Wegner CB, Rice B, Mischler EH Suspected respiratory tract infection in the tracheostomized child: The pediatric pulmonologist's approach. *Chest.* 1998;113(6):1549–1554.

23. Prodhan P, Greenberg B, Bhutta AT, Hyde C, Vankatesan A, Imamura M, Jaquiss RD, Dyamenahalli U. Recombinant human deoxyribonuclease improves atelectasis in mechanically ventilated children with cardiac disease. *Congenit Heart Dis.* 2009;4(3):166–173.

24. Bjornson C, Russell K, Vandermeer B, Klassen TP, Johnson DW. Nebulized epinephrine for croup in children. *Cochrane Database Syst Rev.* 2013;(10):CD006619.

25. Griffin S, Ellis S, Fitzgerald-Barron A, Rose J, Egger M. Nebulised steroid in the treatment of croup: A systematic review of randomised controlled trials. *Br J Gen Pract.* 2000;50(451):135–141.

26. Harless J, Ramaiah R, Bhananker SM. Pediatric airway management. *Int J Crit Illn Inj Sci.* 2014;4(1):65–70.

27. Bergerson PS, JC Shaw. Are infants really obligatory nasal breathers? *Clin Pediatr.* 2001;40:567–569.

28. Chua HL, Collis GG, Newbury AM, Chan K, Bower GD, Sly PD, Le Souef PN. The influence of age on aerosol deposition in children with cystic fibrosis. *Eur Respir J.* 1994;7(12):2185–2191.

29. Fleming S(1), Thompson M, Stevens R, Heneghan C, Plüddemann A, Maconochie I, Tarassenko L, Mant D. Normal ranges of heart rate and respiratory rate in children from birth to 18 years of age: A systematic review of observational studies. *Lancet.* 2011; 377(9770):1011–1018.

30. Azouz W, Chetcuti P, Hosker HS, Saralaya D, Stephenson J, Chrystyn H. The inhalation characteristics of patients when they use different dry powder inhalers. *J Aerosol Med Pulm Drug Deliv.* 2015; 28(1):35–42.

31. Murakami G, Igarashi T, Adachi Y, Matsuno M, Adachi Y, Sawai M, Yoshizumi A, Okada T. Measurement of bronchial hyperreactivity in infants and preschool children using a new method. *Ann Allergy.* 1990;64(4):383–387.

32. Iles R, Lister P, Edmunds AT. Crying significantly reduces absorption of aerosolised drug in infants. *Arch Dis Child.* 1999;81(2):163–165.

33. Amirav I, Newhouse MT. Review of optimal characteristics of face-masks for valved-holding chambers (VHCs). *Pediatr Pulmonol.* 2008;43(3):268–274.

34. Shah SA, Berlinski AB, Rubin BK. Force-dependent static dead space of face masks used with holding chambers. *Respir Care.* 2006;51(2):140–114.

35. Everard ML. Role of inhaler competence and contrivance in "difficult asthma." *Paediatr Respir Rev.* 2003; 4(2):135–142.

36. Collis GG, Cole CH, Le Souëf PN. Dilution of nebulised aerosols by air entrainment in children. *Lancet.* 1990;336(8711):341–343.

37. Mallol J, Rattray S, Walker G, Cook D, Robertson CF. Aerosol deposition in infants with cystic fibrosis. *Pediatr Pulmonol.* 1996;21(5):276–281.

38. Schüepp KG, Devadson S, Roller C, Wildhaber JH. A complementary combination of delivery device and drug formulation for inhalation therapy in preschool children. *Swiss Med Wkly.* 2004; 134(13–14):198–200.

39. Amirav I, Newhouse MT, Minocchieri S, Castro-Rodriguez JA, Schüepp KG. Factors that affect the efficacy of inhaled corticosteroids for infants and young children. *J Allergy Clin Immunol.* 2010; 125(6):1206–1211.

40. A Lowenthal D, Kattan M. Facemasks versus mouthpieces for aerosol treatment of asthmatic children. *Pediatr Pulmonol.* 1992;14(3):192–196.

41. Lipworth BJ, Jackson CM. Comparable efficacy of administration with face mask or mouthpiece of nebulized budesonide suspension for infants and young children with persistant asthma. *Am J Respir Crit Care Med.* 2001;163(5):1277–278.

42. Berlinski A. Effect of mask dead space and occlusion of mask holes on delivery of nebulized albuterol. *Respir Care.* 2014;59(8):1228–1232.

43. Sangwan S, Gurses BK, Smaldone GC. Facemasks and facial deposition of aerosols. *Pediatr Pulmonol.* 2004;37(5):447–452.

44. Harris KW, Smaldone GC. Facial and ocular deposition of nebulized budesonide: Effects of face mask design. *Chest.* 2008;133(2):482–488.

45. Kumar P, Parashette KR and Noronha P. Perioral dermatitis in a child associated with an inhalation steroid. *Dermatol Online J.* 2010;16(4). Retrieved from: http://escholarship.org/uc/item/0tq4z5z9.

46. Nakagawa TA, Guerra L, Storgion SA. Aerosolized atropine as an unusual cause of anisocoria in a child with asthma. *Pediatr Emerg Care.* 1993;9(3):153–154.

47. Amirav I, Luder AS, Halamish A, Raviv D, Kimmel R, Waisman D, Newhouse MT. Design of aerosol face masks for children using computerized 3D face analysis. *J Aerosol Med Pulm Drug Deliv*. 2014; 27(4):272–278.

48. Amirav I, Luder A, Chleechel A, Newhouse MT, Gorenberg M. Lung aerosol deposition in suckling infants. *Arch Dis Child*. 2012;97(6):497–501.

49. Erzinger S, Schueepp KG, Brooks-Wildhaber J, Devadason SG, Wildhaber JH. Facemasks and aerosol delivery in vivo. *J Aerosol Med*. 2007;20 Suppl 1:S78–S83; discussion S83–S84.

50. Amirav I, Balanov I, Gorenberg M, Groshar D, Luder AS. Nebuliser hood compared to mask in wheezy infants: Aerosol therapy without tears! *Arch Dis Child*. 2003;88(8):719–723.

51. Bar-Yishay E, Avital A, Springer C, Amirav I. Lung function response to bronchodilator nebulization via hood in wheezy infants: A pilot study. *Isr Med Assoc J*. 2011;13(1):39–43.

52. Kugelman A, Amirav I, Mor F, Riskin A, Bader D. Hood versus mask nebulization in infants with evolving bronchopulmonary dysplasia in the neonatal intensive care unit. *J Perinatol*. 2006;26(1):31–36.

53. Kim J, Xi J, Si X, Berlinski A, Su WC. Hood nebulization: Effects of head direction and breathing mode on particle inhalability and deposition in a 7-month-old infant model. *J Aerosol Med Pulm Drug Deliv*. 2014;27(3):209–218.

54. Kradjan WA, Lakshminarayan S. Efficiency of air compressor-driven nebulizers. *Chest*. 1985; 87(4):512–516.

55. Nikander K, Nicholls C, Denyer J, Pritchard J. The evolution of spacers and valved holding chambers. *J Aerosol Med Pulm Drug Deliv*. 2014;27 Suppl 1:S4–S23.

56. Geller D and Berlinski A. Aerosol delivery of medication. In: Light MJ, et al. Eds. *Pediatric Pulmonology*. Elk Grove Village, IL: American Academy of Pediatrics;2011.

57. Chavez A, McCracken A, Berlinski A. Effect of face mask dead volume, respiratory rate, and tidal volume on inhaled albuterol delivery. *Pediatr Pulmonol*. 2010;45(3):224–229.

58. Esposito-Festen JE, Ates B, van Vliet FJ, Verbraak AF, de Jongste JC, Tiddens HA. Effect of a facemask leak on aerosol delivery from a pMDI-spacer system. *J Aerosol Med*. 2004;17(1):1–6.

59. Berlinski A, von Hollen D, Pritchard JN, Hatley RH. Delay between actuation and shaking of a hydrofluoroalkane fluticasone pressurized metered-dose inhaler. *Respir Care*. 2018;63(3):289–293.

60. Hatley RH, Parker J, Pritchard JN, von Hollen D. Variability in delivered dose from pressurized metered-dose inhaler formulations due to a delay between shake and fire. *J Aerosol Med Pulm Drug Deliv*. 2017;30(1):71–79.

61. Berlinski A, Pennington D. Effect of interval between actuations of albuterol hydrofluoroalkane pressurized metered-dose inhalers on their aerosol characteristics. *Respir Care*. 2017;62(9):1123–1130.

62. Zar HJ, Brown G, Donson H, Brathwaite N, Mann MD, Weinberg EG. Home-made spacers for bronchodilator therapy in children with acute asthma: A randomized trial. *Lancet*. 1999; 354(9183):979–982.

63. Zar HJ, Weinberg EG, Binns HJ, Gallie F, Mann MD. Lung deposition of aerosol—A comparison of different spacers. *Arch Dis Child*. 2000;82(6):495–498.

64. Tal A, Golan H, Grauer N, Aviram M, Albin D, Quastel MR. Deposition pattern of radiolabeled salbutamol inhaled from a metered-dose inhaler by means of a spacer with mask in young children with airway obstruction. *J Pediatr*. 1996;128(4):479–484.

65. Esposito-Festen J, Ijsselstijn H, Hop W, van Vliet F, de Jongste J, Tiddens H. Aerosol therapy by pressured metered-dose inhaler-spacer in sleeping young children: To do or not to do? *Chest*. 2006; 130(2):487–492.

66. Fok TF, Lam K, Chan CK, Ng PC, Zhuang H, Wong W, Cheung KL. Aerosol delivery to non-ventilated infants by metered dose inhaler: Should a valved spacer be used? *Pediatr Pulmonol*. 1997; 24(3):204–212.

67. Stephen D, Vatsa M, Lodha R, Kabra SK. A randomized controlled trial of 2 inhalation methods when using a pressurized metered dose inhaler with valved holding chamber. *Respir Care*. 2015; 60(12):1743–1748.

68. Roller CM, Zhang G, Troedson RG, Leach CL, Le Souëf PN, Devadason SG. Spacer inhalation technique and deposition of extrafine aerosol in asthmatic children. *Eur Respir J*. 2007;29(2):299–306.

69. Devadason SG, Huang T, Walker S, Troedson R, Le Souëf PN. Distribution of technetium-99m-labelled QVAR delivered using an Autohaler device in children. *Eur Respir J*. 2003;21(6):1007–1011.

70. Berlinski A, von Hollen D, Hatley RHM, Hardaker LEA, Nikander K. Drug delivery in asthmatic children following coordinated and uncoordinated inhalation maneuvers: A randomized crossover trial. *J Aerosol Med Pulm Drug Deliv*. 2017;30(3):182–189.

71. Schultz A, Le Souëf TJ, Venter A, Zhang G, Devadason SG, Le Souëf PN. Aerosol inhalation from spacers and valved holding chambers requires few tidal breaths for children. *Pediatrics*. 2010; 126(6):e1493–e1498.

72. Sanders MJ, Bruin R. Are we misleading users of respiratory spacer devices? *Prim Care Respir J*. 2013; 22(4):466–467.

73. Geller DE. New liquid aerosol generation devices: Systems that force pressurized liquids through nozzles. *Respir Care*. 2002;47(12):1392–404; discussion 1404–1405.

74. Hochrainer D, Hölz H, Kreher C, Scaffidi L, Spallek M, Wachtel H. Comparison of the aerosol velocity and spray duration of Respimat Soft Mist inhaler and pressurized metered dose inhalers. *J Aerosol Med.* 2005;18(3):273–282.

75. Newman SP, Brown J, Steed KP, Reader SJ, Kladders H. Lung deposition of fenoterol and flunisolide delivered using a novel device for inhaled medicines: Comparison of RESPIMAT with conventional metered-dose inhalers with and without spacer devices. *Chest.* 1998;113(4):957–963.

76. Kamin W, Frank M, Kattenbeck S, Moroni-Zentgraf P, Wachtel H, Zielen S. A Handling study to assess use of the Respimat(®) Soft Mist™ inhaler in children under 5 Years old. *J Aerosol Med Pulm Drug Deliv.* 2015;28(5):372–381.

77. Raissy HH, Kelly HW. Tiotropium bromide in children and adolescents with asthma. *Paediatr Drugs.* 2017; 19(6):533–538.

78. Amirav I, Newhouse MT, Luder A, Halamish A, Omar H, Gorenberg M. Feasibility of aerosol drug delivery to sleeping infants: A prospective observational study. *BMJ Open.* 2014;4(3):e004124.

79. Berlinski A, Cooper B. Oronasal and tracheostomy delivery of soft mist and pressurized metered-dose inhalers with valved holding chamber. *Respir Care.* 2016;61(7):913–919.

80. Nielsen KG, Skov M, Klug B, Ifversen M, Bisgaard H. Flow-dependent effect of formoterol dry-powder inhaled from the aerolizer. *Eur Respir J.* 1997; 10(9):2105–2109.

81. Haynes A, Geller D, Weers J, Ament B, Pavkov R, Malcolmson R, Debonnett L, Mastoridis P, Yadao A, Heuerding S. Inhalation of tobramycin using simulated cystic fibrosis patient profiles. *Pediatr Pulmonol.* 2016;51(11):1159–1167.

82. Berlinski A. Assessing new technologies in aerosol medicine: Strengths and limitations. *Respir Care.* 2015;60(6):833–847; discussion 847–849.

83. De Boeck K, Alifier M, Warnier G. Is the correct use of a dry powder inhaler (Turbohaler) age dependent? *J Allergy Clin Immunol.* 1999;103(5 Pt 1):763–767.

84. Adachi YS, Adachi Y, Itazawa T, Yamamoto J, Murakami G, Miyawaki T. Ability of preschool children to use dry powder inhalers as evaluated by In-Check Meter. *Pediatr Int.* 2006;48(1):62–65.

85. Berlinski A. Inhaled drug delivery for children on long-term mechanical ventilation. In Sterni LM and Carroll JL. *Caring for the Ventilator Dependent Child. A Clinical guide.* 1st edition. New York: Humana Press, 2016, pp. 217–239.

86. Berlinski A. Pediatric aerosol therapy. *Respir Care.* 2017;62(6):662–677.

87. Milési C, Boubal M, Jacquot A, Baleine J, Durand S, Odena MP, Cambonie G. High-flow nasal cannula: Recommendations for daily practice in pediatrics. *Ann Intensive Care.* 2014;4:29.

88. Bhashyam AR, Wolf MT, Marcinkowski AL, Saville A, Thomas K, Carcillo JA, Corcoran TE. Aerosol delivery through nasal cannulas: As in vitro study. *J Aerosol Med Pulm Drug Deliv.* 2008;21(2):181–188.

89. Ari A, Harwood R, Sheard M, Dailey P, Fink JB. In vitro comparison of heliox and oxygen in aerosol delivery using pediatric high flow nasal cannula. *Pediatr Pulmonol.* 2011;46(8):795–801.

90. Perry SA, Kesser KC, Geller DE, Selhorst DM, Rendle JK, Hertzog JH. Influences of cannula size and flow rate on aerosol drug delivery through the Vapotherm humidified high-flow nasal cannula system. *Pediatr Crit Care Med.* 2013;14(5):e250–256.

91. Sunbul FS, Fink JB, Harwood R, Sheard MM, Zimmerman RD, Ari A. Comparison of HFNC, bubble CPAP and SiPAP on aerosol delivery in neonates: An in-vitro study. *Pediatr Pulmonol.* 2015;50(11):1099–106.

92. Lin HL, Harwood RJ, Fink JB, Goodfellow LT, Ari A. In vitro comparison of aerosol delivery using different face masks and flow rates with a high-flow humidity system. *Respir Care.* 2015;60(9):1215–1219.

93. Morley SL. Non-invasive ventilation in paediatric critical care. *Paediatr Respir Rev.* 2016;20:24–31.

94. Fauroux B, Itti E, Pigeot J, Isabey D, Meignan M, Ferry G, Lofaso F, Willemot JM, Clément A, Harf A. Optimization of aerosol deposition by pressure support in children with cystic fibrosis: An experimental and clinical study. *Am J Respir Crit Care Med.* 2000; 162(6):2265–2271.

95. Maccari JG, Teixeira C, Savi A, de Oliveira RP, Machado AS, Tonietto TF, Ludwig E, Teixeira PJ, Knorst MM. Nebulization during spontaneous breathing, CPAP, and bi-level positive-pressure ventilation: A randomized analysis of pulmonary radioaerosol deposition. *Respir Care.* 2014;59(4):479–484.

96. Galindo-Filho VC, Brandão DC, Ferreira Rde C, Menezes MJ, Almeida-Filho P, Parreira VF, Silva TN, Rodrigues-Machado Mda G, Dean E, Dornelas de Andrade A. Noninvasive ventilation coupled with nebulization during asthma crises: A randomized controlled trial. *Respir Care.* 2013;58(2):241–249.

97. White CC, Crotwell DN, Shen S, Salyer J, Yung D, Zheng J, DiBlasi RM. Bronchodilator delivery during simulated pediatric noninvasive ventilation. *Respir Care.* 2013;58(9):1459–1466.

98. Velasco J, and Berlinski A. Albuterol delivery efficiency during non-invasive ventilation in a model of a spontaneously breathing child (Abstract). *Am J Respir Crit Care Med.* 2017:A2813.

99. Velasco J, Berlinski A. Albuterol delivery efficiency in a pediatric model of noninvasive ventilation with double-limb circuit. *Respir Care.* 2018;63(2):141–146.

100. Trachsel D, Hammer, J. Indications for tracheostomy in children. *Paediatr Respir Rev.* 2006;7:162–168.

101. Willis LD, Berlinski A. Survey of aerosol delivery techniques to spontaneously breathing tracheostomized children. *Respir Care.* 2012;57(8):1234–1241.

102. Baran D, Dachy A, Klastersky J. Concentration of gentamicin in bronchial secretions of children with cystic fibrosis of tracheostomy. (Comparison between the intramuscular route, the endotracheal instillation and aerosolization). *Int J Clin Pharmacol Biopharm*. 1975;12(3):336–341.

103. O'Callaghan C, Hardy J, Stammers J, Stephenson TJ, Hull D. Evaluation of techniques for delivery of steroids to lungs of neonates using a rabbit model. *Arch Dis Child*. 1992;67(1 Spec No):20–24.

104. O'Callaghan C, Dryden S, Cert DN, Gibbin K. Asthma therapy and a tracheostomy. *J Laryngol Otol*. 1989;103(4):427–428.

105. Subhedar NV, Doyle C, Shaw NJ. Administration of inhaled medication via a tracheostomy in infants with chronic lung disease of prematurity. *Pediatr Rehabil*. 1999;3(2):41–42.

106. Berlinski A, Chavez A. Albuterol delivery via metered dose inhaler in a spontaneously breathing pediatric tracheostomy model. *Pediatr Pulmonol*. 2013; 48(10):1026–1034.

107. Cooper B, Berlinski A. Albuterol delivery via facial and tracheostomy route in a model of a spontaneously breathing child. *Respir Care*. 2015; 60(12):1749–1758.

108. Berlinski A and Cooper B. Oronasal and tracheostomy delivery of soft mist and pressurized metered-dose inhalers with valved holding chamber. *Respir Care*. 2016;61(7):913–919.

109. Berlinski A. Nebulized albuterol delivery in a model of spontaneously breathing children with tracheostomy. *Respir Care*. 2013;58(12):2076–2086.

110. Alhamad BR, Fink JB, Harwood RJ, Sheard MM, Ari A. Effect of aerosol devices and administration techniques on drug delivery in a simulated spontaneously breathing pediatric tracheostomy model. *Respir Care*. 2015;60(7):1026–1032.

111. Wee WB, Tavernini S, Martin AR, Amirav I, Majaesic C, Finlay WH. Dry powder inhaler delivery of tobramycin in in vitro models of tracheostomized children. *J Aerosol Med Pulm Drug Deliv*. 2017;30(1):64–70.

112. Berlinski A, Ari A, Davies P, Fink J, Majaesic C, Reychler G, Tatla T, Amirav I. Workshop report: Aerosol delivery to spontaneously breathing tracheostomized patients. *J Aerosol Med Pulm Drug Deliv*. 2017;30(4):207–222.

113. Ballard J, Lugo RA, Salyer JW. A survey of albuterol administration practices in intubated patients in the neonatal intensive care unit. *Respir Care*. 2002; 47(1):31–38.

114. Watter Watterberg KL, Clark AR, Kelly HW, Murphy S. Delivery of aerosolized medication to intubated babies. *Pediatr Pulmonol*. 1991;10(2):136–141.

115. Grigg J, Arnon S, Jones T, Clarke A, Silverman M. Delivery of therapeutic aerosols to intubated babies. *Arch Dis Child*. 1992;67(1 Spec No):25–30.

116. Fok TF, Monkman S, Dolovich M, Gray S, Coates G, Paes B, Rashid F, Newhouse M, Kirpalani H. Efficiency of aerosol medication delivery from a metered dose inhaler versus jet nebulizer in infants with bronchopulmonary dysplasia. *Pediatr Pulmonol*. 1996;21(5):301–309.

117. Pfenninger J, Aebi C. Respiratory response to salbutamol (albuterol) in ventilator-dependent infants with chronic lung disease: Pressurized aerosol delivery versus intravenous injection. *Intensive Care Med*. 1993;19(5):251–255.

118. Rotschild A, Solimano A, Puterman M, Smyth J, Sharma A, Albersheim S. Increased compliance in response to salbutamol in premature infants with developing bronchopulmonary dysplasia. *J Pediatr*. 1989;115(6):984–991.

119. Fok TF, Lam K, Ng PC, So HK, Cheung KL, Wong W, So KW. Randomised crossover trial of salbutamol aerosol delivered by metered dose inhaler, jet nebuliser, and ultrasonic nebuliser in chronic lung disease. *Arch Dis Child Fetal Neonatal* Ed. 1998; 79(2):F100–F114.

120. Garner SS, Wiest DB, Bradley JW, Habib DM. Two administration methods for inhaled salbutamol in intubated patients. *Arch Dis Child*. 2002;87(1):49–53.

121. Cameron D, Arnot R, Clay M, Silverman M. Aerosol delivery in neonatal ventilator circuits: A rabbit lung model. *Pediatr Pulmonol*. 1991;10(3):208–213.

122. Flavin M, MacDonald M, Dolovich M, Coates G, O'Brodovich H. Aerosol delivery to the rabbit lung with an infant ventilator. *Pediatr Pulmonol*. 1986;2(1):35–39.

123. Fok TF, Al-Essa M, Monkman S, Dolovich M, Girard L, Coates G, Kirpalani H. Pulmonary deposition of salbutamol aerosol delivered by metered dose inhaler, jet nebulizer, and ultrasonic nebulizer in mechanically ventilated rabbits. *Pediatr Res*. 1997;42(5):721–727.

124. Dubus JC, Montharu J, Vecellio L, De Monte M, De Muret A, Goucher A, Cantagrel S, Le Pape A, Mezzi K, Majoral C, Le Guellec S, Diot P. Lung deposition of HFA beclomethasone dipropionate in an animal model of bronchopulmonary dysplasia. *Pediatr Res*. 2007;61(1):21–25.

125. Sood BG, Shen Y, Latif Z, Galli B, Dawe EJ, Haacke EM. Effective aerosol delivery during high-frequency ventilation in neonatal pigs. *Respirology*. 2010;15(3):551–555.

126. Dubus JC, Vecellio L, De Monte M, Fink JB, Grimbert D, Montharu J, Valat C, Behan N, Diot P. Aerosol deposition in neonatal ventilation. *Pediatr Res*. 2005;58(1):10–14.

127. Ferrari F, Liu ZH, Lu Q, Becquemin MH, Louchahi K, Aymard G, Marquette CH, Rouby JJ. Comparison of lung tissue concentrations of nebulized ceftazidime in ventilated piglets: Ultrasonic versus vibrating plate nebulizers. *Intensive Care Med*. 2008; 34(9):1718–1723.

128. Yokoe DS, Anderson DJ, Berenholtz SM, Calfee DP, Dubberke ER, Ellingson KD, Gerding DN et al. A compendium of strategies to prevent healthcare-associated infections in acute care hospitals: 2014 updates. *Infect Control Hosp Epidemiol.* 2014; 35 Suppl 2:S21–S31.

129. Hanhan U, Kissoon N, Payne M, Taylor C, Murphy S De Nicola LK. Effects of in-line nebulization on preset ventilator variables. *Respir Care.* 1993; 38(5):474–478.

130. McPeck M, O'Riordan, TG, and Smaldone GC. Choice of mechanical ventilator: Influence on nebulizer performance. *Respir Care.* 1993; 38(8):887–895.

131. Di Paolo ER, Pannatier A, Cotting J. In vitro evaluation of bronchodilator drug delivery by jet nebulization during pediatric mechanical ventilation. *Pediatr Crit Care Med.* 2005;6(4):462–469.

132. Sidler-Moix AL, Dolci U, Berger-Gryllaki M, Pannatier A, Cotting J, Di Paolo ER. Albuterol delivery in an in vitro pediatric ventilator lung model: Comparison of jet, ultrasonic, and mesh nebulizers. *Pediatr Crit Care Med.* 2013;14(2):e98–e102.

133. Wan GH, Lin HL, Fink JB, Chen YH, Wang WJ, Chiu YC, Kao YY, Liu CJ. In vitro evaluation of aerosol delivery by different nebulization modes in pediatric and adult mechanical ventilators. *Respir Care.* 2014;59(10):1494–1500.

134. Cole CH, Mitchell JP, Foley MP, Nagel MW. Hydrofluoroalkane-beclomethasone versus chlorofluorocarbon-beclomethasone delivery in neonatal models. *Arch Dis Child Fetal Neonatal Ed.* 2004; 89(5):F417–F418.

135. Lugo RA, Kenney JK, Keenan J, Salyer JW, Ballard J, Ward RM. Albuterol delivery in a neonatal ventilated lung model: Nebulization versus chlorofluorocarbon- and hydrofluoroalkane-pressurized metered dose inhalers. *Pediatr Pulmonol.* 2001;31(3):247–254.

136. Avent ML, Gal P, Ransom JL, Brown YL, Hansen CJ. Comparing the delivery of albuterol metered-dose inhaler via an adapter and spacer device in an in vitro infant ventilator lung model. *Ann Pharmacother.* 1999;33(2):141–143.

137. Garner SS, Southgate WM, Wiest DB, Brandeburg S, Annibale DJ. Albuterol delivery with conventional and synchronous ventilation in a neonatal lung model. *Pediatr Crit Care Med.* 2002;3(1):52–56.

138. Avent ML, Gal P, Ransom JL, Brown YL, Hansen CJ, Ricketts WA, Soza F. Evaluating the delivery of nebulized and metered-dose inhalers in an in vitro infant ventilator lung model. *Ann Pharmacother.* 1999; 33(2):144–148.

139. Benson JM, Gal P, Kandrotas RJ, Watling SM, Hansen CJ. The impact of changing ventilator parameters on availability of nebulized drugs in an in vitro neonatallung system. *DICP.* 1991;25(3):272–275.

140. Berlinski A, Kumaran S. Particle size characterization of nebulized albuterol delivered by a vibrating mesh nebulizer through pediatric endotracheal tubes (abstract). *Am J Respir Crit Care Med.* 2016:A2191.

141. Berlinski A, and Kumaran S. Particle size characterization of nebulized albuterol delivered by a jet nebulizer through pediatric endotracheal tubes. *Am J Respir Crit Care Med.* 2017:A2812.

142. DiBlasi RM, Crotwell DN, Shen S, Zheng J, Fink JB, Yung D. Iloprost drug delivery during infant conventional and high-frequency oscillatory ventilation. *Pulm Circ.* 2016;6(1):63–69.

143. Fang TP, Lin HL, Chiu SH, Wang SH, DiBlasi RM, Tsai YH, Fink JB. Aerosol delivery using jet nebulizer and vibrating mesh nebulizer during high frequency oscillatory ventilation: An in vitro comparison. *J Aerosol Med Pulm Drug Deliv.* 2016;29(5):447–453.

144. Parker DK, Shen S, Zheng J, Ivy DD, Crotwell DN, Hotz JC, DiBlasi RM. Inhaled treprostinil drug delivery during mechanical ventilation and spontaneous breathing using two different nebulizers. *Pediatr Crit Care Med.* 2017;18(6):e253–e260.

145. Mazela J, Chmura K, Kulza M, Henderson C, Gregory TJ, Moskal A, Sosnowski TR, Florek E, Kramer L, Keszler M. Aerosolized albuterol sulfate delivery under neonatal ventilatory conditions: In vitro evaluation of a novel ventilator circuit patient interface connector. *J Aerosol Med Pulm Drug Deliv.* 2014;27(1):58–65.

146. Berlinski A, and Kumaran S. Particle size variation of nebulized albuterol occurs while traveling through neonatal mechanical ventilation circuits. *Eur Respir J.* 2017; 50(suppl 61); PA2065.

147. Mazela J, Sosnoski TR, Moscal A, Gadzinowski J. Small neonatal endotracheal tube sizes decrease aerosol penetration—Computational fluid dynamic study. *Respiratory Drug Delivery Europe.* 2001: 401–404.

148. Longest PW, Azimi M, Hindle M. Optimal delivery of aerosols to infants during mechanical ventilation. *J Aerosol Med Pulm Drug Deliv.* 2014;27(5):371–385.

149. Ahrens RC, Ries RA, Popendorf W, Wiese JA. The delivery of therapeutic aerosols through endotracheal tubes. *Pediatr Pulmonol.* 1986;2(1):19–26.

150. Takaya T, Takeyama K, Takiguchi M. The efficiency of beta 2-agonist delivery through tracheal tubes with the metered-dose inhaler: An in vitro study. *J Anesth.* 2002;16(4):284–288.

151. Garner SS, Wiest DB, Bradley JW. Albuterol delivery by metered-dose inhaler in mechanically ventilated pediatric lung model. *Crit Care Med.* 1996; 24(5)870–874.

152. Garner SS, Wiest DB, Bradley JW. Albuterol delivery by metered-dose inhaler with a pediatric mechanical ventilatory circuit model. *Pharmacotherapy.* 1994; 14(2):210–214.

153. Wildhaber JH, Hayden MJ, Dore ND, Devadason SG, LeSouëf PN. Salbutamol delivery from a hydrofluoroalkane pressurized metered-dose inhaler in pediatric ventilator circuits: An in vitro study. *Chest.* 1998; 113(1):186–191.

154. Mandhane P, Zuberbuhler P, Lange CF, Finlay WH. Albuterol aerosol delivered via metered-dose inhaler to intubated pediatric models of 3 ages, with 4 spacer designs. *Respir Care.* 2003;48(10):948–955.

155. Habib DM, Garner SS, Brandeburg S. Effect of helium-oxygen on delivery of albuterol in a pediatric, volume-cycled, ventilated lung model. *Pharmacotherapy.* 1999;19(2):143–149.

156. Garner SS, Wiest DB, Stevens CE, Habib DM. Effect of heliox on albuterol delivery by metered-dose inhaler in pediatric in vitro models of mechanical ventilation. *Pharmacotherapy.* 2006; 26(10):1396–1402.

157. Garner SS, Wiest DB, Bradley JW. Albuterol delivery by metered-dose inhaler in a pediatric high-frequency oscillatory ventilation model. *Crit Care Med.* 2000;28(6):2086–2089.

158. Ari A, Atalay OT, Harwood R, Sheard MM, Aljamhan EA, Fink JB. Influence of nebulizer type, position, and bias flow on aerosol drug delivery in simulated pediatric and adult lung models during mechanical ventilation. *Respir Care.* 2010; 55(7):845–851.

159. Berlinski A, Willis JR. Albuterol delivery by 4 different nebulizers placed in 4 different positions in a pediatric ventilator in vitro model. *Respir Care.* 2013; 58(7):1124–1133.

160. Berlinski A, Willis JR. Effect of tidal volume and nebulizer type and position on albuterol delivery in a pediatric model of mechanical ventilation. *Respir Care.* 2015; 60(10):1424–1430.

161. Berlinski A and Willis JR. Albuterol delivery by intrapulmonary percussive ventilator and jet nebulizer in a pediatric ventilator model. *Respir Care.* 2010; 55(12):1699–1704.

162. Longest PW, Tian G. Development of a new technique for the efficient delivery of aerosolized medications to infants on mechanical ventilation. *Pharm Res.* 2015; 32(1):321–336.

9

Asthma

OMAR S. USMANI

Introduction   161
The history of inhalation aerosols for asthma   161
Asthma pathology, physiology, and pharmacology   162
Factors affecting aerosol deposition and clinical
outcomes   162
    Physicochemical mechanisms   162
    Airway caliber and disease   162
    Breathing maneuver   163

Human factors   163
Inhaler device   163
    pMDIs   163
    DPIs   164
    SMIs   164
    Nebulizers   164
References   164

INTRODUCTION

The delivery of drugs via the inhaled route has been the foundation and mainstay in the therapeutic management of the majority of respiratory disorders, including asthma. In contrast to systemic routes of delivery, the inhaled route targets drug directly to the lungs, utilizing a smaller drug dose, achieving a more rapid onset of pharmacological action, and decreasing the incidence of adverse clinical effects. Indeed, recent interest has seen developments in the utilization of inhaled aerosolized delivery to the respiratory tract as a gateway for systemic drug delivery with a variety of therapeutic compounds (1–3).

THE HISTORY OF INHALATION AEROSOLS FOR ASTHMA

The inhalation of aerosols to treat the cardinal symptoms of asthma has been described through the ages by many ancient civilizations (4–7). In India, in 2000 BC, the practice of Ayurvedic medicine advocated inhaling the vapors of the burning leaves of an anticholinergic plant, Datura stramonium, for the relief of patients with respiratory ailments. The practice of the Ancient Egyptians, described in Eber's papyrus, was the inhalation of the heated vapors of another anticholinergic, Hyoscyamus mutis, to treat the symptoms of wheeze. In Greek medicinal practice, both Hippocrates and Galen described the inhalation of hot vapors as beneficial remedies to alleviate respiratory symptoms. In his *Cannon of Medicine* from the tenth century AD, the Persian physician Ibn Sinna Avicenna described the

inhalation of aerosolized essential oils of eucalyptus and pine to ease patients with symptoms of airway obstruction; these compounds are still used in present-day over-the-counter (OTC) inhalation remedies (8).

During the Industrial Revolution in the early 1800s in the United Kingdom, smoking the leaves of Datura in pipes was employed as a standard approach and remedy to treat asthma patients (9), with the consequence that so-called asthma cigarettes containing Datura-tobacco mixtures were developed and became commonplace in the therapeutic management of the disease. By the 1900s, a variety of aerosolized devices adapted to deliver liquids were being utilized, and with the new discoveries in respiratory pharmacological agents such as adrenaline and cortisone, the nebulized delivery of these agents were popular for the treatment of patients with asthma (10–12).

Modern inhalation therapy for asthma began with the suggestion from Susie Maison, the teenage daughter of Dr. George Maison, who suffered from severe asthma, to aerosolize her asthma medication "like hair spray" (13). Dr. Maison was President of Riker Labs and instructed his chief chemist Irving Porusch to rise to his daughter's challenge and, within a year, the first pressurized metered-dose inhalers (pMDIs) were manufactured with the bronchodilators of isoprotenerol and adrenaline (14). The following decade represented an innovative technological era leading to many advances in inhaled asthma management with both "reliever" (bronchodilator) and "preventer" (corticosteroid) drugs in chlorofluorocarbon (CFC)-propelled pMDIs. By the early 1970s, breath-actuated pMDIs had been developed (15), and spacers and valve-holding chambers were being utilized with pMDIs to enhance inhaled drug delivery to the lungs.

In parallel to these advances, new drugs such as disodium cromoglycate delivered in new devices as a dry powder to atopic patients with asthma saw the advent of the dry powder inhaler (DPI) that was free of propellant and relied on the patient's inspiratory flow to aerosolize drug (16). The phaseout of CFC-pMDIs and transition to the alternative propellant HFA (hydrofluoroalkane) pMDIs was heralded by the Montreal Protocol in 1987.

The last decade has seen many advances in aerosol science for treating patients with asthma, including drug formulations of inhaled corticosteroid to improve their targeting to distal lung regions in patients with asthma (17); enhancing the efficiency of aerosolized devices through sophisticated nebulizers delivering corticosteroids (18); most recently, after being long-established in history, the new indication of inhaled long-acting muscarinic antagonists in asthma (19); and novel inhaled biological treatment for the management of asthmatic patients (20).

ASTHMA PATHOLOGY, PHYSIOLOGY, AND PHARMACOLOGY

Asthma is a chronic inflammatory disease involving the large and small airways, and because of its heterogeneous nature, *asthma* is considered an umbrella term to define several different phenotypes (21) The inflammatory biology in asthma is characterized by mast cells, eosinophils, and CD4+ T-2 cells, with key mediators of histamine; prostaglandins and leukotrienes; and cytokines of interleukin (IL)-5, IL-13, and IL-4 (22). Pathologically the key features are of airway smooth muscle hyperplasia, mucus plugging, and airway inflammation, all contributing to bronchoconstriction, airway hyper-responsiveness and airflow obstruction. The physiological hallmark of asthma is variable airflow obstruction that is usually reversible and rarely progressive, and its variable nature can be diurnal and/or seasonal. Collectively, these pathophysiology features present in the patient with the classical symptoms of wheeze, chest tightness, shortness of breath, and cough.

It is recognized that a good proportion of patients with asthma have poor control of their disease even with optimal treatment and management for their asthma (23). Contributing factors to ongoing poor disease control include environmental exposures (such as house dust mite), associated clinical conditions (such as allergic rhinitis), poor adherence with their medication as prescribed, and the patient's inability to use their inhaled medication correctly (24). Recently, there has been a lot of interest around the inability of current inhaled drugs to target the distal inflamed lung regions as a key contributor to poor disease control (25). The primary aim in the management of asthma is to alleviate symptoms by controlling inflammation and improve disease control.

A variety of inhaled drug classes are available to treat patients with asthma, including short-acting beta$_2$-agonists (SABAs), long-acting beta$_2$-agonists (LABAs), short-acting

muscarinic antagonists (SAMAs), long-acting muscarinic antagonists (LAMAs), inhaled corticosteroids (ICSs), and the dual combination therapy of ICS/LABA. A vast number of inhaler device/drug combinations are available, more than 200 in Europe, where many are available for the treatment of patients with asthma (26). Most recently, the combination of LABA/LAMA/ICS (triple therapy) in one inhaler device has been licensed for use in patients with severe chronic obstructive pulmonary disease (COPD). The main classes of inhaler device are pressurized metered-dose inhalers (pMDIs), dry powder inhalers (DPIs), soft mist inhalers (SMIs), and nebulizers (27).

FACTORS AFFECTING AEROSOL DEPOSITION AND CLINICAL OUTCOMES

Physicochemical mechanisms

The three main physicochemical mechanisms by which inhaled particles deposit in the human airways include inertial impaction, gravitational sedimentation, and diffusional transport (28,29). These mechanisms underlie the key factors that affect the deposition of aerosolized therapeutic drug within the lungs, which are divided into aerosol factors and patient characteristics (Table 9.1). It has been shown that aerosol particle size is a critical factor that determines the amount and distribution of inhaled drug in the lungs of patients with asthma (30,31).

Airway caliber and disease

Airway caliber, particularly in the state of disease, has been shown to affect the deposition of inhaled drug with the lungs; consequently, this will affect the clinical performance of the drug. Bronchial spasm, smooth muscle hypertrophy, luminal mucus plugging, and airway fibrosis are cardinal pathophysiological features present in differing extents in asthma and COPD, and collectively contribute to airway narrowing in these disease states. Imaging studies of radiolabeled drugs show that patents with asthma have lower total lung

Table 9.1 Factors affecting the respiratory deposition of inhaled medical aerosols

Aerosol characteristics	Patient variables
Particle size	Inhalation maneuver
Particle density	1. Inspiratory flow
	2. Breathing frequency
	3. Inhaled aerosol volume
	4. Breath-hold pause
	5. Degree of lung inflation
Aerosol formulation	Airways diameter
1. Hygroscopicity	
2. Charge	
3. Surfactant	
Delivery device	Airway disease and severity
	Pediatric versus adult airways

deposition and poorer distal airways penetration than healthy subjects (32). Studies utilizing experimentally induced bronchoconstriction also show lower levels of lung deposition (33,34). Pharmacokinetic approaches have informed us that a narrow airway caliber leads to decreased total lung deposition of inhaled aerosol. Plasma fenoterol concentrations measured in patients with asthma were shown to be lower than in healthy subjects (35). Indeed, with increasing disease severity, potentially causing greater airway narrowing, peak plasma salbutamol concentrations were shown to be lower in patients with severe asthma compared to those with mild asthma (36,37). Recent data show that a small particle formulation can achieve consistent lung deposition of approximately 33% in healthy subjects (forced expiratory volume in one second [FEV_1] 112% predicted), asthmatic patients (FEV_1 71% predicted) and patients with COPD (FEV_1 44% predicted), suggesting that the formulation can overcome the inherent airway obstruction to achieve consistent deposition (38).

Breathing maneuver

In the patient clinic, the inhalation maneuver adopted by the patient critically affects the ability to effectively achieve an adequate drug dose delivered to the lungs from the inhaler device, and consequently can affect the therapeutic benefit and adverse effect profile of the drug and inhaler device system. It is important to relay to the patients that a relaxed, slow, and deep breathing maneuver over 4–5 seconds followed by a 5-second breath-hold pause will achieve optimal lung deposition from a pMDIs. Unfortunately, a rapid inhalation is often seen in the majority of patients in the clinic, and this will increase oropharyngeal deposition and minimize adequate lung deposition through the physical process of impaction (39). On the contrary, a fast and hard inhalation technique is usually required for the majority of DPIs, as they rely on the negative inspiratory pressure of the patient in order to deaggregate the drug powder from its carrier molecule and achieve aerosolization in order to be inhaled. Such faster inspiratory flows with DPIs are needed for adequate airway deposition compared to a suboptimal slow breathing technique from a DPI that may not achieve device performance and effective drug delivery to the lungs (40,41).

Human factors

The patient's ability to use her or his device is a key human factor and is an aspect that can be controlled with dedicated and effective training. Unfortunately, this aspect of therapeutic management is often overlooked by healthcare professionals, and the patient has to utilize the patient information leaflet accompanying the inhaler device, which can be difficult to follow, or utilize social media to help him or her learn how to use the device. Indeed, regular checking of inhalation technique is vital to achieve optimal deposition of drug from the device and adequate clinical outcomes, where correct inhalation is a cornerstone of successful asthma management and highlighted in global documents on asthma (42). Recent data from a multicenter cross-sectional study of adults with asthma show a number of critical errors in inhaler use were identified, and they were related to worsening asthma control and increased asthma exacerbations (43). Suboptimal inhalation from a DPI device and actuation of a pMDI device before inhalation were shown to worsen asthma control and increase disease exacerbations. It has been shown that if the inhalation maneuver is correctly performed with actuation just after the beginning of inspiration during low lung volumes, this achieves better total lung deposition as well as better deposition in the conducting airways and alveolar lung region (44,45). Another factor to consider in the inhalation maneuver is the inhaled volume, where a greater inhaled aerosol volume will allow more drug particles to achieve distal airway penetration (46,47). A breath-hold pause at the end of inhalation can improve the deposition of inhaled drug reaching the distal airways by achieving adequate airway residence time for the drug particles to deposit on the airway walls by sedimentation or diffusion (48).

Inhaler device

pMDIs

Optimal deposition of inhaled drug in the lungs is achieved from a pMDI when it is actuated at the start of the patient's inhalation using a slow and deep breathing maneuver over 4–5 seconds, followed by a breath-hold pause of 5 seconds at the end of inspiration (45). However, it is clearly recognized that there remain fundamental problems with all inhaler devices that may affect lung deposition and ultimately clinical performance, and these include poor instruction in use (49), failure to understand the technique (50), and errors in using the device (51). Specific to pMDIs is the problem between coordination in the actuation of the device with the start of inhalation, which has been shown to affect clinical outcomes with worsening asthma control (43). The problem of coordination is more noticeable in the elderly and in physically impaired patients, and in order to circumvent poor drug delivery to the lungs, device holding adaptors, add-on spacer attachments, and breath-actuated pMDIs have been developed (52,53). Breath-actuated pMDIs are triggered by the patient's inhalation, which activates the inhaler (54). However, it has been shown that breath-actuated devices offer no added advantage in terms of lung deposition of inhaled aerosol over patients with good conventional pMDI inhaler technique. Newer HFA pMDI with smaller particle size formulations, slower plume velocities, and higher fine particle fraction show better drug deposition to the lungs with les oropharyngeal deposition compared to larger particle pMDIs (25).

pMDIs can be used with spacer devices, which allow space and time for the aerosol cloud to slow down and consequently reduce deposition within the oropharynx, and hence reduce the potential for unwanted local and systemic (through gastrointestinal absorption) adverse effects (55,56). Furthermore, spacers allow time for the propellant within the aerosol to evaporate, leading to smaller drug particles, where it has been shown that smaller particles and a slow inhalation achieve improved deposition within the lungs (31). For patients with difficulty in inhaler actuation and breathing coordination, the use of valve-holding chambers (VHCs) with pMDIs allows a better opportunity to achieve adequate drug deposition in the lungs, where the VHC acts as a reservoir for the aerosolized drug from which the patient breathes tidally (52).

DPIs

DPIs are wholly dependent on the patient's inspiratory effort in order to deaggregate the drug from its carrier particle and achieve adequate dispersion of the aerosol into drug particles of appropriate size to allow delivery to the lungs (57). DPIs are very dependent on a sufficiently generated inspiratory flow by the patient, where studies have shown that optimal drug deposition in the lungs often requires generated inhalation flows of 60 liters/min or greater (58,59). In the clinic, patients may often not be able to generate the requisite inhalation flows to activate DPIs, and studies in patients with asthma and COPD have demonstrated suboptimal inspiratory flows in those using DPIs (60,61). Another important factor that can affect lung deposition and consequently clinical efficacy is the storage of DPIs: the deterioration of the drug within the device may occur in damp and humid conditions, and DPIs should preferably be stored in a dry environment (62). In the last decade, some DPIs have been developed that require less patient effort to activate with lower inspiratory flows of between 15 and 30 liters/min to adequately aerosolize the drug powder (63,64).

SMIs

The SMI Respimat (Boehringer-Ingelheim, Germany), is a multidose nonpropellant-based aerosol device that forces pressurized drug solution (tiotropium, and more recently, tiotropium combined with olodaterol) through nozzles, generating a slow-moving aerosol (65). The aerosol also has a prolonged plume duration and a high fine particle fraction, which together achieve greater lung deposition in contrast to the same long-acting muscarinic antagonist (tiotropium) delivered by a DPI (66). Such innovation in device technology, through its efficient targeting to the airways, is allowing a reduction in the clinically prescribed dose. Similar advances in device engineering are also being realized with nebulizers in order to improve their efficiency.

NEBULIZERS

Conventional nebulizers such as jet nebulizers and ultrasonic nebulizers (67,68) are in widespread clinical use, but they are highly inefficient because, at best, approximately 5% of the delivered dose reaches the lungs. In order to compensate such inefficiency, much higher drug doses are used; for example, 5 mg of salbutamol delivered via a nebulizer versus 200 µg from a pMDI. Indeed, it is well recognized there is great variation in the aerosol output and large variations in the particle size distributions that are generated (69), particularly when nebulizer therapy is given in an acute clinical setting where the patient is in relative distress and has an erratic breathing maneuver. These factors all contribute to the marked inefficiency in drug delivery and deposition within the lungs. Indeed, data show that salbutamol delivered by a pMDI and spacer in patients with an acute asthma attack is as effective clinically in alleviating symptoms as is a nebulizer (70). A newer generation of nebulizers have been developed that offer a marked improvement in the efficiency and precision of pulmonary drug delivery over conventional nebulizer systems and, although the devices are more costly, they may be cost effective, particularly with expensive medication, by employing a reduced drug dose than is currently utilized (71,72). Recent data show that smart nebulizer delivery of budesonide to patients with corticosteroid dependent asthma allowed significant reductions in the dose without worsening the risk of asthma exacerbation in improving lung function (18).

REFERENCES

1. Hickey AJ. Back to the future: Inhaled drug products. *J Pharm Sci.* 2013;102(4):1165–1172.
2. Laube BL. The expanding role of aerosols in systemic drug delivery, gene therapy and vaccination: An update. *Transl Respir Med.* 2014;2:3.
3. Rubin BK. Air and soul: The science and application of aerosol therapy. *Respir Care.* 2010;55(7):911–921.
4. Gandevia B. Historical review of the use of parasympatholytic agents in the treatment of respiratory disorders. *Postgrad Med J.* 1975;51:13–20.
5. Grossman J. The evolution of inhaler technology. *J Asthma.* 1994;31:55–64.
6. Sakula A. 1988. A history of asthma. The FitzPatrick lecture. *J R Coll Physicians Lond.* 1987;22:36–44.
7. Yernault JC. Inhalation therapy: An historical perspective. *Eur Respir Rev.* 1994;4:65–67.
8. Al Aboud K. The founder of Vicks: Lunsford Richardson (1854–1919). *Skin Med.* 2010;8(2):100–101.
9. Sims J. Datura stramonium or thorn apple as a cure or relief of asthma. *Edinburgh Med Surg J.* 1812;8:364–367.
10. Barger G, Dale HH. Chemical structure and sympathomimetic action of amines. *J Physiol.* 1910;41:19.
11. Camps PWL. A note on the inhalation treatment of asthma. *Guy's Hospital Report.* 1929;79:496–498.
12. Gelfand ML. Administration of cortisone by the aerosol method in the treatment of bronchial asthma. *N Engl J Med.* 1951;245:293–294.
13. Fink JB, Rau JL. New horizons in respiratory care. *Resp Care.* 2000;45:824–825.
14. Thiel CG. From Susie's question to CFC free: An inventor's perspective of 40 years of MDI development and regulation. In: *Respiratory Drug Delivery,* Vol. V. Dalby RN, Byron PR, Farr SJ, eds. Buffalo Grove, IL: Interpharm Press, 1996, pp. 115–123.
15. Crompton GK. Breath-activated aerosol. *Br Med J.* 1971;2:652–653.

16. Howell JB, Altounyan RE. A double-blind trial of disodium cromoglycate in the treatment of allergic bronchial asthma. *Lancet*. 1967;2:539–542.

17. Usmani OS. Small-airway disease in asthma: Pharmacological considerations. *Curr Opin Pulm Med*. 2015;21(1):55–67.

18. Vogelmeier C, Kardos P, Hofmann T, Canisius S, Scheuch G, Muellinger B, Nocker K et al. Nebulised budesonide using a novel device in patients with oral steroid-dependent asthma. *Eur Resp J*. 2015;45(5):1273–1282.

19. Rodrigo GJ. Anticholinergics for asthma: A long history. *Curr Opin Allergy Clin Immunol*. 2018;18(1):38–43.

20. Krug N, Hohlfeld JM, Kirsten AM, Kornmann O, Beeh KM, Kappeler D, Korn S et al. Allergen-induced asthmatic responses modified by a GATA3-specific DNAzyme. *N Engl J Med*. 2015;372(21):1987–1995.

21. Perlikos F, Hillas G, Loukides S. Phenotyping and endotyping asthma based on biomarkers. *Curr Top Med Chem*. 2016;16(14):1582–1586.

22. Barnes PJ. Cellular and molecular mechanisms of asthma and COPD. *Clin Sci (Lond)*. 2017;131(13):1541–1558.

23. Demoly P, Gueron B, Annunziata K, Adamek L, Walters RD. Update on asthma control in five European countries: Results of a 2008 survey. *Eur Resp Rev*. 2010;19(116):150–157.

24. Bonini M, Usmani OS. Novel methods for device and adherence monitoring in asthma. *Curr Opin Pulm Med*. 2018;24(1):63–69.

25. Usmani OS, Barnes PJ. Assessing and treating small airways disease in asthma and chronic obstructive pulmonary disease. *Ann Med*. 2012;44(2):146–56.

26. Lavorini F, Corrigan CJ, Barnes PJ, Dekhuijzen PRN et al. Retail sales of inhalation devices in European countries: So much for a global policy. *Resp Med*. 2011;105(7):1099–1103.

27. Lavorini F, Fontana GA, Usmani OS. New inhaler devices—The good, the bad and the ugly. *Respiration*. 2014;88(1):3–15.

28. Agnew JE, Bateman JR, Pavia D, Clarke SW. A model for assessing bronchial mucus transport. *J Nucl Med*. 1984;25:170–176.

29. Yu J, Chien YW. Pulmonary drug delivery: Physiologic and mechanistic aspects. *Crit Rev Ther Drug Carrier Syst*. 1997;14:395–453.

30. Usmani OS, Biddiscombe MF, Nightingale JA, Underwood SR, Barnes PJ. The effects of bronchodilator particle size in asthmatics using monodisperse aerosols. *J Appl Physiol*. 2003;95:2106–2112.

31. Usmani OS, Biddiscombe MF, Barnes PJ. Regional lung deposition and bronchodilator response as a function of $\beta2$-agonist particle size. *Am J Respir Crit Care Med*. 2005;172:1497–1504.

32. Melchor R, Biddiscombe MF, Mak VH, Short MD, Spiro SG. Lung deposition patterns of directly labelled salbutamol in normal subjects and in patients with reversible airflow obstruction. *Thorax*. 1993;48:506–511.

33. Svartengren M, Philipson K, Linnman L, Camner P. Regional deposition of particles in human lung after induced bronchoconstriction. *Exp Lung Res*. 1986;10:223–233.

34. Svartengren M, Anderson M, Philipson K, Camner P. Individual differences in regional deposition of 6-micron particles in humans with induced broncho-constriction. *Exp Lung Res*. 1989;15:139–149.

35. Newnham DM, McDevitt DG, Lipworth BJ. Comparison of the extrapulmonary beta2-adrenoceptor responses and pharmacokinetics of salbutamol given by standard metered dose-inhaler and modified actuator device. *Br J Clin Pharmacol*. 1993; 36:445–450.

36. Lipworth BJ, Newnham DM, Clark RA, Dhillon DP, Winter JH, McDevitt DG. Comparison of the relative airways and systemic potencies of inhaled fenoterol and salbutamol in asthmatic patients. *Thorax*. 1995;50:54–61.

37. Lipworth BJ, Clark DJ. Effects of airway calibre on lung delivery of nebulised salbutamol. *Thorax*. 1997;52:1036–1039.

38. De Backer W, Devolder A, Poli G, Acerbi D, Monno R, Herpich C, Sommerer K et al. Lung deposition of BDP/formoterol HFA pMDI in healthy volunteers, asthmatic, and COPD patients. *J Aerosol Med Pulm Drug Deliv*. 2010;23(3):137–148

39. Farr SJ, Rowe AM, Rubsamen R, Taylor G. Aerosol deposition in the human lung following administration from a microprocessor controlled pressurized metered dose inhaler. *Thorax*. 1995;50:639–644.

40. Hindle M, Byron PR. Dose emissions from marketed dry powder inhalers. *Int J Pharm*. 1995;116:169–177.

41. Tarsin W, Assi KH, Chrystyn H. In-vitro intra- and inter-inhaler flow rate-dependent dosage emission from a combination of budesonide and eformoterol in a dry powder inhaler. *J Aerosol Med*. 2004;17:25–32.

42. Global Initiative for Asthma (GINA). http://gin-asthma.org/.

43. Price DB, Román-Rodríguez M, McQueen RB, Bosnic-Anticevich S, Carter V, Gruffydd-Jones K, Haughney J et al. Inhaler errors in the CRITIKAL study: Type, frequency, and association with asthma outcomes. *J Allergy Clin Immunol Pract*. 2017;5(4):1071–1081.

44. Newman SP, Pavia D, Clarke SW. How should a pressurized beta-adrenergic bronchodilator be inhaled? *Eur J Resp Dis*. 1981;62:3–21.

45. Newman SP, Pavia D, Garland N, Clarke SW. Effects of various inhalation modes on the deposition of radioactive pressurized aerosols. *Eur J Resp Dis Suppl*. 1982;119:57–65.

46. Farr SJ, Gonda I, Licko V. Physiochemical and physiological factors influencing the effectiveness of inhaled insulin. In: *Respiratory Drug Delivery*, Vol. VI. Dalby RN, Byron PR, Farr SJ, eds. Buffalo Grove, IL: Interpharm Press, 1998, pp. 25–33.

47. Pavia D, Thomson M, Shannon HS. Aerosol inhalation and depth of deposition in the human lung. The effect of airway obstruction and tidal volume inhaled. *Arch Environ Health*. 1977;32:131–137.

48. Newman SP, Pavia D, Clarke SW. Improving the bronchial deposition of pressurized aerosols. *Chest*. 1981;80:909–911.

49. Guidry GG, Brown WD, Stogner SW, George RB. Incorrect use of metered dose inhalers by medical personnel. *Chest*. 1992;101:31–33.

50. De Blaquiere P, Christensen DB, Carter WB, Martin TR. Use and misuse of metered-dose inhalers by patients with chronic lung disease. A controlled, randomized trial of two instruction methods. *Am Rev Resp Dis*. 1989;140:910–916.

51. Usmani OS, Lavorini F, Marshall J, Dunlop WCN, Heron L, Farrington E, Dekhuijzen R. Critical inhaler errors in asthma and COPD: A systematic review of impact on health outcomes. *Resp Res*. 2018;19(1):10.

52. Allen SC. Competence thresholds for the use of inhalers in people with dementia. *Age Ageing*. 1997;26:83–86.

53. Larsen JS, Hahn M, Ekholm B, Wick KA. Evaluation of conventional press-and-breathe metered-dose inhaler technique in 501 patients. *J Asthma*. 1994;31:193–199.

54. Hampson NB, Mueller MP. Reduction in patient timing errors using a breath-activated metered dose inhaler. *Chest*. 1994;106:462–465.

55. Newman SP. Spacer devices for metered dose inhalers. *Clin Pharmacokinet*. 2004;43:349–360.

56. Terzano C. Metered dose inhalers and spacer devices. *Eur Rev Med Pharmacol Sci*. 1999;3:159–169.

57. Hickey AJ, Mansour HM, Telko MJ, Xu Z, Smyth HD, Mulder T, McLean R et al. Physical characterization of component particles included in dry powder inhalers. II. Dynamic characteristics. *J Pharm Sci*. 2007;96(5):1302–1319.

58. Assi K, Chrystyn H. The device resistance of recently introduced dry-powder inhalers. *J Pharm Pharmacol*. 2000;52:58.

59. Lavorini F, Pistolesi M, Usmani OS. Recent advances in capsule-based dry powder inhaler technology. *Multidiscip Respir Med*. 2017;12:11.

60. Chodosh S, Flanders JS, Kesten S, Serby CW, Hochrainer D, Witek TJ Jr. Effective delivery of particles with the HandiHaler dry powder inhalation system over a range of chronic obstructive pulmonary disease severity. *J Aerosol Med*. 2001;14:309–315.

61. Hawksworth GM, James L, Chrystyn H. Characterization of the inspiratory manoeuvre when asthmatics inhale through a Turbohaler pre- and post-counselling in a community pharmacy. *Respir Med*. 2000;94:501–504.

62. Janson C, Lööf T, Telg G, Stratelis G, Nilsson F. Difference in resistance to humidity between commonly used dry powder inhalers: An in vitro study. *NPJ Prim Care Respir Med*. 2016;26:16053.

63. Chan HK, Chew NY. Novel alternative methods for the delivery of drugs for the treatment of asthma. *Adv Drug Deliv Rev*. 2003;55:793–805.

64. Corradi M, Chrystyn H, Cosio BG, Pirozynski M, Loukides S, Louis R, Spinola M, Usmani OS. NEXThaler, an innovative dry powder inhaler delivering an extrafine fixed combination of beclometasone and formoterol to treat large and small airways in asthma. *Expert Opin Drug Deliv*. 2014;11(9):1497–1506.

65. Zierenberg B. Optimizing the in vitro performance of Respimat. *J Aerosol Med*. 1999;12:S19–S24.

66. Brand P, Hederer B, Austen G, Dewberry H, Meyer T. Higher lung deposition with Respimat Soft Mist inhaler than HFA-MDI in COPD patients with poor technique. *Int J Chron Obstruct Pulmon Dis*. 2008;3(4):763–770.

67. Kendrick AH, Smith EC, Wilson RS. Selecting and using nebuliser equipment. *Thorax*. 1997;52:S92–S101.

68. Muers MF. Overview of nebuliser treatment. *Thorax*. 1997;52:S25–S30.

69. Loffert DT, Ikle D, Nelson HS. A comparison of commercial jet nebulizers. *Chest*. 1994;106:1788–1792.

70. Boyd R, Stuart P. Pressurised metered dose inhalers with spacers versus nebulisers for beta-agonist delivery in acute asthma in children in the emergency department. *Emerg Med J*. 2005;22(9):641–642.

71. Geller DE. New liquid aerosol generation devices: Systems that force pressurized liquids through nozzles. *Resp Care*. 2002;47:1392–1404.

72. Smaldone GC. Smart nebulizers. *Resp Care*. 2002;47:1434–1441.

10

Drug delivery in pulmonary aspergillosis

SAWITTREE SAHAKIJPIJARN, JAY I. PETERS, AND ROBERT O. WILLIAMS, III

Introduction	167	Preclinical study	173
Pulmonary aspergillosis	167	Clinical study	173
Pathogen	167	Itraconazole	174
Classification	168	Nebulized formulations	174
Aspergilloma	168	Dry powder inhaled formulation	176
Allergic bronchopulmonary aspergillosis	168	Preclinical study	176
Chronic necrotizing aspergillosis	169	Voriconazole	177
Invasive pulmonary aspergillosis	170	Nebulized formulations	177
Therapeutic treatment	171	Dry powder inhaled formulations	177
Delivery of inhaled antifungal agents	172	Preclinical study	178
Amphotericin B	172	Caspofungin	179
Aerosolized formulations	172	Conclusion	179
Dry powder inhaled formulations	172	References	179
Aerosol delivery devices	173		

INTRODUCTION

Pulmonary aspergillosis is a serious pulmonary infection associated with significant morbidity and mortality in immunocompromised patients. Invasive pulmonary aspergillosis produces severe symptoms, including pleuritic chest pain, hemoptysis, thrombosis or infraction of surrounding tissue, and pulmonary or cerebral hemorrhage (1). The global death rate from this type of infection is reported to be over 50% (2), despite the availability of antifungal drugs such as voriconazole (V-Fend®), available since 2002, or posaconazole (Noxafil®), which has been available since 2007 (3). This high mortality rate results mainly from factors such as the severity of comorbidities, difficulty of diagnosis, and the limitations of the drugs currently available.

Most of the antifungal drugs in the pharmaceutical market have been commercialized as oral dosage forms. This leads to some challenges, including drug–drug interactions, low oral bioavailability, high liver metabolism, and low oral bioavailability that increases the variability of systemic drug concentrations (4). For this reason, pulmonary delivery of antifungal drugs to treat or prevent these severe pulmonary infections is a promising option because these drugs can be delivered to the site of action with minimal systemic exposure. This chapter summarizes the pulmonary drug delivery systems currently available for the treatment of pulmonary aspergillosis.

PULMONARY ASPERGILLOSIS

Pathogen

Aspergillus spp. are commonly found in the outdoor environment, including soil, dust, compost, foods, and plant debris (1). They are also found in indoor environments, including hospitals (1,5). Among the large number of *Aspergillus* species, four species are the major cause of Aspergillosis diseases: *A. fumigatus* (65%–75%), *A. flavus* (5%–10%), *A. terreus* (2%–3%), and *A. niger* (1.5%–3%) (6). *Aspergillus* spores, which are in the respirable size (1.9–6.0 µm), can be inhaled and deposited deep in the lung (7,8). Although all individuals inhale several hundred airborne *Aspergillus* spores each day (6), this deep intrusion can be eliminated through the mucociliary escalator, alveolar macrophages, and the immune system (6,8–10). In contrast, immunocompromised patients, or patients who have bronchial diseases, cannot effectively eliminate *Aspergillus* spores (11). Consequently, in these individuals, *Aspergillus* spores can germinate into hyphae-inducing pulmonary aspergillosis (12).

Classification

The degree of immunosuppression of the host is associated with the clinical symptoms and the prognosis of aspergillosis infections (13). The clinical syndromes tend to develop based on the relationship between the pathogen and the host's immune dysfunction or immune hyperactivity (Figure 10.1) (13). In terms of pulmonary aspergillosis, there are four primary spectra of clinical syndromes: (1) *aspergilloma*, (2) *chronic necrotizing aspergillosis* (CNA) or *chronic pulmonary aspergillosis* (CPA), (3) *invasive aspergillosis* (IA), and (4) *allergic bronchopulmonary aspergillosis* (ABPA) (12). CPA is commonly found in patients who have underlying lung diseases, while IA mainly occurs in immunocompromised patients, such as hematopoietic stem cell transplant recipients, solid organ transplant recipients, patients who are undergoing chemotherapy (resulting in neutropenia), or patients who are taking corticosteroids (13).

ASPERGILLOMA

Aspergilloma is the most common form of aspergillosis infection and also one of the noninvasive forms of *Aspergillus* lung disease (1). In cases of aspergilloma, a *fungus ball* is described as a chronic, extensive colonization of *Aspergillus* in a pulmonary cavity and rarely in an area of cystic bronchiectasis. A fungus ball is composed of inflammatory cells, fibrin, mucus, tissue debris, and fungal hyphae (13). The fungus ball generally develops in cavities affected by preexisting cavitary lung diseases such as tuberculosis, sarcoidosis, bronchiectasis, bronchial cysts and bulla, ankylosing spondylitis, neoplasm, or pulmonary infection (14,15). Inadequate drainage leads to the growth of *Aspergillus* on the wall of these cavities, which in turn causes the movement of the fungus ball within the cavity (15). This movement does not invade the surrounding lung parenchyma or blood vessels (15–17). However, local invasion may occur in rare cases, and this leads to invasive pulmonary aspergillosis or a subacute, chronic necrotizing aspergillosis (6,14).

In many patients, aspergilloma is asymptomatic for years. However, when symptoms present, hemoptysis is the most frequent, accounting for 70%–90% (18). Hemoptysis is generally mild, but severe hemoptysis sometimes occurs, especially in patients who have underlying tuberculosis (14,19).

Aspergilloma is diagnosed by radiography. A computerized tomography (CT) scan of an aspergilloma presents as an ovoid or round opacity within the lung cavity and a thickening of localized pleura (20). A solid, round, or oval mass is separated from the wall of the cavity by a crescent of air. This is called an *air crescent sign* or *monod sign* (Figure 10.2) (21,22). In addition, this change of intracavitary mass from images taken in different positions determines the mobility of the mass within the cavity (22). This solid mass within the lung cavity changes lung physiology, causing poor drug penetration into the mycetomal cavities. Consequently, systemic antifungal drugs are not effective enough for the treatment of the disease (22,23). Definitive surgical therapy is often not possible secondary to severe underlying lung disease, and bronchial embolization may be required to treat significant hemoptysis (24,25). However, alternative therapies are currently needed for this disorder (25).

ALLERGIC BRONCHOPULMONARY ASPERGILLOSIS

ABPA is a noninvasive form of aspergillosis that occurs after *Aspergillus* spores are deposited and grow on the bronchial mucosa (6). ABPA is a hypersensitivity reaction in the lung to the *Aspergillus* antigen, most often due to *A. fumigatus* in particular (12). The pathogenesis of ABPA is sometimes associated with *Aspergillus*-specific IgE-mediated type I hypersensitivity reactions, specific IgG-mediated type III

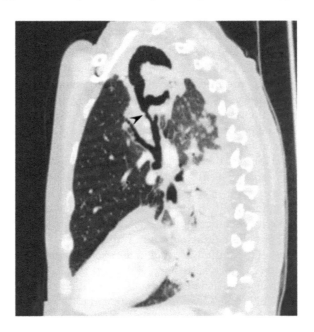

Figure 10.2 Sagittal CT image of a patient with aspergilloma, demonstrating solitary left upper lobe aspergilloma, left lower lobe consolidation, and broncho-cavity communication (black arrowhead). (Reprinted with permission from Tunnicliffe, G., *Respir. Med.*, 107, 1113–1123, 2013.)

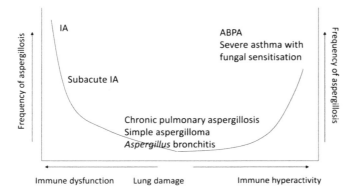

Figure 10.1 Relationship between the pathogen and severity of pulmonary aspergillosis. (Reprinted with permission from Kosmidis, C. and Denning, D.W., *Thorax.*, 70, 270–277, 2015.)

hypersensitivity reactions, and abnormal T-lymphocyte cellular immune responses (15). The allergic inflammatory response results in eosinophilic infiltration, which causes tissue lesion and damage to the bronchial wall (6).

ABPA is commonly found in patients who have chronic asthma or cystic fibrosis and who have concomitant atopy. However, the incidence of ABPA in these patients is not high (1,6). Only 2% of patients with asthma and only 2%–15% of patients with cystic fibrosis develop ABPA (26,27). Almost all patients with ABPA have clinical symptoms of asthma, including episodic wheezing, expectoration of sputum, brown plugs, pleuritic chest pain, and fever (15). ABPA has five stages: (1) acute, (2) remission, (3) exacerbation, (4) steroid-dependent asthma, and (5) fibrosis. During the first stage, the recommended treatment is corticosteroid therapy, which leads to a period of asymptomatic remission. By the fifth stage, however, the patient shows symptoms of pulmonary fibrosis, which leads to the reduction of pulmonary function (14,28).

There are multiple radiological features of ABPA in chest CT scans. First, central airway dilation with thickened walls are usually seen as rings or linear opacities in the upper and central regions of the lung (29). Other signs of endobronchial impaction include transient bronchocentric opacities, lobar collapse, and small peripheral lung nodules (29). The "hyperdense bronchial mucous plugging sign" is also present in some cases (Figure 10.3). This finding is felt to be pathognomonic for ABPA (30).

CHRONIC NECROTIZING ASPERGILLOSIS

CNA is called a *semi-invasive* or *subacute invasive* aspergillosis (6). CNA is a destructive infectious process in the parenchyma of the lung. This process originates from the local invasion of *Aspergillus* species (6,29). Unlike invasive aspergillosis, CNA gives rise to slow, progressive symptoms with no vascular invasion and no subsequent dissemination to other organs (6,12). CNA is commonly found in middle-aged and elderly patients who have altered local pulmonary defense mechanisms (31). It has been reported in patients who have pulmonary resection or pulmonary radiation treatment (29). It is also found in patients who have chronic lung diseases such as chronic obstructive pulmonary disease (COPD), bronchiectasis, pneumoconiosis, cystic fibrosis, lung infarction, lung sarcoidosis, or previous pulmonary tuberculosis (32). CNA also occurs in patients who have had thoracic surgery (6,12,32). In addition, CNA is found in immunocompromised patients such as individuals with diabetes mellitus, alcoholism, chronic liver disease, low-dose corticosteroid therapy, malnutrition, or connective tissue diseases such as rheumatoid arthritis and ankylosing spondylitis (12). It is a form of subacute or chronic pneumonia, often suspected when patients fail to respond to antibiotics, and usually requires bronchoscopy for definitive diagnosis.

The symptoms of CNA include weight loss, malaise, fatigue, sweats, anorexia, and fever. Patients may also experience chronic coughing, breathlessness, chest discomfort, and sometimes mild to severe hemoptysis (12,13).

Imaging studies (e.g., chest x-rays, chest CT scans) show that infiltration is commonly present in the upper lobes. Also, as the disease progresses, imaging shows consolidation, adjacent pleural thickening, and cavitary lesions in the upper lung lobes that progress over time (13) (Figure 10.4). The adjacent pleural thickening may develop to form a bronchopleural fistula, which is an early indication of a locally invasive process (33,34).

Figures 10.5 and 10.6 show the radiological evolution, which is a slow process. If CNA is not treated, pulmonary fibrosis develops over time and may expand to the entire lung (13).

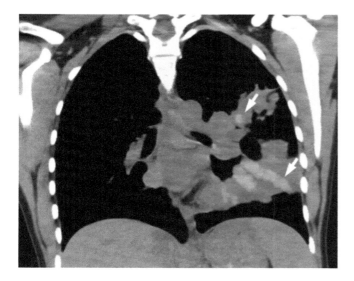

Figure 10.3 Coronal CT image of a patient with allergic bronchopulmonary aspergillosis showing the hyperdense bronchial mucous plugging sign and high attenuation mucoid impaction in the abnormally dilated bronchi (white arrows). (Reprinted with permission from Tunnicliffe, G., *Respir. Med.*, 107, 1113–1123, 2013.)

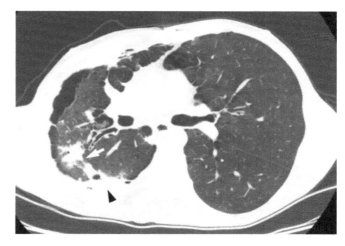

Figure 10.4 Axial CT image of a patient with chronic pulmonary necrotizing aspergillosis demonstrating consolidative opacities, areas of cystic change, and pleural thickening (black arrowhead). (Reprinted with permission from Tunnicliffe, G., *Respir. Med.*, 107, 1113–1123, 2013.)

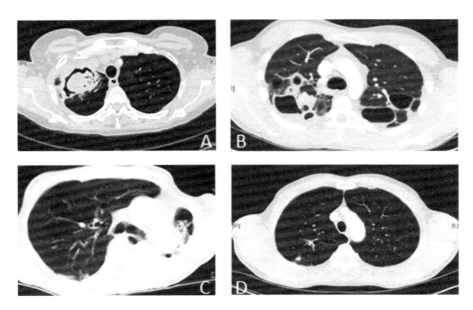

Figure 10.5 CT scan showing different forms of chronic pulmonary aspergillosis: Simple aspergilloma (A), chronic cavitary pulmonary aspergillosis (B), chronic fibrosing pulmonary aspergillosis (C), and an *Aspergillus* nodule (D). (Reprinted with permission from Kosmidis, C. and Denning, D.W., *Thorax.*, 70, 270–277, 2015.)

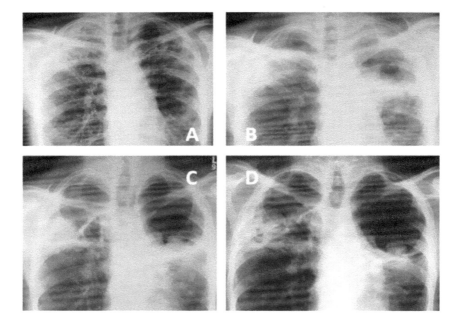

Figure 10.6 Serial chest x-rays of a patient with chronic cavitary pulmonary aspergillosis, demonstrating the disease progression in January 2001 (A), February 2002 (B), April 2003 (C), and July 2003 (D). (Reprinted with permission from Kosmidis, C. and Denning, D.W., *Thorax.*, 70, 270–277, 2015.)

INVASIVE PULMONARY ASPERGILLOSIS

Invasive pulmonary aspergillosis (IPA) is a common and serious manifestation of pulmonary aspergillosis. IPA is a potentially lethal infection that mainly affects immunocompromised patients such as transplant recipients (bone marrow and lung); patients with hematological malignancies, prolonged neutropenia, AIDS, or chronic granulomatous disease; and patients who are undergoing chronic corticosteroid treatment or cytotoxic therapy (1,35,36). In addition to diseases of compromised immunity, IPA is found in patients with critical illnesses, patients with COPD, patients who are undergoing anti-tumor necrosis factor (anti-TNF) therapy, and patients who have had cardiothoracic and vascular surgeries (6,12,15).

When *Aspergillus* spores are inhaled into the lower respiratory tract, the primary defense mechanism against *Aspergillus* conidia is the recognition of the cell wall of the pathogen by the receptors in the lung and the subsequent production of cytokines that stimulate neutrophil recruitment (37). The symptoms of IPA are similar to bronchopneumonia (38). The main symptoms include cough, sputum production, dyspnea, and fever that is unresponsive to antibiotics. Some patients may also have pleuritic chest pain, pneumothorax, and hemoptysis (12,14,38). In addition, patients with IPA may present similar to a pulmonary embolism with sudden chest pain and breathing difficulty (22).

In the initial stage, a plain chest radiograph shows diffuse nodular pulmonary infiltrates and other pulmonary lesions such as pleural-based, wedge-shaped densities and cavities (39). A common finding in chest radiography is pulmonary macronodules that are surrounded by a halo of ground-glass capacity and perilesional hemorrhage associated with alveolar invasion (Figure 10.7) (22,29).

Therapeutic treatment

Only three groups of antifungal drugs are useful in the treatment of *Aspergillus*, including polyenes, azoles, and echinocandins (15). According to the Infectious Disease Society of America (IDSA), guidelines for the diagnosis and management of aspergillosis, voriconazole is the primary treatment for invasive pulmonary aspergillosis and chronic necrotizing aspergillosis (15,40). Alternative therapies of these indications (e.g., itraconazole, posaconazole, caspofungin, micafungin) are used in combination with the primary treatment to avoid drug resistance (40).

The current recommended therapies on the market are mostly developed as oral dosage forms (e.g., voriconazole, itraconazole, posaconazole) or parenteral administration

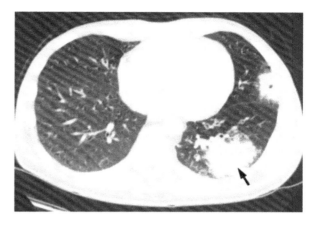

Figure 10.7 Axial CT image of a patient with invasive pulmonary aspergillosis demonstrating a large subpleural "target lesion" in the left lower lobe (arrow) and a smaller nodule in the lingual. (Reprinted with permission from Tunnicliffe, G., *Respir. Med.*, 107, 1113–1123, 2013.)

(e.g., voriconazole, itraconazole, amphotericin B, caspofungin, micafungin) (4). However, the high risk of treatment failure is felt to be related to low oral bioavailability, high liver metabolism, the hepatic first-pass effect, and low blood flow to the target area due to the angio-invasive hyphae of the fungus (41).

Since the fungal infection occurs in the lower respiratory tract, the treatment of pulmonary aspergillosis is more challenging. Drug concentration of oral and parenteral formulations are often increased to achieve plasma concentration and thus maintain the therapeutic level of concentration at the pulmonary sites of infection; however, higher plasma concentration leads to serious toxicity. To address this difficulty, more attention has been given to adjunctive pulmonary drug delivery of antifungal drugs for the treatment of pulmonary aspergillosis (4) (Table 10.1).

Table 10.1 Antifungal agents for the treatment of pulmonary aspergillosis

Drug groups	Drug name	Dosage form	Route
Polyene	Amphotericin B	Injectable, liposome Injectable, lipid complex	Intravenous (Infusion)
Triazole	Itraconazole	Capsule, tablet, solution, suspension	Oral
	Voriconazole	Suspension, tablet	Oral
		Injectable, powder	Intravenous (Infusion)
	Posaconazole	Suspension, Delayed release tablet	Oral
		Injectable, solution	Intravenous
	Isavuconazole	Capsule	Oral
		Injectable, powder	Intravenous
Echinocandins	Micafungin	Injectable, powder	Intravenous (Infusion)
	Caspofungin	Injectable, powder	Intravenous (Infusion)
	Anidulafungin	Injectable, powder	Intravenous (Infusion)

Source: Hope, W.W. et al., *Curr. Opin. Infect Dis.*, 21, 580–586, 2008; Drew, R.H., *Med. Mycol.*, 47, S355–S361, 2009.

DELIVERY OF INHALED ANTIFUNGAL AGENTS

Amphotericin B

Amphotericin B (AMB) is a systemic antifungal agent that has a broad spectrum of applications against various yeasts, molds, and dimorphic fungi, including *Aspergillus* species (3). It has been administered through many routes, including oral, endobronchial, intrathecal, intra-articular, intraperitoneal, and ophthalmic routes (43). AMB became the drug of choice for the treatment of many fungal diseases in the late 1950s due to its broad spectrum of application and administration and also because of its availability for parenteral preparations (44). AMB is considered a concentration-dependent drug in which the increase of drug concentration is associated with pharmacodynamics and fungicidal activity (45). However, poor systemic distribution to the lung leads to a higher dose requirement, which increases the risk of adverse drug effects (46–48). Therefore, the pulmonary delivery of AMB has been developed to improve drug concentration in the lung and reduce the required dose.

AEROSOLIZED FORMULATIONS

Pulmonary application of injectable formulations

Intravenous formulations of AMB have been used for pulmonary delivery. The low solubility and the aggregation of drug molecules in aqueous solutions are minimized by forming a complex with deoxycholate; however, amphotericin B deoxycholate (AMBd) is still highly aggregated and causes severe nephrotoxicity and other dose-limiting adverse effects (49). Other formulations of AMB were developed to avoid toxicity by forming lipid-carrier systems such as submicronic colloidal systems, liposomes, and lipid complexes (49–51). Although the toxicity of AMBd has been reported, pulmonary administration allows lower required doses in aerosolized formulations. Intravenous formulations of AMB have been reformed as aerosolized formulations for the treatment of pulmonary aspergillosis. These aerosolized formulations currently include AMBd, liposomal amphotericin B (L-AMB), amphotericin B lipid complex (ABLC), and amphotericin B colloidal dispersion (ABCD). Several studies have reported the ability of intravenous formulations to generate aerosols for pulmonary delivery utilizing different types of nebulizers (52–54).

Macrophage targeting system

An important strategy to develop inhaled AMB is to improve the penetration of the drug into the macrophage. If the drug targets the macrophages, the interaction between the free drug and nontarget tissues can be minimized. Subsequently, the required dose of liposomal AMB for the treatment of aspergillosis can be lowered (55,56). AMB has been encapsulated in liposomes with surfaces modified by anchoring alveolar macrophage-specific ligands (e.g., O-palmitoyl mannan [OPM], O-palmitoyl pullulan [OPP]). Aerosolized liposomes prepared in chlorofluorocarbon aerosol propellants can reach the peripheral regions of the lung. The ligand-anchored liposomal aerosols exhibit rapid delivery to the lung with a high population of alveolar macrophages, and these aerosols maintained a high drug concentration in the lungs for up to 24 h (57).

Micellar delivery system

Polymeric micelles have been used as vehicles for the delivery of AMB, since the amphiphilic structure of the micelle improves drug solubility and lessens the aggregation of AMB (58–60). Gilani et al. introduced chitosan-based micelles as a carrier for the pulmonary delivery of AMB. Depolymerized chitosan-stearic acid (DC-SA) micelles significantly enhanced drug solubility. These aerosols demonstrated optimal aerodynamic properties. Polymeric nanomicelles were stable during nebulization using air-jet nebulizers and during characterization using a twin-impinger apparatus. The fine particle fraction ranged from 40%–52%, and the nebulization efficacy was up to 56% (61).

Nanoparticle delivery system

Nanoparticles made from functional polymers using synthetic chemistry have been applied for pulmonary delivery. Anionic hydrogels based on polymethacrylic acid have the mucoadhesive property to sustain the drug in the respiratory tract more than 8 h (62). Shirkhani et al. introduced AMB-polymethacrylic acid nanoparticles that are not toxic to the lung epithelium and monocyte-derived macrophages in both healthy mouse lungs and in lungs infected with *Aspergillus*. They found that AMB-polymethacrylic acid nanoparticles could be effectively delivered to the lung using an AeroEclipse II nebulizer, and this prevented both fungal growth and lung inflammation (63).

DRY POWDER INHALED FORMULATIONS

A liposomal dry powder inhaler (DPI) was developed to control drug release at the localized site. Multilamellar vesicles of AMB were prepared by reverse phase evaporation using an organic solvent and water. The ratio of the aqueous phase to organic phases was optimized to produce liposomes with a high percentage of drug entrapment. The drug was mixed with hydrogenated soy phosphatidylcholine, cholesterol, and either saturated soy phosphatidylglycerol or stearylamine in an ethanol-ethyl acetate solvent system to prepare negatively (AMB1) and positively charged liposomes (AMB2), respectively. The formed liposomal dispersion was extruded through a 2 µm polycarbonate membrane above the phase transition temperature to produce liposomes that have a mean particle size less than 5 µm. The AMB liposomes were mixed with sucrose in a mass lipid:sucrose ratio of 1:5 followed by lyophilization. Lactose was used as a carrier to prepare the liposomal DPI formulation. Lyophilized AMB powder was blended with lactose in a liposome:carrier ratio of 1:6. The fine particle fractions of AMB1 and AMB2 were 22.6% ± 2.2% and 16.8% ± 2.2%, respectively. It was reported that small multilamellar AMB liposomes were stable for over one year under refrigerated storage conditions (2°C–8°C). The formulation of AMB in the anhydrous state would be an attractive formulation for the treatment of pulmonary aspergillosis. Preclinical and clinical studies will be evaluated (64).

AEROSOL DELIVERY DEVICES

Several studies have evaluated the performance of various nebulizers in generating AMB aerosols for pulmonary delivery (52–54). Ultrasonic nebulizers (Fisoneb® or DP100®) and jet nebulizers (Respirgard II®) were compared in order to study drug deposition and pharmacokinetics in patients with pulmonary mycetoma. The Fisoneb nebulizer showed the greatest concentration of inhaled drug in the inspiratory filter (26.5% and 28.3%) with a mass median aerodynamic diameter MMAD 4.82 μm ± 0.78 μm. The Fisoneb nebulizer delivered AMB more efficiently to the central airways, the lung periphery, and the mycetoma lung regions. No unfavorable effects were found in patients during the 4-week trial. This study concluded that the AMB suspension can be effectively nebulized by a variety of nebulizers and is well tolerated by human subjects (52).

Corcoran et al. compared the aerosol size and output rates of 12 types of nebulizer delivery systems to select the optimal nebulizer delivery system for lipid complex AMB (Abelcet; ABLC). Corcocan et al. showed that the AeroEclipse® Nebulizer with a DeVilbiss® 8650D compressor provided the highest pulmonary dose (5.7 mg) and highest pulmonary delivery rate (0.23 mg/min). This delivery system was used to deliver ABLC (35 mg) and to measure the aerosol deposition in lung transplant recipients. It was found that, with this system, the drug was well distributed in the lungs; however, due to inadequate ventilation, the drug was delivered suboptimally to the native lung of single-lung transplant recipients. This study indicated that the detailed clinical research and development of aerosol drug delivery techniques was necessary for special populations (53).

Recently, Lambros et al. compared the performance of three commercial jet nebulizer systems (Pulmo-Aide/Micromist, Envoy/Sidestream, and Proneb/Pari LC Star) in the production of ABLC aerosols at two concentrations, 5 mg/mL and 10 mg/mL. They found that the higher ABLC concentration increased the nebulizer output rate. Pulmo-Aide/Micromist and Envoy/Sidestream exhibited high output rates. The different nebulizers exhibited different particle size distributions, leading to various deposition sites in the airways. The aerosols prepared by Proneb/Pari LC star and Envoy/Sidestream had a droplet size of 1.0–3.5 μm, while aerosols prepared by Pulmo-Aide/Micromist had a droplet size 3.5–6.0 μm (54).

This study raised some concerns about the optimal nebulizers for the delivery of the drug to the infection site of pulmonary aspergillosis (54). Moreover, the nebulizer delivery system was developed for certain populations. An appropriate delivery system of aerosolized liposomal AMB for children using a breath-actuated nebulizer (AeroEclipse by Trudell Medical International, Canada) was developed without any changes to the liposome after nebulization. By using a breath-actuated nebulizer, drug loss can be minimized, and liposomal AMB aerosols can maintain a respirable size range without disruption of the liposomes (65).

PRECLINICAL STUDY

The efficacy of pulmonary administration of AMB was compared to the intravenous route. By using a murine model of pulmonary aspergillosis, the efficacy of nebulized AMBd and liposomal AMB was compared to conventional intravenous formulations. It was found that both nebulized formulations reached a satisfactory concentration in the lungs, and this concentration was higher than conventional intravenous formulations (66). The concentration of AMB from the liposomal AMB formulation was 46.7 μg/g ± 10.5 μg/g in the lung tissue, which was much higher than the minimum inhibitory concentration (MIC) for *Aspergillus fumigatus* (0.4–0.8 mg/L). On the other hand, the concentration of AMB after intravenous administration was only 16.4 μg/g ± 2.4 μg/g (67).

In a subsequent study, four commercial AMB formulations, including AMB deoxycholate (AMBd), liposomal AMB (L-AMB), AMB lipid complex (ABLC), and AMB colloidal dispersion (ABCD), were evaluated in rats with granulocytopenia who had invasive pulmonary aspergillosis. All the aerosols of the four nebulized formulations had optimal respirable size. The AMB concentration of aerosols in the lungs was higher than the minimum inhibitory concentration of *Aspergillus fumigatus*. All four formulations significantly prolonged survival of the rats; however, only L-AMB showed prolonged antifungal activity after treatment given at 6 weeks before inoculation. Although all four commercial formulations were nebulized efficiently in rats, with optimal aerosol particle sizes and lung deposition, the lipid formulation is safer because AMBd has a detrimental effect due to deoxycholate on the surfactant function of the respiratory tract (68). Therefore, the aerosolization of AMB is a useful approach to control the drug in the lung and improve the efficacy of the treatment of invasive aspergillosis (66–68).

CLINICAL STUDY

The efficacy of aerosolized AMB for the prophylaxis and treatment of pulmonary aspergillosis was studied in many groups of patients, especially in patients who have undergone lung transplantation or have hematologic malignancies. The safety and efficacy of nebulized liposomal AMBd in the prevention of aspergillus infections in lung transplant patients has been studied (69–71). A prospective, nonrandomized, uncontrolled study reported that patients who received 120 mg of nebulized AMBd for 120 d after transplantation had a significantly reduced risk of developing aspergillosis (69).

The efficacy of other formulations, including nebulized liposomal AMB, has been studied in terms of their prophylaxis against pulmonary aspergillosis (72,73). Only 8 of

104 lung transplant patients (7.7%) developed *Aspergillus* infections after they received nebulized liposomal AMB prophylaxis (73). AMB achieved sufficient concentrations in the lung for 14 d. The administration of nebulized liposomal AMB every 2 weeks is a promising regimen for prophylaxis against aspergillosis (72). Perfect et al. reported that the aerosols of a lipid formulation of AMB were safer and better tolerated in lung transplant recipients compared to AMBd (74). The efficacy of aerosolized liposomal AMB for the prevention of IPA was also studied in patients who received chemotherapy with expected duration of neutropenia for greater than 10 days. In the intent-to-treat population, the incidence of IPA was significantly lower in patients receiving the aerosolized liposomal AMB compared with placebo (odds ratio 0.26%, 95% confidence interval [CI] 0.09–0.72). Although aerosolized liposomal AMB significantly reduced the incidence of IPA in patients with chemotherapy-induced neutropenia from 14% to 4%, the reduction in IPA-related mortality was not significant (75).

Moreover, ABLC has been evaluated in a few clinical studies. Aerosolized ABLC was tolerated in 50 of 51 patients (98%) who had received heart–lung transplants (76). The efficacy of aerosolized ABLC for the prevention of aspergillosis was evaluated in lung transplant patients. After lung transplantation, patients received aerosolized ABLC once every 2 days for 2 weeks and then once per week for at least 13 weeks. Only 1 of 60 lung transplant recipients (2%) who received aerosolized ABLC developed invasive fungal infections during the 6-month follow-up period. Additionally, aerosolized ABLC was safe and well tolerated for the prophylaxis of aspergillosis in lung transplant patients during 6 months of study. Only four patients (6.4%) reported nausea and vomiting, and no significant bronchospasm was reported (77). The efficacy of aerosolized AMBd and ABLC for the prevention of fungal infections was studied in lung recipient transplants. No significant difference in disease progression between the two formulations was reported within 2 months (70). Moreover, aerosolized AMBd and ABLC were also evaluated in terms of their ABPA treatment efficacy in seven patients who had cystic fibrosis with recurrent ABPA and a failure to taper systemic corticosteroid. Successful therapy was reported in six of seven patients; these six patients were able to discontinue their steroid use without relapsing after several years of recurrent ABPA episodes (78).

Studies have reported the efficacy of aerosolized AMB formulations in the prophylaxis of pulmonary aspergillosis (69–75). The mortality rate and incidence of IPA were analyzed from six animal studies and two clinical trials involving 768 high-risk patients. The meta-analysis showed the lower mortality rate in animals receiving aerosolized AMB compared with placebo (odds ratio 0.13, 95% CI 0.08–0.21). In addition, the incidence of IPA was lower in patients who receive aerosolized AMB compared with placebo. The systemic review and meta-analysis proved that the aerosolized AMB was effective for the prophylaxis of IPA (79). However, clinical trials which involve large sample sizes

are still needed to confirm the drug efficacy (79). Moreover, the IDSA does not recommend the routine use of nebulized AMB due to insufficient clinical evidence (40,51).

Itraconazole

Itraconazole (ITZ) is a triazole antifungal agent that is classified as a Biopharmaceutical Classification System (BCS) class II drug. Itraconazole was developed to broaden the range of antifungal activity against *Aspergillus* spp. (80). Although many ITZ products are available in the market, oral formulations of ITZ have many limitations. Since ITZ has poor and pH-dependent solubility, it exhibits poor and variable absorption characteristics that lead to low bioavailability (81). Undissolved ITZ particles are rapidly eliminated by the mucocilliary escalator and macrophage phagocytosis (82). Low concentrations of ITZ in the lung limit its pharmacological action, causing therapeutic failure. Another limitation is drug–drug interaction. Itraconazole is highly bonded to plasma protein and metabolized mainly by the hepatic cytochrome P450 3A4. Due to its properties as a CYP 450 and CYP 3A4 inhibitor, ITZ can strongly interact with other drugs metabolized by these enzymes (e.g., warfarin, rifampin, tacrolimus) (83). Furthermore, oral ITZ formulations cause many adverse effects, such as nausea and vomiting (24%), hepatotoxicity (8.5%), and skin rash (5%–19%) (81). And systemic therapy with ITZ may not be an optimal choice for pulmonary infections because of insufficient drug diffusion into the pulmonary lumen and tissues (84). Pulmonary delivery is a promising approach to compensate for poor diffusion and to achieve effective concentration in the lungs (84,85). To develop inhaled ITZ, many techniques have been used to improve drug solubility, such as complexation, particle size reduction, solid dispersion, and the formation of nanostructured lipid-based carriers and polymeric micelles.

NEBULIZED FORMULATIONS
Solid dispersion system

Solid dispersion has been applied to improve ITZ solubility in water. Nebulized ITZ was developed as nanoparticles by using particle-engineering technologies. Itraconazole was dissolved in an organic solvent with the combination of polysorbate 20 (AIP-1) or polysorbate 80 and poloxamer 407 (AIP-2 and CIP). The evaporative precipitation into aqueous solution (EPAS) technology was used to prepare the crystalline ITZ powder (CIP), while the spray freezing into liquid (SFL) technology generated the amorphous ITZ powder (AIP-1 and AIP-2). The addition of poloxamer 407 and polysorbate 80 improved the dissolution of both amorphous and crystalline ITZ. The ITZ nanostructured particles were dispersed in an aqueous solution and then delivered to the lung using a nebulizer. The AIP-2 and CIP formulations showed a similar concentration (C_{max}) in the mouse lung after nebulization. After a single nebulization, both AIPs and CIP demonstrated a drug concentration higher than

0.5 µg/g for at least 24 h. However, the AIP-1 formulation exhibited a shorter half-life and a higher elimination rate due to its lower dissolution rate and more rapid clearance by the mucocilliary escalator. Furthermore, the aqueous droplets of the formulation showed optimal aerodynamic properties of 2.76–2.82 µm MMAD and 71%–85% FPF. Therefore, this study suggests that particle engineering is an effective method for the development of poorly water-soluble drugs for inhalation (85).

Surfactants increase drug solubility and bioavailability, but they may also interfere with cell lipid bilayer membranes, leading to long-term safety issues (86). Yang et al. developed a nebulized ITZ formulation without adding any synthetic polymers or surfactants. In their formulations, they used mannitol and lecithin, which are biodegradable materials and acceptable excipients for inhaled products (87). They used the ultra-spray freezing (USF) process to prepare nanostructured aggregates of ITZ:mannitol:lecithin (1:0.5:2, w/w). Using the ultra-rapid freezing (URF) process, a solid dispersion or solution that contained a mixture of the drug and polymer was rapidly frozen after it was sprayed directly into liquid nitrogen (88). The aerosol of a colloidal dispersion of ITZ exhibited optimal aerodynamic characteristics, with a mean diameter of 230 nm, a large surface area of 71 m²/g, and a wettable surface. Thermal analysis and XRD patterns showed the absence of crystallinity in the drug, which indicates that ITZ is fully miscible with the excipients and is molecularly dispersed in a solid solution. A solid solution increases the exposure area of the drug to the dissolution media, which significantly improves dissolution and bioavailability. It was shown that the ITZ nanoparticles dissolved rapidly in the simulated lung fluid and reached a supersaturation level that was 27 times higher than the crystalline solubility. *In vivo* single-dose 24-hour pharmacokinetics reported substantial lung deposition and systemic absorption that achieved 1.6 g/mL in serum in 2 h (89). Compared to the SFL-ITZ formulation in Vaughn's study, the URF-ITZ formulation exhibited a faster absorption rate, a shorter T_{max}, a C_{max} twice as high in the lung tissue, and a C_{max} 10 times as high in the blood (89,90). In addition, bioavailability increased due to the addition of lecithin, which functions as a permeability enhancer (89).

Yang et al. further evaluated the impact of the *in vitro* solubility advantage of amorphous versus crystalline ITZ nanoparticles on *in vivo* bioavailability after nebulization. Amorphous nanostructured aggregates of ITZ were prepared by URF, while the nanocrystalline ITZ, which contained the same composition, was prepared by wet milling. The *in vivo* bioavailability of the nebulized amorphous ITZ nanoparticles was compared to the nebulized nanocrystalline ITZ. The authors found that the extent of supersaturation in the stimulated lung fluid of the URF-ITZ colloidal dispersion was 4.7 times greater than the wet-milled ITZ colloidal dispersion, due to an increase in the surface area for dissolution obtained by solid dispersion. Although both aqueous colloidal dispersions have comparable aerodynamic performance, the area under the plasma drug concentration-time curve (AUC) of URF-ITZ was 3.8 times greater than that of wet-milled ITZ due to an increase of supersaturation in the simulated lung fluid. Furthermore, the high supersaturation and the rapid dissolution of amorphous nanoparticles minimized the crystallization of undissolved particles of URF-ITZ in the lung fluid, which could reduce the clearance of ITZ by the lung defense system. This study confirmed that the lung administration of amorphous ITZ nanoparticles has potential advantages for both local and systemic therapy (91).

ß-cyclodextrin complexation

An aqueous ITZ solution was developed by forming an inclusion complex with 2-hydroxypropyl-cyclodextrin (HPβCD-ITZ) without other excipients. The aerodynamic properties and *in vitro* pharmacokinetics of the aerosols of an HPβCD-ITZ solution and a URF-ITZ colloidal dispersion were compared in mice using an Aeroneb® micropump nebulizer. It was found that aerosols of both formulations exhibited optimal aerodynamic properties and similar ITZ lung deposition. The nebulized HPβCD-ITZ solution exhibited a similar C_{max}, a lower elimination rate, and a higher lung AUC_{0-24h} compared to the nebulized URF-ITZ colloidal dispersion. Since the URF-ITZ nanoparticle colloidal dispersion required the elimination of the phase-to-phase transition, solubilized ITZ exhibited a faster systemic absorption across the lung epithelium. However, URF-ITZ colloidal dispersion showed a faster absorption rate in the serum compared to the HPβCD-ITZ solution because of the permeation properties of lecithin in the formulation (92).

Nano-size reduction

Size reduction is another strategy to improve drug solubility. A nebulized ITZ nanosuspension was prepared by a wet-milling process that used milling beads. By adding a surfactant (e.g., polysorbate 80), the particle size of the nanosuspension was reduced to as low as 180–200 nm. The ITZ nanosuspension was stable without particle growth for up to 3 months at 8°C. The ITZ nanosuspension was compatible with vibrating mesh (Pari eFlow®) and pressurized air nebulizers (Pari LC Plus® and MedelJet Basic®). A single-dose inhalation resulted in a very high and long-lasting exposure of the lung tissue with minimal systemic exposure. The total lung concentration was 21.4 µg/g, and the clearance half-life in the tissue was 25.4 h. The tissue concentration remained at 14.3 µg/g after 24 h, which was 28 times higher than the MIC of *Aspergillus fumigatus* of 0.5 µg/mL. This study concludes that ITZ nanosuspension is an attractive inhaled formulation (93).

Lipid nanoparticle delivery system

Lipid nanoparticles provide several advantages, such as low toxicity, the ability to incorporate both lipophilic and hydrophilic drugs, and the ability to control drug release (94–96). In the case of pulmonary delivery, the small size of the lipid nanoparticles increases the lung deposition; in addition, the particles' bioadhesive properties also prolong the residence time in the lung (97). Recently, Pardeike et al. introduced an itraconazole-loaded nanostructured lipid carrier (NLC) formulation that could be administered by nebulization. The particle matrix of NLC was prepared by mixing solid lipid Precrol ATO 5 with liquid lipid oleic acid in a ratio of 9:1, while polysorbate 20 was selected as a stabilizer for the system due to its high wettability. It was found that the lipid carriers could entrap the drug up to 98.78%. The ITZ-loaded NLC exhibited good long-term stability without particle aggregation due to the electrostatic repulsion between particles and the steric hindrance of the surfactant. During nebulization using a jet stream and an ultrasonic nebulizer, the ITZ-loaded NLC was stable, with no significant change in particle sizes (98). The drug deposition of loaded NLC was further evaluated in falcons. The particle size of ITZ-loaded NLC did not change after nebulization. Gamma scintigraphic images revealed that the fine aerosol droplet of ITZ-loaded NLC reached the two main areas of infection (i.e., the lung and caudal air sacs), which indicates the successful pulmonary delivery of ITZ for the treatment of aspergillosis in falcons (99). NLC is a promising carrier system to deliver ITZ in the deep lung (98,99).

Micellar delivery system

Polymeric micelles have been used as an alternative carrier system for the delivery of poorly soluble drugs. Moazeni et al. studied the potential of chitosan-based polymeric micelles, which were used as a nanocarrier system for the pulmonary delivery of ITZ. Through the conjugation of stearic acid and hydrophilic depolymerized chitosan, the modified polymer form micelles in the nanosize range (120–200 nm). The polymeric micelles entrapped ITZ up to 43.2 µg/mL ± 2.27 µg/mL, which is 1000 times greater than ITZ solubility. The shear force that was induced by the air jet nebulizer (Hudson®, UK) did not affect the stability of ITZ polymeric micelles. The fine particle fraction was 38%–47%. An in vitro nebulization study revealed that 49% of the drug was released from the outer surface of the polymeric micelles in the first 12 h, and the remaining drug was gradually released within 60 h. This study concluded that the stearic acid–grafted, chitosan-based polymeric micelles can be used as nanocarriers to deliver ITZ to the lung by nebulization (100).

DRY POWDER INHALED FORMULATION

Solid dispersion system

More recently, Duret et al. developed a dry powder inhaled formulation of ITZ. The solubility of ITZ was increased by reducing the size to the nanometer scale using the amorphous state and improving wettability utilizing a surfactant. A solid dispersion containing amorphous ITZ, mannitol, and d-alpha tocopherol polyethylene glycol 1000 succinate (TPGS) was prepared using spray drying with hydroalcoholic solutions. The dry powder of the solid dispersion containing amorphous ITZ and mannitol exhibited optimal aerosol properties and a higher dissolution rate compared to bulk ITZ. The addition of a surfactant (TGPS) to the formulation improved drug dissolution, but it also dramatically decreased the fine particle fraction, thus decreasing the aerosol performance (101).

In the subsequent study, hydrogenated soy lecithin was selected for the ITZ-based solid dispersions instead of TPGS. This study found that the increase in the dissolution rate corresponded to the increase in the phospholipid concentration because the amphiphilic structure of the phospholipid improved the wettability of the hydrophobic ITZ in aqueous media. The best formulation, containing 10% phospholipid (by weight of ITZ), exhibited the fastest dissolution profile and an optimal aerosol performance. The formulation resulted in an emitted dose of 81.9% and a fine particle fraction of 46.9%–67.0%. Furthermore, the phospholipid did not affect the aerodynamic performance of the formulation. Hence, this study demonstrated an alternative DPI formulation that contains acceptable inhalation excipients for the treatment of invasive pulmonary aspergillosis (102).

Nanoparticle delivery system

The development of nanoparticles for inhalation has been limited due to the high aggregation of nanoparticles. Particle engineering techniques such as spray drying have been applied to prepare a stable formulation of micronized dry powder containing ITZ nanoparticles. The chitosan-based nanoparticle containing chitosan and tripolyphosphate in a ratio of 1:3 was prepared by a modified ionic gelation method. The complex of ITZ–HPβCD was encapsulated into the chitosan-based nanoparticles. The nanoparticles showed optimal respirable sizes that ranged from 190–240 nm. The nanoparticles were co–spray dried with lactose and mannitol to produce inhalable microparticles. The addition of mannitol and leucine during co–spray drying significantly improved the aerosolization properties of the drug (103).

Aghdam et al. introduced ITZ-loaded nanotransfersomal DPI formulations. They found that the nanotransfersomal formulation containing lecithin and span in a ratio of 90:10 exhibited a narrow size distribution and an optimal respirable particle size (171 nm MMAD). In addition, co–spray dried formulations containing mannitol and tranfersomes in the ratio of 2:1 exhibited the best aerosolization efficiency (37% FPF). This study concludes that the nanotranfersome, which is a novel biocompatible vesicular system, can be used in DPI formulations for pulmonary delivery (104).

PRECLINICAL STUDY

The efficacy of the aerosolized nanostructured ITZ in the prevention of invasive pulmonary aspergillosis has been reported (105,106). The in vivo efficacy of the aerosolized nanostructured ITZ formulations (AIP-2 and CIP) was compared to the Sporanox oral liquid (Janssen) using a murine model of invasive pulmonary aspergillosis. Each formulation was administered to mice for 12 days. This administration began one day before spore inoculation with *Aspergillus flavus*. It was shown that the SFL (AIP-2) and EPAS (CIP) formulations resulted in higher median survival than Sporanox oral liquid and the control groups. Moreover, the SFL formulation showed the longest median survival: up to 20 days, which was due to higher lung exposure and lower lung elimination compared to CIP and Sporanox (107).

Alvarez et al. assessed the efficacy of the aerosolized SFL formulation in the prevention of invasive pulmonary aspergillosis due to *Aspergillus fumigatus*. The aerosolized SFL formulation exhibited a longer survival time (7.5 days) and a higher survival rate (35%) compared to the mice that received Sporanox oral liquid (5 days, 0%) or the controls (6.5 days, 10%). This result is consistent with Hoebon's study, which indicates that the amorphous nanostructured ITZ allows for a greater survival rate against *Aspergillus flavus*. Although no statistically significant reduction in pulmonary fungal burden was observed in any formulations, a higher lung colony forming unit (CFU) was found in the control animals. The histopathology revealed that the number of necrotic foci and vascular lesions were reduced in the mice that received aerosolized nanostructured ITZ (106). These two studies confirm that the aerosols of amorphous nanostructured ITZ may effectively limit the disease progression of pulmonary aspergillosis (105,106).

Additionally, the systemic exposure and toxicity of the novel nanostructured ITZ formulation was evaluated (90,107). The oral and pulmonary administrations of amorphous nanoparticulate ITZ and the Sporanox oral solution (Janssen) were compared in terms of the lung and serum concentrations in mice. This study found that the pulmonary-dosed amorphous ITZ nanoparticles showed a greater lung tissue concentration and a higher lung level per unit serum concentration compared to the orally dosed ITZ compositions. No significant difference was found between these two oral formulations. The pulmonary application of the amorphous nanoparticulate ITZ could sustain a high concentration in lung tissue, while the serum levels remained above the minimum lethal concentration (MLC) of *Aspergillus fumigatus* over 24 h (90).

The safety of an amorphous nanostructured ITZ dispersion was also evaluated in mice after nebulization every 12 hours for 12 days. The results of the lung histology, immunogenic potential, and cellular uptake revealed that the airway remained clear, with no evidence of epithelial ulceration or inflammation in the bronchia, peribronchia, or perivascular tissue. No IL-12 was found in any groups, which indicates that no cytokine induction occurred in the lung. Hence, the inhalation of amorphous ITZ or the excipients does not cause immunogenic inflammation or changes in pulmonary histology (107).

As for dry powder inhaled formulations, three itraconazole DPI formulations in a mannitol solution were prepared using spray drying. One formulation contained crystalline ITZ (F1), one contained amorphous ITZ with a phospholipid (F2), and the third contained amorphous ITZ with no phospholipid (F3). The pharmacokinetic profiles of these three

formulations were compared in mice. The solubility of amorphous ITZ-based solid dispersion (F2 and F3) reached the supersaturation point in the lung fluid, which enhanced the systemic bioavailability and increased the absorption rate into the systemic compartment compared to micronized crystalline ITZ. The plasmatic $AUC_{0-24\,h}$ of F1, F2, and F3 were 182.0, 491.5, and 376.8 ng h/mL, respectively. The T_{max} of F1, F2, and F3 were 60, 30, and 5 min, respectively (108).

This pharmacokinetic study revealed that the amorphous ITZ-based solid dispersion formulations extended pulmonary retention and maintained the drug concentration in the lung at a higher concentration than the MIC for *Aspergillus fumigatus* (2 g/g lung) after endotracheal administration for 24 hours. However, the addition of phospholipid increased the dissolution rate and elimination rate of ITZ from the lung. The faster absorption rate and the greater extent of drug absorption may lead to a rapid elimination from the lung and side effects related to peak concentration in plasma (108).

Voriconazole

Voriconazole (VCZ) has been developed to increase potency and a broader spectrum of antifungal activity (109). VCZ has been reported as causing a successful outcome in 52.8% of patients, which is higher than the success rate of patients who received AMBd (110). However, the limitations of the systemic administration of VCZ include high interpatient and intrapatient pharmacokinetic variability, potential drug interactions, and a narrow therapeutic range with adverse effects such as neurological toxicity and hepatotoxicity (111–113). To overcome the limitations of oral or intravenous delivery, targeted lung delivery of VCZ has been developed to increase the drug concentration at the site of infection and reduce the dose required for therapy.

NEBULIZED FORMULATIONS

The commercial VCZ injection (Vfend®) has been used for pulmonary delivery. In the injectable formulation, drug solubility was improved by forming the inclusion complex with sulfobutyl ether-ß-cyclodextrin. The commercial VCZ injection (Vfend) was evaluated in terms of its ability to generate an aerosol using an Aeroneb Pro micro pump nebulizer. The aerosolized aqueous VCZ solution was isotonic. The aerosol exhibited an optimal mass median aerodynamic diameter of 2.98 mm and a fine particle fraction of 71.7%. This study concluded that the commercial VCZ injection can be applied for pulmonary delivery (114).

DRY POWDER INHALED FORMULATIONS

Particle engineering has been applied to develop inhaled formulations of poorly soluble drugs because they provide several advantages for pulmonary delivery (115). For example, nanoparticles and large porous particles can improve the fine particle fraction and lung deposition (116). Recently, dry powder compositions of crystalline and amorphous VCZ were prepared using thin film freezing (TFF). This thin film–frozen VCZ (TFF-VCZ) formulation with no stabilizing agent formed a microstructured crystalline morphology, while a TFF-VCZ-PVP K25 (1:3) formulation formed nanostructured amorphous VCZ. A Handihaler® DPI device was selected to aerosolize the low-density aggregate particles of both TFF formulations. Both TFF-processed powders exhibited low densities and high surface areas. However, the microstructured crystalline TFF-VCZ showed better aerodynamic properties. The aerodynamic diameters of microstructured crystalline and nanostructured amorphous VCZ were 4.2 μm and 5.2 μm, respectively. The fine particle fractions of microstructured crystalline and nanostructured amorphous VCZ were 37.8% and 32.4%, respectively (117).

To prolong residency time in the lung, Sinha et al. introduced a sustained-release formulation of VCZ. The poly(lactic-co-glycolic) acid (PLGA) nanoparticles containing VCZ were prepared using a multiple-emulsification technique and freeze drying. The effervescent mixture of citric acid and sodium bicarbonate was added to the emulsion during the multiple-emulsification process. The resulting effervescent salts released carbon dioxide to produce porous VCZ nanoparticles. Compared to nonporous particles, the porous particles exhibited a lower mass median aerodynamic diameter (MMAD) and a higher initial drug deposition (approximately 120 μg/g of tissue). The drug was released from the porous particles at a higher concentration than the nonporous particles due to the larger diffusion surface of the porous structure. The drug release study revealed that 20% of the drug was released from the nanoparticles within 2 hours, and this was followed by a sustained release over 15 days (118).

The drug was sustained in the lung after administration for up to 5 days for the nonporous nanoparticles and up to 7 days for the porous nanoparticles. Although the nanoparticles exhibited a low entrapment efficiency of 8%–60%, the biodegradable PLGA nanoparticles could sustain the drug level in the lung over a longer period of time (118). Das et al. further investigated the effect of PLGA on drug release in the lung by radiolabeling and gamma scintigraphy. The VCZ-loaded PLGA nanoparticles containing 3% w/w of VCZ were prepared by multiple emulsion solvent evaporation. It was found that the radiolabeled particles accumulated in the lung at a higher rate compared to the free drug. The free drug was excreted at a higher rate than the nanoparticles. This study confirms that the VCZ-encapsulated PLGA nanoparticles via pulmonary delivery is a better delivery system to sustain a high concentration of VCZ in the deep lung, which is expected to provide a greater antifungal effect (119).

To improve entrapment efficiency, Arora et al. developed a controlled-release VCZ dry powder formulation that was prepared using a one-step processing technique. Spray drying was used to prepare VCZ (pure drug) and VCZ-loaded polyactide microparticles (VLM). VCZ was entrapped in the nanoparticles with up to 98.56% ± 3.75% efficiency. Due to the amorphous form and the spherical morphology of the VLM powder, VLM exhibited smaller MMAD (3.68 μm ± 0.05 μm) and higher FPF (43.56% ± 0.13%) compared to spray-dried VCZ. However, both formulations can be delivered to the middle and lower regions of the lungs. The drug release profiles revealed that the polyactide microparticles sustained the drug release up to 2 days. Therefore, the sustained-release DPI formulation of VCZ prepared using spray drying is an alternative option for the treatment of pulmonary aspergillosis (120).

The use of biodegradable polymers in inhaled formulations is still questionable, despite the fact that a few studies have reported the potential of inhaled VCZ-loaded PLGA nanoparticles for the treatment of pulmonary aspergillosis. Arora et al. developed leucine-modified VCZ microparticles that were prepared using spray drying. The spray-dried powder containing 80% w/w VCZ and 20% w/w leucine exhibited an optimal particle size and aerodynamic properties. The spray-dried dry powder was chemically stable after three months of storage both under room conditions (25°C, 60% RH) and under accelerated conditions (40°C, 75% RH). The formulation was safe for pulmonary epithelial tissue, and leucine did not affect the transport kinetics of VCZ. This VCZ formulation was effectively delivered and maintained in the lung for 8 h at a higher concentration than the MIC for Aspergillus (121).

PRECLINICAL STUDY

The pharmacokinetics of the commercial VCZ injection (Vfend) after nebulization was evaluated in mice. High concentrations of VCZ were detected in the lung tissue and plasma for 30 minutes after nebulization. However, after one single dose, the VCZ concentration in the lung was low to undetectable after 6–8 hours, while VCZ was detectable in the plasma for up to 24 hours after nebulization. After a single dose, the maximum concentrations were 11.0 ± 1.6 μg/g of wet lung weight and 7.9 ± 0.68 μg/mL of plasma. After multiple doses, the peak concentration in lung tissue was 6.73 ± 3.64 μg/g wet lung weight, and the peak concentration in plasma was 2.32 ± 1.52 μg/mL. Although pulmonary delivery of VCZ exhibited low lung deposition, high concentrations in the lung tissue and plasma could be beneficial for the treatment of invasive pulmonary aspergillosis (122).

Tolman et al. evaluated the efficacy of inhaled VCZ in the prevention of invasive pulmonary aspergillosis caused by *Aspergillus fumigatus* in a murine model. It was found that pulmonary application of commercial intravenous VCZ (Vfend) exhibited a higher survival in mice and a lesser extent of invasive disease. The survival of mice that received aerosolized VCZ (92%) was significantly higher than the control group (25%, p <0.05) and higher than those treated with AMB (31%, p <0.05). In addition, the mice in the aerosolized VCZ prophylaxis group showed a longer median survival time (>12 days) than the mice that received the control application (7.5 days) or amphotericin B (7 days). Mice that received either the control or AMB developed a more severe invasive disease that exhibited abnormalities in the lung such as epithelial disruption, congestion, necrosis, angioinvasion, and vascular lesions in the small airways.

These lung injuries and inflammatory changes were not found in mice that received aerosolized VCZ. This study also suggested that aerosolized VCZ is a promising strategy for the prevention and treatment of IPA (114).

As for dry powder inhalation, Beinborn et al. evaluated the single-dose 24-hour pharmacokinetics of both an amorphous VCZ formulation and a crystalline VCZ formulation in mice. They reported that the microstructured crystalline TFF-VRC remained in the lung longer compared to the nanostructured amorphous TFF-VRC-PVP K25. This is because the faster dissolution of the nanostructured amorphous formulation leads to a more rapid partition of the drug into the plasma, a shorter retention, and a lower exposure in the lung tissue. This study concludes that inhalation of microstructured crystalline VRC could be an attractive formulation for the treatment of invasive pulmonary aspergillosis (117).

Caspofungin

Caspofungin, an antifungal drug in echinocandins, has been approved as an alternative treatment for aspergillosis, especially in patients who fail to benefit from AMB or itraconazole (123–125). In the past, the efficacy of aerosolized caspofungin was investigated in a rat model of pulmonary aspergillosis. It was shown that aerosolized caspofungin was effective in delaying mortality from invasive pulmonary aspergillosis in rats (126). Caspofungin has been considered a promising drug for aerosol administration due to its broad spectrum of applications against *Aspergillus* spp. and its low toxicity compared to other available drugs (123,124). Beringer et al. evaluated the suitability of caspofungin for pulmonary delivery via nebulization. The commercial caspofungin (Cancidas®, Merck), which was developed as a lyophilized powder, was reconstituted with 0.9% NaCl to produce a 10 mg/mL solution and a 30 mg/mL solution. Although the caspofungin solutions were acidic (pH <6.3), the addition of 0.3 N NaOH can adjust the pH of the reconstituted solution to neutral, which is in the physiological pH range. The osmolality of caspofungin solutions is in the tolerable range for inhalation. In addition, the viscosity of the solutions was similar to water and was not dependent on the drug concentration. Therefore, the drug solutions achieved optimal physicochemical properties for airway tolerability (127).

Beringer et al. also evaluated the ability of the drug solutions to generate aerosols that target the lung using three commercial jet nebulizer systems: Micromist (Hudson RCI, Temecula, CA), Sidestream MS 2400 (Invacare, Elyria, OH), and Pari LC Star (Pari Respiratory Equipment, Midlothian, VA). They found that the drug output rate increased as the drug concentration increased. The Proneb Ultra/Pari-LC star system showed the highest respirable fraction for both high and low concentrations (93% versus 83%) compared to the other two nebulizers. Furthermore, they compared the efficacy of the three jet nebulizer systems by considering the least drug waste and the shortest time required to deliver the target dose. They demonstrated that the Pulmo-Aide/Micromist system was the most efficient disposable nebulizer system because only 59 mg of caspofungin was required for nebulization over 15 minutes in a 10 mg/mL concentration. In contrast, the Proneb Ultra/Pari-LC star system was the most efficient reusable nebulizer system because only 54 mg of caspofungin was required for nebulization over 5 minutes in a 30 mg/mL concentration to achieve the target dose. This study confirmed that nebulization is a promising method for the delivery of caspofungin to the lung (127).

CONCLUSION

The development of inhaled antifungal agents remains a promising strategy for the prevention and treatment of pulmonary aspergillosis infections. Inhaled AMB has been proven effective against *Aspergillus*; however, the long-term use of aerosolized AMB requires further study. Triazole antifungal agents (e.g., itraconazole, voriconazole) have been developed using several techniques as both nebulized formulations and dry powder inhalation formulations, but more preclinical and clinical studies are needed to confirm their efficacy and safety in pulmonary applications.

REFERENCES

1. Soubani AO, Chandrasekar PH. The clinical spectrum of pulmonary aspergillosis. *Chest*. 2002;121(6):1988–1999. Epub 2002/06/18. PubMed PMID: 12065367.
2. Lin SJ, Schranz J, Teutsch SM. Aspergillosis case-fatality rate: Systematic review of the literature. *Clin Infect Dis*. 2001;32(3):358–366. Epub 2001/02/15. doi:10.1086/318483. PubMed PMID: 11170942.
3. Desoubeaux G, Bailly E, Chandenier J. Diagnosis of invasive pulmonary aspergillosis: Updates and recommendations. *Med Mal Infect*. 2014;44(3):89–101. doi:10.1016/j.medmal.2013.11.006. PubMed PMID: 24548415.
4. Merlos R, Amighi K, Wauthoz N. Recent developments in inhaled triazoles against invasive pulmonary aspergillosis. *Curr Fungal Infect Rep*. 2014;8(4):331–342. doi:10.1007/s12281-014-0199-5.
5. Lehrnbecher T, Frank C, Engels K, Kriener S, Groll AH, Schwabe D. Trends in the postmortem epidemiology of invasive fungal infections at a university hospital. *J Infect*. 2010;61(3):259–265. doi:10.1016/j.jinf.2010.06.018. PubMed PMID: 20624423.
6. Díaz Sánchez C, López Viña A. Pulmonary aspergillosis. *Archivos de Bronconeumología* (English Edition). 2004;40(3):114–122. doi:10.1016/S1579-2129(06)70076-3.
7. Pasqualotto AC. Differences in pathogenicity and clinical syndromes due to *aspergillus fumigatus* and *aspergillus flavus*. *Med Mycol*. 2009;47(1):261–270. Epub 2008/07/26. doi:10.1080/13693780802247702. PubMed PMID: 18654921.

8. Morris G, Kokki MH, Anderson K, Richardson MD. Sampling of aspergillus spores in air. *J Hosp Infect.* 2000;44(2):81–92. Epub 2000/02/09. doi:10.1053/jhin.1999.0688. PubMed PMID: 10662557.

9. Hasenberg M, Behnsen J, Krappmann S, Brakhage A, Gunzer M. Phagocyte responses towards Aspergillus fumigatus. *Int J Med Microbiol.* 2011;301(5):436–444. Epub 2011/05/17. doi:10.1016/j.ijmm.2011.04.012. PubMed PMID: 21571589.

10. Dagenais TR, Keller NP. Pathogenesis of *Aspergillus fumigatus* in invasive aspergillosis. *Clin Microbiol Rev.* 2009;22(3):447–465. Epub 2009/07/15. doi:10.1128/cmr.00055-08. PubMed PMID: 19597008; PMCID: PMC2708386.

11. Thompson GR, TF P. Pulmonary aspergillosis: Recent advances. *Semin Respir Crit Care Med.* 2011;32(6):673–681. doi:10.1055/s-0031-1295715. PubMed PMID: 22167395.

12. Kousha M, Tadi R, Soubani AO. Pulmonary aspergillosis: A clinical review. *Eur Respir Rev.* 2011;20(121):156–174. doi:10.1183/09059180.00001011. PubMed PMID: 21881144.

13. Kosmidis C, Denning DW. The clinical spectrum of pulmonary aspergillosis. *Thorax.* 2015;70(3):270–277. Epub 2014/10/31. doi:10.1136/thoraxjnl-2014-206291. PubMed PMID: 25354514.

14. Patterson TF. Aspergillosis. In *Essential of Clinical Mycology.* 2nd ed., 2011. pp. 243–263. New York: Springer.

15. Zmeili OS, Soubani AO. Pulmonary aspergillosis: A clinical update. *QJM.* 2007;100(6):317–334. doi:10.1093/qjmed/hcm035. PubMed PMID: 17525130.

16. Tomee J, Mannes GM, van der Bij W et al. Serodiagnosis and monitoring of *aspergillus* infections after lung transplantation. *Ann Intern Med.* 1996;125(3):197–201. doi:10.7326/0003-4819-125-3-199608010-00006.

17. Rafferty P, Biggs BA, Crompton GK, Grant IW. What happens to patients with pulmonary aspergilloma? Analysis of 23 cases. *Thorax* 1983;38(8):579–583. PubMed PMID: PMC459614.

18. Sharma OP, Chwogule R. Many faces of pulmonary aspergillosis. *Eur Respir J.* 1998;12(3):705–715. PubMed PMID: 9762804.

19. Amchentsev A, Kurugundla N, Saleh AG. Aspergillus-related lung disease. *Respir Med CME.* 2008;1(3):205–215. doi:10.1016/j.rmedc.2008.08.008.

20. Sansom HE, Baque-Juston M, Wells AU, Hansell DM. Lateral cavity wall thickening as an early radiographic sign of mycetoma formation. *Eur Radiol.* 2000;10(2):387–390. doi:10.1007/s003300050061. PubMed PMID: 10663774.

21. Sah SK, Li Y, Ganganah O, Shi X, Li Y. An update of clinical characteristics and imaging findings of pulmonary aspergillosis. *IJDI.* 2015;3(1). doi:10.5430/ijdi.v3n1p8.

22. Tunnicliffe G, Schomberg L, Walsh S, Tinwell B, Harrison T, Chua F. Airway and parenchymal manifestations of pulmonary aspergillosis. *Respir Med.* 2013;107(8):1113–1123. doi:10.1016/j.rmed.2013.03.016. PubMed PMID: 23702091.

23. Glimp RA, Bayer AS. Pulmonary aspergilloma: Diagnostic and therapeutic considerations. *Arch Intern Med.* 1983;143(2):303–308. Epub 1983/02/01.

24. Khalil A, Fedida B, Parrot A, Haddad S, Fartoukh M, Carette MF. Severe hemoptysis: From diagnosis to embolization. *Diagn Interv Imaging.* 2015;96(7–8):775–788. doi:10.1016/j.diii.2015.06.007.

25. Regnard JF, Icard P, Nicolosi M, Spagiarri L, Magdeleinat P, Jauffret B, Levasseur P. Aspergilloma: A series of 89 surgical cases. *Ann Thorac Surg.* 2000;69(3):898–903. Epub 2000/04/06. PubMed PMID: 10750780.

26. Stevens DA, Moss RB, Kurup VP, Knutsen AP, Greenberger P, Judson MA, Denning DW et al., Participants in the Cystic Fibrosis Foundation Consensus C. Allergic bronchopulmonary aspergillosis in cystic fibrosis—State of the art: Cystic Fibrosis Foundation Consensus Conference. *Clin Infect Dis.* 2003;37 Suppl 3:S225–S264. doi:10.1086/376525. PubMed PMID: 12975753.

27. Patterson K, Strek ME. Allergic bronchopulmonary aspergillosis. *Proc Am Thorac Soc.* 2010;7(3):237–244. doi:10.1513/pats.200908-086AL. PubMed PMID: 20463254.

28. Agarwal R. Allergic bronchopulmonary aspergillosis. *Chest.* 2009;135(3):805–826. Epub 2009/03/07. doi:10.1378/chest.08-2586. PubMed PMID: 19265090.

29. Franquet T, Müller NL, Giménez A, Guembe P, Torre Jdl, Bagué S. Spectrum of pulmonary aspergillosis: Histologic, clinical, and radiologic findings. *RadioGraphics.* 2001;21(4):825–837. doi:10.1148/radiographics.21.4.g01jl03825. PubMed PMID: 11452056.

30. Molinari M, Ruiu A, Biondi M, Zompatori M. Hyperdense mucoid impaction in allergic bronchopulmonary aspergillosis: CT appearance. *Monaldi Arch Chest Dis.* 2004;61(1):62–64. PubMed PMID: 15366339.

31. Kaymaz D, Ergun P, Candemir I, Cicek T. Chronic necrotizing pulmonary aspergillosis presenting as transient migratory thoracic mass: A diagnostic dilemma. *Respir Med Case Rep.* 2016;19:140–142. Epub 2016/10/19. doi:10.1016/j.rmcr.2016.09.007. PubMed PMID: 27752463; PMCID: PMC5061306.

32. Grahame-Clarke CN, Roberts CM, Empey DW. Chronic necrotizing pulmonary aspergillosis and pulmonary phycomycosis in cystic fibrosis. *Respir Med.* 1994;88(6):465–468. Epub 1994/07/01. PubMed PMID: 7938799.

33. Cabral FC, Marchiori E, Zanetti G, Takayassu TC, Mano CM. Semi-invasive pulmonary aspergillosis in an immunosuppressed patient: A case report. *Cases J.* 2009;2(1):40. Epub 2009/01/14. doi:10.1186/ 1757-1626-2-40. PubMed PMID: 19138387; PMCID: PMC2633327.

34. Kim SY, Lee KS, Han J, Kim J, Kim TS, Choo SW, Kim SJ. Semi-invasive pulmonary aspergillosis. *AJR Am J Roentgenol.* 2000;174(3):795–798. doi:10.2214/ ajr.174.3.1740795.

35. Gerson SL, Talbot GH, Hurwitz S, Strom BL, Lusk EJ, Cassileth PA. Prolonged granulocytopenia: The major risk factor for invasive pulmonary aspergillosis in patients with acute leukemia. *Ann Intern Med.* 1984;100(3):345–351. Epub 1984/03/01. PubMed PMID: 6696356.

36. Segal BH, Walsh TJ. Current approaches to diagnosis and treatment of invasive aspergillosis. *Am J Respir Crit Care Med.* 2006;173(7):707–717. Epub 2006/01/03. doi:10.1164/rccm.200505-727SO. PubMed PMID: 16387806.

37. Schaffner A, Douglas H, Braude A. Selective protection against conidia by mononuclear and against mycelia by polymorphonuclear phagocytes in resistance to Aspergillus. Observations on these two lines of defense in vivo and in vitro with human and mouse phagocytes. *J Clin Invest.* 1982;69(3):617–631. Epub 1982/03/01. PubMed PMID: 7037853; PMCID: PMC371019.

38. Albelda SM, Talbot GH, Gerson SL, Miller WT, Cassileth PA. Pulmonary cavitation and massive hemoptysis in invasive pulmonary aspergillosis. *Am Rev Respir Dis.* 1985;131(1):115–120. doi:10.1164/ arrd.1985.131.1.115. PubMed PMID: 3966697.

39. Caillot D, Casasnovas O, Bernard A, Couaillier JF, Durand C, Cuisenier B, Solary E et al., Improved management of invasive pulmonary aspergillosis in neutropenic patients using early thoracic computed tomographic scan and surgery. *J Clin Oncol.* 1997;15(1):139–147. doi:10.1200/ JCO.1997.15.1.139. PubMed PMID: 8996135.

40. Patterson TF, Thompson III GR, Denning DW, Fishman JA, Hadley S, Herbrecht R, Kontoyiannis DP et al., Practice guidelines for the diagnosis and management of aspergillosis: 2016 Update by the infectious diseases society of america. *Clin Infect Dis.* 2016;63(4):1–60. doi:10.1093/cid/ciw326. PubMed PMID: 27365388; PMCID: PMC4967602.

41. Hope WW, Billaud EM, Lestner J, Denning DW. Therapeutic drug monitoring for triazoles. *Curr Opin Infect Dis.* 2008;21(6):580–586. Epub 2008/11/04. doi:10.1097/QCO.0b013e3283184611. PubMed PMID: 18978525.

42. Approved Drug Products with Therapeutic Equivalence Evaluations (Orange Book). Silver Spring, MD: Food and Drug Administration [cited 2017]. Available from https://www.fda.gov/drugs/ informationondrugs/ucm129662.htm.

43. Drew RH. Aerosol and other novel administrations for prevention and treatment of invasive aspergillosis. *Med Mycol.* 2009;47 Suppl 1:S355–S361. doi:10.1080/13693780802247710. PubMed PMID: 18654913.

44. Arthur RR, Drew RH, Perfect JR. Novel modes of antifungal drug administration. *Expert Opin Investig Drugs.* 2004;13(8):903–932. doi:10.1517/13543784.13.8.903. PubMed PMID: 15268632.

45. Lepak AJ, Andes DR. Antifungal pharmacokinetics and pharmacodynamics. *Cold Spring Harb Perspect Med.* 2014;5(5):a019653. doi:10.1101/cshperspect. a019653. PubMed PMID: 25384765; PMCID: PMC4448584.

46. Lewis RE, Liao G, Hou J, Chamilos G, Prince RA, Kontoyiannis DP. Comparative analysis of amphotericin B lipid complex and liposomal amphotericin B kinetics of lung accumulation and fungal clearance in a murine model of acute invasive pulmonary aspergillosis. *Antimicrob Agents Chemother.* 2007;51(4):1253–1258. doi:10.1128/AAC.01449-06. PubMed PMID: 17261624; PMCID: PMC1855500.

47. Olson JA, Adler-Moore JP, Schwartz J, Jensen GM, Proffitt RT. Comparative efficacies, toxicities, and tissue concentrations of amphotericin B lipid formulations in a murine pulmonary aspergillosis model. *Antimicrob Agents Chemother.* 2006;50(6):2122–2131. doi:10.1128/AAC.00315-06. PubMed PMID: 16723574; PMCID: PMC1479157.

48. Vogelsinger H, Weiler S, Djanani A, Kountchev J, Bellmann-Weiler R, Wiedermann CJ, Bellmann R. Amphotericin B tissue distribution in autopsy material after treatment with liposomal amphotericin B and amphotericin B colloidal dispersion. *J Antimicrob Chemother.* 2006;57(6):1153–1160. doi:10.1093/jac/dkl141. PubMed PMID: 16627591.

49. Torrado JJ, Espada R, Ballesteros MP, Torrado-Santiago S. Amphotericin B formulations and drug targeting. *J Pharm Sci.* 2008;97(7):2405–2425. doi:10.1002/jps.21179. PubMed PMID: 17893903.

50. Kuiper L, Ruijgrok EJ. A review on the clinical use of inhaled amphotericin B. *J Aerosol Med Pulm Drug Deliv.* 2009;22(3):213–227. doi:10.1089/ jamp.2008.0715. PubMed PMID: 19466905.

51. Le J, Schiller DS. Aerosolized delivery of antifungal agents. *Curr Fungal Infect Rep.* 2010;4(2):96–102. doi:10.1007/s12281-010-0011-0. PubMed PMID: 20502511; PMCID: PMC2868999.

52. Diot P, Rivoire B, Le Pape A, Lemarie E, Dire D, Furet Y, Breteau M, Smaldone GC. Deposition of amphotericin B aerosols in pulmonary aspergilloma. *Eur Respir J* 1995;8(8):1263–1268. doi:10.1183/09031936. 95.08081263.

53. Corcoran TE, Venkataramanan R, Mihelc KM, Marcinkowski AL, Ou J, McCook BM, Weber L et al., Aerosol deposition of lipid complex amphotericin-B (Abelcet) in lung transplant recipients. *Am J Transplant*. 2006;6(11):2765–2773. Epub 2006/10/20. doi:10.1111/j.1600-6143.2006.01529.x. PubMed PMID: 17049064.

54. Lambros MP, Beringer PM, Wong-Beringer A. Nebulizer choice affects the airway targeting of amphotericin B lipid complex aerosols. *J Pharm Technol*. 2013;29(5):199–204. doi:10.1177/8755122513500905.

55. De Marie S., Janknegt R., A. B-WI. Clinical use of liposomal and lipid-complexed amphotericin B. *J Antimicrob Chemother*. 1994;33(5):907–916. Epub 1994/05/01. PubMed PMID: 8089064.

56. Janknegt R, de Marie S, Bakker-Woudenberg IA, Crommelin DJ. Liposomal and lipid formulations of amphotericin B. *Clin Pharmacokinet*. 1992;23(4):279–291. doi:10.2165/00003088-199223040-00004.

57. Vyas SP, Quraishi S, Gupta S, Jaganathan KS. Aerosolized liposome-based delivery of amphotericin B to alveolar macrophages. *Int J Pharm*. 2005;296(1–2):12–25. doi:10.1016/j.ijpharm.2005.02.003. PubMed PMID: 15885451.

58. Croy SR, Kwon GS. Polymeric micelles for drug delivery. *Curr Pharm Des*. 2006;12(36):4669–4684. Epub 2006/12/16. PubMed PMID: 17168771.

59. Jones M, Leroux J. Polymeric micelles—A new generation of colloidal drug carriers. *Eur J Pharm Biopharm*. 1999;48(2):101–111. Epub 1999/09/02. PubMed PMID: 10469928.

60. Kwon GS. Polymeric micelles for delivery of poorly water-soluble compounds. *Crit Rev Ther Drug Carrier Syst*. 2003;20(5):357–403. Epub 2004/02/13. PubMed PMID: 14959789.

61. Gilani K, Moazeni E, Ramezanli T, Amini M, Fazeli MR, Jamalifar H. Development of respirable nano-micelle carriers for delivery of amphotericin B by jet nebulization. *J Pharm Sci*. 2011;100(1):252–259. Epub 2010/07/06. doi:10.1002/jps.22274. PubMed PMID: 20602350.

62. Bertelli M, Gallo S, Buda A, Cecchin S, Fabbri A, Lapucci C, Andrighetto G, Sidoti V, Lorusso L, Pandolfo M. Novel mutations in the arylsulfatase A gene in eight Italian families with metachromatic leukodystrophy. *J Clin Neurosci*. 13(4):443–448. doi:10.1016/j.jocn.2005.03.039.

63. Shirkhani K, Teo I, Armstrong-James D, Shaunak S. Nebulised amphotericin B-polymethacrylic acid nanoparticle prophylaxis prevents invasive aspergillosis. *Nanomedicine*. 2015;11(5):1217–1226. doi:10.1016/j.nano.2015.02.012.

64. Shah SP, Misra A. Development of liposomal amphotericin B dry powder inhaler formulation. *Drug Deliv*. 2004;11(4):247–253. Epub 2004/09/17. doi:10.1080/10717540490467375. PubMed PMID: 15371106.

65. Kamalaporn H, Leung K, Nagel M, Kittanakom S, Calvieri B, Reithmeier RA, Coates AL. Aerosolized liposomal Amphotericin B: A potential prophylaxis of invasive pulmonary aspergillosis in immunocompromised patients. *Pediatr Pulmonol*. 2014;49(6):574–580. doi:10.1002/ppul.22856. PubMed PMID: 23843366.

66. Gavalda J, Martin MT, Lopez P, Gomis X, Ramirez JL, Rodriguez D, Len O, Puigfel Y, Ruiz I, Pahissa A. Efficacy of nebulized liposomal amphotericin B in treatment of experimental pulmonary aspergillosis. *Antimicrob Agents Chemother*. 2005;49(7):3028–3030. doi:10.1128/AAC.49.7.3028-3030.2005. PubMed PMID: 15980392; PMCID: PMC1168712.

67. Ruijgrok EJ, Fens MH, Bakker-Woudenberg IA, van Etten EW, Vulto AG. Nebulized amphotericin B combined with intravenous amphotericin B in rats with severe invasive pulmonary aspergillosis. *Antimicrob Agents Chemother*. 2006;50(5):1852–1854. doi:10.1128/AAC.50.5.1852-1854.2006. PubMed PMID: 16641459; PMCID: PMC1472188.

68. Ruijgrok EJ, Fens MH, Bakker-Woudenberg IA, van Etten EW, Vulto AG. Nebulization of four commercially available amphotericin B formulations in persistently granulocytopenic rats with invasive pulmonary aspergillosis: Evidence for long-term biological activity. *J Pharm Pharmacol*. 2005;57(10):1289–1295. doi:10.1211/jpp.57.10.0007. PubMed PMID: 16259757.

69. Monforte Vc, Roman A, Gavalda J, Bravo C, Tenorio L, Ferrer A, Maestre J, Morell F. Nebulized amphotericin B prophylaxis for *Aspergillus* infection in lung transplantation: Study of risk factors. *J Heart Lung Transplant*. 2001;20(12):1274–1281. doi:10.1016/S1053-2498(01)00364-3.

70. Drew RH, Dodds Ashley E, Benjamin DK, Jr., Duane Davis R, Palmer SM, Perfect JR. Comparative safety of amphotericin B lipid complex and amphotericin B deoxycholate as aerosolized antifungal prophylaxis in lung-transplant recipients. *Transplantation*. 2004;77(2):232–237. Epub 2004/01/27. doi:10.1097/01.TP.0000101516.08327.A9. PubMed PMID: 14742987.

71. Lowry CM, Marty FM, Vargas SO, Lee JT, Fiumara K, Deykin A, Baden LR. Safety of aerosolized liposomal versus deoxycholate amphotericin B formulations for prevention of invasive fungal infections following lung transplantation: A retrospective study. *Transpl Infect Dis*. 2007;9(2):121–125. Epub 2007/04/28. doi:10.1111/j.1399-3062.2007.00209.x. PubMed PMID: 17461997.

72. Monforte V, Ussetti P, Lopez R, Gavalda J, Bravo C, de Pablo A, Pou L, Pahissa A, Morell F, Roman A. Nebulized liposomal amphotericin B prophylaxis for *Aspergillus* infection in lung transplantation: Pharmacokinetics and safety. *J Heart Lung Transplant.* 2009;28(2):170–175. Epub 2009/02/10. doi:10.1016/j.healun.2008.11.004. PubMed PMID: 19201343.

73. Monforte V, Ussetti P, Gavalda J, Bravo C, Laporta R, Len O, Garcia-Gallo CL, Tenorio L, Sole J, Roman A. Feasibility, tolerability, and outcomes of nebulized liposomal amphotericin B for *Aspergillus* infection prevention in lung transplantation. *J Heart Lung Transplant.* 2010;29(5):523–530. Epub 2010/01/12. doi:10.1016/j.healun.2009.11.603. PubMed PMID: 20061165.

74. Perfect JR, Ashley ED, Drew R. Design of aerosolized amphotericin B formulations for prophylaxis trials among lung transplant recipients. *Clin Infect Dis.* 2004;39(Supplement_4):S207–S210. doi:10.1086/421958.

75. Rijnders BJ, Cornelissen JJ, Slobbe L, Becker MJ, Doorduijn JK, Hop WC, Ruijgrok EJ et al., Aerosolized liposomal amphotericin B for the prevention of invasive pulmonary aspergillosis during prolonged neutropenia: A randomized, placebo-controlled trial. *Clin Infect Dis.* 2008;46(9):1401–1408. doi:10.1086/586739. PubMed PMID: 18419443.

76. Palmer SM, Drew RH, Whitehouse JD, Tapson VF, Duane Davis R, McConnell RR, Kanj SS, Perfect JR. Safety of aerosolized amphotericin B lipid complex in lung transplant recipients 12. *Transplantation.* 2001;72(3):545–548. PubMed PMID: 00007890-200108150-00036.

77. Borro JM, Solé A, de la Torre M, Pastor A, Fernandez R, Saura A, Delgado M, Monte E, Gonzalez D. Efficiency and safety of inhaled amphotericin B lipid complex (Abelcet) in the prophylaxis of invasive fungal infections following lung transplantation. *Transplant Proc.* 40(9):3090–3093. doi:10.1016/j.transproceed.2008.09.020.

78. Proesmans M, Vermeulen F, Vreys M, De Boeck K. Use of nebulized amphotericin B in the treatment of allergic bronchopulmonary aspergillosis in cystic fibrosis. *Int J Pediatr.* 2010;2010:376287. Epub 2011/01/15. doi:10.1155/2010/376287. PubMed PMID: 21234103; PMCID: PMC3014676.

79. Xia D, Sun WK, Tan MM, Zhang M, Ding Y, Liu ZC, Su X, Shi Y. Aerosolized amphotericin B as prophylaxis for invasive pulmonary aspergillosis: A meta-analysis. *Int J Infect Dis.* 2015;30:78–84. doi:10.1016/j.ijid.2014.11.004. PubMed PMID: 25461661.

80. Stewart E, Thompson G. Treatment of primary pulmonary aspergillosis: An assessment of the evidence. *J Fungi.* 2016;2(3):25. doi:10.3390/jof2030025.

81. Smith D, van de Velde V, Woestenborghs R, Gazzard BG. The pharmacokinetics of oral itraconazole in AIDS patients. *J Pharm Pharmacol.* 1992;44(7):618–619. Epub 1992/07/01. PubMed PMID: 1357148.

82. Williams HD, Trevaskis NL, Charman SA, Shanker RM, Charman WN, Pouton CW, Porter CJ. Strategies to address low drug solubility in discovery and development. *Pharmacol Rev.* 2013;65(1):315–499. Epub 2013/02/07. PubMed PMID: 23383426.

83. Domínguez-Gil Hurlé A, Sánchez Navarro A, García Sánchez MJ. Therapeutic drug monitoring of itraconazole and the relevance of pharmacokinetic interactions. *Clin Microbiol Infect.* 2006;12:97–106. doi:10.1111/j.1469-0691.2006.01611.x.

84. Li J, Rayner CR, Nation RL, Owen RJ, Spelman D, Tan KE, Liolios L. Heteroresistance to colistin in multidrug-resistant acinetobacter baumannii. *Antimicrob Agents Chemother.* 2006;50(9):2946–2950. Epub 2006/08/31. doi:10.1128/AAC.00103-06. PubMed PMID: 16940086; PMCID: PMC1563544.

85. McConville JT, Overhoff KA, Sinswat P, Vaughn JM, Frei BL, Burgess DS, Talbert RL, Peters JI, Johnston KP, Williams III RO. Targeted high lung concentrations of itraconazole using nebulized dispersions in a murine model. *Pharm Res.* 2006;23(5):901–911. doi:10.1007/s11095-006-9904-6. PubMed PMID: 16715380.

86. Patton JS, McCabe JG, Hansen SE, Daugherty AL. Absorption of human growth hormone from the rat lung. *Biotechnol Ther.* 1989;1(3):213–228. PubMed PMID: 2562650.

87. Bosquillon C LC, Preat V, Vanbever R. Influence of formulation excipients and physical characteristics of inhalation dry powders on their aerosolization performance. *J Control Release.* 2001;70(3):329–339.

88. Vaughn JM, Gao X, Yacaman MJ, Johnston KP, Williams III RO. Comparison of powder produced by evaporative precipitation into aqueous solution (EPAS) and spray freezing into liquid (SFL) technologies using novel Z-contrast STEM and complimentary techniques. *Eur J Pharm Biopharm.* 2005;60(1):81–89. doi:10.1016/j.ejpb.2005.01.002. PubMed PMID: 15848060.

89. Yang W, Tam J, Miller DA, Zhou J, McConville JT, Johnston KP, Williams III RO. High bioavailability from nebulized itraconazole nanoparticle dispersions with biocompatible stabilizers. *Int J Pharm.* 2008;361(1–2):177–188. doi:10.1016/j.ijpharm.2008.05.003. PubMed PMID: 18556158.

90. Vaughn JM, McConville JT, Burgess D, Peters JI, Johnston KP, Talbert RL, Williams III RO. Single dose and multiple dose studies of itraconazole nanoparticles. *Eur J Pharm Biopharm.* 2006;63(2):95–102. doi:10.1016/j.ejpb.2006.01.006. PubMed PMID: 16516450.

91. Yang W, Johnston KP, Williams III RO. Comparison of bio-availability of amorphous versus crystalline itraconazole nanoparticles via pulmonary administration in rats. *Eur J Pharm Biopharm*. 2010;75(1):33–41. doi:10.1016/j.ejpb.2010.01.011. PubMed PMID: 20102737.

92. Yang W, Chow KT, Lang B, Wiederhold NP, Johnston KP, Williams III RO. In vitro characterization and pharmacokinetics in mice following pulmonary delivery of itraconazole as cyclodextrin solubilized solution. *Eur J Pharm Sci*. 2010;39(5):336–347. doi:10.1016/j.ejps.2010.01.001. PubMed PMID: 20093186.

93. Rundfeldt C, Steckel H, Scherliess H, Wyska E, Wlaz P. Inhalable highly concentrated itraconazole nano-suspension for the treatment of bronchopulmonary aspergillosis. *Eur J Pharm Biopharm*. 2013;83(1):44–53. doi:10.1016/j.ejpb.2012.09.018. PubMed PMID: 23064325.

94. Weyhers H, Ehlers S, Hahn H, Souto EB, Muller RH. Solid lipid nanoparticles (SLN)--effects of lipid composition on in vitro degradation and in vivo toxicity. *Pharmazie*. 2006;61(6):539–544. Epub 2006/07/11. PubMed PMID: 16826974.

95. Müller RH MK, Gohla S. Solid lipid nanoparticles (SLN) for controlled drug delivery–a review of the state of the art. *Eur J Pharm Biopharm* 2000;50(1):161–177.

96. Müller RH RM, Wissing SA. Nanostructured lipid matrices for improved microencapsulation of drugs. *Int J Pharm* 2002;242(1):121–128.

97. Jaques PA, Kim CS. Measurement of total lung deposition of inhaled ultrafine particles in healthy men and women. *Inhal Toxicol*. 2000;12(8):715–731. Epub 2000/07/06. doi:10.1080/08958370050085156. PubMed PMID: 10880153.

98. Pardeike J, Weber S, Haber T, Wagner J, Zarfl HP, Plank H, Zimmer A. Development of an itraconazole-loaded nanostructured lipid carrier (NLC) formulation for pulmonary application. *Int J Pharm*. 2011;419(1–2):329–338. doi:10.1016/j.ijpharm.2011.07.040. PubMed PMID: 21839157.

99. Pardeike J, Weber S, Zarfl HP, Pagitz M, Zimmer A. Itraconazole-loaded nanostructured lipid carriers (NLC) for pulmonary treatment of aspergillosis in falcons. *Eur J Pharm Biopharm*. 2016;108:269–276. doi:10.1016/j.ejpb.2016.07.018. PubMed PMID: 27449629.

100. Moazeni E, Gilani K, Najafabadi AR, Reza Rouini M, Mohajel N, Amini M, Barghi MA. Preparation and evaluation of inhalable itraconazole chitosan based polymeric micelles. *Daru*. 2012;20(1):85. doi:10.1186/2008-2231-20-85. PubMed PMID: 23351398; PMCID: PMC3555998.

101. Duret C, Wauthoz N, Sebti T, Vanderbist F, Amighi K. Solid dispersions of itraconazole for inhalation with enhanced dissolution, solubility and dispersion properties. *Int J Pharm*. 2012;428(1–2):103–113. doi:10.1016/j.ijpharm.2012.03.002. PubMed PMID: 22414388.

102. Duret C, Wauthoz N, Sebti T, Vanderbist F, Amighi K. New respirable and fast dissolving itraconazole dry powder composition for the treatment of invasive pulmonary aspergillosis. *Pharm Res*. 2012;29(10):2845–2859. doi:10.1007/s11095-012-0779-4. PubMed PMID: 22644590.

103. Jafarinejad S, Gilani K, Moazeni E, Ghazi-Khansari M, Najafabadi AR, Mohajel N. Development of chitosan-based nanoparticles for pulmonary delivery of itraconazole as dry powder formulation. *Powder Technology*. 2012;222:65–70. doi:10.1016/j.powtec.2012.01.045.

104. Hassanpour Aghdam M, Ghanbarzadeh S, Javadzadeh Y, Hamishehkar H. Aggregated nanotransfersomal dry powder inhalation of itraconazole for pulmonary drug delivery. *Adv Pharm Bull*. 2016;6(1):57–64. Epub 2016/04/29. doi:10.15171/apb.2016.009. PubMed PMID: 27123418; PMCID: PMC4845537.

105. Hoeben BJ, Burgess DS, McConville JT, Najvar LK, Talbert RL, Peters JI, Wiederhold NP et al., In vivo efficacy of aerosolized nanostructured itraconazole formulations for prevention of invasive pulmonary aspergillosis. *Antimicrob Agents Chemother*. 2006;50(4):1552–1554. doi:10.1128/AAC.50.4.1552-1554.2006. PubMed PMID: 16569882; PMCID: PMC1426984.

106. Alvarez CA, Wiederhold NP, McConville JT, Peters JI, Najvar LK, Graybill JR, Coalson JJ et al., Aerosolized nanostructured itraconazole as prophylaxis against invasive pulmonary aspergillosis. *J Infect*. 2007;55(1):68–74. doi:10.1016/j.jinf.2007.01.014. PubMed PMID: 17360039.

107. Vaughn JM, Wiederhold NP, McConville JT, Coalson JJ, Talbert RL, Burgess DS, Johnston KP, Williams III RO, Peters JI. Murine airway histology and intracellular uptake of inhaled amorphous itraconazole. *Int J Pharm*. 2007;338(1–2):219–224. doi:10.1016/j.ijpharm.2007.02.014. PubMed PMID: 17368772.

108. Duret C, Merlos R, Wauthoz N, Sebti T, Vanderbist F, Amighi K. Pharmacokinetic evaluation in mice of amorphous itraconazole-based dry powder formulations for inhalation with high bioavailability and extended lung retention. *Eur J Pharm Biopharm*. 2014;86(1):46–54. doi:10.1016/j.ejpb.2013.03.005. PubMed PMID: 23523546.

109. Shalini K, Kumar N, Drabu S, Sharma PK. Advances in synthetic approach to and antifungal activity of triazoles. *Beilstein J Org Chem*. 2011;7:668–677. Epub 2011/08/02. doi:10.3762/bjoc.7.79. PubMed PMID: 21804864; PMCID: PMC3135122.

110. Herbrecht R, Denning DW, Patterson TF, Bennett JE, Greene RE, Oestmann J-W, Kern WV et al., Voriconazole versus amphotericin B for primary therapy of invasive aspergillosis. *N Engl J Med*. 2002;347(6):408–415. doi:10.1056/NEJMoa020191. PubMed PMID: 12167683.

111. Hyland R, Jones BC, Smith DA. Identification of the cytochrome P450 enzymes involved in the N-oxidation of voriconazole. *Drug Metabolism and Disposition: The Biological Fate of Chemicals.* 2003;31(5):540–547. Epub 2003/04/16. PubMed PMID: 12695341.

112. Pascual A, Calandra T, Bolay S, Buclin T, Bille J, Marchetti O. Voriconazole therapeutic drug monitoring in patients with invasive mycoses improves efficacy and safety outcomes. *Clin Infect Dis.* 2008;46(2):201–211. Epub 2008/01/04. doi:10.1086/524669. PubMed PMID: 18171251.

113. Trifilio S, Pennick G, Pi J, Zook J, Golf M, Kaniecki K, Singhal S et al., Monitoring plasma voriconazole levels may be necessary to avoid subtherapeutic levels in hematopoietic stem cell transplant recipients. *Cancer.* 2007;109(8):1532–1535. Epub 2007/03/14. doi:10.1002/cncr.22568. PubMed PMID: 17351937.

114. Tolman JA, Wiederhold NP, McConville JT, Najvar LK, Bocanegra R, Peters JI, Coalson JJ, Graybill JR, Patterson TF, Williams III RO. Inhaled voriconazole for prevention of invasive pulmonary aspergillosis. *Antimicrob Agents Chemother.* 2009;53(6): 2613–2615. doi:10.1128/AAC.01657-08. PubMed PMID: 19289523; PMCID: PMC2687213.

115. Chow AH, Tong HH, Chattopadhyay P, Shekunov BY. Particle engineering for pulmonary drug delivery. *Pharm Res.* 2007;24(3):411–437. Epub 2007/01/25. doi:10.1007/s11095-006-9174-3. PubMed PMID: 17245651.

116. Edwards DA, Hanes J, Caponetti G, Hrkach J, Ben-Jebria A, Eskew ML, Mintzes J, Deaver D, Lotan N, Langer R. Large porous particles for pulmonary drug delivery. *Science.* 1997;276(5320):1868–1871. Epub 1997/06/20. PubMed PMID: 9188534.

117. Beinborn NA, Du J, Wiederhold NP, Smyth HD, Williams RO, 3rd. Dry powder insufflation of crystalline and amorphous voriconazole formulations produced by thin film freezing to mice. *Eur J Pharm Biopharm.* 2012;81(3):600–608. doi:10.1016/j.ejpb.2012.04.019. PubMed PMID: 22569473.

118. Sinha B, Mukherjee B, Pattnaik G. Poly-lactide-co-glycolide nanoparticles containing voriconazole for pulmonary delivery: In vitro and in vivo study. *Nanomedicine.* 2013;9(1):94–104. doi:10.1016/j.nano.2012.04.005. PubMed PMID: 22633899.

119. Das PJ, Paul P, Mukherjee B, Mazumder B, Mondal L, Baishya R, Debnath MC, Dey KS. Pulmonary delivery of voriconazole loaded nanoparticles providing a prolonged drug level in lungs: A promise for treating fungal infection. *Mol Pharm.* 2015;12(8):2651–2664. Epub 2015/05/06. doi:10.1021/acs.molpharmaceut.5b00064. PubMed PMID: 25941882.

120. Arora S, Haghi M, Loo CY, Traini D, Young PM, Jain S. Development of an inhaled controlled release voriconazole dry powder formulation for the treatment of respiratory fungal infection. *Mol Pharm.* 2015;12(6):2001–2009. doi:10.1021/mp500808t. PubMed PMID: 25923171.

121. Arora S, Haghi M, Young PM, Kappl M, Traini D, Jain S. Highly respirable dry powder inhalable formulation of voriconazole with enhanced pulmonary bioavailability. *Expert Opin Drug Deliv.* 2016;13(2):183–193. doi:10.1517/17425247.2016.1114603. PubMed PMID: 26609733.

122. Tolman JA, Nelson NA, Son YJ, Bosselmann S, Wiederhold NP, Peters JI, McConville JT, Williams III RO. Characterization and pharmacokinetic analysis of aerosolized aqueous voriconazole solution. *Eur J Pharm Biopharm.* 2009;72(1):199–205. doi:10.1016/ j.ejpb.2008.12.014. PubMed PMID: 19348016.

123. Deresinski SC, Stevens DA. Caspofungin. *Clin Infect Dis.* 2003;36(11):1445–1457. Epub 2003/05/27. doi:10.1086/375080. PubMed PMID: 12766841.

124. Wong-Beringer A, Kriengkauykiat J. Systemic antifungal therapy: New options, new challenges. *Pharmacotherapy.* 2003;23(11):1441–1462. Epub 2003/11/19. PubMed PMID: 14620391.

125. Walsh TJ, Teppler H, Donowitz GR, Maertens JA, Baden LR, Dmoszynska A, Cornely OA et al., Caspofungin versus liposomal amphotericin B for empirical antifungal therapy in patients with persistent fever and neutropenia. *N Engl J Med.* 2004;351(14):1391–1402. Epub 2004/10/02. doi:10.1056/NEJMoa040446. PubMed PMID: 15459300.

126. Kurtz MB, Bernard EM, Edwards FF, Marrinan JA, Dropinski J, Douglas CM, Armstrong D. Aerosol and parenteral pneumocandins are effective in a rat model of pulmonary aspergillosis. *Antimicrob Agents Chemother.* 1995;39(8):1784–1789. doi:10.1128/aac.39.8.1784.

127. Wong-Beringer A, Lambros MP, Beringer PM, Johnson DL. Suitability of caspofungin for aerosol delivery: Physicochemical profiling and nebulizer choice. *Chest.* 2005;128(5):3711–3716. Epub 2005/11/24. doi:10.1378/chest.128.5.3711. PubMed PMID: 16304338.

11

Lung cancer inhalation therapeutics

RAJIV DHAND

Introduction	187	Chemotherapy	196
Lung cancer	188	Pharmacokinetics	196
Delivery of inhaled anticancer agents	189	Preclinical efficacy	197
Aerosol deposition	189	Inhaled chemotherapeutic agents	197
Targeting airway deposition of drugs	190	Gene therapy	199
Formulations	191	Antisense therapy	200
Solutions	191	Bacteria/cells	200
Dry powders	191	Clinical use of inhaled anticancer agents	201
Liposomes	192	Immunologics/cytokines	201
Microparticles	192	Chemotherapy	201
Nanoparticles	193	Gene therapy	201
Swellable hydrogels	193	Adverse effects	201
Micelles	193	Limitations of inhaled anticancer agents	202
Inorganic nanocarriers	193	Environmental contamination	202
Aerosol delivery devices	194	Unanswered questions	202
Inhaled anticancer agents	194	Conclusion	203
Immunologics/cytokines	194	References	203
Monoclonal antibodies	195		

INTRODUCTION

In parallel with the rising rates of tobacco consumption, lung cancer has become a major worldwide public health problem over the course of the last century. In 2012, there were an estimated 1.8 million new cases of lung cancer and over 1.6 million deaths worldwide, accounting for 19% of all cancer deaths (1). Worldwide mortality from lung cancer is expected to approximately double in both men and women by 2035 (2). In the United States, lung cancer is the most common cause of death in both men and women (3). Despite significant advances in prevention, screening, and treatment, approximately 234,030 new cases and approximately 154,050 deaths are expected from lung cancer in 2018 (4), accounting for about 14% of all new cases and about 26% of all cancer deaths, in the United States (1,4). It is noteworthy that incidence rates of lung cancer in the United States are declining, about twice as fast in men as in women, probably due to the declining rates of tobacco smoking (1).

The broad categories of lung cancer are non-small-cell lung cancer (NSCLC); small cell lung cancer (SCLC); and other tumors, including carcinoid tumors. NSCLC accounts for 85% of cases, and there are three major subtypes: adenocarcinoma, squamous cell carcinoma, and large cell anaplastic carcinoma, with adenocarcinoma being the most prevalent type of NSCLC (Table 11.1). SCLC, which is a highly malignant tumor derived from cells exhibiting neuroendocrine characteristics, accounts for approximately 15% of lung cancer cases. Carcinoid tumors represent less than 5% of all lung cancers. In addition, other common tumors, such as carcinomas of the breast, head and neck, colon, kidney, stomach, and prostate, and sarcomas and melanoma often metastasize to the lungs.

Table 11.1 Histological classification of lung cancers[a]

Primary	Metastatic
Epithelial tumors	**Local spread**
Adenocarcinoma	Lung cancer
Squamous cell carcinoma	**Airway spread**
Neuroendocrine tumors	Breast cancer
Small cell carcinoma	Renal cancer
Large cell neuroendocrine carcinoma	Colon cancer
	Melanoma
Carcinoid tumors	**Lymphatic spread**
Preinvasive lesion	Breast cancer
Large cell carcinoma	Stomach cancer
Adenosquamous carcinoma	Pancreatic cancer
Sarcomatoid carcinomas	Prostate cancer
Other and unclassified carcinomas	
Salivary gland-type tumors	
Papillomas	
Adenomas	
Mesenchymal tumors	**Hematogenous**
Lymphohistiocytic tumors	**spread**
Tumors of ectopic origin	Breast cancer
	Kidney cancer
	Head and neck
	cancer
	Hepatic cancer
	Gastric cancer
	Choriocarcinoma
	Melanoma
	Sarcoma
	Spread from pleural
	space
	Ovarian cancer
	Mesothelioma
	Lymphoma

Source: Travis, W.D., et al. *WHO Classification of Tumors of the Lung, Pleura, Thymus and Heart*, Lyon, France, International Agency for Research on Cancer, 2015.
[a] Based on the 2015 WHO Classification of Lung Tumors.

LUNG CANCER

In patients with suspected lung cancer, histopathologic diagnosis and disease staging require a detailed clinical evaluation followed by noninvasive testing and invasive procedures. Staging depends on the anatomical extent of the tumor, and it determines the appropriate surgical and medical treatment plan. Staging of NSCLC, based on the TNM classification proposed by the American Joint Committee on Cancer, depends on the size of the main (primary) tumor (T) and whether it has grown into adjacent tissues, whether the cancer has spread to nearby (regional) lymph nodes (N), and whether the cancer has spread (metastasized; M) to other organs of the body. Metastasis occurs by several routes, including blood-borne, or via lymphatics, airways, and air spaces (Table 11.1). The most common sites of metastasis

from lung cancer are the brain, bones, adrenal glands, liver, kidneys, and the other lung. In the revised TNM staging system (8th edition) adopted in 2018 (5), tumors that are completely surrounded by lung parenchyma, are more than 2 cm away from the carina, do not invade the visceral or parietal pleura, and have no associated lymph node or metastatic disease are categorized as Stage I (early disease). These patients have the best prognosis, but only 15% of all lung cancer patients present with early (Stage I) disease. Patients with Stage II tumors have features intermediate between Stage I and Stage III NSCLC; they have tumors localized to the lung and nodal disease that does not involve the mediastinum. Patients with tumors larger than 5 cm in diameter that show pleural, mediastinal, or chest wall invasion or smaller tumors that are associated with mediastinal lymph node disease are categorized as Stage III, and tumors exhibiting metastasis are designated as Stage IV disease (6).

The treatment for many patients with early-stage disease (Stages I and II) is primarily surgical; however, the role for systemic chemotherapy has been gradually expanding, now playing an important role in the treatment of both early stage (Stage II disease with positive lymph nodes) and locally advanced NSCLC (Stage III) (7). Oncologists commonly employ chemotherapy or a combination of chemotherapy, immunotherapy, and radiation therapy for treatment of late stage or advanced (Stage III and IV) lung cancers. Notably, systemic treatment with cytotoxic chemotherapy has the potential to produce serious adverse effects, and a significant proportion of patients may not be candidates for such therapy because of comorbidities and poor performance status.

Despite the availability of new diagnostic and genetic technologies, advancements in surgical techniques, and the development of new biologic treatments, the overall 5-year survival rate for lung cancer in the United States remains at a poor 19.5% (8). The estimated 5-year survival rate in Europe, China, and developing countries is only 8.9%. Lung cancer stage is often advanced at the time of diagnosis; up to 40% of cases of NSCLC have Stage IV (metastatic disease) at presentation (9). Patients with Stage I disease at diagnosis have a 5-year survival rate of approximately 50%. In stark contrast, patients with advanced stage disease and distant metastasis at diagnosis have a dismal 5-year survival rate of only 4%, emphasizing the need for better screening methods to detect early-stage cancers (1).

The continuing search for alternative therapies for patients with surgically unresectable lung cancer provides newer approaches, including specific oral tyrosine kinase inhibitors that target driver mutations in the epidermal growth factor receptor (EGFR), and monoclonal antibodies directed against specific markers on the cancer cells (10,11). Mutations in EGFR are commonly observed in nonsmokers with adenocarcinoma (12). Another driver mutation, which involves a rearrangement in the anaplastic lymphoma kinase (ALK) gene, occurs in a smaller proportion of patients with adenocarcinoma. Agents that target this mutation have also shown efficacy and ability to prolong survival in patients with advanced lung cancer (13). The newest treatment modality for treatment of NSCLC involves immunotherapy with immune checkpoint inhibitors targeting key modulators of the immune regulation system that allow cancers to escape the body's immune system. Three monoclonal antibodies directed against the programmed death (PD-1) or programmed death ligand-1 (PDL-1) proteins have been approved for use in patients with lung cancer (10,14). Patients with advanced lung cancer have longer survival with these therapies, and a small number of patients achieve prolonged remissions.

The field is rapidly moving toward personalized therapy for patients with lung cancer employing various combinations of chemotherapy, targeted molecular approaches, immunotherapy, and radiation therapy. However, the majority of new cases of lung cancer now arise in the developing regions of the world that have large populations of individuals who smoke cigarettes and are therefore at risk of developing lung cancer (1). Thus, there is a pressing need to develop newer, cost effective, and well-tolerated treatments that can prolong survival among patients with lung cancer.

Currently, oncologists employ oral administration or intravenous (IV) infusions to deliver the newer anticancer agents for the treatment of lung cancer. Only a small fraction of the systemically administered dose, given orally or by IV route, is distributed to the lungs, and drug concentrations achieved within lung tumors are low (15). Inhalation therapy has intuitive advantages over systemic routes of administration because it is possible to achieve high local concentrations of therapeutic agents with minimal systemic effects (16). Bronchoalveolar tumors are accessible endobronchially and are potentially targetable with aerosolized therapies. Most studies of inhaled anticancer treatments focus on patients with NSCLC because SCLC has often spread beyond the lungs at the time of diagnosis. The ability to target aerosols to specific lung regions combined with formulation of inhaled anticancer therapies with lower toxicity and prolonged effects have both made significant progress in recent years (16,17). Such advances make it feasible to treat patients with NSCLC with inhaled aerosols.

DELIVERY OF INHALED ANTICANCER AGENTS

Aerosol deposition

Regional administration of immunotherapy, chemotherapy, and genetic manipulation successfully treats a variety of solid tumors. Inhalational delivery, a noninvasive method of regional drug delivery, achieves high pulmonary concentrations of the delivered agent, with low systemic toxicity and the potential to target therapy, and avoids hepatic metabolism of drugs (16,17). Inhalation offers a pain- and needle-free delivery method that could be self-administered and frequently repeated. The ability to achieve high concentrations of chemotherapeutic agents within lung tumors may be a critical factor in reducing treatment failures as well as emergence of resistance to treatment (18). With this

approach, tumors that have become refractory to systemic chemotherapy could respond to inhalation treatment (19,20). Newer aerosol delivery methods significantly increase the efficiency of drug delivery to the lungs (21,22). The development of novel, locally administered anticancer agents may help to better target the tumors and potentially reduce occurrence of adverse effects due to systemically administered therapies. Inhalation therapy therefore has the potential to become an effective and safe treatment for patients with lung cancer (16). However, to be effective in treating lung cancers, drug aerosols have to circumvent several barriers: aerosolized agents must dissolve in the lining fluid of the airways and alveoli, penetrate tumors, cause cytotoxic effects without producing drug resistance, and avoid rapid clearance or degradation by enzymes. Ideally, such agents should effectively eradicate tumors without producing bystander effects and toxicity to healthy tissues, and without causing environmental contamination. These complex requirements necessitate new approaches and novel formulations to provide effective therapy.

Aerosol particle size, inspiratory flow rate, tidal volume, and airway geometry are among several factors that influence aerosol deposition in the lungs (17). The optimal site for inhaled drug deposition may vary depending on the site of the tumor. Aerosols with larger mass median aerodynamic diameter (MMAD) of 4–5 µm target centrally located lung tumors, whereas slow inhalation of aerosols containing drug particles of 1–3 µm in diameter increases the likelihood of drug deposition in peripheral airways and alveoli, and is more appropriate for targeting peripheral tumors (e.g., adenocarcinoma and pulmonary metastasis). Airway obstruction by the tumor or the presence of associated obstructive lung disease could influence aerosol deposition patterns. Likewise, the high humidity environment in the lung could alter the particle size of some drugs and change their deposition. Other physical properties of the aerosol particles, such as pH, electrostatic charge, and osmolarity, also play a role in drug deposition (23).

After deposition, drugs undergo dissolution and transport across the epithelial membranes for absorption into the circulation. In the conducting airways, mucociliary clearance mechanisms transport particulate matter up to the oropharynx, whereas in the alveoli, the principal mechanisms of clearance are by alveolar macrophage phagocytosis and absorption into the pulmonary circulation. A variety of techniques could enhance the local concentration of therapeutic agents in the lung (24,25). In patients with lung cancer, mucociliary clearance may not rapidly remove drugs depositing on the conducting airways in the tumor vicinity because tumor cells lack functioning cilia, allowing for a longer residence time and greater opportunity for the drug to reach the tumor by direct local penetration. Moreover, regional distribution of drugs depositing on the airways occurs via a rich plexus of bronchial capillaries that have pre- and post-capillary connections with the pulmonary circulation (26). Due to these communications between the bronchial and pulmonary circulations, drugs administered by inhalation could achieve adequate drug concentrations even within small tumors that are located in the lung parenchyma and lack direct communication with a major airway.

The chemical characteristics and biological effects of drugs have a strong influence on their efficacy as anticancer agents. In addition, the delivery of adequate concentrations of anticancer agents to all cancer cells in solid tumors is strongly dependent on the structure and function of the vasculature, drug transport properties in tissue, and tumor size. Drugs show variable penetration into tumors; drugs such as 5-fluorouracil (5-FU), which bind macromolecules minimally, readily penetrate and are uniformly cytotoxic throughout the tumor. In contrast, the efficacy of other drugs, such as paclitaxel, depend on tumor cellularity, density of the tumor interstitium, and apoptotic activity of the drug. Tumor endothelial cells proliferate faster but form less tight junctions than endothelial cells in normal tissue (27), which may be attributed to production of vascular endothelial growth factor (VEGF) by tumor cells (28). As a result, the endothelial barrier of tumor microvessels demonstrates a tenfold higher permeability of tumor vessel walls to albumin than that of continuous normal capillaries (29) and allows passage of nanoparticles (NPs) with a diameter of approximately 100 nm (30). These characteristics of macromolecule and nanoparticle transport have been termed the enhanced permeability and retention (EPR) effect (31). Human cancers vary in the magnitude of the EPR effect (32,33).

Human tumors also contain different amounts of extracellular matrix (ECM). ECM can increase the diffusion distance for a drug to reach target tumor cells, and binding to ECM components could reduce the amount of free drug (34). ECM can take up space (35,36) and present a steric barrier to diffusion of NPs (36). Moreover, tumor microvessels can collapse if the ECM is very dense (37,38) or if there is uncontrolled proliferation of tumor cells (39).

In normal tissues, reabsorption into the lymphatic circulation balances the net outward flow of fluid from blood vessels. Tumors lack functional lymphatics, and increased permeability of tumor microvessels leads to the accumulation of fluid and high interstitial fluid pressure (IFP), which can reach 5–10 mmHg or higher compared to near zero or even slightly negative in normal tissues (40,41). As the elevated IFP approaches the intravascular pressure, the pressure gradient in the interstitial space could be almost near zero, thereby hindering the transport of macromolecules and NPs for which convection is normally the dominant transport mechanism in tissue. Diffusion, the remaining major transport process, is very slow for macromolecules and NPs (41). Moreover, rapid absorption of drugs into the systemic circulation across the thin pulmonary epithelial barrier could further limit the efficacy of anticancer agents against lung tumors. Thus, inhaled therapies could achieve higher drug concentrations in the tumor vicinity, but the ability of these agents to eradicate cancer cells depends on the tumor environment and clearance mechanisms. Targeting drugs to lung tumors could more effectively treat lung cancers.

Targeting airway deposition of drugs

Many lung tumors localize to one lobe or segment of the lung; therefore selective targeting of tumors could exponentially enhance local concentrations within the tumor while avoiding exposure of uninvolved areas of the lung to potentially toxic agents. Appropriate targeting of anticancer agents enhances the chances of inducing a remission and eradication of cancers by subsequent surgery or radiation therapy. *Passive* and *active* targeting approaches deliver inhaled agents to specific sites in the lung. In the *passive targeting* approach, deposition at specific sites within the lung is achieved by modifications of aerosol droplet size, breathing pattern, depth and duration of breath-hold, timing of the aerosol bolus in relation to inspiratory airflow, and density of the inhaled gas (42). However, variations in patient's lung volumes and airway geometry make it difficult to achieve precise regional targeting even with a specified breathing pattern and size of aerosol particles (43). Thus, it is not possible to define a single set of parameters to target specific lung regions that are applicable to all patients. Newer devices (e.g., the Akita system® or I-neb adaptive aerosol delivery [AAD] system®) provide attractive options for delivery of inhaled anticancer agents. With these devices, the ability to synchronize aerosol generation with the patient's breathing and regulate the inhalation flow rate enhances aerosol delivery efficiency with more precise control over the delivered dose (44,45). A unique feature of the I-neb AAD system is the target inhalation mode (TIM), which guides the user to longer inhalations. The aims of the TIM are to reduce the treatment time by increasing the total inhalation time per minute and to increase lung deposition by reducing impaction in the upper airways through slow and deep inhalations (46). The AAD technology also provides visual, audible, and tactile signals to guide the patient on delivery performance.

Enhanced condensation growth is another technique to bypass upper airway deposition and achieve optimal lower respiratory tract deposition (47). In this technique, a submicrometer aerosol passes through one nostril at slightly subsaturated humidification, whereas a humidified airstream saturated with water vapor passes through the other nostril with a temperature maintained at a few degrees above *in vivo* wall conditions. The nasal septum physically separates the two airstreams, and minimal nasal deposition occurs as the submicrometer aerosol traverses the nose. The two airstreams combine in the nasopharynx with condensational growth of the aerosol particles as the airstream moves downward into the lungs. In a bench nose, mouth, and throat model, mean drug deposition was reduced from 72.6% to 14.8%, whereas aerosol size increased from an initial MMAD of 900 nm to approximately 2 μm at the exit of the model (48). This technique overcomes the barrier imposed to aerosol particles by the nasal passages and could be employed to enhance lung deposition of agents delivered by inhalation while breathing through the nose.

In addition, NP-based drug delivery is enhanced by the EPR effect in tumors. The leaky microvessels within tumors allow extravasation of NPs, and the lack of lymphatic drainage promotes their long-term retention within tumors (49). Modifications of the size of the drug particles could enhance selective uptake by tumors with increased vascular endothelial permeability. However, the EPR effect provides less than a twofold increase in nanodrug delivery compared with normal organs, and the drug concentrations achieved are not sufficient for curing most cancers (50). These passive targeting techniques could result in enhanced drug uptake within lung cancers by customizing the inhalation device and manipulating the formulation to generate droplets of optimum size and aerodynamic properties, especially for those cancers located in the trachea and major bronchi (51,52).

In the *active targeting* approach, the drug targets a diseased area of lung or the tumor by some specific molecular or biological recognition that allows its binding to the target cells. For this purpose, an intracorporeal nebulizing catheter (INC) could deliver therapy to a specific area of the lung (53). Active targeting can be achieved by target-specific receptor ligands such as EGFR (54), luteinizing hormone releasing hormone (LHRH) (55), transferrin (56), or folate (57), or target-specific anti-EGFR antibodies coupled with chemotherapy drugs (58). TNF-related apoptosis-inducing ligand (TRAIL) is a protein functioning as a ligand that induces apoptosis. It causes apoptosis, primarily in tumor cells, by binding to certain death receptors. Particles coated with TRAIL could be employed to specifically target death receptors that are overexpressed in cancer cells but not healthy cells (59). Employing beta-agonist receptors as target ligands enhances gene delivery to lungs (60). An external magnetic field that guides inert superparamagnetic iron oxide NPs (SPIONs) to a desired lung region has been employed (17,61). These active targeting techniques offer promising and novel approaches, and extensive research is being conducted to develop formulations that specifically employ this approach for treatment of lung cancers.

Formulations

SOLUTIONS

Nebulizers commonly deliver solution formulations of inhaled anticancer agents to the lungs. In the past, solution formulations employed in nebulizers were not specifically prepared for inhalation and had the potential to produce local irritant effects. However, the active moiety in the solution retained efficacy after nebulization. Repeated inhalations of the IV formulations of cisplatinum and gemcitabine were shown to be well tolerated in anesthetized, mechanically ventilated dogs (53,62). No signs of significant local or systemic toxicity were observed after administration of escalating doses of cisplatin (10, 15, 20, and 30 mg/m^2 given by INC every 2 weeks for 10 weeks; cumulative dose 75 mg/m^2) (53). In a follow-up

study, administration of escalating doses of combination chemotherapy (gemcitabine [GEM] 1,2,3, or 6 mg/Kg and cisplatin 10 mg/m^2 given by INC every 2 weeks for 10 weeks) also did not produce significant clinical or biochemical side effects (62). All the dogs developed focal pneumonitis radiologically limited to the treated lobe, which increased in severity over time following increasing doses of chemotherapy. At autopsy, these radiologic changes correlated with chronic pneumonitis with fibrosis. Other investigators employed a freeze-dried powder of GEM or carboplatin solution reconstituted with normal saline for inhalation (63,64). Because of problems in maintaining stability of solution formulations, dry powders, especially in a nanoparticle form, are preferred for many newer inhaled anticancer agents.

DRY POWDERS

Dry powders are more stable than solutions and powder formulations may be preferable to aqueous solutions for delivery of inhaled anticancer agents. Ideal formulations of dry powders have the majority of drug particles in the range of 1 to 5 μm in size, and they exhibit desirable flow properties, low agglomeration tendency, and good batch-to-batch uniformity. Carrier particles (e.g., lactose or mannitol) added as excipients and a dispersibility enhancer, such as magnesium stearate or leucine, improve handling and dispensing of the active agent, and reduce cohesiveness between particles. Small particles of the active agent adhere to the surface of the larger carrier particles to form agglomerates. In the absence of excipients, dry powders formulated as loose agglomerates disperse into small particles with application of energy from a patient's breath or other active source. Micronization involving milling techniques, commonly air jet milling, or by *in situ* micronization utilizing various forms of controlled precipitation commonly achieves production of particles of the active agent in the desired size range (65,66). Spray drying is a widely used technique to manufacture particles by forcing a solution (less commonly a suspension) under pressure into a drying chamber through a spray nozzle. The dried particles that remain after the solvent or liquid evaporates are collected through a cyclone separator. Spray drying allows various compounds to be incorporated into a single particle, and to produce porous particles with density <0.1 g/cm^3.

Porous particles (e.g., Pulmospheres, Nektar Therapeutics) have a larger particle size but their aerodynamic diameter is smaller (because of their lower density), and their deposition in the respiratory tract is similar to smaller particles of unit density. The larger size and surface area of porous particles allows them to carry a higher drug payload. Such porous particles avoid ingestion by alveolar macrophages, they have a prolonged residence time within the deep lung, and they could potentially release their payload over extended periods of time (67). Inhalable doxorubicin (DOX)-loaded, highly porous polylactic-co-glycolic acid (PLGA) microparticles prepared by using ammonium bicarbonate, a gas forming porogen, remained in the lungs of mice for 14 days and produced significant decrease in numbers and mass of

B16–F10 melanoma tumors (68). Co-loading of miRNA (miR-519c) with DOX into inhaled PLGA porous microparticles downregulated the overexpressed ABCG2 that is responsible for outflux of anticancer drugs in resistant tumors (69). Likewise, attachment of TRAIL to the surface of inhaled DOX PLGA porous microparticles provided synergistic activity against lung cancer (59).

Inhaled agents could also be incorporated into the matrix of biodegradable synthetic polymers polylactic acid (PLA); PLGA; natural polymers such as albumin, gelatin, chitosan, or sodium hyaluronate; and poly(ether-anhydrides). Polymers modify the surface properties of particles, have high drug encapsulation efficiency, protect the drug from degradation and macrophage phagocytosis, and prolong its effect due to sustained drug release. Because of limitations to the amount of drug loading in such particles, achieving optimum drug concentrations in the lung requires frequent dosing. After repetitive dosing, the incompletely degraded polymer could accumulate in the lung (70). Biodegradable polymers are safer and are preferred over synthetic polymers because the latter have the potential to activate cytokines.

Supercritical fluid technology is another promising method for preparing dry powders for inhalation (71). Particle replication in nonwetting templates (PRINT) technology has the advantage of preparing particles of uniform size and shape. In this technique, a silicon master template fabricated with photolithography creates a polymeric mold that has cavities of the precise particle size and shape required. Capillary forces fill the cavities with the drug or excipient, and an adhesive layer extracts the solidified particles in the mold. After dissolving the adhesive layer, a liquid suspension of the recovered particles or a dry free-flowing powder prepared by lyophilization or evaporation could be employed (72).

LIPOSOMES

Liposomes of a variety of drugs, with a wide range of lipophilicities, including small molecules, nucleotides, deoxyribonucleic acid (DNA) constructs, peptides, and proteins, are prepared by encapsulating an aqueous solution within a hydrophobic phospholipid membrane (73). Natural or synthetic phospholipids that may be electrically neutral or carry a net positive or negative charge typically form liposome membranes. Based on their size and morphology, liposomes are classified as multilamellar vesicles (0.1–20 μm), large unilamellar vesicles (0.1–1.0 μm), or small unilamellar vesicles (25–100 nm). Liposomes are able to carry hydrophilic anticancer agents within the aqueous cores and hydrophobic agents within the lipid bilayers. Their site of deposition within the respiratory tract and rate of drug release depend on their composition, size, charge, drug/lipid ratio, and method of delivery.

Liposome formulations have the combined advantages of minimal toxicity and prolonged drug effect compared to aqueous solutions. Liposomes of approximately 100 nm size are able to take advantage of the EPR effect; they pass through tumor blood vessels and accumulate within cancerous tissue where they release their payload (49). For example, CsA liposomes prepared for pulmonary delivery had a prolonged drug release compared to the free drug (74). Liposome absorption into lymphatic vessels (a common route for the spread of lung tumors) allows targeting of cancer cells that have metastasized to lymph nodes. Attaching monoclonal antibodies or ligands to the liposome surface allows targeting to specific cell surface receptors (stealth liposomes), or liposomes may be designed to release the drug on encountering a specific environment, such as the lower pH within cancers (pH-sensitive liposomes).

Liposomes are delivered to the airways by direct instillation or microspray, or by jet or ultrasonic nebulization. Leakage of drugs from liposomes due to high shear stresses encountered during nebulization alters the therapeutic response to the drug depending on the magnitude of leakage (75). Compared to jet nebulization, use of vibrating mesh nebulizers customized with large mesh apertures could reduce drug leakage from liposomes, especially those smaller than 1 μm in size. Ultrasonic nebulizers are not suitable for delivering liposomes (76), whereas soft mist inhalers (SMIs), such as the AERx (Aradigm Corp., Novo Nordisk, Hayward, CA) are able to deliver liposome DNA complexes as respirable aerosols (77).

Polymer coating of liposome surface with polyethylene glycol (PEG) avoids selective uptake by alveolar macrophages and prolongs the effect of the payload, but it may reduce bilayer stability during nebulization and promote drug leakage (78). In contrast, incorporation of cholesterol or high phase transition phospholipids in liposome formulations improves their stability during nebulization (79–81). Another technique to avoid leakage of encapsulated drug or active agent during rehydration of dry powders is to create liposomes *in situ* in the airways from the individual dried components (lipids, drug, and a powder-dispersing agent such as lactose). Proliposomes are powdered phospholipid formulations that generate liposomes when they contact an aqueous environment (82,83). In addition, dispersion of a physical mixture of phospholipid(s) and drug in saline produced liposomes spontaneously, thereby creating reservoirs for the encapsulation of drugs. These liposomes are administered by nebulization, with the nebulization properties depending on the phospholipid mixture and drug (84).

Thus, aerosolized delivery of anticancer agents as liposomes requires consideration of several factors such as liposome size, formulation stability, the type of nebulizer, and targeting the aerosol to the tumor site. Encapsulation of anticancer agents within liposomes allows modulation of their release profile; prolonged residence time in the lung; enhanced drug dose per inhalation, especially for poorly soluble drugs; masking the taste; and reducing local irritation with inhaled drugs, besides cellular targeting.

MICROPARTICLES

Microparticles (size range 0.1–500 μm), produced from naturally occurring or synthetic polymers, are physically and chemically more stable than liposomes and are capable of carrying a higher drug payload. Natural synthetic biocompatible and biodegradable polymers such as chitosan, PLGA, PLA, poly(butylcyanoacrylate) and poly(lactic-co-lysine graft lysine) are commonly employed in producing such particles (85,86). Coating these particles with PEG enhances their sustained release property. Other techniques, including addition of dipalmitoylphosphatidylcholine, chitosan, or hydroxypropylcellulose, also prolong residence of particles in the lung. Microparticles produced by these techniques have higher stability, are able to carry a higher drug load, release the drug slowly, and have longer pharmacological activity than liposomal formulations (87). For example, docetaxel-loaded microspheres demonstrated sustained drug release, increased lung bioavailability, and reduced systemic toxicity (88). Modulation of the morphology, size, and porosity of these microparticles could enhance their application for specific pulmonary indications (87).

NANOPARTICLES

The therapeutic effects of nebulized anticancer agents depend on their ability to penetrate into tumors and reach cancer cells in sufficient concentrations to have a therapeutic effect. NPs are attractive because they optimize drug solubility, encapsulation efficacy, and drug release profiles. After release from an aerosol, NPs form aggregates in the micrometer size range. These aggregates have sufficient mass to deposit by sedimentation. NPs deposit in the deep lung lining fluid and escape mucociliary clearance, they are not engulfed by alveolar macrophages, and they have a more prolonged residence time in the lung (89). NPs retain the encapsulated drug and, because of enhanced intracellular uptake, they can specifically target tumor cells and provide controlled and prolonged drug release within the tumor cells (90). The advantage of NP formulations is that they require once or twice daily dosing. However, particle accumulation within alveoli could occur after repeated dosing. Carrier particles enhance the lung deposition of inhaled NPs in the size range 10–100 nm.

Lipid-coated NPs have less local toxicity than microspheres. Biodegradable polymeric nanocarriers such as gelatin-based NPs containing cisplatin have shown activity against adenocarcinoma cells (91,92). In experimental models, paclitaxel-loaded solid lipid NPs (93) and DOX-loaded NPs effectively reduced the number and size of tumors in mice (94). Investigators employed direct covalent coupling of drugs to a polymeric carrier such as human serum albumin (95), hyaluronan (96), or PEGylated poly-L-lysine dendrimer (97) to enhance the efficacy of chemotherapeutic agents. Abraxane®, an injectable suspension of albumin NPs with bound paclitaxel, has been in clinical use but is not available as an inhaled formulation.

Drug-loaded or antibody-containing NPs encapsulated within microparticles (so-called Trojan particles) by spray drying of NPs followed by assembly into hollow porous particles have been delivered into the deep lung to provide sustained drug release (98,99). NPs could concurrently deliver drugs and genes to the same cells, and the ability to coat them with a variety of targeting molecules allows for greater therapeutic choices. Solid lipid NPs (SLNs) have a solid hydrophobic core and a single-layer phospholipid shell. With the aim of reducing their toxicity, these formulations use physiological lipids, primarily triglycerides and phospholipids. Drug-loaded SLNs administered within microparticles have greater stability and controlled release, enhanced bioavailability, and greater therapeutic effectiveness (100). However, the drug loading capacity within such particles is low, and drug expulsion may occur during storage (101,102). Nevertheless, nebulized paclitaxel SLNs achieved greater suppression of lung metastasis compared to IV paclitaxel in a mouse model (93).

Nanostructured lipid carriers consist of an unstructured solid lipid matrix that contains solid and liquid lipids and an aqueous phase containing surfactant. Such carriers have a higher drug-loading capacity and less drug leakage than SLNs (103). Nanostructured lipid carriers loaded with celecoxib, a cyclooxygenase-2 (COX2) inhibitor, demonstrated controlled release up to 72 hours and time and concentration-dependent cytotoxicity against A549 cells (104).

SWELLABLE HYDROGELS

Another approach to delivery of inhaled anticancer agents is to employ 1–5 μm particles in the dry state that swell to form larger particles in the warm and humid environment of the lung. Such formulations evade being engulfed by alveolar macrophages and could be employed as carriers for drug-loaded NPs (105).

MICELLES

Amphipathic surfactant molecules self-assemble to a core shell nanostructure in aqueous solution at a certain concentration and temperature to form polymeric micelles. At low concentrations, these amphiphilic molecules exist separately as unimers; however, at a critical micelle concentration (CMC), they aggregate to form almost spherical micelles. Micelles represent colloidal dispersions with a particle size from 5 to 50–100 nm. The hydrophobic fragments of amphiphilic molecules form the core of a micelle, allowing carriage of poorly soluble pharmaceuticals within the core. Chemical alteration of the structure of these micelles allows development of formulations with greater drug stability, controlled release, and targeted drug delivery (106).

INORGANIC NANOCARRIERS

Limiting the exposure time and modulating the size and concentration of inhalable metal NPs control their toxicity to lung tissues. Magnetic hyperthermia is an alternative approach that works by generating heat when magnetic components, including SPIONs, are exposed to an interchanging magnetic field (107). In mice carrying an orthotopic lung cancer model, administration of EGFR-targeted SPIONs for targeted hyperthermia produced enhanced tumor retention and significantly reduced lung tumor growth compared to appropriate controls (61). In human lungs, the use of such techniques requires particles that are highly responsive to electromagnetic fields and have high-distance mobility (108).

Mesoporous silica NPs have large pore volume and surface area. Trapping the drugs in the pores protects them from degradation, or agents are conjugated by covalent or electrostatic interactions to the available surface functional groups (109). The mesoporous silica NPs had higher lung deposition compared to IV administration. Complex particles could be generated with mesoporous silica NPs that combine local delivery of chemotherapy; siRNA to prevent or suppress resistance; and a surface-engineering approach to target cancer cells, such as PEG-LHRH (Figure 11.1). With the aim of enhancing drug cytotoxicity, one group of investigators used mesoporous silica NPs containing DOX and cisplatin and (MRP1 and BCL2 mRNA) targeted siRNA attached to the surface to suppress pump and non-pump-mediated resistance (110).

Aerosol delivery devices

Traditionally, pressurized metered-dose inhalers (pMDIs), dry powder inhalers (DPIs), SMIs, or nebulizers are used to generate aerosols, but pMDIs and DPIs are rarely employed for delivery of anticancer agents, and SMIs are currently employed only for delivery of bronchodilators. Dry powder aerosols formulated alone or with phospholipids are under development for delivery of anticancer agents ("Dry powders"). More modern technologies generate aerosols by passing a solution through a vibrating mesh (e.g., Aeroneb®, or e Flow®), by producing a soft mist from a drug solution (e.g., Respimat® and AERx®), or by evaporative condensation of a drug powder (e.g., Staccato inhaler®) (17). A Microsprayer® could target aerosols to specific intrapulmonary sites. Nebulizers can deliver larger doses than other aerosol delivery devices, but the characteristics of the aerosol produced by a jet nebulizer depend on the viscosity, surface tension, pH, ionic strength, and osmolarity of the formulation. Significant patient coordination or training in breathing techniques is not required to use conventional nebulizers, a noteworthy advantage over other aerosol delivery devices. Breath-actuated nebulizers are preferable for administration of anticancer agents in order to minimize waste and avoid contamination of the environment.

INHALED ANTICANCER AGENTS

Inhalation is used to administer several types of therapies directed against lung cancer, including (1) activators of the local immune response and cytokines, (2) monoclonal antibodies, (3) chemotherapeutic agents, (4) genes, (5) antisense nucleotides, and (6) bacteria/cellular carriers.

Immunologics/cytokines

Tumors evade or overwhelm the host's immune system, and the lungs are particularly vulnerable in this regard because constant exposure to the external environment creates an immunosuppressive environment that allows cancer to grow. Exogenous stimulation of the immune system or

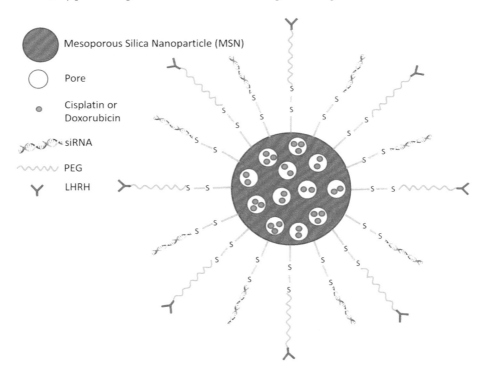

Figure 11.1 Co-delivery of siRNA and anticancer agents using mesoporous silica nanoparticles (MSNs). The surface engineered approach consists of surface-bound siRNA and PEG-LHRH. (Reproduced from Youngren-Ortiz, S.R., et al. *Kona.*, 2017, 34, 44–69. doi:10.14356/kona.2017005.)

removal of inhibitory signals from immunosuppressive cells or both in combination could lyse tumor cells. The clinical success of immune checkpoint inhibitors mentioned earlier clearly demonstrates that targeting immune cells in addition to attacking the malignant cells within the tumor is a viable strategy for treating lung cancer (10).

The main immunosuppressor cells of the innate immune system are resident pulmonary macrophages and myeloid-derived suppressor cells (MDSCs). The physiological role of resident macrophages is to downregulate immune responses to antigens depositing on respiratory epithelial surfaces. MDSCs are a heterogeneous population of bone marrow–derived cells that progressively accumulate within tumors and suppress the function of effector cells, including T cells and NK cells (111). Bidirectional cross-talk between the pulmonary macrophages and MDSCs further amplifies the immunosuppressive activity. Thus, optimizing immune function in the lung requires modulation of both the effector cell–refractory tumor microenvironment and the potency of the effector cells (112).

Tumor-associated macrophages have a significant role in controlling the tumor microenvironment, and inhalation of granulocyte macrophage colony stimulating factor (GM-CSF) could activate these cells. In humans, inhaled GM-CSF (500 µg/day in 2 divided doses) has modest effects in patients with pulmonary metastasis (113). In patients with metastatic melanoma, aerosol delivery of GM-CSF may induce melanoma specific immunity, similarly to an *in vivo* dendritic cell vaccination (114). In experimental and human studies, destruction of tumor cells by activated macrophages could prolong survival.

Interleukin 2 (IL-2), Interleukin 12 (IL-12), and GM-CSF sustain the recruitment, activation, and availability of cytotoxic cells such as natural killer (NK) cells or T cells that ultimately exert antitumor activity (115,116). In experimental animals, liposomal encapsulation enhances the anticancer activity of inhaled (IL-2) compared to free IL-2. Inhalation two or three times a day of 1×10^6 units of IL-2 was found to be effective for treatment of canine osteosarcoma lung metastases (117). In metastatic renal carcinoma in humans, which can lead to death due to respiratory insufficiency, high-dose inhaled IL-2 in combination with low-dose subcutaneous IL-2 and subcutaneous IFN-α improved median survival (118). However, inhaled IL-2 alone did not achieve significant efficacy in treatment of patients with renal cancer and NSCLC. Inhaled IL-2 also had only modest effects against human metastatic lung cancers (119). A combination of low-dose inhaled IL-2 (3 × 3 million IU once daily) and monthly bolus dacarbazine injections was clinically effective in 20 patients with pulmonary metastasis from malignant melanoma (120). In five patients, inhaled IL-2 administered after resection of pulmonary metastasis (prophylaxis group) prevented development of new lung metastasis during treatment for a median duration of 24.5 months in four of them. In a preclinical model of lung metastasis induced by IV administration of osteosarcoma cells,

inhaled IL-2 combined with NK cell infusion produced significantly more regression of lung metastasis than phosphate-buffered saline (PBS) inhalation, IL-2 alone, or PBS with NK cells infusion (121).

Interferons (IFNs) are important mediators of immunity against tumors, and low doses of cIFNs stimulate the immune system against cancer cells. IFN-γ is most potent, and its effects are augmented by co-administration of Tumor Necrosis Factor-α (TNF-α) (122). Inhaled IFN-α had no efficacy in treating diffuse or locally advanced bronchoalveolar carcinoma (123).

Toll-like receptor (TLR) agonists are effective in preclinical models and in patients with malignant melanoma, renal carcinoma, and recurrent or refractory lymphoma (124). Intrapulmonary insufflation of lipopolysaccharides, TLR4 ligands, in mouse lungs induced IL-12 production by alveolar M1 macrophages without systemic effects and demonstrated antitumor effects against a Lewis carcinoma model (125).

Other investigators employed a combination of TLR3 and TLR9 agonists. Poly(I:C) is a TLR3 agonist that converts tumor-associated macrophages from a tumor-supporting (M2) to tumor counteracting (M1) function. Aerosolized Poly(I:C) combined with aerosolized CpG-ODN, a TLR 9 agonist that activates NK cells, effectively suppressed tumor growth in a B16 murine melanoma lung metastasis model (126). In a subsequent study, the investigators added an inhaled antibody directed to Ly6G and Ly6C markers to deplete MDSCs locally or inhaled IFN-γ to activate NK cells and macrophage innate cells in the lung to the inhaled TLR3/TLR9 agonist combination in an attempt to further enhance antitumor activity (127). Addition of the antibody or IFN-γ to CpG-ODN/Poly(I:C) resulted in significantly improved antitumor effects, but the combination of the antibody, IFN-γ, and CpG-ODN/Poly(I:C) did not produce additive effects to those seen with the agents administered individually with CpG-ODN/Poly(I:C) (127). Utilizing the innate immune function to modulate the tumor microenvironment offers a fresh approach to destroying tumors by immune mechanisms.

Monoclonal antibodies

Monoclonal antibodies have shown efficacy against cancer in preclinical models. Inhaled cetuximab, a chimeric IgG1 antibody targeting EGFR, accumulated within intrabronchially implanted A431 cells in mice and led to regression of tumors (128). A combination of aerosolized biotinylated cetuximab (bCet) with AvidinOX was administered to mice bearing A549 metastatic lung cancer. Prenebulization of AvidinOX followed 4 hours later by nebulized bCet produced greater reduction in tumor growth compared to mice treated with nebulized bCet alone, and tumor growth could be controlled with a bCet dose that was 1/25,000 times lower than the effective IV dose (129).

Two major concerns need to be addressed for use of inhaled monoclonal antibodies. First, although they achieve higher concentrations in the lungs, including cancerous tissues, they are rapidly cleared from the lungs within 1 to 2 days, whereas full-length antibodies administered IV have a plasma half-life of up to 3 weeks or more (130). Engineered antibody fragments have the advantages of enhanced tissue penetration, binding to cryptic epitopes, multi-specific actions, and relatively economical production within bacteria (131). However, engineered fragments, such as F(ab')2 or Fab antibody, are just as rapidly cleared from the lungs after inhalation as full-length antibodies. The residence time of such antibody fragments within the lung could be increased by PEGylation (132). Second, degradation and concentration of monoclonal antibodies occurs during aerosolization. The use of mesh nebulizers helps to preserve monoclonal antibodies compared to jet or ultrasonic nebulizers (133,134), and addition of surfactant further reduces the effects of mesh nebulization on the integrity and activity of monoclonal antibodies (134).

Chemotherapy

Systemic chemotherapy is the primary treatment option for patients with advanced-stage lung cancer. However, with systemic chemotherapy, less than 6% of the administered dose distributes to the lungs, and this may limit the concentrations of chemotherapy that are achieved in the lung (135). Inhalation of chemotherapeutic agents could greatly enhance the concentrations achieved in the lung (53,136). However, the peak blood levels achieved after inhalation are much lower than those after IV administration (53,135).

Proof-of-concept preclinical studies in animal models of primary and metastatic lung cancer demonstrate the efficacy, safety, and favorable pharmacokinetics of several inhaled chemotherapeutic agents, including DOX, cisplatin, GEM, and liposomal encapsulated forms of paclitaxel and 9-nitro-20(s)-camptothecin (9-NC) (24,137,138). In dogs with spontaneous primary and metastatic lung cancers, including sarcoma, carcinomas, and malignant melanoma, partial responses were observed to inhaled paclitaxel or DOX administered every 2 weeks. Inhalation of liposomal camptothecin and 9-NC reduced the size of human breast, colon, and lung cancer cells implanted subcutaneously in mice. Likewise, liposomal 9-NC effectively reduced metastasis in a murine malignant melanoma model, and in a nude mice model with pulmonary metastasis of human osteosarcoma cells (139). Inhalation of liposomal paclitaxel (3 days per week) was effective in reducing lung metastasis and prolonging survival in a murine renal cell carcinoma pulmonary metastasis model (140).

GEM aerosol (given two or three times a week) after osteosarcoma tumor cell inoculation in mice inhibited the growth of lung metastasis and reduced subcutaneous tumor growth, indicating a possible systemic effect of aerosolized GEM. Furthermore, in an orthotopic model of large cell undifferentiated primary lung cancer produced by implantation of NCI-H460 cancer cells in Bagg Albino (BALB/c) nude mice, administration of GEM with an endotracheal sprayer

completely inhibited tumor growth in about one-third of animals and partially inhibited growth in the remainder. While higher doses of inhaled GEM produced more profound tumor suppression, lower doses were safer and were not associated with any observed clinical or histological signs of toxicity (141). Concomitant systemic and inhaled therapy could enhance the efficacy of treatment without increasing overall toxicity.

PHARMACOKINETICS

Following aerosol administration of ^{14}C-labeled DOX in dogs, levels of radioactivity achieved in the lungs with aerosol delivery were higher, seemed to persist for longer periods, and produced significantly lower systemic radioactivity levels than those observed after IV administration (15). Similarly, liquid chromatography identified higher concentrations and slower clearance of paclitaxel from lung tissue extracts in dogs treated with inhaled liposomal paclitaxel versus IV administration of the same drug (140).

Cisplatin administered by an INC to the right caudal lung lobe of healthy dogs produced high platinum concentrations in the lung parenchyma (53). Immediately following a single inhaled dose, mean platinum levels in the lung were 44 times greater than in most other tissues, and peak blood levels were 15.6 times lower than those observed after IV infusion of a comparable dose. Later studies with inhaled liposomal cisplatin corroborated these findings (20). Kelsen and colleagues reported that serum levels of cisplatin 5 minutes after an IV dose of 100–120 mg/m^2, the dose commonly employed for treatment of osteosarcoma, ranged from 1600 to 9500 ng/mL (median 5500 ng/mL) (142). After 24 hours of IV dosing, the serum cisplatin levels ranged from 400 to 3500 ng/mL (median 1400 ng/mL) (142). In contrast, following inhalation of cisplatin, serum levels after 30 minutes ranged from 43.6 to 157.4 ng/mL (median 84.6 ng/mL) and at 18–24 hours post-dose, the levels were 47.0 to 153.5 ng/mL (median 81.9 ng/mL) (20). As expected, cisplatin levels in the lung after inhalation were much higher than after IV cisplatin administration. In three patients who had bronchoalveolar lavage (BAL) performed within 24 hours of receiving inhaled lipid cisplatin (ILC), the levels in BAL (9.4, 2951.9, and 11,201.6 ng/mL) tended to be variable but generally higher than the corresponding levels in serum (61.9, 50.2, and 80.4 ng/mL) (20). Similarly, 24 and 96 hours after instillation of cisplatin conjugated with hyaluronan into the lungs of rats, platinum levels in the lung were 5.7 times and 1.2 times higher, respectively, compared to rats receiving IV cisplatin (96). The levels of platinum in the draining lymph nodes were higher and plasma levels more sustained with a reduced peak plasma concentration after instillation compared to IV administration. After instillation, however, the animals developed patchy areas of moderate inflammation, suggesting that aerosolization may be preferable to instillation for delivering such cisplatin conjugates to the lung (96).

Resistance to anticancer agents could develop by several mechanisms, including decreased drug influx, increased drug efflux, activation of DNA repair, detoxification, and inactivation of apoptosis. A large family of transmembrane proteins, ATP-binding cassette (ABC) transporters, are ATP-dependent efflux systems that expel anticancer drugs from the cytoplasm out of the cells and reduce their intracellular concentration. These transmembrane efflux proteins include P-glycoprotein (P-gp), multidrug resistance-associated proteins (MRPs), and breast cancer resistant protein (BRCP) and appear to account for most of the reported multidrug resistance in humans. The overexpression of specific ABC transporters in cancer cell lines and tumors produces multidrug resistance, which is the major factor contributing to the failure of chemotherapy (143).

PRECLINICAL EFFICACY

The aerosolization process does not affect the cytotoxic effect of the chemotherapy as shown by similar levels of growth inhibition with nebulized and non-nebulized gemcitabine in NCI-H460 and A549 NSCLC cell lines (144). *In vivo* efficacy of aerosol chemotherapy has been evaluated in mouse models for lung metastasis treated with inhaled liposomal 9-nitrocamptothecin (L-9NC) (139), inhaled GEM (145), or inhaled liposomal paclitaxel (140). Weekly inhalation of GEM achieved complete or partial inhibition of tumor growth after intrabronchial implantation of large cell undifferentiated primary lung cancer cells (NCI-H460) in BALB/c nude mice (141). Aerosolized azacytidine not only suppressed the growth of lung tumors engrafted in nude rats, it exhibited a longer half-life within tumors after inhalation compared to systemic administration (146).

In dogs with primary lung cancer or lung metastases, inhaled paclitaxel and DOX resulted in tumor shrinkage in 25% of the dogs, without producing adverse effects commonly seen with IV chemotherapy (19). Aerosol administration of GEM to dogs who naturally developed lung metastases from osteosarcoma was well tolerated, but did not produce any cures and did not prolong survival among the treated dogs (147).

While earlier studies demonstrated the feasibility and relative safety of targeted direct local administration of chemotherapeutic agents to the lung, employing formulations designed specifically for inhalation rather than the IV formulations of cisplatin and GEM employed in the previous investigations could alleviate concerns about local toxicity. More recently developed formulations are suitable for inhalation and do not cause local toxicity. For example, Feng and colleagues insufflated freeze-dried porous microspheres of PLGA loaded with DOX and paclitaxel into the lungs of C57BL/6J mice implanted with B16-F10 melanoma cells (148). The combination of DOX and paclitaxel had a synergistic effect in reducing the number of tumor lesions in the lungs of the mice without causing histological evidence of damage to healthy alveoli. Other novel formulations that could enhance the safety of inhaled chemotherapeutic agents while preserving their efficacy for treating lung cancers are under active investigation (149,150).

INHALED CHEMOTHERAPEUTIC AGENTS

Treatment with aerosolized 5-FU, GEM, azacytidine, DOX, L-9NC, liposomal paclitaxel and platinum agents has shown activity against lung cancer and metastasis to the lung in preclinical studies. Subsequent phase I/II clinical trials have assessed the safety and anticancer effect of several chemotherapeutic agents, including inhaled 5-FU, GEM, L-9NC, DOX, and platinum agents (Table 11.2).

Nucleoside analogs

5-FU is a fluoropyrimidine that acts as an antimetabolite inhibiting DNA and ribonucleic acid (RNA) synthesis. In the first study of inhaled chemotherapy in humans, Tatsumura and colleagues observed that 5-FU concentrations in the airways and regional lymph nodes were at therapeutic levels while the serum contained only trace levels of the drug (136). Interestingly, the levels of 5-FU were significantly higher in the tumor tissue than in the normal lung tissue. Six of ten patients with unresectable lung cancer who were previously untreated and received inhaled 5-FU responded to therapy with no significant adverse effects from these treatments (136).

GEM belongs to the same class of drugs as 5-FU. Inhaled GEM administered once a week for 9 weeks to 11 patients with lung cancer resulted in a partial response in one patient and stable disease in four patients (63).

Doxorubicin

Inhaled DOX has shown preclinical activity against both primary lung cancer and lung metastasis. A phase I trial evaluated the safety of increasing doses of inhaled DOX in 53 patients with lung metastases (151). Pulmonary toxicities were the most frequently reported adverse events, and five patients had severe adverse effects ($\geq$ Grade 3). One patient had a partial response and eight patients had stable disease.

In a subsequent phase I/II study, patients with treatment-naive advanced stage NSCLC were treated with the maximal tolerated dose (MTD) for inhaled DOX (6 mg/m^2) along with IV cisplatin and docetaxel (152). The investigators reported a 29% response rate (7 responders out of 24 evaluable patients) and stable disease rate of 54%. Toxicities were primarily due to systemic chemotherapy, and pulmonary toxicities were generally mild (grades 1–2). In this study, the addition of inhaled DOX to IV chemotherapy did not result in significant improvement in treatment outcomes, and the authors did not recommend further evaluation of this combination (152).

Liposomal-9-nitro camptothecin

A Phase I trial evaluated the feasibility and safety of inhaled L-9NC in the treatment of patients with primary or metastatic lung cancer (153). Patients tolerated a dose of 13.3 μg/kg/day of L-9NC administered on days 1–5 every week for a period of 6 weeks. The maximally tolerated dose was 20 μg/kg/day. Two patients with metastatic endometrial cancer had partial response to treatment, and the therapy was

Table 11.2 Clinical studies of inhaled chemotherapy

First author	Year	Chemotherapy agent/delivery device	Disease state	Evaluation	Outcome
Tatsumura, T	1993	5-FU nebulizer	Lung cancer	Bronchoscopy, HPLC, histopathology	Aerosolized 5-FU accumulated at therapeutic concentrations in airways and regional lymph nodes. Partial responses in 60% of patients without significant pulmonary or systemic side effects.
Verschraegen, CF	2004	9-NC liposomal nebulizer	Primary lung cancer or metastases to lung	HRCT, blood, BAL, urine analysis	Chemical pharyngitis was dose-limiting. Other side effects included nausea, vomiting, cough, bronchial irritation, fatigue, and reversible fall in FEV_1. Partial remissions observed in some patients.
Wittgen, BP	2007	Cis liposomal nebulizer	Lung cancer	Blood, pulmonary function, chest x-ray, chest CT, PK, RECIST	Dose-escalating study in 17 patients with primary or metastatic lung cancer. No dose-limiting toxicity at maximum delivered dose. Generally reversible fall in pulmonary function, nausea and vomiting, but no other systemic toxicity was reported. Stability of disease was observed in 12 patients.
Otterson, GA	2007	DOX nebulizer	Metastases to lung	CT, RECIST, HPLC, V/Q, blood	Phase I study of 53 patients with cancer metastatic to lungs. Increasing doses of doxorubicin (0.4–9.4 mg/m^2) were given every 3 weeks. Pulmonary toxicity was dose-limiting. Partial responses observed in some patients.
Otterson, GA	2010	DOX nebulizer	Advanced NSCLC	CT, RECIST, V/Q	Phase I/II dose escalation study of inhaled DOX in combination with i.v. docetaxel and cisplatin. 43 patients with metastatic NSCLC were treated, with partial responses in 6 patients and complete response in 1 patient, some patients developed late decreases in pulmonary function.
Lemarie, E	2011	GEM vibrating mesh nebulizer with a vertical chamber spacer	NSCLC	Gamma scintigraphy, blood, chest x-ray, chest CT, head CT, pulmonary function tests, PK	Patients with NSCLC (n = 11) unresponsive to chemotherapy were treated with inhaled GEM doses between 1 and 4 mg/Kg body weight. A maximum dose of 3 mg/Kg/week was safe. Side-effects included cough, dyspnea, vomiting, and bronchospasm. Partial responses observed in some patients.
Zarogoulidis, P	2011	CARBO nebulizer	NSCLC	HRCT, RECIST, blood	Sixty patients with untreated NSCLC received i.v. docetaxel and either inhaled carbo, inhaled and i.v. carbo, or i.v. carbo. The combination of inhaled and i.v. carbo prolonged survival. Fever and cough were common side effects.
Chou, AJ	2013	Cis liposomal nebulizer	Recurrent osteosarcoma with metastases to the lungs	PFT, blood, urine, V/Q scan, CT	19 children with high-grade metastatic osteosarcoma. Nausea, vomiting, dyspnea, wheezing, and cough.

5 FU: 5 fluorouracil; 9NC: 9-nitro camptothecin; BAL: bronchoalveolar lavage; CARBO: carboplatin; Cis: cisplatin; CT: computer tomography; DOX: doxorubicin; FEV_1: forced expiratory volume in 1 second; GEM: gemcitabine; HPLC: high-performance liquid chromatography; HRCT: high-resolution computer tomography; NSCLC: non-small-cell lung cancer; PK: pharmacokinetics; RECIST: response evaluation criteria in solid tumors; V/Q: ventilation/perfusion scan.

effective in treating tumors outside the lung (153). Overall, inhaled L-9NC was well tolerated with an acceptable safety profile; however, no further clinical development of this formulation has been reported.

Platinum agents

Cisplatin and carboplatin are the primary treatment agents used in several combination chemotherapy regimens for systemic treatment of lung cancer. In a Phase I study, patients showed good tolerance to inhaled cisplatin encapsulated in microscopic phospholipid spheres or Sustained Release Lipid Inhalation Targeting (SLIT)™ (154). The serum levels of cisplatin varied between low to undetectable in most patients. At the time of evaluation, 12 of 17 patients achieved stable disease (138). Cisplatin lipid complex was administered to 19 pediatric patients with pulmonary metastases from recurrent osteosarcoma in a Phase I/II study (20). In the eight patients with non-bulky disease (size of lesions ≤2 cm), one had partial response and two patients had stable disease. Because dose-limiting toxicity was not reported in the clinical trials reported with SLIT™ (20,154), further studies are needed to determine if higher doses or use of alternative formulations of cisplatin could improve the efficacy of treatment.

Carboplatin is one of the frontline agents for treatment of advanced stage NSCLC. Sixty patients with advanced stage NSCLC were randomized into 3 groups. The first group received IV carboplatin and docetaxel (control arm), whereas the second group received IV docetaxel, two-thirds of the calculated carboplatin IV, and one-third carboplatin dose as an inhalant. The third group received the entire dose of carboplatin administered in the aerosol form along with IV docetaxel. Patients receiving both IV and inhaled carboplatin (group 2) had better survival outcomes compared to the control arm—275 days versus 211 days (64). There was a trend toward improvement in the median overall survival for patients receiving inhaled carboplatin with IV docetaxel.

Development of resistance to chemotherapeutic agents is a frequent cause of treatment failure and tumor recurrence. Several approaches to reduce the development of resistance, such as adding pump and nonpump suppressors to inhaled chemotherapy (155) or combining an active agent with an appropriate drug carrier that can specifically target sites in the respiratory tract where drug transporter genes are highly expressed are under active investigation.

Paclitaxel

Paclitaxel is a hydrophobic drug that achieves high concentrations in the lung after aerosolization. In liposomal formulations, paclitaxel could leak and form crystals on the surface. Likewise, the stress of freeze drying could induce leakage of paclitaxel from liposomes. However, inhalation of paclitaxel alone did not produce complete arrest of tumor growth (140), whereas co-administration with cyclosporine A, which has a high affinity for P-glycoprotein and prevents active elimination of other drugs, produced

significant reduction in the size and number of tumors (156). Pulmonary administration of polymeric micelles of paclitaxel-loaded poly (ethylene oxide)-block-distearoylphosphatidylethanolamine (PEG-DSPE) produced much greater accumulation of drug in the lung with lower systemic distribution compared to IV administration of the same formulation or intratracheal administration of Taxol (a commercially available formulation of paclitaxel) (157). Formulation of paclitaxel with an amphiphilic block copolymer using poly-glycolide-ε-caprolactone with PEG and tocopherol succinate produced greater cytoxicity in an *in vitro* A549 model compared to a commercial taxol compound or free paclitaxel (158). A pH-responsive liposomal formulation of paclitaxel employed DPPC and 1,2-dioleoyl-*sn*-glycero-3-phosphoethanolamine (DOPE), an unsaturated phospholipid that functions similarly to surfactant protein B in endogenous surfactant. DOPE acts as a fusogenic lipid that is able to release the drug at the lower pH environment in tumors or inside cytosolic endosome/lysosome organelles. Nebulization of this nanoformulation was superior in inhibiting the growth of pulmonary metastasis of melanoma (B16-F10) in mice compared to IV treatment with two commercial formulations of paclitaxel (Taxol and Abraxane). Moreover, the inhaled formulation was not associated with significant pulmonary toxicity (159).

Gene therapy

Specialized constructs of DNA delivered to cancer cells could correct specific abnormalities in mutated genes that are responsible for development of cancer or those conferring resistance to chemotherapy. Other approaches target genes that induce immune response to tumors, or those inducing apoptosis in tumor cells. Liquid suspended gene particles are difficult to nebulize at concentrations of DNA >5 mg/mL because of their viscosity. Moreover, naked DNA undergoes fragmentation with the shear stresses during nebulization; vectors protect DNA from degradation and facilitate direct transfer of genes to the patient's tissues. These vectors are typically composed of viral capsid, or cationic lipids, polymers, or peptides carry genes within plasmid DNA. Removal of genes required for replication from viral delivery systems enhances their safety. Although these replication-deficient viruses are efficient at transfection, their clinical use is challenging because they are inherently immunogenic. In Phase I and Phase II studies of patients with lung cancer, replacing p53 tumor suppressor gene using an adenoviral vector by intratumoral injection did not produce promising results (160,161).

Nonviral carriers are safer than viral carriers, but they have lower transfection efficiency. Among the several cationic polymers, polyethyleinimine (PEI) achieves higher transfection efficiency both in tissue culture and *in vivo*. Selective gene expression occurs in the lungs of mice after IL-12 gene administration in PEI-based polyplexes for treatment of osteosarcoma lung metastasis (162). The growth of lung metastasis was inhibited by aerosolized PEI-p53 complexes, and animals survived longer than the control group (163). Similarly, a modified PEI-p53 complex (p53CD[1–366]) or PEI-IL12 interfered with the growth of osteosarcoma lung metastasis without producing toxicity or signs of inflammation even after repeated exposures (162,164). However, the cytotoxicity of PEI depends on its molecular weight and configuration (165,166). Several cationic lipids, such as dioleoyltrimethylammonium propane (DOTAP) and dioleyloxypropyltrimethylammonium (DOTMA), have been employed as gene carriers, with DOTMA having higher transfection efficiency than DOTAP. Mixing cationic lipids with neutral lipids facilitates formation of liposomes and enhances their disassembly after uptake into the cell. Notably, a significant drawback of cationic lipoplexes is that high doses could trigger inflammatory responses in the lung. To avoid such toxicity, investigators employed biodegradable polymer-based NPs, which have a prolonged residence time in the lung, as gene carriers.

Several investigators have successfully delivered genes by inhalation using these nonviral carriers. Inhalation of p53 tumor suppressor gene in lipoplexes containing polylysine and protamine reduced lung metastasis in a murine model of malignant melanoma (167). Likewise, upregulation of beclin-1, a tumor suppressor gene involved in autophagy, sensitized tumor cells to radiation therapy (168). Another approach involves transfection of tumors with a gene that codes for a specific enzyme that transforms a benign drug into a toxic metabolite that causes cell death ("suicide gene"). For example, transduction of herpes simplex virus 1 thymidine kinase (HSVtk) gene makes cells susceptible to ganciclovir, a nucleoside analogue, which is normally poorly metabolized by mammalian cells. HSVtk converts ganciclovir to a metabolite that causes cell death by interfering with DNA replication. Clinical trials have employed an adenoviral vector to transduce HSVtk by intratumoral injection into mesothelioma with partial success (169). Inhalation of phosphatase and tensin homologue deleted on chromosome 10 (PTEN) tumor suppressor gene with glycosylated conjugated PEI resulted in expression of a functional PTEN protein in the lung with reduced phosphorylation of its target protein and apoptosis in transduced lung cells (170).

Various other physical techniques to facilitate DNA uptake into cells by transiently increasing membrane permeability involve application of electrical impulses (electroporation) or ultrasound energy (sonoporation).

The combination of conventional chemotherapy with inhaled gene therapy has additive effects. For example, sequential administration of aerosolized PEI-p53 and 9NC-DLPC (dilauroylphosphatidylcholine liposome form of 9NC) showed additive activity in inhibiting the growth of B16-F10 tumor lung metastasis in mice (171). The transfer of ABCA 10 transgene, a membrane protein that modulates drug absorption, using adenoviral type 5 (dEI/E3), a cytomegalovirus promoter, increased the concentration and efficacy of inhaled cisplatin (155).

Despite recent advances, gene therapy for lung cancer needs to overcome several barriers to achieve meaningful success. Efficient delivery of the therapeutic gene to specific dysfunctional tumor cells is a significant hurdle. Carriers that target specific cells by utilizing receptor-ligand interactions must recognize receptors on the apical airway epithelial cell surface because receptors on the basal-lateral surface may not be accessible *in vivo*. Even after cellular uptake, the genetic material must overcome several intracellular barriers before protein translation occurs. Finally, effective suppression of tumors may require repeated dosing, and vectors employed for gene delivery must be safe for both acute and chronic administration.

Antisense therapy

In this approach, a targeted oligonucleotide that reduces transcription of complementary messenger ribonucleic acid (mRNA) inhibits gene expression (172). Plasmid or viral vector mediated transfer of small interfering RNA (siRNA) or short hairpin RNA (shRNA) precursors was reported in animal models. A chitosan-graft 1.8 K PEI copolymer has the advantage of reducing toxicity of PEI and enhancing transfection efficacy of chitosan (57). In a B16-F10 model of lung metastasis, nebulized PEI-WTI (Wilms tumor gene) RNAi complexes reduced the number and size of lung metastasis, probably through inhibition of angiogenesis (173). Use of poly(amidoamine) (PAMAM) dendrimers (G4NH2) as carriers to complex siRNA efficiently target and silence genes expressed in A549 cells (174).

Delivery of a lung cancer cell-target shRNA to inhibit the Akt signaling pathway suppressed the growth of lung tumors in mice. In mice bearing breast cancer pulmonary metastasis, inhalation of small hairpin osteopontin downregulated osteopontin expression, and reduced migration, angiogenesis, and invasion of breast cancer cells (175). Moreover, aerosolized delivery of shAkt1 complexed with a biocompatible hyperbranched polyspermine (HSPSE) reduced tumor size in a mouse k-RAS^{LAI} lung cancer model (176). However, it is difficult to achieve adequate concentrations of these molecules within tumors, and nontransduced cells within the tumor show limited bystander effects (177).

Combining inhaled chemotherapy and antisense therapy (178) is another attractive approach. LHRH-targeted nanolipid carriers combining delivery of DOX or paclitaxel with siRNA targeted to MRP1 and BCL2, as inhibitors of both pump and nonpump drug resistance, significantly enhanced the cytotoxicity of the complex (178).

Bacteria/cells

DNA could be effectively delivered by employing the innate ability of bacteria to invade cells. Delivery of genetic material by bacteria is achieved by either of two approaches: (1) specific replication of bacteria within tumors or (2) intracellular transfer of plasmids within cancer cells (bactofection) by various bacterial species, such as *Salmonella, Escherichia coli,* and *Listeria* species. Anaerobic and facultatively anaerobic bacteria specifically target the relative hypoxic environment within tumors. Bacteria also show chemotaxis to necrotic regions within tumors, and bacterial entry and colonization within tumors is facilitated by aberrant "leaky" vasculature and local immune suppression. Several bacterial species (*Bifidobacterium, Salmonella, Escherichia coli, Vibrio cholera*, and *Listeria monocytogenes*) are capable of tumor-specific growth after IV administration, and they transport and amplify genes within tumors (179). However, the inhalation of bacteria has not been employed for DNA delivery and the potential for environmental spread of the vector will need to be carefully addressed if such a delivery mechanism is employed in clinical practice.

Although normal cell drug uptake is generally considered a barrier to drug transport efficiency, tumor-associated macrophages and stem cells have been harnessed for drug delivery (180,181). For example, resident macrophages preferentially take up a systemically administered polymer–platinum prodrug NP in an HT1080 fibrosarcoma xenograft in nude mice (181). Slow drug release from these cells contributed to the antitumor effect of this NP. At the experimental endpoint, tumors of animals treated with the NP were two times smaller than control-treated tumors. Selective depletion of macrophages reduced drug uptake by two and reduced the inhibition of tumor growth by the NP.

CLINICAL USE OF INHALED ANTICANCER AGENTS

Immunologics/cytokines

Selective activation of local immunity in the lungs to control metastases is an active line of investigation. Inhaled IL-2 alone given for treatment of patients with renal cancer and NSCLC did not produce impressive results, but it was more effective when combined with systemic low dose IL-2 and IFN-α, high dose systemic IL-2, or chemotherapy (182). In patients with metastatic melanoma, aerosol delivery of GM-CSF has modest clinical effects, but it may induce melanoma specific immunity. The use of inhaled monoclonal antibodies, such as cetuximab, merits further study because they retain activity after aerosolization and are able to penetrate into orthotopic lung tumors in Balb/c nude mice.

Chemotherapy

The efficacy of inhaled chemotherapy in a clinical setting has been reported by a few investigators (Table 11.2). Inhaled 5-fluorouracil (5-FU) achieved tumor tissue levels that were 5 to 15 times higher than those in normal lung; the levels were higher than those needed for anti-neoplastic activity, and 5-FU alone or in combination with other chemotherapy agents was partially effective in patients with NSCLC (136). Inhaled liposomal 9-NC produced partial responses in lung tumors and liver metastasis in patients

with pulmonary metastasis from a variety of tumors (153). A liposomal formulation of cisplatin (sustained release lipid inhalation targeting [SLIT]) given over 1–4 consecutive days in 21-day treatment cycles to patients with lung cancer stabilized the disease in 12 out of 17 patients and was not associated with systemic side effects (154). In 11 patients with NSCLC (including 6 patients with diffuse bronchoalveolar carcinoma) who were unresponsive to previous chemotherapy, weekly inhalation of GEM (0.5 or 1 mg/Kg) produced a minor response in one patient and stable disease in 4 patients (63). Likewise, a survival benefit was noted in NSCLC patients after use of inhaled carboplatin in addition to systemic carboplatin in combination with IV docetaxel (64). In early stage (Stage II) NSCLC patients who received inhaled cisplatin 2 hours prior to surgery, the subcarinal lymph node had higher concentrations of cisplatin than those in blood (183). Thus, inhaled drugs could diffuse from the alveoli into the lymphatic circulation and regional lymph nodes. Whether inhaled drugs could achieve adequate concentration to lyse cancer cells within lymph nodes needs further evaluation.

In patients with metastatic osteosarcoma limited to the lungs, inhalation of liposomal cisplatin produced sustained benefit in some patients with less bulky disease without producing toxic effects that commonly occur after IV cisplatin administration (20).

Gene therapy

There has been much progress in developing vectors for gene delivery, and several promising experimental approaches have not yet been effectively applied in clinical practice. Replacement of a mutated or absent tumor suppressor gene should lead to suppression of tumor growth or tumor cell death. Several early phase clinical trials have evaluated restoration of wild type p53 in lung tumor cells. These approaches have employed direct intratumoral injection with adenoviral vectors and have shown partial responses, but the benefits over chemotherapy or radiotherapy alone have not been convincing. Promising gene therapy approaches involve stimulation of an endogenous immune response to the tumor, and combining antisense therapy with chemotherapy (178).

ADVERSE EFFECTS

Most adverse events of inhaled chemotherapy are due to direct local effects of the chemotherapeutic agents on the upper and lower respiratory tract. After IV administration, chemotherapeutic agents have the potential to produce a variety of pulmonary toxic effects, including some that are severe and life threatening. After inhaled chemotherapy, nonpulmonary side effects are infrequent. The observed side effects include metallic taste, cough, weight loss, neurotoxicity, and cardiotoxicity (Table 11.3).

Among a variety of agents given by inhalation, dose-limiting pulmonary toxicity occurred only with DOX.

Table 11.3 Adverse effects with inhaled chemotherapy

Type of adverse effect	Symptoms	Severity	Remarks
Respiratory	Cough, hoarseness, bronchoconstriction, dyspnea, fall in pulmonary function, acute lung injury	Dose-limiting lung toxicity can occur but is uncommon	Pre-treatment with bronchodilators and corticosteroids is recommended
Gastrointestinal (GI)	Glossitis, pharyngitis, nausea, vomiting,	Glossitis and pharyngitis could be dose limiting	GI side effects are common
Hematological	Anemia, cytopenias	Hematological effects are uncommon	Neutropenia may occur with repeated dosing
Biochemical	No significant changes	Biochemical changes are rare	Inhalation of chemotherapy is associated with very few biochemical derangements
Miscellaneous	Metallic taste, fever, fatigue	Usually not dose limiting	These side effects are more frequent. Other systemic side effects, e.g., ototoxicity, occur infrequently

Several symptoms such as cough, wheezing, shortness of breath, bronchospasm, and chest pain occur with varying frequency after inhalation of chemotherapy. An alveolar interstitial pattern on radiographs is associated with histological findings of moderate fibrosis (53,62). Occasionally, bilateral ground glass opacities and hypoxemia are reported after inhaled chemotherapy. Severe pulmonary toxicity has been observed with inhaled DOX (151), GEM (63), and liposomal cisplatin (20). Prior administration of inhaled bronchodilators and corticosteroids could mitigate bronchoconstriction and drop in pulmonary function (20,63,151,152). Nebulized liposomal 9-NC did not produce significant toxic effects in patients with lung cancer (153).

Adverse effects due to inhaled nonchemotherapeutic agents include reduction in forced vital capacity, bilateral infiltrates, pleural effusion, and bronchospasm with inhaled GM-CSF in patients with metastatic disease (113,114). In contrast, other investigators have reported only minor toxicity in patients who received inhaled GM-CSF. Inhalation of IL-2 is limited by the development of pulmonary vascular leakage, which is dose-, route-, and formulation-dependent (182). Adenoviral vectors tend to create neutralizing antibodies and can be associated with significant local and systemic inflammation involving neutralizing antibodies and cytotoxic lymphocytes. In contrast, adeno-associated virus has not been associated with any significant toxicity. Nonviral vectors and polymers exhibit cytotoxicity that is mainly due to their strong electrostatic charge. The molecular weight of the polymers plays an important role, with higher molecular weight polymers producing higher incidence of adverse respiratory effects (165,166). Systemic absorption of inhaled NPs and their distribution to various body organs raises concerns about toxicity. Cytotoxicity, allergic, and inflammatory reactions are more likely with particles smaller than 100 nm in size compared to larger particles with similar composition. NPs composed of endogenous chemicals, such as dipalmitoylphosphatidyl-choline, have less potential for toxicity.

LIMITATIONS OF INHALED ANTICANCER AGENTS

Environmental contamination

To minimize occupational exposure of healthcare workers or others who are administering inhaled chemotherapeutic agents, a well-ventilated room with a HEPA filter air cleaning system for aerosol administration is mandatory. However, Verschraegen and colleagues allowed patients to take their inhaled chemotherapy at home (153). Establishing the safety of domiciliary chemotherapy could have enormous implications for convenience and cost of treatment.

Unanswered questions

Investigations are ongoing to establish the optimal drug regimens, formulations, and methods of inhaled drug delivery for treatment of patients with lung cancer. When inhaled agents are used as adjuncts, whether they should be given before (neo-adjuvant), concurrently with, or after (adjuvant) other forms of treatment has not been established. Future investigations will need to clarify if inhalation targeted only to the tumor site is more effective and less toxic compared to drug deposition in both lungs. Focused investigations could elucidate which tumor types (primary/secondary) respond best to inhalational treatment, whether such therapy is more effective at an early or late stage of the disease, and if inhaled therapy effectively treats micrometastases in the lungs and at other sites following lymphatic or vascular spread of the tumor. Successfully addressing these questions with well-designed clinical trials will aid in clarifying the role of inhalational anticancer therapy in clinical practice.

CONCLUSION

- Several different agents, including immunologics/cytokines, monoclonal antibodies, chemotherapy, gene therapy, antisense therapy, or gene transfer by bacterial infection, alone or in combination, have been employed for treatment of primary or metastatic cancer in the lung.
- Aerosolized chemotherapy could target centrally located tumors with limited invasion or tumors that have relapsed after surgery as an adjunct to other well-established methods of treating lung malignancies.
- Inhaled chemotherapy also appears to be an attractive option for treatment of bronchoalveolar carcinoma, a peripheral tumor that can be multifocal and spreads along alveolar walls, or multiple pulmonary metastases.
- Challenges to using inhaled anticancer formulations include the need for relatively large doses that lead to long administration times; delivering aerosol to the site of the tumor, especially past areas of airway obstruction; achieving adequate drug release within or in close proximity to the tumor; and adequate drug penetration into larger tumors. If the drug is rapidly absorbed into the systemic circulation, it may need frequent administration or it may need to be reformulated to prolong its residence time in the lung.
- Patients recruited in many oncology trials are often those who have failed other standard treatments and have a poor outcome. Although this is appropriate from a safety viewpoint, efficacy may be better demonstrated in patients with an early disease (TNM Stage I or Stage II). However, surgical resection is the preferred treatment for early stage lung cancer; other treatment modalities are the exception rather than the rule. Alternative options are generally considered only for patients who are not surgical candidates.
- The effects of inhaled drugs in combination should be tested in human studies because doublet therapy is the cornerstone of systemic therapy for lung cancer. Targeted inhalation therapy of lung tumors could improve the duration and quality of life, even if the patient ultimately succumbs to the disease.
- Inhaled anticancer agents preserve their efficacy after aerosolization, and have minimal toxicity on the respiratory tract.
- Future innovations in inhaled formulations of anticancer agents hope to achieve targeted deposition at the site of the tumor with agents that readily permeate tumor cells and show prolonged effects within tumors. Such approaches could significantly improve the prognosis for patients with advanced NSCLC.

REFERENCES

1. Siegel RL, Miller KD, Jemal A. Cancer Statistics 2017. *CA: A Cancer Journal for Clinicians* 2017;6791. Epub 7–30. doi:10.3322/caac.21387.

2. Didkowska J, Wojciechowska U, Manczuk M, Lobaszewski J. Lung cancer epidemiology: Contemporary and future challenges worldwide. *Annals of Translational Medicine.* 2016;4(8):150. Epub 2016/05/20. doi:10.21037/atm.2016.03.11. PubMed PMID: 27195268; PMCID: PMC4860480.

3. Torre LA, Siegel RL, Jemal A. Lung cancer statistics. *Advances in Experimental Medicine and Biology.* 2016;893:1–19. Epub 2015/12/17. doi:10.1007/978-3-319-24223-1_1. PubMed PMID: 26667336.

4. American Cancer Society . Key statistics for lung cancer. Available at https://www.cancer.org/cancer/non-small-cell-lung-cancer/about/key-statistics.html.

5. Rami-Porta R, Asamura H, Travis WD, Rusch VW. Lung cancer—Major changes in the American Joint Committee on Cancer eighth edition cancer staging manual. *CA: A Cancer Journal for Clinicians.* 2017;67(2):138–155. Epub 2017/02/01. doi:10.3322/caac.21390. PubMed PMID: 28140453.

6. Detterbeck FC. The eighth edition TNM stage classification for lung cancer: What does it mean on main street? *The Journal of Thoracic and Cardiovascular Surgery.* 2018;155(1):356–359. Epub 2017/10/25. doi:10.1016/j.jtcvs.2017.08.138. PubMed PMID: 29061464.

7. Leong D, Rai R, Nguyen B, Lee A, Yip D. Advances in adjuvant systemic therapy for non-small-cell lung cancer. *World Journal of Clinical Oncology.* 2014;5(4):633–645. Epub 2014/10/11. doi:10.5306/wjco.v5.i4.633. PubMed PMID: 25302167; PMCID: PMC4129528.

8. SEER Cancer Statistics Review: National Cancer Institute; 1975–2014. Available from https://seer.cancer.gov/csr/1975_2014.

9. Du L, S. Herbst R, Morgensztern D. Immunotherapy in lung cancer *Hematology/Oncology Clinics.* 2017;31:131–141. doi:10.1016/j.hoc.2016.08.004.

10. Vachani A, Sequist LV, Spira A. AJRCCM: 100-Year anniversary. The shifting landscape for lung cancer: Past, present, and future. *American Journal of Respiratory and Critical Care Medicine.* 2017;195(9):1150–1160. Epub 2017/05/02. doi:10.1164/rccm.201702-0433CI. PubMed PMID: 28459327; PMCID: PMC5439022.

11. Patel JD, Hensing TA, Rademaker A, Hart EM, Blum MG, Milton DT, Bonomi PD. Phase II study of pemetrexed and carboplatin plus bevacizumab with maintenance pemetrexed and bevacizumab as first-line therapy for nonsquamous non-small-cell lung cancer. *Journal of Clinical Oncology: Official Journal of the American*

Society of Clinical Oncology. 2009;27(20):3284–3289. Epub 2009/05/13. doi:10.1200/jco.2008.20.8181. PubMed PMID: 19433684.

12. Li C, Fang R, Sun Y, Han X, Li F, Gao B, Iafrate AJ, Liu XY, Pao W, Chen H, Ji H. Spectrum of oncogenic driver mutations in lung adenocarcinomas from East Asian never smokers. *PLoS One.* 2011;6(11):e28204. Epub 2011/12/06. doi:10.1371/journal.pone.0028204. PubMed PMID: 22140546; PMCID: PMC3227646.

13. Solomon BJ, Mok T, Kim DW, Wu YL, Nakagawa K, Mekhail T, Felip E et al. First-line crizotinib versus chemotherapy in ALK-positive lung cancer. *The New England Journal of Medicine.* 2014;371(23):2167–2177. Epub 2014/12/04. doi:10.1056/NEJMoa1408440. PubMed PMID: 25470694.

14. Hirsch FR, Suda K, Wiens J, Bunn PA, Jr. New and emerging targeted treatments in advanced non-small-cell lung cancer. *Lancet.* 2016;388(10048):1012–1024. Epub 2016/09/07. doi:10.1016/s0140-6736(16)31473-8. PubMed PMID: 27598681.

15. Sharma S, White D, Imondi AR, Placke ME, Vail DM, Kris MG. Development of inhalational agents for oncologic use. *Journal of Clinical Oncology: Official Journal of the American Society of Clinical Oncology.* 2001;19(6):1839–1847. Epub 2001/03/17. doi:10.1200/jco.2001.19.6.1839. PubMed PMID: 11251016.

16. Dhand R. Inhaled anticancer agents. In: *Advances in Pulmonary Drug Delivery*, H.-K. Chan, H.K. and Kwok, P. (Eds.). CRC Press, LLC, Taylor & Francis Group, Boca Raton, FL, 2016, Chapter 5, pp. 67–92.

17. Dolovich MB, Dhand R. Aerosol drug delivery: Developments in device design and clinical use. *Lancet.* 2011;377(9770):1032–1045. Epub 2010/11/03. doi:10.1016/s0140-6736(10)60926-9. PubMed PMID: 21036392.

18. Minchinton AI, Tannock IF. Drug penetration in solid tumours. *Nature Reviews Cancer.* 2006;6(8):583–592. Epub 2006/07/25. doi:10.1038/nrc1893. PubMed PMID: 16862189.

19. Hershey AE, Kurzman ID, Forrest LJ, Bohling CA, Stonerook M, Placke ME, Imondi AR, Vail DM. Inhalation chemotherapy for macroscopic primary or metastatic lung tumors: Proof of principle using dogs with spontaneously occurring tumors as a model. *Clinical Cancer Research: An Official Journal of the American Association for Cancer Research.* 1999;5(9):2653–2659. Epub 1999/09/28. PubMed PMID: 10499645.

20. Chou AJ, Gupta R, Bell MD, Riewe KO, Meyers PA, Gorlick R. Inhaled lipid cisplatin (ILC) in the treatment of patients with relapsed/progressive osteosarcoma

metastatic to the lung. *Pediatric Blood & Cancer.* 2013;60(4):580–586. Epub 2012/12/21. doi:10.1002/pbc.24438. PubMed PMID: 23255417.

21. Roche N, Dekhuijzen PN. The evolution of pressurized metered-dose inhalers from early to modern devices. *Journal of Aerosol Medicine and Pulmonary Drug Delivery.* 2016;29(4):311–327. Epub 2016/01/30. doi:10.1089/jamp.2015.1232. PubMed PMID: 26824873.

22. Stein SW, Thiel CG. The history of therapeutic aerosols: A chronological review. *Journal of Aerosol Medicine and Pulmonary Drug Delivery.* 2017;30(1):20–41. Epub 2016/10/18. doi:10.1089/jamp.2016.1297. PubMed PMID: 27748638; PMCID: PMC5278812.

23. Darquenne C. Aerosol deposition in health and disease. *Journal of Aerosol Medicine and Pulmonary Drug Delivery.* 2012;25(3):140–147. Epub 2012/06/13. doi:10.1089/jamp.2011.0916. PubMed PMID: 22686623; PMCID: PMC3417302.

24. Gagnadoux F, Hureaux J, Vecellio L, Urban T, Le Pape A, Valo I, Montharu J, Leblond V, Boisdron-Celle M, Lerondel S, Majoral C, Diot P, Racineux JL, Lemarie E. Aerosolized chemotherapy. *Journal of Aerosol Medicine and Pulmonary Drug Delivery.* 2008;21(1):61–70. Epub 2008/06/04. doi:10.1089/jamp.2007.0656. PubMed PMID: 18518832.

25. Patton JS, Brain JD, Davies LA, Fiegel J, Gumbleton M, Kim KJ, Sakagami M, Vanbever R, Ehrhardt C. The particle has landed—characterizing the fate of inhaled pharmaceuticals. *Journal of Aerosol Medicine and Pulmonary Drug Delivery.* 2010;23 Suppl 2:S71–S87. Epub 2010/12/08. doi:10.1089/jamp.2010.0836. PubMed PMID: 21133802.

26. Deffebach ME, Charan NB, Lakshminarayan S, Butler J. The bronchial circulation. Small, but a vital attribute of the lung. *The American Review of Respiratory Disease.* 1987;135(2):463–481. Epub 1987/02/01. doi:10.1164/arrd.1987.135.2.463. PubMed PMID: 3544986.

27. Ribatti D, Nico B, Crivellato E, Vacca A. The structure of the vascular network of tumors. *Cancer Letters.* 2007;248(1):18–23. Epub 2006/08/02. doi:10.1016/j.canlet.2006.06.007. PubMed PMID: 16879908.

28. Dewhirst MW, Ashcraft KA. Implications of increase in vascular permeability in tumors by VEGF: A commentary on the pioneering work of Harold Dvorak. *Cancer Research.* 2016;76(11):3118–3120. Epub 2016/06/03. doi:10.1158/0008-5472.can-16-1292. PubMed PMID: 27251086.

29. Levick JR. *An Introduction to Cardiovascular Physiology.* London, UK: Hodder Arnold, 2003.

30. Yuan F, Leunig M, Huang SK, Berk DA, Papahadjopoulos D, Jain RK. Microvascular permeability and interstitial penetration of sterically

stabilized (stealth) liposomes in a human tumor xenograft. *Cancer Research*. 1994;54(13):3352–3356. Epub 1994/07/01. PubMed PMID: 8012948.

31. Maeda H, Wu J, Sawa T, Matsumura Y, Hori K. Tumor vascular permeability and the EPR effect in macromolecular therapeutics: A review. *Journal of Controlled Release: Official Journal of the Controlled Release Society*. 2000;65(1–2):271–284. Epub 2000/03/04. PubMed PMID: 10699287.

32. Miller MA, Gadde S, Pfirschke C, Engblom C, Sprachman MM, Kohler RH, Yang KS, et al. Predicting therapeutic nanomedicine efficacy using a companion magnetic resonance imaging nanoparticle. *Science Translational Medicine*. 2015;7(314):314ra183. Epub 2015/11/20. doi:10.1126/scitranslmed.aac6522. PubMed PMID: 26582898; PMCID: PMC5462466.

33. Bertrand N, Wu J, Xu X, Kamaly N, Farokhzad OC. Cancer nanotechnology: The impact of passive and active targeting in the era of modern cancer biology. *Advanced Drug Delivery Reviews*. 2014;66:2–25. Epub 2013/11/26. doi:10.1016/j.addr.2013.11.009. PubMed PMID: 24270007; PMCID: PMC4219254.

34. Chang Q, Ornatsky OI, Siddiqui I, Straus R, Baranov VI, Hedley DW. Biodistribution of cisplatin revealed by imaging mass cytometry identifies extensive collagen binding in tumor and normal tissues. *Scientific Reports*. 2016;6:36641. Epub 2016/11/05. doi:10.1038/srep36641. PubMed PMID: 27812005; PMCID: PMC5095658 invented, developed and manufactures mass cytometry technologies, including the Helios CyTOF system, the Imaging Mass Cytometer and metal-conjugated reagents.

35. Krol A, Maresca J, Dewhirst MW, Yuan F. Available volume fraction of macromolecules in the extravascular space of a fibrosarcoma: Implications for drug delivery. *Cancer Research*. 1999;59(16):4136–4141. Epub 1999/08/27. PubMed PMID: 10463619.

36. Yuan F, Krol A, Tong S. Available space and extracellular transport of macromolecules: Effects of pore size and connectedness. *Annals of Biomedical Engineering*. 2001;29(12):1150–1158. Epub 2002/02/21. PubMed PMID: 11853267.

37. Provenzano PP, Cuevas C, Chang AE, Goel VK, Von Hoff DD, Hingorani SR. Enzymatic targeting of the stroma ablates physical barriers to treatment of pancreatic ductal adenocarcinoma. *Cancer Cell*. 2012;21(3):418–429. Epub 2012/03/24. doi:10.1016/j.ccr.2012.01.007. PubMed PMID: 22439937; PMCID: PMC3371414.

38. Stylianopoulos T, Martin JD, Chauhan VP, Jain SR, Diop-Frimpong B, Bardeesy N, Smith BL et al. Causes, consequences, and remedies for growth-induced solid stress in murine and human tumors.

Proceedings of the National Academy of Sciences of the United States of America. 2012;109(38):15101–15108. Epub 2012/08/31. doi:10.1073/pnas.1213353109. PubMed PMID: 22932871; PMCID: PMC3458380.

39. Chauhan VP, Boucher Y, Ferrone CR, Roberge S, Martin JD, Stylianopoulos T, Bardeesy N. et al. Compression of pancreatic tumor blood vessels by hyaluronan is caused by solid stress and not interstitial fluid pressure. *Cancer Cell*. 2014;26(1):14–15. Epub 2014/07/16. doi:10.1016/j.ccr.2014.06.003. PubMed PMID: 25026209; PMCID: PMC4381566.

40. Jain RK. The Eugene M. Landis Award Lecture 1996: Delivery of molecular and cellular medicine to solid tumors. *Microcirculation* (New York, NY: 1994). 1997;4(1):1–23. Epub 1997/03/01. PubMed PMID: 9110280.

41. Jain RK. Normalization of tumor vasculature: An emerging concept in antiangiogenic therapy. *Science* (New York, NY). 2005;307(5706):58–62. Epub 2005/01/08. doi:10.1126/science.1104819. PubMed PMID: 15637262.

42. Kleinstreuer C, Zhang Z, Donohue JF. Targeted drug-aerosol delivery in the human respiratory system. *Annual Review of Biomedical Engineering*. 2008;10:195–220. Epub 2008/04/17. doi:10.1146/annurev.bioeng.10.061807.160544. PubMed PMID: 18412536.

43. Clark AR HM. Regional lung deposition: Can it be controlled and have an impact on safety and efficacy? *Respiratory Drug Delivery* 2012 1:89–100.

44. Diaz KT, Skaria S, Harris K, Solomita M, Lau S, Bauer K, Smaldone GC, Condos R. Delivery and safety of inhaled interferon-gamma in idiopathic pulmonary fibrosis. *Journal of Aerosol Medicine and Pulmonary Drug Delivery*. 2012;25(2):79–87. Epub 2012/03/01. doi:10.1089/jamp.2011.0919. PubMed PMID: 22360317.

45. Scheuch G, Siekmeier R. Novel approaches to enhance pulmonary delivery of proteins and peptides. *Journal of Physiology and Pharmacology: An Official Journal of the Polish Physiological Society*. 2007;58 Suppl 5(Pt 2):615–625. Epub 2008/03/28. PubMed PMID: 18204175.

46. Denyer J, Dyche T. The Adaptive Aerosol Delivery (AAD) technology: Past, present, and future. *Journal of Aerosol Medicine and Pulmonary Drug Delivery*. 2010;23 Suppl 1:S1–S10. Epub 2010/04/14. doi:10.1089/jamp.2009.0791. PubMed PMID: 20373904; PMCID: PMC3116630.

47. Longest PW, Walenga RL, Son YJ, Hindle M. High-efficiency generation and delivery of aerosols through nasal cannula during noninvasive ventilation. *Journal of Aerosol Medicine and Pulmonary Drug Delivery*. 2013;26(5):266–279. Epub 2013/01/01.

doi:10.1089/jamp.2012.1006. PubMed PMID: 23273243; PMCID: PMC3826475.

48. Longest PW, Tian G, Hindle M. Improving the lung delivery of nasally administered aerosols during noninvasive ventilation-an application of enhanced condensational growth (ECG). *Journal of Aerosol Medicine and Pulmonary Drug Delivery*. 2011;24(2):103–118. Epub 2011/03/18. doi:10.1089/jamp.2010.0849. PubMed PMID: 21410327; PMCID: PMC3123840.

49. Torchilin VP. Passive and active drug targeting: Drug delivery to tumors as an example. *Handbook of Experimental Pharmacology*. 2010(197):3–53. Epub 2010/03/11. doi:10.1007/978-3-642-00477-3_1. PubMed PMID: 20217525.

50. Nakamura Y, Mochida A, Choyke PL, Kobayashi H. Nanodrug delivery: Is the enhanced permeability and retention effect sufficient for curing cancer? *Bioconjugate Chemistry*. 2016;27(10):2225–2238. Epub 2016/10/21. doi:10.1021/acs.bioconjchem.6b00437. PubMed PMID: 27547843.

51. Ghazanfari T, Elhissi AM, Ding Z, Taylor KM. The influence of fluid physicochemical properties on vibrating-mesh nebulization. *International Journal of Pharmaceutics*. 2007;339(1–2):103–111. Epub 2007/04/25. doi:10.1016/j.ijpharm.2007.02.035. PubMed PMID: 17451896.

52. Najlah M, Vali A, Taylor M, Arafat BT, Ahmed W, Phoenix DA, Taylor KM, Elhissi A. A study of the effects of sodium halides on the performance of air-jet and vibrating-mesh nebulizers. *International Journal of Pharmaceutics*. 2013;456(2):520–527. Epub 2013/08/27. doi:10.1016/j.ijpharm.2013.08.023. PubMed PMID: 23973409.

53. Selting K, Waldrep JC, Reinero C, Branson K, Gustafson D, Kim DY, Henry C, Owen N, Madsen R, Dhand R. Feasibility and safety of targeted cisplatin delivery to a select lung lobe in dogs via the AeroProbe intracorporeal nebulization catheter. *Journal of Aerosol Medicine and Pulmonary Drug Delivery*. 2008;21(3):255–268. Epub 2008/09/02. doi:10.1089/jamp.2008.0684. PubMed PMID: 18759657.

54. Tseng CL, Wu SY, Wang WH, Peng CL, Lin FH, Lin CC, Young TH, Shieh MJ. Targeting efficiency and biodistribution of biotinylated-EGF-conjugated gelatin nanoparticles administered via aerosol delivery in nude mice with lung cancer. *Biomaterials*. 2008;29(20):3014–3022. Epub 2008/04/26. doi:10.1016/j.biomaterials.2008.03.033. PubMed PMID: 18436301.

55. Kuzmov A, Minko T. Nanotechnology approaches for inhalation treatment of lung diseases. *Journal of Controlled Release: Official Journal of the Controlled Release Society*. 2015;219:500–518. Epub 2015/08/25. doi:10.1016/j.jconrel.2015.07.024. PubMed PMID: 26297206.

56. Gaspar MM, Radomska A, Gobbo OL, Bakowsky U, Radomski MW, Ehrhardt C. Targeted delivery of transferrin-conjugated liposomes to an ortho-topic model of lung cancer in nude rats. *Journal of Aerosol Medicine and Pulmonary Drug Delivery*. 2012;25(6):310–318. Epub 2012/08/04. doi:10.1089/jamp.2011.0928. PubMed PMID: 22857016.

57. Jiang HL, Xu CX, Kim YK, Arote R, Jere D, Lim HT, Cho MH, Cho CS. The suppression of lung tumorigenesis by aerosol-delivered folate-chitosan-graft-polyethylenimine/Akt1 shRNA complexes through the Akt signaling pathway. *Biomaterials*. 2009;30(29):5844–5852. Epub 2009/07/31. doi:10.1016/j.biomaterials.2009.07.017. PubMed PMID: 19640582.

58. Schiller JH. Anti-EGFR monoclonal antibodies in lung cancer treatment. *The Lancet Oncology*. 2015;16(7):738–739. Epub 2015/06/06. doi:10.1016/s1470-2045(15)00020-0. PubMed PMID: 26045341.

59. Kim I, Byeon HJ, Kim TH, Lee ES, Oh KT, Shin BS, Lee KC, Youn YS. Doxorubicin-loaded porous PLGA microparticles with surface attached TRAIL for the inhalation treatment of metastatic lung cancer. *Biomaterials*. 2013;34(27):6444–6453. Epub 2013/06/13. doi:10.1016/j.biomaterials.2013.05.018. PubMed PMID: 23755831.

60. Luo Y, Zhai X, Ma C, Sun P, Fu Z, Liu W, Xu J. An inhalable beta(2)-adrenoceptor ligand-directed guanidinylated chitosan carrier for targeted delivery of siRNA to lung. *Journal of Controlled Release: Official Journal of the Controlled Release Society*. 2012;162(1):28–36. Epub 2012/06/16. doi:10.1016/j.jconrel.2012.06.005. PubMed PMID: 22698944.

61. Sadhukha T, Wiedmann TS, Panyam J. Inhalable magnetic nanoparticles for targeted hyperthermia in lung cancer therapy. *Biomaterials*. 2013;34(21):5163–5171. Epub 2013/04/18. doi:10.1016/j.biomaterials.2013.03.061. PubMed PMID: 23591395; PMCID: PMC4673896.

62. Selting K, Essman S, Reinero C, Branson KR, Henry CJ, Owen N, Guntur VP, Waldrep JC, Kim DY, Dhand R. Targeted combined aerosol chemotherapy in dogs and radiologic toxicity grading. *Journal of Aerosol Medicine and Pulmonary Drug Delivery*. 2011;24(1):43–48. Epub 2010/12/21. doi:10.1089/jamp.2010.0822. PubMed PMID: 21166584.

63. Lemarie E, Vecellio L, Hureaux J, Prunier C, Valat C, Grimbert D, Boidron-Celle M et al. Aerosolized gemcitabine in patients with carcinoma of the lung: Feasibility and safety study. *Journal of Aerosol Medicine and Pulmonary Drug Delivery*. 2011;24(6):261–270. Epub 2011/07/29. doi:10.1089/jamp.2010.0872. PubMed PMID: 21793717.

64. Zarogoulidis P, Eleftheriadou E, Sapardanis I, Zarogoulidou V, Lithoxopoulou H, Kontakiotis T, Karamanos N et al. Feasibility and effective-ness of inhaled carboplatin in NSCLC patients.

Investigational New Drugs. 2012;30(4):1628–1640. Epub 2011/07/09. doi:10.1007/s10637-011-9714-5. PubMed PMID: 21739158.

65. Weers JG, Tarara TE, Clark AR. Design of fine particles for pulmonary drug delivery. *Expert Opinion on Drug Delivery.* 2007;4(3):297–313. Epub 2007/05/11. doi:10.1517/17425247.4.3.297. PubMed PMID: 17489656.

66. Chan H KP. *Novel Particle Production Technologies for Inhalation Products.* Inhalation Drug Delivery: Techniques and Products. Chichester, UK: John Wiley & Sons, 2013, pp. 47–62.

67. Edwards DA, Hanes J, Caponetti G, Hrkach J, Ben-Jebria A, Eskew ML, Mintzes J, Deaver D, Lotan N, Langer R. Large porous particles for pulmonary drug delivery. *Science* (New York, NY). 1997;276(5320):1868–1871. Epub 1997/06/20. PubMed PMID: 9188534.

68. Kim I, Byeon HJ, Kim TH, Lee ES, Oh KT, Shin BS, Lee KC, Youn YS. Doxorubicin-loaded highly porous large PLGA microparticles as a sustained-release inhalation system for the treatment of metastatic lung cancer. *Biomaterials.* 2012;33(22):5574–5583. Epub 2012/05/15. doi:10.1016/j.biomaterials.2012.04.018. PubMed PMID: 22579235.

69. Wu D, Wang C, Yang J, Wang H, Han H, Zhang A, Yang Y, Li Q. Improving the intracellular drug concentration in lung cancer treatment through the codelivery of doxorubicin and miR-519c mediated by porous PLGA microparticle. *Molecular Pharmaceutics.* 2016;13(11):3925–3933. Epub 2016/09/30. doi:10.1021/acs.molpharmaceut.6b00702. PubMed PMID: 27684197.

70. Hitzman CJ, Elmquist WF, Wattenberg LW, Wiedmann TS. Development of a respirable, sustained release microcarrier for 5-fluorouracil I: In vitro assessment of liposomes, microspheres, and lipid coated nanoparticles. *Journal of Pharmaceutical Sciences.* 2006;95(5):1114–1126. Epub 2006/03/30. doi:10.1002/jps.20591. PubMed PMID: 16570302.

71. Okuda T, Kito D, Oiwa A, Fukushima M, Hira D, Okamoto H. Gene silencing in a mouse lung metastasis model by an inhalable dry small interfering RNA powder prepared using the supercritical carbon dioxide technique. *Biological & Pharmaceutical Bulletin.* 2013;36(7):1183–1191. Epub 2013/07/03. PubMed PMID: 23811567.

72. Garcia A, Mack P, Williams S, Fromen C, Shen T, Tully J, Pillai J, Kuehl P, Napier M, Desimone JM, Maynor BW. Microfabricated engineered particle systems for respiratory drug delivery and other pharmaceutical applications. *Journal of Drug Delivery.* 2012;2012:941243. Epub 2012/04/21. doi:10.1155/2012/941243. PubMed PMID: 22518316; PMCID: PMC3307013.

73. Cipolla D, Gonda I, Chan HK. Liposomal formulations for inhalation. *Therapeutic Delivery.* 2013;4(8):1047–1072. Epub 2013/08/08. doi:10.4155/tde.13.71. PubMed PMID: 23919478.

74. Arppe J VM, Waldrep J. Pulmonary pharmacokinetics of cyclosporine A liposomes. *International Journal of Pharmaceutics* 1998;161:205–214.

75. Gaspar M, Bakowsky U, Ehrhardt C. Inhaled liposomes-current strategies and future challenges. *Journal of Biomedical Nanotechnology.* 2008;4:245–257. doi:10.1166/jbn.2008.334.

76. Elhissi A, Taylor KMG. Delivery of liposomes generated from proliposomes using air-jet, ultrasonic, and vibrating-mesh nebulisers. *Journal of Drug Delivery Science and Technology.* 2005;15:261–265. doi:10.1016/S1773-2247(05)50047-59.

77. Deshpande D, Blanchard J, Srinivasan S, Fairbanks D, Fujimoto J, Sawa T, Wiener-Kronish J, Schreier H, Gonda I. Aerosolization of lipoplexes using AERx pulmonary delivery system. *American Association of Pharmaceutical Scientists.* 2002;4(3):E13. Epub 2002/11/09. doi:10.1208/ps040313. PubMed PMID: 12423062; PMCID: PMC2751352.

78. Lehofer B, Bloder F, Jain PP, Marsh LM, Leitinger G, Olschewski H, Leber R, Olschewski A, Prassl R. Impact of atomization technique on the stability and transport efficiency of nebulized liposomes harboring different surface characteristics. *European Journal of Pharmaceutics and Biopharmaceutics: Official Journal of Arbeitsgemeinschaft fur Pharmazeutische Verfahrenstechnik eV.* 2014;88(3):1076–1085. Epub 2014/12/03. doi:10.1016/j.ejpb.2014.10.009. PubMed PMID: 25460154.

79. Elhissi AM, Faizi M, Naji WF, Gill HS, Taylor KM. Physical stability and aerosol properties of liposomes delivered using an air-jet nebulizer and a novel micropump device with large mesh apertures. *International Journal of Pharmaceutics.* 2007;334(1–2):62–70. Epub 2006/11/25. doi:10.1016/j.ijpharm.2006.10.022. PubMed PMID: 17123757.

80. Taylor KMG, Taylor G, Kellaway IW, Stevens J. The stability of liposomes to nebulisation. *International Journal of Pharmaceutics.* 1990;58(1):57–61. doi:10.1016/0378-5173(90)90287-E.

81. Niven RW, Schreier H. Nebulization of liposomes. I. Effects of lipid composition. *Pharmaceutical Research.* 1990;7(11):1127–1133. Epub 1990/11/01. PubMed PMID: 2293210.

82. Payne NI, Timmins P, Ambrose CV, Ward MD, Ridgway F. Proliposomes: A novel solution to an old problem. *Journal of Pharmaceutical Sciences.* 1986;75(4):325–329. Epub 1986/04/01. PubMed PMID: 3723351.

83. Rojanarat W, Changsan N, Tawithong E, Pinsuwan S, Chan HK, Srichana T. Isoniazid proliposome powders for inhalation-preparation, characterization and cell

culture studies. *International Journal of Molecular Sciences*. 2011;12(7):4414–4434. Epub 2011/08/17. doi:10.3390/ijms12074414. PubMed PMID: 21845086; PMCID: PMC3155359.

84. Desai TR, Hancock RE, Finlay WH. A facile method of delivery of liposomes by nebulization. *Journal of Controlled Release: Official Journal of the Controlled Release Society*. 2002;84(1–2):69–78. Epub 2002/10/26. PubMed PMID: 12399169.

85. Smola M, Vandamme T, Sokolowski A. Nanocarriers as pulmonary drug delivery systems to treat and to diagnose respiratory and non respiratory diseases. *International Journal of Nanomedicine*. 2008;3(1):1–19. Epub 2008/05/21. PubMed PMID: 18488412; PMCID: PMC2526354.

86. Kaur G, Narang RK, Rath G, Goyal AK. Advances in pulmonary delivery of nanoparticles. *Artificial Cells, Blood Substitutes, and Immobilization Biotechnology*. 2012;40(1–2):75–96. Epub 2011/08/03. doi:10.3109/10731199.2011.592494. PubMed PMID: 21806501.

87. Feng SS CS. Chemotherapeutic engineering. Application and further development of chemical engineering principles for chemotherapy of cancer and other diseases. *Chemical Engineering Science*. 2003;58:4087–4114.

88. Wang H, Xu Y, Zhou X. Docetaxel-loaded chitosan microspheres as a lung targeted drug delivery system: In vitro and in vivo evaluation. *International Journal of Molecular Sciences*. 2014;15(3):3519–3532. Epub 2014/03/01. doi:10.3390/ijms15033519. PubMed PMID: 24577314; PMCID: PMC3975351.

89. Ehrhardt C, Fiegel J, Fuchs S, Abu-Dahab R, Schaefer UF, Hanes J, Lehr CM. Drug absorption by the respiratory mucosa: Cell culture models and particulate drug carriers. *Journal of Aerosol Medicine: The Official Journal of the International Society for Aerosols in Medicine*. 2002;15(2):131–139. Epub 2002/08/20. doi:10.1089/089426802320282257. PubMed PMID: 12184863.

90. Wicki A, Witzigmann D, Balasubramanian V, Huwyler J. Nanomedicine in cancer therapy: Challenges, opportunities, and clinical applications. *Journal of Controlled Release: Official Journal of the Controlled Release Society*. 2015;200:138–157. Epub 2014/12/30. doi:10.1016/j.jconrel.2014.12.030. PubMed PMID: 25545217.

91. Tseng CL, Su WY, Yen KC, Yang KC, Lin FH. The use of biotinylated-EGF-modified gelatin nanoparticle carrier to enhance cisplatin accumulation in cancerous lungs via inhalation. *Biomaterials*. 2009;30(20):3476–3485. Epub 2009/04/07. doi:10.1016/j.biomaterials.2009.03.010. PubMed PMID: 19345990.

92. Elzoghby AO. Gelatin-based nanoparticles as drug and gene delivery systems: Reviewing three decades of research. *Journal of Controlled Release: Official Journal of the Controlled Release Society*. 2013;172(3):1075–1091. Epub 2013/10/08. doi:10.1016/j.jconrel.2013.09.019. PubMed PMID: 24096021.

93. Videira M, Almeida AJ, Fabra A. Preclinical evaluation of a pulmonary delivered paclitaxel-loaded lipid nanocarrier antitumor effect. *Nanomedicine: Nanotechnology, Biology, and Medicine*. 2012;8(7):1208–1215. Epub 2011/12/31. doi:10.1016/j.nano.2011.12.007. PubMed PMID: 22206945.

94. Roa WH, Azarmi S, Al-Hallak MH, Finlay WH, Magliocco AM, Lobenberg R. Inhalable nanoparticles, a non-invasive approach to treat lung cancer in a mouse model. *Journal of Controlled Release: Official Journal of the Controlled Release Society*. 2011;150(1):49–55. Epub 2010/11/10. doi:10.1016/j.jconrel.2010.10.035. PubMed PMID: 21059378.

95. Sabra S, Abdelmoneem M, Abdelwakil M, Mabrouk MT, Anwar D, Mohamed R, Khattab S et al. Self-Assembled nanocarriers based on amphiphilic natural polymers for anti-cancer drug delivery applications. *Current Pharmaceutical Design*. 2017;23(35):5213–5229. Epub 2017/05/30. doi:10.2174/1381612823666170526111029. PubMed PMID: 28552068.

96. Xie Y, Aillon KL, Cai S, Christian JM, Davies NM, Berkland CJ, Forrest ML. Pulmonary delivery of cisplatin-hyaluronan conjugates via endotracheal instillation for the treatment of lung cancer. *International Journal of Pharmaceutics*. 2010;392(1–2):156–163. Epub 2010/04/07. doi:10.1016/j.ijpharm.2010.03.058. PubMed PMID: 20363303; PMCID: PMC2873163.

97. Kaminskas LM, McLeod VM, Ryan GM, Kelly BD, Haynes JM, Williamson M, Thienthong N, Owen DJ, Porter CJ. Pulmonary administration of a doxorubicin-conjugated dendrimer enhances drug exposure to lung metastases and improves cancer therapy. *Journal of Controlled Release: Official Journal of the Controlled Release Society*. 2014;183:18–26. Epub 2014/03/19. doi:10.1016/j.jconrel.2014.03.012. PubMed PMID: 24637466.

98. Tsapis N, Bennett D, Jackson B, Weitz DA, Edwards DA. Trojan particles: Large porous carriers of nanoparticles for drug delivery. *Proceedings of the National Academy of Sciences of the United States of America*. 2002;99(19):12001–12005. Epub 2002/08/30. doi:10.1073/pnas.182233999. PubMed PMID: 12200546; PMCID: PMC129387.

99. Kaye RS, Purewal TS, Alpar HO. Simultaneously manufactured nano-in-micro (SIMANIM) particles for dry-powder modified-release delivery of antibodies. *Journal of Pharmaceutical Sciences*.

2009;98(11):4055–4068. Epub 2009/02/04. doi:10.1002/jps.21673. PubMed PMID: 19189420.

100. Weber S, Zimmer A, Pardeike J. Solid Lipid Nanoparticles (SLN) and nanostructured lipid carriers (NLC) for pulmonary application: A review of the state of the art. *European Journal of Pharmaceutics and Biopharmaceutics: Official Journal of Arbeitsgemeinschaft fur Pharmazeutische Verfahrenstechnik eV*. 2014;86(1):7–22. Epub 2013/09/07. doi:10.1016/j.ejpb.2013.08.013. PubMed PMID: 24007657.

101. Mehnert W, Mader K. Solid lipid nanoparticles: Production, characterization and applications. *Advanced Drug Delivery Reviews*. 2001;47(2–3):165–196. Epub 2001/04/20. PubMed PMID: 11311991.

102. Subedi RK, Kang KW, Choi HK. Preparation and characterization of solid lipid nanoparticles loaded with doxorubicin. *European Journal of Pharmaceutical Sciences: Official Journal of the European Federation for Pharmaceutical Sciences*. 2009;37(3–4):508–513. Epub 2009/05/02. doi:10.1016/j.ejps.2009.04.008. PubMed PMID: 19406231.

103. Paranjpe M, Muller-Goymann CC. Nanoparticle-mediated pulmonary drug delivery: A review. *International Journal of Molecular Sciences*. 2014;15(4):5852–5873. Epub 2014/04/11. doi:10.3390/ijms15045852. PubMed PMID: 24717409; PMCID: PMC4013600.

104. Patlolla RR, Chougule M, Patel AR, Jackson T, Tata PN, Singh M. Formulation, characterization and pulmonary deposition of nebulized celecoxib encapsulated nanostructured lipid carriers. *Journal of Controlled Release: Official Journal of the Controlled Release Society*. 2010;144(2):233–241. Epub 2010/02/16. doi:10.1016/j.jconrel.2010.02.006. PubMed PMID: 20153385; PMCID: PMC2868936.

105. El-Sherbiny IM, McGill S, Smyth HD. Swellable microparticles as carriers for sustained pulmonary drug delivery. *Journal of Pharmaceutical Sciences*. 2010;99(5):2343–2356. Epub 2009/12/08. doi:10.1002/jps.22003. PubMed PMID: 19967777; PMCID: PMC3654803.

106. Lavasanifar A, Samuel J, Kwon GS. Poly(ethylene oxide)-block-poly(L-amino acid) micelles for drug delivery. *Advanced Drug Delivery Reviews*. 2002;54(2):169–190. Epub 2002/03/19. PubMed PMID: 11897144.

107. Ahmad J, Akhter S, Rizwanullah M, Amin S, Rahman M, Ahmad MZ, Rizvi MA, Kamal MA, Ahmad FJ. Nanotechnology-based inhalation treatments for lung cancer: State of the art. *Nanotechnology Science and Applications*. 2015;8:55–66. Epub 2015/12/08. doi:10.2147/nsa.s49052. PubMed PMID: 26640374; PMCID: PMC4657804.

108. Upadhyay D, Scalia S, Vogel R, Wheate N, Salama RO, Young PM, Traini D, Chrzanowski W. Magnetised thermo responsive lipid vehicles for targeted and controlled lung drug delivery. *Pharmaceutical Research*. 2012;29(9):2456–2467. Epub 2012/05/16. doi:10.1007/s11095-012-0774-9. PubMed PMID: 22584949.

109. Vivero-Escoto JL, Slowing, II, Trewyn BG, Lin VS. Mesoporous silica nanoparticles for intracellular controlled drug delivery. *Small* (Weinheim an der Bergstrasse, Germany). 2010;6(18):1952–1967. Epub 2010/08/07. doi:10.1002/smll.200901789. PubMed PMID: 20690133.

110. Taratula O, Garbuzenko OB, Chen AM, Minko T. Innovative strategy for treatment of lung cancer: Targeted nanotechnology-based inhalation co-delivery of anticancer drugs and siRNA. *Journal of Drug Targeting*. 2011;19(10):900–914. Epub 2011/10/11. doi:10.3109/1061186x.2011.622404. PubMed PMID: 21981718.

111. Keskinov AA, Shurin MR. Myeloid regulatory cells in tumor spreading and metastasis. *Immunobiology*. 2015;220(2):236–242. Epub 2014/09/03. doi:10.1016/j.imbio.2014.07.017. PubMed PMID: 25178934.

112. Ostrand-Rosenberg S, Sinha P, Beury DW, Clements VK. Cross-talk between myeloid-derived suppressor cells (MDSC), macrophages, and dendritic cells enhances tumor-induced immune suppression. *Seminars in Cancer Biology*. 2012;22(4):275–281. Epub 2012/02/09. doi:10.1016/j.semcancer.2012.01.011. PubMed PMID: 22313874; PMCID: PMC3701942.

113. Anderson PM, Markovic SN, Sloan JA, Clawson ML, Wylam M, Arndt CA, Smithson WA, Burch P, Gornet M, Rahman E. Aerosol granulocyte macrophage-colony stimulating factor: A low toxicity, lung-specific biological therapy in patients with lung metastases. *Clinical Cancer Research: An Official Journal of the American Association for Cancer Research*. 1999;5(9):2316–2323. Epub 1999/09/28. PubMed PMID: 10499599.

114. Markovic SN, Suman VJ, Nevala WK, Geeraerts L, Creagan ET, Erickson LA, Rowland KM, Jr., Morton RF, Horvath WL, Pittelkow MR. A dose-escalation study of aerosolized sargramostim in the treatment of metastatic melanoma: An NCCTG Study. *American Journal of Clinical Oncology*. 2008;31(6):573–579. Epub 2008/12/09. doi:10.1097/COC.0b013e318173a536. PubMed PMID: 19060590; PMCID: PMC2694721.

115. Zhang C, Zhang J, Niu J, Zhou Z, Zhang J, Tian Z. Interleukin-12 improves cytotoxicity of natural killer cells via upregulated expression of NKG2D. *Human Immunology*. 2008;69(8):490–500. Epub 2008/07/16. doi:10.1016/j.humimm.2008.06.004. PubMed PMID: 18619507.

116. Kiany S, Gordon N. Aerosol delivery of interleukin-2 in combination with adoptive transfer of natural killer cells for the treatment of lung metastasis: Methodology and effect. *Methods in Molecular Biology* (Clifton, NJ). 2016;1441:285–295. Epub 2016/05/15. doi:10.1007/978-1-4939-3684-7_24. PubMed PMID: 27177675.

117. Khanna C, Anderson PM, Hasz DE, Katsanis E, Neville M, Klausner JS. Interleukin-2 liposome inhalation therapy is safe and effective for dogs with spontaneous pulmonary metastases. *Cancer*. 1997;79(7):1409–1421. Epub 1997/04/01. PubMed PMID: 9083164.

118. Huland E, Heinzer H, Huland H. Treatment of pulmonary metastatic renal-cell carcinoma in 116 patients using inhaled interleukin-2 (IL-2). *Anticancer Research*. 1999;19(4a):2679–2683. Epub 1999/09/02. PubMed PMID: 10470219.

119. Skubitz KM, Anderson PM. Inhalational interleukin-2 liposomes for pulmonary metastases: A phase I clinical trial. *Anti-cancer Drugs*. 2000;11(7):555–563. Epub 2000/10/19. PubMed PMID: 11036958.

120. Posch C, Weihsengruber F, Bartsch K, Feichtenschlager V, Sanlorenzo M, Vujic I, Monshi B, Ortiz-Urda S, Rappersberger K. Low-dose inhalation of interleukin-2 bio-chemotherapy for the treatment of pulmonary metastases in melanoma patients. *British Journal of Cancer*. 2014;110(6):1427–1432. Epub 2014/02/13. doi:10.1038/bjc.2014.62. PubMed PMID: 24518593; PMCID: PMC3960625.

121. Guma SR, Lee DA, Yu L, Gordon N, Hughes D, Stewart J, Wang WL, Kleinerman ES. Natural killer cell therapy and aerosol interleukin-2 for the treatment of osteosarcoma lung metastasis. *Pediatric Blood & Cancer*. 2014;61(4):618–626. Epub 2013/10/19. doi:10.1002/pbc.24801. PubMed PMID: 24136885; PMCID: PMC4154381.

122. Debs RJ, Fuchs HJ, Philip R, Montgomery AB, Brunette EN, Liggitt D, Patton JS, Shellito JE. Lung-specific delivery of cytokines induces sustained pulmonary and systemic immunomodulation in rats. *Journal of Immunology* (Baltimore, MD: 1950). 1988;140(10):3482–3488. Epub 1988/05/15. PubMed PMID: 3283235.

123. Kinnula V, Cantell K, Mattson K. Effect of inhaled natural interferon-alpha on diffuse bronchioalveolar carcinoma. *European Journal of Cancer* (Oxford, England: 1990). 1990;26(6):740–741. Epub 1990/01/01. PubMed PMID: 2168196.

124. Krieg AM. Toll-like receptor 9 (TLR9) agonists in the treatment of cancer. *Oncogene*. 2008;27(2):161–167. Epub 2008/01/08. doi:10.1038/sj.onc.1210911. PubMed PMID: 18176597.

125. Hirota K, Oishi Y, Taniguchi H, Sawachi K, Inagawa H, Kohchi C, Soma G, Terada H. Antitumor effect of inhalatory lipopolysaccharide and synergetic effect in combination with cyclophosphamide. *Anticancer Research*. 2010;30(8):3129–3134. Epub 2010/09/28. PubMed PMID: 20871031.

126. Le Noci V, Tortoreto M, Gulino A, Storti C, Bianchi F, Zaffaroni N, Tripodo C, Tagliabue E, Balsari A, Sfondrini L. Poly(I:C) and CpG-ODN combined aerosolization to treat lung metastases and counter the immunosuppressive microenvironment. *Oncoimmunology*. 2015;4(10):e1040214. Epub 2015/10/10. doi:10.1080/2162402x.2015.1040214. PubMed PMID: 26451303; PMCID: PMC4589046.

127. Le Noci V, Sommariva M, Tortoreto M, Zaffaroni N, Campiglio M, Tagliabue E, Balsari A, Sfondrini L. Reprogramming the lung microenvironment by inhaled immunotherapy fosters immune destruction of tumor. *Oncoimmunology*. 2016;5(11):e1234571. Epub 2016/12/22. doi:10.1080/2162402x.2016.1234571. PubMed PMID: 27999750; PMCID: PMC5139640.

128. Maillet A, Guilleminault L, Lemarie E, Lerondel S, Azzopardi N, Montharu J, Congy-Jolivet N, et al. The airways, a novel route for delivering monoclonal antibodies to treat lung tumors. *Pharmaceutical Research*. 2011;28(9):2147–2156. Epub 2011/04/15. doi:10.1007/s11095-011-0442-5. PubMed PMID: 21491145.

129. De Santis R, Rosi A, Anastasi AM, Chiapparino C, Albertoni C, Leoni B, Pelliccia A et al. Efficacy of aerosol therapy of lung cancer correlates with EGFR paralysis induced by AvidinOX-anchored biotinylated Cetuximab. *Oncotarget*. 2014;5(19):9239–9255. Epub 2014/09/23. doi:10.18632/oncotarget.2409. PubMed PMID: 25238453; PMCID: PMC4253431.

130. Guilleminault L, Azzopardi N, Arnoult C, Sobilo J, Herve V, Montharu J, Guillon A, et al. Fate of inhaled monoclonal antibodies after the deposition of aerosolized particles in the respiratory system. *Journal of Controlled Release: Official Journal of the Controlled Release Society*. 2014;196:344–354. Epub 2014/12/03. doi:10.1016/j.jconrel.2014.10.003. PubMed PMID: 25451545.

131. Nelson AL, Reichert JM. Development trends for therapeutic antibody fragments. *Nature Biotechnology*. 2009;27(4):331–337. Epub 2009/04/09. doi:10.1038/nbt0409-331. PubMed PMID: 19352366.

132. Koussoroplis SJ, Paulissen G, Tyteca D, Goldansaz H, Todoroff J, Barilly C, Uyttenhove C, Van Snick J, Cataldo D, Vanbever R. PEGylation of antibody fragments greatly increases their local residence time

following delivery to the respiratory tract. *Journal of Controlled Release: Official Journal of the Controlled Release Society*. 2014;187:91–100. Epub 2014/05/23. doi:10.1016/j.jconrel.2014.05.021. PubMed PMID: 24845126.

133. Maillet A, Congy-Jolivet N, Le Guellec S, Vecellio L, Hamard S, Courty Y, Courtois A, et al. Aerodynamical, immunological and pharmacological properties of the anticancer antibody cetuximab following nebulization. *Pharmaceutical Research*. 2008;25(6):1318–1326. Epub 2007/11/22. doi:10.1007/s11095-007-9481-3. PubMed PMID: 18030605.

134. Respaud R, Marchand D, Parent C, Pelat T, Thullier P, Tournamille JF, Viaud-Massuard MC et al. Effect of formulation on the stability and aerosol performance of a nebulized antibody. *MABS*. 2014;6(5):1347–1355. Epub 2014/12/18. doi:10.4161/mabs.29938. PubMed PMID: 25517319; PMCID: PMC4623101.

135. Litterst CL, Gram TE, Dedrick RL, Leroy AF, Guarino AM. Distribution and disposition of platinum following intravenous administration of cis-diamminedichloroplatinum(II) (NSC 119875) to dogs. *Cancer Research*. 1976;36(7 pt 1):2340–2344. Epub 1976/07/01. PubMed PMID: 1277140.

136. Tatsumura T, Koyama S, Tsujimoto M, Kitagawa M, Kagamimori S. Further study of nebulisation chemotherapy, a new chemotherapeutic method in the treatment of lung carcinomas: Fundamental and clinical. *British Journal of Cancer*. 1993;68(6):1146–1149. Epub 1993/12/01. PubMed PMID: 8260366; PMCID: PMC1968665.

137. Carvalho TC, Carvalho SR, McConville JT. Formulations for pulmonary administration of anticancer agents to treat lung malignancies. *Journal of Aerosol Medicine and Pulmonary Drug Delivery*. 2011;24(2):61–80. Epub 2011/03/18. doi:10.1089/jamp.2009.0794. PubMed PMID: 21410326.

138. Zarogoulidis P, Chatzaki E, Porpodis K, Domvri K, Hohenforst-Schmidt W, Goldberg EP, Karamanos N, Zarogoulidis K. Inhaled chemotherapy in lung cancer: Future concept of nanomedicine. *International Journal of Nanomedicine*. 2012;7:1551–1572. Epub 2012/05/24. doi:10.2147/ijn.s29997. PubMed PMID: 22619512; PMCID: PMC3356182.

139. Koshkina NV, Kleinerman ES, Waidrep C, Jia SF, Worth LL, Gilbert BE, Knight V. 9-Nitrocamptothecin liposome aerosol treatment of melanoma and osteosarcoma lung metastases in mice. *Clinical Cancer Research: An Official Journal of the American Association for Cancer Research*. 2000;6(7):2876–2880. Epub 2000/07/29. PubMed PMID: 10914737.

140. Koshkina NV, Waldrep JC, Roberts LE, Golunski E, Melton S, Knight V. Paclitaxel liposome aerosol treatment induces inhibition of pulmonary metastases in murine renal carcinoma model. *Clinical Cancer Research: An Official Journal of the American Association for Cancer Research*. 2001;7(10):3258–3262. Epub 2001/10/12. PubMed PMID: 11595722.

141. Gagnadoux F, Pape AL, Lemarie E, Lerondel S, Valo I, Leblond V, Racineux JL, Urban T. Aerosol delivery of chemotherapy in an orthotopic model of lung cancer. *The European Respiratory Journal*. 2005;26(4):657–661. Epub 2005/10/06. doi:10.1183/09031936.05.00017305. PubMed PMID: 16204597.

142. Kelsen DP, Alcock N, Young CW. Cisplatin nephrotoxicity. Correlation with plasma platinum concentrations. *American Journal of Clinical Oncology*. 1985;8(1):77–80. Epub 1985/02/01. PubMed PMID: 4039530.

143. Dlugosz A, Janecka A. ABC transporters in the development of multidrug resistance in cancer therapy. *Current Pharmaceutical Design*. 2016;22(30):4705–4716. Epub 2016/10/30. PubMed PMID: 26932159.

144. Gagnadoux F, Leblond V, Vecellio L, Hureaux J, Le Pape A, Boisdron-Celle M, Montharu J, Majoral C, Fournier J, Urban T, Diot P, Racineux JL, Lemarie E. Gemcitabine aerosol: In vitro antitumor activity and deposition imaging for preclinical safety assessment in baboons. *Cancer Chemotherapy and Pharmacology*. 2006;58(2):237–244. Epub 2005/12/06. doi:10.1007/s00280-005-0146-9. PubMed PMID: 16328414.

145. Koshkina NV, Kleinerman ES. Aerosol gemcitabine inhibits the growth of primary osteosarcoma and osteosarcoma lung metastases. *International Journal of Cancer*. 2005;116(3):458–463. Epub 2005/04/01. doi:10.1002/ijc.21011. PubMed PMID: 15800950.

146. Reed MD, Tellez CS, Grimes MJ, Picchi MA, Tessema M, Cheng YS, March TH, Kuehl PJ, Belinsky SA. Aerosolised 5-azacytidine suppresses tumour growth and reprogrammes the epigenome in an orthotopic lung cancer model. *British Journal of Cancer*. 2013;109(7):1775–1781. Epub 2013/09/21. doi:10.1038/bjc.2013.575. PubMed PMID: 24045660; PMCID: PMC3790193.

147. Rodriguez CO, Jr., Crabbs TA, Wilson DW, Cannan VA, Skorupski KA, Gordon N, Koshkina N, Kleinerman E, Anderson PM. Aerosol gemcitabine: Preclinical safety and in vivo antitumor activity in osteosarcoma-bearing dogs. *Journal of Aerosol Medicine and Pulmonary Drug Delivery*. 2010;23(4):197–206. Epub 2009/10/07. doi:10.1089/jamp.2009.0773. PubMed PMID: 19803732; PMCID: PMC2888930.

148. Feng T, Tian H, Xu C, Lin L, Xie Z, Lam MH, Liang H, Chen X. Synergistic co-delivery of doxorubicin and paclitaxel by porous PLGA microspheres for pulmonary inhalation treatment. *European Journal of Pharmaceutics and Biopharmaceutics: Official Journal of Arbeitsgemeinschaft fur Pharmazeutische*

Verfahrenstechnikev. 2014;88(3):1086–1093. Epub 2014/10/12. doi:10.1016/j.ejpb.2014.09.012. PubMed PMID: 25305583.

149. Meenach SA, Anderson KW, Zach Hilt J, McGarry RC, Mansour HM. Characterization and aerosol dispersion performance of advanced spray-dried chemotherapeutic PEGylated phospholipid particles for dry powder inhalation delivery in lung cancer. *European Journal of Pharmaceutical Sciences: Official Journal of the European Federation for Pharmaceutical Sciences*. 2013;49(4):699–711. Epub 2013/05/28. doi:10.1016/j.ejps.2013.05.012. PubMed PMID: 23707466; PMCID: PMC5818719.

150. Meenach SA, Anderson KW, Hilt JZ, McGarry RC, Mansour HM. High-performing dry powder inhalers of paclitaxel DPPC/DPPG lung surfactant-mimic multifunctional particles in lung cancer: Physicochemical characterization, in vitro aerosol dispersion, and cellular studies. *American Association of Pharmaceutical Scientists*. 2014;15(6):1574–1587. Epub 2014/08/21. doi:10.1208/s12249-014-0182-z. PubMed PMID: 25139763; PMCID: PMC4245438.

151. Otterson GA, Villalona-Calero MA, Sharma S, Kris MG, Imondi A, Gerber M, White DA et al. Phase I study of inhaled Doxorubicin for patients with metastatic tumors to the lungs. *Clinical Cancer Research: An Official Journal of the American Association for Cancer Research*. 2007;13(4):1246–1252. Epub 2007/02/24. doi:10.1158/1078-0432.ccr-06-1096. PubMed PMID: 17317836.

152. Otterson GA, Villalona-Calero MA, Hicks W, Pan X, Ellerton JA, Gettinger SN, Murren JR. Phase I/II study of inhaled doxorubicin combined with platinum-based therapy for advanced non-small cell lung cancer. *Clinical Cancer Research: An Official Journal of the American Association for Cancer Research*. 2010;16(8):2466–2473. Epub 2010/04/08. doi:10.1158/1078-0432.ccr-09-3015. PubMed PMID: 20371682; PMCID: PMC4262532.

153. Verschraegen CF, Gilbert BE, Loyer E, Huaringa A, Walsh G, Newman RA, Knight V. Clinical evaluation of the delivery and safety of aerosolized liposomal 9-nitro-20(s)-camptothecin in patients with advanced pulmonary malignancies. *Clinical Cancer Research: An Official Journal of the American Association for Cancer Research*. 2004;10(7):2319–2326. Epub 2004/04/10. PubMed PMID: 15073107.

154. Wittgen BP, Kunst PW, van der Born K, van Wijk AW, Perkins W, Pilkiewicz FG, Perez-Soler R, Nicholson S, Peters GJ, Postmus PE. Phase I study of aerosolized SLIT cisplatin in the treatment of patients with carcinoma of the lung. *Clinical Cancer Research: An Official Journal of the American Association for Cancer Research*. 2007;13(8):2414–2421. Epub 2007/04/18. doi:10.1158/1078-0432.ccr-06-1480. PubMed PMID: 17438100.

155. Hohenforst-Schmidt W, Zarogoulidis P, Linsmeier B, Kioumis I, Li Q, Huang H, Sachpatzidou D et al. Enhancement of aerosol cisplatin chemotherapy with gene therapy expressing ABC10 protein in respiratory system. *Journal of Cancer*. 2014;5(5):344–350. Epub 2014/04/12. doi:10.7150/jca.9021. PubMed PMID: 24723977; PMCID: PMC3982181.

156. Koshkina NV, Golunski E, Roberts LE, Gilbert BE, Knight V. Cyclosporin A aerosol improves the anticancer effect of paclitaxel aerosol in mice. *Journal of Aerosol Medicine: The Official Journal of the International Society for Aerosols in Medicine*. 2004;17(1):7–14. Epub 2004/05/04. doi:10.1089/089426804322994415. PubMed PMID: 15120008.

157. Gill KK, Nazzal S, Kaddoumi A. Paclitaxel loaded PEG(5000)-DSPE micelles as pulmonary delivery platform: Formulation characterization, tissue distribution, plasma pharmacokinetics, and toxicological evaluation. *European Journal of Pharmaceutics and Biopharmaceutics: Official Journal of Arbeitsgemeinschaft fur Pharmazeutische Verfahrenstechnik eV*. 2011;79(2):276–284. Epub 2011/05/18. doi:10.1016/j.ejpb.2011.04.017. PubMed PMID: 21575719.

158. Zhao T, Chen H, Dong Y, Zhang J, Huang H, Zhu J, Zhang W. Paclitaxel-loaded poly(glycolide-co-epsilon-caprolactone)-b-D-alpha-tocopheryl polyethylene glycol 2000 succinate nanoparticles for lung cancer therapy. *International Journal of Nanomedicine*. 2013;8:1947–1957. Epub 2013/05/23. doi:10.2147/ijn.s44220. PubMed PMID: 23696703; PMCID: PMC3658437.

159. Joshi N, Shirsath N, Singh A, Joshi K, Banerjee R. Endogenous lung surfactant inspired pH responsive nanovesicle aerosols: Pulmonary compatible and site-specific drug delivery in lung metastases. *Scientific Reports* 2014;4:7085. doi:10.1038/srep07085.

160. Schuler M, Rochlitz C, Horowitz JA, Schlegel J, Perruchoud AP, Kommoss F, Bolliger CT, et al. A phase I study of adenovirus-mediated wild-type p53 gene transfer in patients with advanced non-small cell lung cancer. *Human Gene Therapy*. 1998;9(14):2075–2082. Epub 1998/10/06. doi:10.1089/hum.1998.9.14-2075. PubMed PMID: 9759934.

161. Schuler M, Herrmann R, De Greve JL, Stewart AK, Gatzemeier U, Stewart DJ, Laufman L et al. Adenovirus-mediated wild-type p53 gene transfer in patients receiving chemotherapy for advanced non-small-cell lung cancer: Results of a multicenter phase II study. *Journal of Clinical Oncology: Official Journal of the American Society of Clinical Oncology*. 2001;19(6):1750–1758. Epub 2001/03/17. doi:10.1200/jco.2001.19.6.1750. PubMed PMID: 11251006.

162. Jia SF, Worth LL, Densmore CL, Xu B, Duan X, Kleinerman ES. Aerosol gene therapy with PEI: IL-12 eradicates osteosarcoma lung metastases. *Clinical Cancer Research: An Official Journal of the American Association for Cancer Research*. 2003;9(9):3462–3468. Epub 2003/09/10. PubMed PMID: 12960138.

163. Gautam A, Densmore CL, Waldrep JC. Inhibition of experimental lung metastasis by aerosol delivery of PEI-p53 complexes. *Molecular Therapy: The Journal of the American Society of Gene Therapy*. 2000;2(4):318–323. Epub 2000/10/06. doi:10.1006/mthe.2000.0138. PubMed PMID: 11020346.

164. Densmore CL, Kleinerman ES, Gautam A, Jia SF, Xu B, Worth LL, Waldrep JC, Fung YK, T'Ang A, Knight V. Growth suppression of established human osteosarcoma lung metastases in mice by aerosol gene therapy with PEI-p53 complexes. *Cancer Gene Therapy*. 2001;8(9):619–627. Epub 2001/10/11. doi:10.1038/sj.cgt.7700343. PubMed PMID: 11593330.

165. Nayerossadat N, Maedeh T, Ali PA. Viral and non-viral delivery systems for gene delivery. *Advanced Biomedical Research*. 2012;1:27. Epub 2012/12/05. doi:10.4103/2277-9175.98152. PubMed PMID: 23210086; PMCID: PMC3507026.

166. Hong SH, Park SJ, Lee S, Cho CS, Cho MH. Aerosol gene delivery using viral vectors and cationic carriers for in vivo lung cancer therapy. *Expert Opinion on Drug Delivery*. 2015;12(6):977–991. Epub 2014/11/26. doi:10.1517/17425247.2015.986454. PubMed PMID: 25423167.

167. Zou Y, Tornos C, Qiu X, Lia M, Perez-Soler R. p53 aerosol formulation with low toxicity and high efficiency for early lung cancer treatment. *Clinical Cancer Research: An Official Journal of the American Association for Cancer Research*. 2007;13(16):4900–4908. Epub 2007/08/19. doi:10.1158/1078-0432.ccr-07-0395. PubMed PMID: 17699870.

168. Shin JY, Lim HT, Minai-Tehrani A, Noh MS, Kim JE, Kim JH, Jiang HL et al. Aerosol delivery of beclin1 enhanced the anti-tumor effect of radiation in the lungs of K-rasLA1 mice. *Journal of Radiation Research*. 2012;53(4):506–515. Epub 2012/07/31. doi:10.1093/jrr/rrs005. PubMed PMID: 22843615; PMCID: PMC3393344.

169. Sterman DH, Treat J, Litzky LA, Amin KM, Coonrod L, Molnar-Kimber K, Recio A. et al. Adenovirus-mediated herpes simplex virus thymidine kinase/ganciclovir gene therapy in patients with localized malignancy: Results of a phase I clinical trial in malignant mesothelioma. *Human Gene Therapy*. 1998;9(7):1083–1092. Epub 1998/06/02. doi:10.1089/hum.1998.9.7-1083. PubMed PMID: 9607419.

170. Kim HW, Park IK, Cho CS, Lee KH, Beck GR, Jr., Colburn NH, Cho MH. Aerosol delivery of gluco-sylated polyethylenimine/phosphatase and tensin homologue deleted on chromosome 10 complex suppresses Akt downstream pathways in the lung of K-ras null mice. *Cancer Research*. 2004;64(21):7971–7976. Epub 2004/11/03. doi:10.1158/0008-5472.can-04-1231. PubMed PMID: 15520204.

171. Gautam A, Waldrep JC, Densmore CL, Koshkina N, Melton S, Roberts L, Gilbert B, Knight V. Growth inhibition of established B16-F10 lung metastases by sequential aerosol delivery of p53 gene and 9-nitrocamptothecin. *Gene Therapy*. 2002;9(5):353–357. Epub 2002/04/09. doi:10.1038/sj.gt.3301662. PubMed PMID: 11938455.

172. Kim YD, Park TE, Singh B, Maharjan S, Choi YJ, Choung PH, Arote RB, Cho CS. Nanoparticle-mediated delivery of siRNA for effective lung cancer therapy. *Nanomedicine* (London, England). 2015;10(7):1165–1188. Epub 2015/05/02. doi:10.2217/nnm.14.214. PubMed PMID: 25929572.

173. Zamora-Avila DE, Zapata-Benavides P, Franco-Molina MA, Saavedra-Alonso S, Trejo-Avila LM, Resendez-Perez D, Mendez-Vazquez JL, Isaias-Badillo J, Rodriguez-Padilla C. WT1 gene silencing by aerosol delivery of PEI-RNAi complexes inhibits B16-F10 lung metastases growth. *Cancer Gene Therapy*. 2009;16(12):892–899. Epub 2009/05/23. doi:10.1038/cgt.2009.35. PubMed PMID: 19461674.

174. Conti DS, Brewer D, Grashik J, Avasarala S, da Rocha SR. Poly(amidoamine) dendrimer nanocarriers and their aerosol formulations for siRNA delivery to the lung epithelium. *Molecular Pharmaceutics*. 2014;11(6):1808–1822. Epub 2014/05/09. doi:10.1021/mp4006358. PubMed PMID: 24811243; PMCID: PMC4051247.

175. Yu KN, Minai-Tehrani A, Chang SH, Hwang SK, Hong SH, Kim JE, Shin JY. et al. Aerosol delivery of small hairpin osteopontin blocks pulmonary metastasis of breast cancer in mice. *PLoS One*. 2010;5(12):e15623. Epub 2011/01/05. doi:10.1371/journal.pone.0015623. PubMed PMID: 21203518; PMCID: PMC3008732.

176. Xie RL, Jang YJ, Xing L, Zhang BF, Wang FZ, Cui PF, Cho MH, Jiang HL. A novel potential biocompatible hyperbranched polyspermine for efficient lung cancer gene therapy. *International Journal of Pharmaceutics*. 2015;478(1):19–30. Epub 2014/12/03. doi:10.1016/j.ijpharm.2014.11.014. PubMed PMID: 25448566.

177. Vachani A, Moon E, Wakeam E, Haas AR, Sterman DH, Albelda SM. Gene therapy for lung neoplasms. *Clinics in Chest Medicine*. 2011;32(4):865–885. Epub 2011/11/08. doi:10.1016/j.ccm.2011.08.006. PubMed PMID: 22054892; PMCID: PMC3210443.

178. Taratula O, Kuzmov A, Shah M, Garbuzenko OB, Minko T. Nanostructured lipid carriers as multifunctional nanomedicine platform for pulmonary

co-delivery of anticancer drugs and siRNA. *Journal of Controlled Release: Official Journal of the Controlled Release Society*. 2013;171(3):349–357. Epub 2013/05/08. doi:10.1016/j.jconrel.2013.04.018. PubMed PMID: 23648833; PMCID: PMC3766401.

179. Baban CK, Cronin M, O'Hanlon D, O'Sullivan GC, Tangney M. Bacteria as vectors for gene therapy of cancer. *Bioengineered Bugs*. 2010;1(6):385–394. Epub 2011/04/07. doi:10.4161/bbug.1.6.13146. PubMed PMID: 21468205; PMCID: PMC3056088.

180. Bago JR, Alfonso-Pecchio A, Okolie O, Dumitru R, Rinkenbaugh A, Baldwin AS, Miller CR, Magness ST, Hingtgen SD. Therapeutically engineered induced neural stem cells are tumour-homing and inhibit progression of glioblastoma. *Nature Communications*. 2016;7:10593. Epub 2016/02/03. doi:10.1038/ncomms10593. PubMed PMID: 26830441; PMCID: PMC4740908.

181. Miller MA, Zheng YR, Gadde S, Pfirschke C, Zope H, Engblom C, Kohler RH et al. Tumour-associated macrophages act as a slow-release reservoir of nano-therapeutic Pt(IV) pro-drug. *Nature Communications*. 2015;6:8692. Epub 2015/10/28. doi:10.1038/ncomms9692. PubMed PMID: 26503691; PMCID: PMC4711745.

182. Huland E, Heinzer H, Huland H, Yung R. Overview of interleukin-2 inhalation therapy. *The Cancer Journal From Scientific American*. 2000;6 Suppl 1:S104–S112. Epub 2000/02/24. PubMed PMID: 10685669.

183. Zarogoulidis P, Darwiche K, Krauss L, Huang H, Zachariadis GA, Katsavou A, Hohenforst-Schmidt W et al. Inhaled cisplatin deposition and distribution in lymph nodes in stage II lung cancer patients. *Future Oncology* (London, England). 2013;9(9):1307–1313. Epub 2013/08/29. doi:10.2217/fon.13.111. PubMed PMID: 23980678.

184. Travis WD, Brambilla, E., Burke, A.P., Marx, A., Nicholson, A. G. *WHO Classification of Tumours of the Lung, Pleura, Thymus and Heart*. Fourth edition ed. Lyon, France: International Agency for Research on Cancer, 2015.

185. Youngren-Ortiz SR, Gandhi NS, Espana-Serrano L, Chougule MB. Aerosol delivery of siRNA to the lungs. Part 2: Nanocarrier-based delivery systems. *Kona: Powder Science and Technology in Japan*. 2017;34:44–69. Epub 2017/04/11. doi:10.14356/kona.2017005. PubMed PMID: 28392618; PMCID: PMC5381822.

12

Inhaled therapeutics in chronic obstructive pulmonary disease

TEJAS SINHA, PAUL DEJULIO, AND PHILIP DIAZ

Background 215
COPD pathophysiology 215
Airway pharmacology 216
Effects of disease on aerosol penetrance 217
Clinical considerations of drug classes 217
    Long-acting muscarinic antagonists 217
    Long-acting beta agonists 217
Inhaled corticosteroids 218
Long-acting muscarinic antagonist/long-acting
    beta agonist combinations 218
Inhaled devices and implications for clinical care 218
    Technology-based clinical outcomes 219
    Future technology 219
References 220

BACKGROUND

Chronic obstructive pulmonary disease (COPD) is defined as a "common preventable and treatable disease, characterized by persistent respiratory symptoms and airflow limitation due to airway and/or alveolar abnormalities that is usually caused by significant exposure to noxious particles or gases" (1). The disease represents a major source of morbidity and mortality in the United States and worldwide. In the United States, it is estimated that 6.3% of adults have COPD, and it is now the third leading cause of death; annual direct and indirect costs attributed to COPD in the United States are approximately $50 billion (2,3). COPD is projected to be the third leading cause death worldwide by the year 2020. By far, the major risk factor for COPD development is a history of regular cigarette smoking. Other risk factors contributing to disease development including the use of biomass fuel for indoor heating and cooking, occupational dust exposure, human immunodeficiency virus (HIV) infection, and a history of early childhood respiratory infections. The pathogenesis of COPD remains an area of active investigation and key molecular elements of disease development in humans is limited by the long-time course of disease development. There is evidence that a number of mechanistic pathways may contribute to disease development, including protease/antiprotease imbalance, oxidant stress, disordered tissue repair, dysregulated immune function, and unchecked pulmonary inflammation (4). The major diagnostic criteria for COPD include identification of risk factors; the presence of respiratory symptoms, including dyspnea and/or cough; and the finding of airflow obstruction on spirometry (1).

COPD PATHOPHYSIOLOGY

The major source of airflow obstruction in COPD occurs at the level of the small airways (approximately 2 mm or less) resulting in an obstructive bronchiolitis (5). Important pathophysiologic features affecting airway caliber include inflammatory infiltrates, mucus hypersecretion, and smooth muscle contraction (5). In addition to small airway abnormalities, patients with COPD typically have lung parenchymal destruction in the form of emphysema. This results in loss of alveolar attachments as well as diminished elastic recoil; these factors contribute to expiratory airflow limitation (6).

Airway and parenchymal abnormalities contribute to abnormal gas exchange and to ventilation perfusion mismatch resulting in hypoxemia. In addition, expiratory airflow limitation leads to air-trapping and hyperinflation. With increased ventilator demands and increased respiratory rate associated with activity or exercise, the air-trapping can become more severe, resulting in "dynamic hyperinflation" (7). This altered mechanics of breathing is a major source of dyspnea and exercise intolerance in this patient population (7).

Recommendations for treatment regimens are driven by the degree of respiratory symptoms and the frequency of acute exacerbations of disease (1). As such, inhaled therapy is central to disease management in COPD. Inhaled bronchodilators can improve respiratory symptoms, exercise tolerance, and health-related quality of life by increasing expiratory airflow and decreasing dynamic hyperinflation (7,8). In addition, inhaled long-acting bronchodilators as well as inhaled corticosteroids have all demonstrated effectiveness in reducing acute exacerbations of disease (9,10).

The following review will focus on the major therapeutic agents used for maintenance therapy in COPD, including long-acting antimuscarinic antagonists (LAMAs), long-acting β-agonists (LABAs), and inhaled corticosteroids (ICSs).

AIRWAY PHARMACOLOGY

Smooth muscle tone of the respiratory tract is largely determined by the activity of the parasympathetic nervous system, with acetylcholine acting as the mediator on muscarinic receptors in the large airways. There are five G protein–coupled muscarinic receptors (M1-M5), but only the first three are found in the airways and are of pharmacologic significance (11). Muscarinic receptor density is greatest in the larger airways and diminishes peripherally (12). The M1 receptor is found in parasympathetic ganglia, and activation facilitates neurotransmission of acetylcholine and consequent bronchoconstriction. The M2 receptor is located on postganglionic nerve terminals; it functions as an auto-receptor and inhibits further release of acetylcholine. Activation of M2 receptors also leads to a reduction in beta-2 receptor signaling and causes a subsequent reduction in airway smooth muscle relaxation. The M3 receptor is the major receptor on submucosal glands and airway vascular endothelium; activation leads to a series of intracellular reactions that eventually causes smooth muscle constriction and increased mucus secretion (12). Given the properties of these receptor subtypes, the optimally constructed anticholinergic agent for COPD patients should antagonize M1 and M3 with minimal affinity for M2 (13).

In addition to bronchodilator effects, there is evidence that LAMAs may have important inflammatory effects in the lung, including attenuating neutrophil chemotaxis and decreasing the concentration of inflammatory cytokines (14).

Autoradiographic studies of human lung have demonstrated that muscarinic receptors of human lung show dense labeling over airway ganglia and submucosal glands (15). In submucosa glands, M3 receptors and M1 receptors can both be found in an approximate 2:1 ratio. Less intense labeling is demonstrated over nerves in intrapulmonary bronchi and airway smooth muscle of both large and small airways. Notably, the muscarinic receptors of human lung smooth muscle are almost entirely of the M3 subtype. M1 receptors can be found throughout the alveolar walls, a finding of unclear functional significance (15). *In situ* hybridization studies have demonstrated there is generally good correlation between receptor subtype mRNA and the distribution of receptor subtypes by autoradiographic methods (15).

β-agonists, including short-acting and long-acting agents, enhance airflow by relaxing airway smooth muscle (16).

The onset and duration of LABA therapy depends on the time it takes for the drug to achieve and maintain effective concentration at the β-2 receptor. Time to effective concentration is affected directly by the concentration of the drug in the airway as well as the receptor selectivity of the agent (17). Activation of the β-2 receptor stimulates the activity of intracellular adenyl cyclase. This enzyme subsequently facilitates synthesis of cyclic 3′5′ adenosine monophosphate (cAMP), which mediates the relaxation of smooth muscle cells (18). The unique pharmacologic properties of each LABA agent dictate its duration and onset of action. For example, formoterol has higher water solubility and lower lipophilicity relative to salmeterol, explaining why it has a more rapid onset of action but slightly shorter duration of action (19). Newer, very long-acting beta agonists such as vilanterol are highly lipophilic (20). There is evidence that LABAs may have anti-inflammatory effects in the lung (21). However, the clinical significance of such effects is not clear (22).

Similar to muscarinic receptors, beta receptors are widely distributed throughout the lung, with autoradiographic studies demonstrating dense labeling over airway epithelium, alveolar walls, and subepithelial glands (23). Less intense labeling was noted in lung airway and vascular smooth muscle. Consistent with functional studies, the large and small airways smooth muscle beta receptors are entirely of the β-2 receptor subtype (23).

The anti-inflammatory effect of corticosteroids (CSs) on target cells is mediated through the binding of the steroid molecules to the cytoplasmic glucocorticoid receptor (GR) (24). This CS-GR complex then reduces inflammation through two mechanisms. One binds directly to genes that activate transcription factors that downregulate pro-inflammatory cytokines and upregulate the release of anti-inflammatory compounds. Second, the CS-GR complex binds directly to signal-dependent pro-inflammatory transcription factors minimizing the ability of these transcription factors to activate more genes that produce pro-inflammatory cytokines (25). One example of relevant pharmacologic differences among specific preparations includes the increased lipophilicity of fluticasone relative to budesonide. This increased lipophilicity leads to a wider volume of distribution with a prolonged duration of action (26). On the other hand, the more balanced hydro- and lipophilicity of budesonide may explain its more rapid onset of anti-inflammatory activity seen in multiple *in vitro* and *in vivo* models (27).

In situ hybridization studies have demonstrated that the highest concentrations of glucocorticoid receptors in the lung are in the vascular smooth muscle, vascular endothelium, and alveolar walls (28). GR receptors are also found in airway epithelium and airway smooth muscle, but in lower concentrations. *In situ* hybridization studies show similar concentrations of GR receptors in normal and asthmatic lungs. Similarly studies evaluating GR function in human alveolar macrophages demonstrate similar function in COPD patients compared to normal (28).

EFFECTS OF DISEASE ON AEROSOL PENETRANCE

Radioactive aerosol studies have documented that smokers, and especially smokers with COPD, have substantially different lung deposition of aerosol compared to normal nonsmokers (29). Central airway and peripheral airway distribution of aerosol in normal is fairly evenly divided in normal, with a ratio of close to 1:1. In smokers, there is greater central airway deposition compared to peripheral, with the ratio of central to peripheral distribution of approximately 1.6:1 (29). In subjects with COPD, central deposition is far greater than peripheral with a nearly threefold greater deposition in the central airways compared to the periphery. Similar data examining the clearance of saline aerosol in subjects with airway obstruction document that the magnitude of bronchial obstruction significantly decreases peripheral deposition of inhaled particles (29).

CLINICAL CONSIDERATIONS OF DRUG CLASSES

Long-acting muscarinic antagonists

Anticholinergic inhalational agents are a backbone of both COPD maintenance and rescue therapy. In fact, the use of anticholinergic agents can be traced back over two centuries; *Datura Stramonium* and other members of the nightshade family contain mixtures of muscarinic antagonists and were smoked for relief of asthma symptoms (30). Much progress has been made in the last century, initially with the isolation of atropine, followed by the development of inhaled ipratropium bromide with respiratory system selectivity, and finally the advent of LAMA therapy with specific subreceptor selectivity (31). The first LAMA agent commercially available was tiotropium bromide. Its preferential long-lasting binding to muscarinic receptor subtypes and ease of once daily use have been considered to be the primary reasons for its clinical success relative to its shorter-acting counterpart, ipratropium bromide (32,33). The efficacy of tiotropium was delineated in the UPLIFT trial, which demonstrated beneficial effects on respiratory symptoms, quality of life, lung function, and exacerbation rate (34). The success of tiotropium has led to the development of additional LAMAs, including glcopyrronium bromide, aclidinium bromide, and umeclidinum bromide with the aim of reproducing the similar clinical effects while also aspiring to concomitantly optimize safety, efficacy, and ease of use.

Despite statistical differences in some outcomes, none of the comparisons between different LAMAs achieve clinically important thresholds for lung function, quality of life, or dyspnea (35). Notably, inhaler technique and compliance has been strictly enforced in most studies. It has been argued that it may be beneficial in the design of future comparison studies to focus on effectiveness versus efficacy, thus allowing for device-handling errors and other patient factors. This would offer the opportunity to further differentiate LAMA agents (and other inhaler-based therapy) on the basis of device preference. Such studies could offer important insight into optimal drug delivery design, information that could be invaluable as more and more agents come to market (36).

Generally, LAMAs have a limited side effect profile with a very low risk for adverse effects as the majority of the drug is active only in the respiratory tract. However, the M3 receptor is also present on a variety of extrapulmonary tissue, including the myocardium, salivary glands, gastrointestinal tract, bladder, and the eye. When systemically available, LAMA agents can subsequently cause tachycardia/tachyarrhythmia, dry mouth from inhibition of salivary secretion, constipation, urinary retention, and increased intraocular pressure with blurry vision. Fortunately, the LAMA agents are quaternary ammonium compounds with low lipid solubility (37). The low lipid solubility prevents absorption across lipid membranes, thereby reducing systemic bioavailability (37). A pooled safety analysis of studies involving LAMAs did show an increased risk of classic anticholinergic effects, including dry mouth, constipation, and urinary retention, but did not show an increased risk of serious adverse events, major adverse events, or fatal events, regardless of inhaler type (38). The safety of glycopyrronium was studied in the GLOW1 and GLOW2 trials. There was no increased risk of significant adverse effects or mortality in either study. Umeclidinium and its combination LABA agent umeclidinium/vilanterol did not show an increased risk for major adverse events or fatal events relative to placebo in a phase IIIb trial (39). Anticholinergic symptoms were present in less than 1%–2% of patients, and the most common side effects noted were headaches and nasopharyngitis (39). Similarly multiple clinical trials have shown that aclidinum bromide is generally well tolerated with no increased incidence of serious adverse effects relative to placebo and minimal anticholinergic side effects (<1%–2%). The most common side effects were headaches and nasopharyngitis (40).

Long-acting beta agonists

Long-acting beta agonist therapy has been an important component of COPD therapy since the 1980s; the modality of inhalational therapy has been critical to the success of LABA therapy, allowing targeted delivery to the lung and maximizing drug safety. LABA agents have numerous clinical benefits, including reducing acute exacerbations of disease, improving airflow, and decreasing dyspnea (18,41,42). LABA agents have been utilized for monotherapy, but there are also known synergistic benefits when they are utilized as combination agents with LAMAs and ICSs (43,44). Formoterol and salmeterol are two of the oldest and most common agents utilized. More recently, very long-acting beta agonists (VLABAs) have become available (45). Such agents are available for once daily dosing and include indacaterol, vilanterol, and olodaterol (45–47).

In the TORCH trial, salmeterol, the best studied LABA, significantly decreased exacerbation rates, improved lung function, and improved health-related quality of life compared to placebo (48). A meta-analysis comparing salmeterol and formoterol showed that formoterol had an 80%–90% chance of offering symptom relief at six months relative to salmeterol, as measured by the St. George's Respiratory Questionnaire (49). A number of studies suggest that VLABAs may be superior at improving lung function and providing symptom relief relative compared to LABAs (50,51).

LABA monotherapy in patients with asthma is considered contraindicated as such treatment has been linked to an increased risk of life-threatening exacerbations and respiratory-related death. However, LABA monotherapy is considered potential first-line therapy in COPD and such concerns do not exist (48). The theoretical safety concern with LABA therapy is that inhaled beta agonists effect could act systemically and cause tachycardia, arrhythmias, and adverse cardiovascular events. The TORCH trial did not show increased cardiovascular events or mortality in patients on LABA monotherapy relative to placebo (48).

Inhaled corticosteroids

Increased airway inflammation is central to COPD pathogenesis (5). As such, inhaled corticosteroids, which target a number of inflammatory pathways, are commonly prescribed. However, while ICS agents are considered first-line controller therapy in asthma patients, they are not indicated for all COPD patients (1). For most COPD patients, maintenance bronchodilator regimens should be prioritized prior to initiation of ICS therapy (1). Nevertheless, nearly 40%–50% patients with COPD are prescribed ICS therapy (52). Subgroups of COPD patients felt to benefit from ICS-containing regimens in COPD include those with COPD/asthma overlap syndrome as well as those with two or more acute exacerbations of disease (1). Multiple studies have demonstrated the efficacy of inhaled corticosteroids in preventing acute COPD exacerbations (10). Notably, when prescribed for COPD, ICS should be used in conjunction with LABA as combination ICS/LABA therapy is superior to ICS monotherapy for COPD (1).

While systemic corticosteroids carry the risk of systemic side effects, including adrenocortical suppression, osteoporosis, bone fractures, skin thinning, diabetes, glaucoma, cataracts, and weight gain (53), inhaled glucocorticoids do not have widespread systemic bioavailability (26). It should be noted that despite relatively low systemic bioavailability, several randomized controlled trials (RCTs) have shown an increased risk for pneumonia in those receiving ICS therapy (54). A meta-analysis of 11 RCTs has also shown that patients on the highest doses of ICS therapy are the greatest risk for pneumonia (54). Despite these risks, observational studies of ICS therapy have not shown increased overall mortality in COPD patients or pneumonia-related mortality (55,56).

Long-acting muscarinic antagonist/long-acting beta agonist combinations

LAMA and LABA inhalational therapy as discussed above are mainstays in the management of COPD given their minimal adverse side effects and well-documented clinical efficacy. Each agent has a distinct mechanism of action on the airway. Combining these bronchodilators appears to have a synergistic effect in improving lung function, leading to better efficacy relative to monocomponent therapy (57). Furthermore, recent data has demonstrated that LAMA/LABA treatment is safe and has superior efficacy in preventing acute exacerbations of COPD compared to ICS/LABA therapy (9). As such, LAMA/LABA treatment is considered first-line therapy among COPD patients with a high symptoms burden and an increased risk of acute exacerbations of disease.

INHALED DEVICES AND IMPLICATIONS FOR CLINICAL CARE

Currently, a number of devices are available for inhaled therapeutics for COPD patients, including nebulizers, pressurized metered dose inhalers (pMDIs), breath-activated pMDIs (BA-MDIs), dry powder inhalers (DPIs), and soft mist inhalers (SMIs) (58). Nebulizers function by converting a liquid in solution or suspension into small droplets (59). In the past, their large size and requirement for accessory equipment (e.g., facemask) made them cumbersome. However, they have undergone significant revisions in design over the years and are now more compact. There are a variety of nebulizers used for COPD treatment, including vibrating mesh, jet, and ultrasonic (58). The pMDI, introduced in 1956, incorporates a propellant, under pressure, to generate a metered-dose of an aerosol through an atomization nozzle (60). pMDIs require coordination of actuation and inhalation for proper delivery of aerosolized medication. These agents can be used with spacers or holding chambers, which allow the velocity of medication particles to decrease before reaching the mouth (61). These holding chambers can facilitate coordination and decrease the amount of oropharyngeal deposition of medication. In addition, BA-MDIs are available that may be helpful for patients with poor coordination of actuation and inhalation. Today, pMDIs are the most commonly used inhalers in COPD management. DPIs are breath-actuated and require the patient to create turbulent inspiratory forces to disaggregate powder medication into fine particles (62). These devices do not require coordination of actuation and inhalation, but they do require an adequate inspiratory flow to ensure proper delivery of inhaled medication. The most recent advancement in handheld inhaler technology is that of the SMI. It is a propellant-free liquid inhaler that creates an aerosol cloud; this may facilitate higher lung drug deposition and lower oropharyngeal deposition when compared to pMDIs or DPIs (63).

Technology-based clinical outcomes

Numerous clinical trials, literature reviews, and expert panel guidelines inform the choice of inhalational drugs; however, in many cases there is no evidence-based rationale for choosing one aerosol device over another (64). A comprehensive special report published in 2005 compared the efficacy of treatment using nebulizers versus pMDIs with or without a spacer/holding chamber versus DPIs. The aim of the report was to provide recommendations to clinicians in selecting a particular aerosol delivery device for their patients (65). Pooled meta-analyses of randomized controlled trials failed to show a significant difference between devices in efficacy outcomes, and it was concluded that each of the devices studied can work equally well in patients who can use them appropriately (64). Similarly, a 2016 Cochrane review article comparing nebulizers to pMDIs and to DPIs concluded that there was a lack of evidence in favor of one mode of delivery over another for bronchodilator treatment during acute exacerbations of COPD (66).

It is worth noting that the conclusions from the above noted reviews were based on pooled studies in which patients received proper education on inhaler use and their ability to execute the technique was confirmed. The equivalence of device technology may therefore only exist in the setting of ideal use. Clearly, patient factors may lead to suboptimal use and differences in outcomes based on inhaler choice. Indeed, numerous studies have demonstrated that patients commonly use their inhalers incorrectly (67,68). COPD is a disease of the elderly and often associated with numerous comorbidities. In addition, problems with proper inspiratory flow generation and coordination become more acute as the disease progresses and as the patient develops more airflow limitation. As such, incorrect inhaler technique has been reported in a very high proportion of COPD patients (67). This leads to inadequate disease control and unnecessary disease morbidity and mortality. It has also been estimated that there are marked economic consequences related in inhaler misuse among patient with obstructive lung disease (69).

Common sources of error include failure to properly prime a pMDI, exhaling into the DPI mouthpiece, and actuating more than one dose into a spacer or holding chamber. However, the two most important patient factors affecting inhaler use in COPD patients include the inability of patients to coordinate breath actuation in pMDIs and the inability to generate sufficient inspiratory flow to actuate a BA-pMDI or a DPI. In light of these two main considerations, recommendations for appropriate delivery devices according to patient characteristics have been published by a European Respiratory Society and International Society for Aerosols in Medicine task force (61). These recommendations suggest that patients with poor inspiratory flow capabilities (< 30 liters/min) be prescribed either a pMDI or a nebulizer. If these patients have poor actuation-inhalation coordination as well, pMDIs should be used with a spacer.

Patients with acceptable inspiratory flows (> 30 liters/min) can be prescribed pMDIs, BA-MDIs, DPIs, or nebulizers. Again, patients with poor actuation-inhalation coordination should be given a spacer when a pMDI is prescribed (61).

Given the importance of patient factors, patient education in proper technique is critical to device function and medication delivery. A 2017 review of 39 randomized control trials concluded that educational interventions on inhaler technique were successful and may result in improved clinical outcomes for patients with COPD (70). These findings may be especially relevant for patients using multiple types of inhalers. There are now over 250 different device–drug combinations available (61). Understanding the proper use of these devices can be challenging for both patients and providers alike. A 2016 survey of pulmonologists revealed that only 54% of respondents were "extremely or very knowledgeable" about treatment devices, and 83% were interested in receiving additional education on COPD treatment devices (62). Naturally, improved training of providers will result in better patient education on proper inhaler technique.

Future technology

The development of future inhaled therapeutics for COPD management should consider aspects most relevant to this population. Such considerations should include methods to facilitate adequate drug delivery to the peripheral airways, especially in patients with severe airflow limitation. In addition, inhalers that facilitate optimal coordination of device actuation and inhalation as well as those that promote adherence to therapy would represent significant advances. Inhaled therapy that optimizes particle size and mass median aerodynamic diameter to promote peripheral distribution of drug should also be considered. The further development of slow-moving velocity aerosols may promote increased lung deposition and peripheral distribution (58). In addition, the development of lipid-based carriers and nanoparticles may be very effective in enhancing distribution of aerosolized medication (71).

Some vibrating mesh nebulizers use smart technology with microchips that can be adaptive and pulse the nebulized drug delivery during the inhalation phase, thus facilitating adherence. Other smart devices such as those utilizing an electronic smart card may facilitate accurate aerosol dosing and delivery, also promoting adherence. Digital inhalers appear to be on the horizon. Electronic systems are being designed to help patients with their care management via electronic dose counting, calendar reminders, and measurement of physiological parameters (71). Inhalers that record and store data on the patient's lung function will help providers guide current and future treatment. Given the global burden of COPD and the critical nature of inhaled therapy in disease management, such new technologies have the potential for substantial impact on worldwide public health.

REFERENCES

1. Vogelmeier CF, Criner GJ, Martinez FJ, Anzueto A, Barnes PJ, Bourbeau J, Celli BR et al. Global strategy for the diagnosis, management, and prevention of chronic obstructive lung disease 2017 report: GOLD executive summary. *Eur Respir J*. 2017;49:1700214. doi:10.1183/13993003.50214-2017.

2. Miniño AM, Murphy S, Xu J, Kochanek KD. Deaths: Final data for 2008. *National Vital Statistics Reports: Centers for Disease Control and Prevention*. 2011;59:1–26.

3. Morbidity & Mortality: 2012 Chart book on cardio-vascular, lung, and blood diseases. Bethesda, MD: National Heart, Lung, and Blood Institute, National Institute of Health; 2012.

4. Drummond MB, Buist AS, Crapo JD, Wise RA, Rennard SI. Chronic obstructive pulmonary dis-ease: NHLBI workshop on the primary preven-tion of chronic lung diseases. *Ann Am Thorac Soc*. 2014;11(Suppl 3):S154–S160. doi:10.1513/AnnalsATS.201312-432LD.

5. Stewart JI, Criner GJ. The small airways in chronic obstructive pulmonary disease: Pathology and effects on disease progression and survival. *Curr Opin Pulm Med*. 2013;19(2):109–115. doi:10.1097/MCP.0b013e32835ceefc.

6. Timmins SC, Diba C, Farrow CE, Schoeffel RE, Berend N, Salome CM, King GG. The relation-ship between airflow obstruction, emphysema extent, and small airways function in COPD. *Chest*. 2012;142(2):312–319. doi:10.1378/chest.11-2169.

7. O'Donnell DE, Webb KA. The major limitation to exercise performance in COPD is dynamic hyperinfla-tion. *J Appl Physiol (1985)*. 2008;105(2):753–755; dis-cussion 5–7. doi:10.1152/japplphysiol.90336.2008b.

8. O'Donnell DE, Casaburi R, Frith P, Kirsten A, De Sousa D, Hamilton A, Xue W, Maltais F. Effects of combined tiotropium/olodaterol on inspiratory capacity and exercise endurance in COPD. *Eur Resp J*. 2017;49(4). doi:10.1183/13993003.01348-2016.

9. Wedzicha JA, Banerji D, Chapman KR, Vestbo J, Roche N, Ayers RT, Thach C et al. Indacaterol-glycopyrronium versus salmeterol-fluticasone for COPD. *N Engl J Med*. 2016;374(23):2222–2234. doi:10.1056/NEJMoa1516385.

10. Nannini LJ, Lasserson TJ, Poole P. Combined corticosteroid and long-acting beta(2)-agonist in one inhaler versus long-acting beta(2)-ago-nists for chronic obstructive pulmonary disease. *Cochrane Database Syst Rev*. 2012;9:CD006829. doi:10.1002/14651858.CD006829.pub2.

11. Barnes PJ. Muscarinic receptor subtypes in airways. *Life Sci*. 1993;52(5–6):521–527.

12. Barnes PJ. Distribution of receptor targets in the lung. *Proc Am Thorac Soc*. 2004;1(4):345–351. doi:10.1513/pats.200409-045MS.

13. Restrepo RD. Use of inhaled anticholinergics in obstructive airway disease. *Resp care*. 2007;52:833–851.

14. Bucher H, Duechs MJ, Tilp C, Jung B, Erb KJ. Tiotropium attenuates virus-induced pulmonary inflammation in cigarette smoke-exposed mice. *J Pharmacol Exp Ther*. 2016;357(3):606–618. doi:10.1124/jpet.116.232009.

15. Mak JC, Barnes PJ. Autoradiographic visualization of muscarinic receptor subtypes in human and guinea pig lung. *Am Rev Resp Dis*. 1990;141(6):1559–1568. doi:10.1164/ajrccm/141.6.1559.

16. Johnson M. Molecular mechanisms of beta(2)-adrenergic receptor function, response, and regulation. *J Allergy Clin Immunol*. 2006;117(1):18–24; quiz 5. doi:10.1016/j.jaci.2005.11.012.

17. Roux FJ, Grandordy B, Douglas JS. Functional and binding characteristics of long acting Beta-2 ago-nists in lung and heart. *Am J Respir Crit Care Med*. 1996;153:1489–1495.

18. Cazzola M, Page CP, Calzetta L, Matera MG. Pharmacology and therapeutics of bronchodilators. *Pharmacol Rev*. 2012;64(3):450–504. doi:10.1124/pr.111.004580.

19. Anderson GP, Linden A, Rabe KF. Why are long-acting beta-adrenoceptor agonists long acting? *Eur Resp J*. 1994;7:435–441.

20. Crisafulli E, Frizzelli A, Fantin A, Manco A, Mangia A, Pisi G, Fainardi V et al. Next generation beta adr-enoreceptor agonists for the treatment of asthma. *Expert Opin Pharmacother*. 2017;18(14):1499–1505. doi:10.1080/14656566.2017.1378348.

21. Gill SK, Marriott HM, Suvarna SK, Peachell PT. Evaluation of the anti-inflammatory effects of β-adrenoceptor agonists on human lung mac-rophages. *Eur J Pharmacol*. 2016;793:49–55. doi:10.1016/j.ejphar.2016.11.005.

22. Theron AJ, Steel HC, Tintinger GR, Feldman C, Anderson R. Can the anti-inflammatory activities of β2-agonists be harnessed in the clinical setting? *Drug Des Devel Ther*. 2013;7:1387–1398. doi:10.2147/DDDT.S50995.

23. Carstairs JR, Nimmo AJ, Barnes PJ. Autoradiographic visualization of beta-adreno-ceptor subtypes in human lung. *Am Rev Resp Dis*. 1985;132(3):541–547. doi:10.1164/arrd.1985.132.3.541.

24. Vandewalle J, Luypaert A, De Bosscher K, Libert C. Therapeutic mechanisms of glucocorticoids. *Trends Endocrinol Metab*. 2018;29(1):42–54. doi:10.1016/j.tem.2017.10.010.

25. Raissy HH, Kelly HW, Harkins M, Szefler SJ. Inhaled corticosteroids in lung diseases. *Am J Resp Crit Care Med*. 2013;187(8):798–803.

26. Dalby C, Polanowski T, Larsson T, Borgstrom L, Edsbacker S, Harrison TW. The bioavailability and airway clearance of the steroid component of budesonide/formoterol and salmeterol/fluticasone

after inhaled administration in patients with COPD and healthy subjects: A randomized controlled trial. *Resp Res.* 2009;10:104–114.

27. Long F, Wang Y, Qi HH, Zhou X, Jin XQ. Rapid non-genomic effects of glucocorticoids on oxidative stress in a guinea pig model of asthma. *Respirology.* 2008;13:227–232.

28. Adcock IM, Gilbey T, Gelder CM, Chung KF, Barnes PJ. Glucocorticoid receptor localization in normal and asthmatic lung. *Am J Respir Crit Care Med.* 1996;154(3 Pt 1):771–782. doi:10.1164/ajrccm.154.3.8810618.

29. Laube BL, Swift DL, Wagner HN, Norman PS, Adams GK. The effect of bronchial obstruction on central airway deposition of a saline aerosol in patients with asthma. *Am Rev Respir Dis.* 1986;133(5):740–743.

30. Barnes PJ. Pulmonary pharmacology. In: Brunton LL, Chabner BA, Knollmann BC (Eds.), *Goodman & Gilman's The pharmacological Basis of Therapeutics.* 12th ed. New York: McGraw-Hill, 2011.

31. Mastrodicasa MA, Droege CA, Mulhall AM, Ernst NE, Panos RJ, Zafar MA. Long acting muscarinic antagonists for the treatment of chronic obstructive pulmonary disease: A review of current and developing drugs. *Expert Opin Inv Drug.* 2017;26(2):161–174.

32. Koumis T, Samuel S. Tiotropium bromide: A new long-acting bronchodilator for the treatment of chronic obstructive pulmonary disease. *Clin Ther.* 2005;27:377–392.

33. Cheyne L, Irvin-Sellers M, White J. Tiotropium versus ipratropium bromide for chronic obstructive pulmonary disease. *Cochrane Database Syst Rev.* 2013;9:CD009552.

34. Tashkin DP, Celli B, Senn S, Burkhart D, Kesten S, Menjoge S, Decramer M, Investigators US. A 4-year trial of tiotropium in chronic obstructive pulmonary disease. *N Engl J Med.* 2008;359(15):1543–1554. doi:10.1056/NEJMoa0805800.

35. Jones P, Beeh K, Chapman KR, Decramer M, Mahler DA, Wedzicha JA. Minimal clinically important differences in pharmacological trials. *Am J Resp Crit Care Med.* 2014;189:250–255.

36. Ismaila AS, Huisman E, Punekar YS, Karabis A. Comparative efficacy of long-acting muscarinic antagonist monotherapies in COPD: A systematic review and network meta-analysis. *Int J Chron Obstruct Pulmon Dis.* 2015;10:2495–2517.

37. Pappano AJ. Cholinoceptor blocking drugs. In: Katzung BG, Trevor AJ (Eds.), *Basic and Clinical Pharmacology.* 13th ed. New York: McGraw-Hill Education Companies, Inc, 2015, pp. 121–132.

38. Halpin D, Dahl R, Hallmann C, Mueller A, Tashkin D. Tiotropium HandiHaler® and Respimat® in COPD: A pooled safety analysis. *Int J Chronic Obstructive Pulmon Dis.* 2015;10:239–259.

39. Donohue JF, Niewoehner D, Brooks J, O'Dell D, Church A. Safety and tolerability of once-daily umeclidinium/vilanterol 125/25 mcg and umeclidinium 125 mcg in patients with chronic obstructive pulmonary disease: Results from a 52-week, randomized, double-blind, placebo-controlled study. *Respir Res.* 2014;15:78. doi:10.1186/1465-9921-15-78.

40. Armstrong E, Wright B. The role of aclidinium bromide in the treatment of chronic obstructive pulmonary disease. *Hosp Pract.* 2014;42(4):99–110.

41. Wang J, Nie B, Xiong W, Xu Y. Effect of long-acting beta-agonists on the frequency of COPD exacerbations: A meta-analysis. *J Clin Pharm Ther.* 2012;37(2):204–211. doi:10.1111/j.1365-2710.2011.01285.x.

42. Barnes PJ, Pedersen S, Busse WW. Efficacy and safety of inhaled corticosteroids. New developments. *Am J Respir Crit Care Med.* 1998;157(3 Pt 2):S1–S53. doi:10.1164/ajrccm.157.3.157315.

43. Schmidt M, Michel MC. How can 1 + 1 = 3? β2-adrenergic and glucocorticoid receptor agonist synergism in obstructive airway diseases. *Mol Pharmacol.* 2011;80(6):955–958. doi:10.1124/mol.111.075481.

44. Cohen JS, Miles MC, Donohue JF, Ohar JA. Dual therapy strategies for COPD: The scientific rationale for LAMA + LABA. *Int J Chron Obstruct Pulmon Dis.* 2016;11:785–797. doi:10.2147/COPD.S54513.

45. Ridolo E, Montagni M, Olivieri E, Riario-Sforza GG, Incorvaia C. Role of indacaterol and the newer very long-acting β2-agonists in patients with stable COPD: A review. *Int J Chron Obstruct Pulmon Dis.* 2013;7:425–432.

46. Beier J, Chanez P, Martinot JB, Schreurs AJ, Tkácová R, Bao W, Jack D, Higgins M. Safety, tolerability and efficacy of indacaterol, a novel once-daily beta(2)-agonist, in patients with COPD: A 28-day randomised, placebo controlled clinical trial. *Pulm Pharmacol Ther.* 2007;20(6):740–749. doi:10.1016/j.pupt.2006.09.001.

47. Slack RJ, Barrett VJ, Morrison VS, Sturton RG, Emmons AJ, Ford AJ, Knowles RG. In vitro pharmacological characterization of vilanterol, a novel long-acting β2-adrenoceptor agonist with 24-hour duration of action. *J Pharmacol Exp Ther.* 2013;344(1):218–230. doi:10.1124/jpet.112.198481.

48. Calverley PM, Anderson JA, Celli B, Ferguson GT, Jenkins C, Jones PW, Yates JC, Vestbo J. Salmeterol and fluticasone propionate and survival in chronic obstructive pulmonary disease. *N Engl J Med.* 2007;356(8):775–789. doi:10.1056/NEJMoa063070.

49. Cope S, Donohue JF, Jansen JP, Kraemer M, Capkun-Niggli G, Baldwin M, Buckley F et al. Comparative efficacy of long-acting bronchodilators for COPD: A network meta-analysis. *Respir Res.* 2013;14:100. doi:10.1186/1465-9921-14-100.

50. Bauwens O, Ninane V, Van de Maele B, Firth R, Dong F, Owen R, Higgins M. 24-hour bronchodilator efficacy of single doses of indacaterol in subjects with COPD: Comparison with placebo and formoterol. *Curr Med Res Opin.* 2009;25(2):463–470. doi:10.1185/03007990802675096.

51. Beier J, Beeh KM, Brookman L, Peachey G, Hmissi A, Pascoe S. Bronchodilator effects of indacaterol and formoterol in patients with COPD. *Pulm Pharmacol Ther.* 2009;22(6):492–496. doi:10.1016/j.pupt.2009.05.001.

52. Van Andel AE, Reisner C, Menjoge SS, Witek TJ. Analysis of inhaled corticosteroid and oral theophylline use among patients with stable COPD from 1987 to 1995. *Chest.* 1999;115(3):703–707.

53. Saag K, Furst D, Barnes P. Major Side Effects of Inhaled Glucocorticoids: UpToDate; 2017 [cited November 2, 2018].

54. Drummond MB, Dasenbrook EC, Pitz MW, Murphy DJ, Fan E. Inhaled corticosteroids in patients with stable chronic obstructive pulmonary disease: A systematic review and meta-analysis. *JAMA.* 2008;300(20):2407–2416. doi:10.1001/jama.2008.717.

55. Singanayagam A, Chalmers JD, Akram AR, Hill AT. Impact of inhaled corticosteroid use on outcome in COPD patients admitted with pneumonia. *Eur Resp J.* 2011;38(1):36–41. doi:10.1183/09031936.00077010.

56. Chen D, Restrepo MI, Fine MJ, Pugh MJ, Anzueto A, Metersky ML, Nakashima B et al. Observational study of inhaled corticosteroids on outcomes for COPD patients with pneumonia. *Am J Respir Crit Care Med.* 2011;184(3):312–316. doi:10.1164/rccm.201012-2070OC.

57. Cazzola M, Molimard M. The scientific rationale for combining long-acting beta2-agonists and muscarinic antagonists in COPD. *Pulm Pharmacol Ther.* 2010;23(4):257–267. doi:10.1016/j.pupt.2010.03.003.

58. Rogliani P, Calzetta L, Coppola A, Cavalli F, Ora J, Puxeddu E, Matera MG, Cazzola M. Optimizing drug delivery in COPD: The role of inhaler devices. *Respir Med.* 2017;124:6–14. doi:10.1016/j.rmed.2017.01.006.

59. Dolovich MB, Dhand R. Aerosol drug delivery: Developments in device design and clinical use. *Lancet.* 2011;377(9770):1032–1045. doi:10.1016/S0140-6736(10)60926-9.

60. Smyth HD. The influence of formulation variables on the performance of alternative propellant-driven metered dose inhalers. *Adv Drug Deliv Rev.* 2003;55(7):807–828.

61. Laube BL, Janssens HM, de Jongh FH, Devadason SG, Dhand R, Diot P, Everard ML et al. What the pulmonary specialist should know about the new inhalation therapies. *Eur Respir J.* 2011;37(6):1308–1331. doi:10.1183/09031936.00166410.

62. Braman S, Carlin BW, Hanania DA, Mahler DA, Ohar JA, Pinto-Plata V, Shah T, Eubanks D, Dhand R. Results of a pulmonologist survey regarding knowledge and practices with inhalation devices for COPD *Respir Care.* 2018;63(7):840–848.

63. Anderson P. Use of respimat soft mist inhaler in COPD patients. *Int J Chron Obstruct Pulmon Dis.* 2006;1(3):251–259.

64. Sims MW. Aerosol therapy for obstructive lung diseases: Device selection and practice management issues. *Chest.* 2011;140(3):781–788. doi:10.1378/chest.10-2068.

65. Dolovich MB, Ahrens RC, Hess DR, Anderson P, Dhand R, Rau JL, Smaldone GC, Guyatt G, Physicians ACoC, American College of Asthma AI, Immunology. Device selection and outcomes of aerosol therapy: Evidence-based guidelines: American College of Chest Physicians/American College of Asthma, Allergy, and Immunology. *Chest.* 2005;127(1):335–371. doi:10.1378/chest.127.1.335.

66. van Geffen WH, Douma WR, Slebos DJ, Kerstjens HA. Bronchodilators delivered by nebuliser versus pMDI with spacer or DPI for exacerbations of COPD. *Cochrane Database Syst Rev.* 2016;8:CD011826. doi:10.1002/14651858.CD011826.pub2.

67. Molimard M, Raherison C, Lignot S, Balestra A, Lamarque S, Chartier A, Droz-Perroteau C et al. Chronic obstructive pulmonary disease exacerbation and inhaler device handling: Real-life assessment of 2935 patients. *Eur Resp J.* 2017;49(2). doi:10.1183/13993003.01794-2016.

68. Molimard M, Raherison C, Lignot S, Depont F, Abouelfath A, Moore N. Assessment of handling of inhaler devices in real life: An observational study in 3811 patients in primary care. *J Aerosol Med.* 2003;16(3):249–254. doi:10.1089/089426803769017613.

69. Usmani OS, Lavorini F, Marshall J, Dunlop WCN, Heron L, Farrington E, Dekhuijzen R. Critical inhaler errors in asthma and COPD: A systematic review of impact on health outcomes. *Resp Res.* 2018;19(1):10. doi:10.1186/s12931-017-0710-y.

70. Klijn SL, Hiligsmann M, Evers SM, Román-Rodríguez M, van der Molen T, van Boven JF. Effectiveness and success factors of educational inhaler technique interventions in asthma & COPD patients: A systematic review. *NPJ Prim Care Resp Med.* 2017;27(1):24. doi:10.1038/s41533-017-0022-1.

71. Bailey MM, Berkland CJ. Nanoparticle formulations in pulmonary drug delivery. *Med Res Rev.* 2009;29(1):196–212. doi:10.1002/med.20140.

13

Cystic fibrosis infection and biofilm busters

JENNIFER FIEGEL AND SACHIN GHARSE

Introduction 223
CF and pulmonary infections 223
  Progression and prevalence of airway pathogens
  in people with CF 224
Current treatments for CF infections 226
  Mucolytic agents 226
  Antibiotic therapies for CF airway infections 226
  Limitations of current treatment strategies 227
Bacterial biofilms in CF 228
  Antibiotic resistance in biofilms 228

Biofilm busters: Novel strategies to eradicate
bacterial biofilms 229
  Antimicrobial peptides 229
  Bacteriophage therapy 230
  Chelating agents 231
  Dispersion compounds 231
  Quorum sensing inhibitors (QSIs) 232
  Silver 232
Conclusion 232
References 233

INTRODUCTION

Cystic fibrosis (CF), one of the most fatal genetic disorders in the world, is a multi-organ disorder caused by mutations in the cystic fibrosis transmembrane conductance regulator (CFTR) gene. The disorder is predominantly observed in Caucasian populations of European ancestry, affecting more than 70,000 people worldwide, with approximately 1000 new CF cases diagnosed every year (1). It is estimated that nearly 10 million people carry the defective CFTR gene, which can be passed on to offspring (2). CF is associated with significant morbidity and early mortality (3).

Up to 95% of people with CF die due to respiratory failure caused by chronic bacterial infections, airway inflammation, and the resulting severe lung damage (4,5). Current clinical therapy is primarily focused on managing the disease through a regular treatment routine to ease symptoms and reduce complications. The treatment regimen includes airway clearance therapy, inhaled mucoactive agents, antibiotic therapy, and nutrient therapy. These strategies have significantly improved the quality of life for CF patients and increased their median age from less than 5 years in the early 1950s, before the introduction of airway clearance and antibiotic treatments, to almost 40 years today (3).

A primary goal of current therapy is to control infections in the lungs, often through aggressive antibiotic therapy. However, bacterial infections remain difficult to treat using conventional antibiotics due to inefficient drug dosing and delivery, the development of antibiotic resistance, and formation of bacterial biofilms in CF lungs. As a result, a number of strategies are being investigated to enhance bacterial susceptibility to traditional antibiotics or to overcome bacterial survival strategies. This chapter will provide a summary of CF pulmonary infections and current treatment strategies, then delve into the role of bacterial biofilms in therapy failure and new strategies to bust bacterial biofilms.

CF AND PULMONARY INFECTIONS

While CF is a multi-organ disorder, the majority of morbidity and mortality associated with the disorder is caused by its manifestation in the lungs. CFTR is a c-AMP-regulated anion channel located on the surfaces of airway epithelial cells (Figure 13.1). It regulates chloride and bicarbonate conduction and sodium absorption across the airway epithelia. Since active ion transport across the epithelium is accompanied by water flow, CFTR regulates water levels in the airway surface liquid (ASL), keeping the epithelial surface hydrated. Mutations in CFTR cause an ion transport defect, resulting in reduced anion secretion and enhanced sodium absorption at the airway epithelium. More than 1900 mutations in the CFTR gene have been identified to cause CF, with different molecular consequences such as defective gating or conductance of CFTR channels.

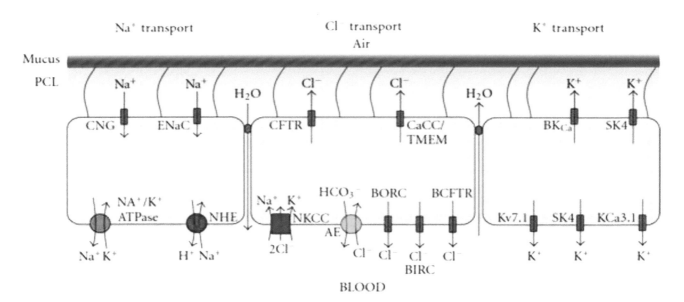

Figure 13.1 Schematic drawing of ciliated airway epithelial cells with Na+, Cl-, and K+channels and transporters. On the apical side, the airway epithelium is covered by the airway surface liquid that consists of the periciliary liquid (PCL) surrounding the cilia and the mucus layer lying atop the PCL. The composition of the PCL is regulated by ion transport processes, mainly apical Na+ reabsorption and Cl- secretion, with H$_2$O following passively along the osmotic gradient. Epithelia display a prominent apical Cl- secretion that is mainly mediated by the cystic fibrosis transmembrane conductance regulator (CFTR) in humans (middle cell). (Reprinted without changes from: Monika I. Hollenhorst, Katrin Richter, and Martin Fronius, "Ion Transport by Pulmonary Epithelia," *Journal of Biomedicine and Biotechnology*, vol. 2011, Article ID 174306, 16 pages, 2011. Copyright © 2011. doi:10.1155/2011/174306. Monika I. Hollenhorst et al. This is an open access article distributed under the Creative Commons Attribution License 3.0 (https://creativecommons.org/licenses/by/3.0/.)

Defective ion transport across the airway epithelium results in increased water flow out of the ASL into the epithelium, leading to dehydration of the airway surface (Figure 13.2) (5). Compression of the periciliary liquid (PCL) layer and an increase in the viscosity of the mucus layer follows, inhibiting ciliary motion and reducing mucociliary clearance. As the disease progresses, mucus plugs are formed that obstruct the airways (3,5). CFTR also mediates bicarbonate secretion, which plays a crucial role in host defense. Defective bicarbonate secretion reduces the pH of the ASL, which in turn renders the host antimicrobial peptides less effective (5,6). Due to these clinical manifestations, CF lungs fail to clear or kill bacteria that enter the airways, providing sufficient residence time for bacteria to colonize the airways. Progression of the disease results in continued lung damage, which further provides bacterial pathogens a pathway to invade the epithelium (7).

Bacterial infection of CF airways is accompanied by an intense inflammatory response. Neutrophils are attracted to the site of inflammation and initial infections can be cleared by the neutrophil response. Thus, in the first few years of life of a CF patient, intermittent colonization is typically observed. As the age of CF patients progresses, persisting bacteria cause a recurrence of infections, and airway inflammation becomes dominated by persistent neutrophils. This inflammatory response is a prolonged version of the response seen in acute infections, as opposed to a macrophage-driven response typically observed in chronic infections. Over time, neutrophils break down and release high molecular weight DNA that further increases the viscosity of mucus and contributes to reduced mucociliary clearance. Inflammatory products secreted by the neutrophils cause structural damage to lung airways and ultimately lead to bronchiectasis. Eventually, most CF patients develop a vicious cycle of airway obstruction, bacterial infection, and excessive inflammation that leads to severe damage to lung airways, reduced clearance processes, and ultimately respiratory failure (8,9).

Progression and prevalence of airway pathogens in people with CF

A host of bacteria infect CF airways over the duration of patients' lives in an age-dependent manner (Figure 13.3) (8). Colonization of the airways begins in infancy or early childhood. Bacteria associated with the nose and skin, such as *Staphylococcus aureus* and *Haemophilus influenzae*, colonize CF airways in early stages. Over time, these organisms are replaced primarily by *Pseudomonas aeruginosa*, which is acquired via patient-to-patient or environmental transmission. *P. aeruginosa* is the main perpetrator of chronic pulmonary infections that adversely affects lung function (8,10–12). The prevalence of *P. aeruginosa* increases with age, and up

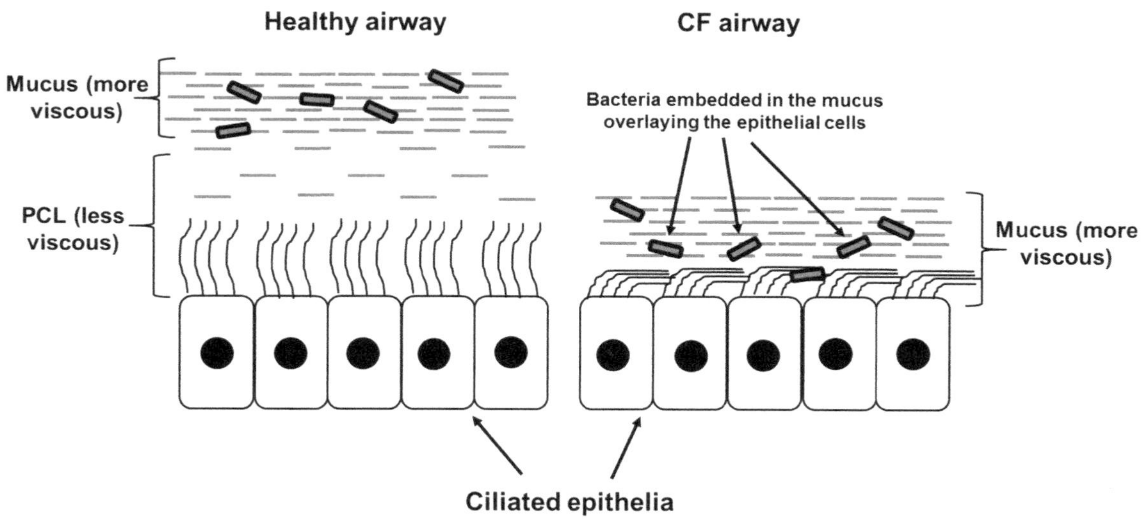

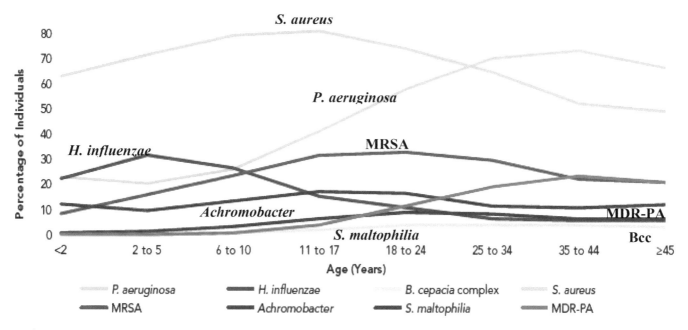

Figure 13.2 Schematic of airway mucosa in healthy (left) and CF airways (right). In healthy airways, the airway surface liquid (ASL) consists of two layers, the upper viscous mucus layer and the less viscous periciliary layer (PCL). The ASL traps pathogens and other inhaled foreign material, which is then cleared through the coordinated beating of cilia on the epithelial surface. In CF airways, water depletion in the airway surface liquid results in a compression of the PCL and cilia, as well as a more viscous mucus phase, causing impaired mucociliary clearance.

Figure 13.3 Prevalence of respiratory microorganisms in patients with CF by age cohort in 2015. Overall percentage of patients (all ages) who had at least one respiratory tract culture (sputum, bronchoscopy, oropharyngeal, or nasal) performed in 2015 that was positive for the following organisms: 47.5%; *Staphylococcus aureus* (green line), 70.6%; *Pseudomonas aeruginosa* (light blue line), *Haemophilus influenzae* (brown line), 15.5%; MRSA (red line), 26.0%; *Stenotrophomonas maltophilia* (purple line), 13.6%; MDR-*Pseudomonas aeruginosa* MDR-PA (dark blue line), 9.2%; *Achromobacter xylosoxidans* (black line), 6.1%; *Burkholderia cepacia* complex (yellow line). (Organisms reported to the U.S. Cystic Fibrosis Patient Registry, 2015. Source of data: Cystic fibrosis patients under care at CF Foundation-accredited care centers in the United States, who consented to have their data entered. Reprinted with permission from Foundation, C.F., *Patient Registry Annual Data Report*, Bethesda, MD, 2015. Copyright 2016 Cystic Fibrosis Foundation.)

to 80% of CF patients are ultimately infected. Smaller numbers of CF patients become infected with other organisms such as *Stenotrophomonas maltophilia* (approximately 30%), *Achromobacter xylosoxidans* (2%–18%) and *Burkholderia cepacia* complex (Bcc) (approximately 3%) (4,8,13–15).

The presence of several organisms has been associated with deterioration of lung function. *Burkholderia cepacia* complex (Bcc) is a group of gram-negative bacterial strains that are often highly resistant to antibiotics. Infections with Bcc have been associated with high fever, severe necrotizing pneumonia (also known as Cepacia syndrome), rapid decline in lung function, and death (8,17–19). *Achromobacter xylosoxidans* is an opportunistic human pathogen associated with a number of infections in individuals with weak immune system or with underlying diseases. The role of this organism with pathogenicity in CF is unclear, with only one study linking chronic infection of CF lungs by *A. xylosoxidans* to reduced lung function (13,20).

Multidrug resistance (MDR) is a bacterial trait that results from multiple resistance mechanisms, with most studies defining MDR as resistance to at least three antibiotics from different classes. MDR infections are much more difficult to treat because the number of antibiotics currently available is limited, resulting in poor therapeutic outcomes and higher mortality (21–23). The prevalence of bacterial strains exhibiting MDR rose substantially from 2000 to 2015, with approximately 25% of individuals culturing positive for methicillin-resistant *S. aureus* (MRSA) or MDR-*pseudomonas aeruginosa* (PA) (Figure 13.4). The number of reported cases has plateaued possibly due to "enhanced awareness and infection prevention and control strategies" (24). Nontuberculosis mycobacteria (NTM) (prevalence of 7%–24%) such as *Mycobacterium abcessus*

complex (MABSC) and *Mycobacterium avium-intracellulare* (MAC) are acquired from the environment and are commonly isolated from older CF patients. NTM are naturally resistant to many antibiotics, making their eradication difficult. MABSC (predominantly found in Europe), in particular, has been associated with a decline in lung function in CF patients (25).

CURRENT TREATMENTS FOR CF INFECTIONS

Because of *P. aeruginosa* prevalence and known pathogenicity, antimicrobial therapy in CF has focused on the eradication of *P. aeruginosa* from CF lungs (4). Genetic and phenotypic flexibility has allowed *P. aeruginosa* to adapt and persist in the CF airways. Current treatments for CF infections focus on aiding the mucociliary escalator to clear pathogens and antimicrobial therapy to kill the pathogens.

Mucolytic agents

Inhaled mucolytic agents reduce the viscosity and elasticity of CF airway mucus by breaking down the structural components of mucus. This results in an improved mucociliary clearance rate from the airways, which can aid the clearance of pathogens from the lungs. For example, dornase alfa, a recombinant human DNase, has been associated with reducing the frequency and severity of airway infections (26,27).

Antibiotic therapies for CF airway infections

Infection eradication in CF airways aims to eliminate *P. aeruginosa* bacteria once they have colonized the airways.

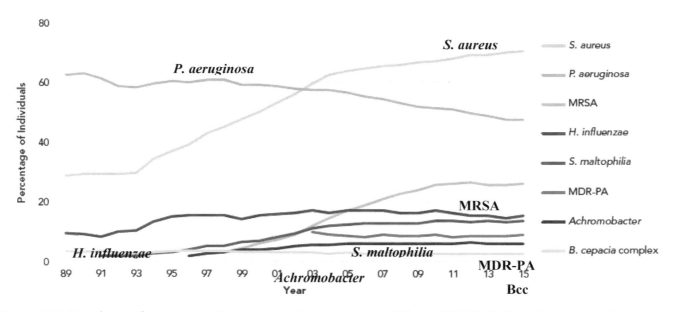

Figure 13.4 Prevalence of respiratory microorganisms in patients with CF from 1989–2015. (Organisms reported to the U.S. Cystic Fibrosis Patient Registry, 2015. Source of data: Cystic fibrosis patients under care at CF Foundation-accredited care centers in the United States, who consented to have their data entered. Reprinted with permission from Foundation, C.F., *Patient Registry Annual Data Report*, Bethesda, MD, 2015.)

The timing of treatment and choice of antibiotics depends upon the patient's age, susceptibility of the bacterium, and the severity of the infection (24). Antibiotics are administered individually or in combination via the oral route in the case of mild infections and via the intravenous or inhalation routes in case of moderate to severe infections (4,28). Prophylactic administration of antibiotics has not been adopted in the United States based on the guidelines provided by the Pulmonary Clinical Practice Guidelines Committee of the Cystic Fibrosis Foundation (29). Prior studies have observed that prophylactic administration of antibiotics via oral delivery, inhalation, or both routes together did not delay the rate of acquisition of *P. Aeruginosa* (30). Furthermore, prophylaxis treatment against initial *S. aureus* infections was observed to lead to earlier colonization and infection by *P. aeruginosa* and therefore did not prevent progression of infections (28,31). As a result, treatment has been focused on eradicating infections once bacteria colonize the airways.

Current treatment strategies against established pulmonary bacterial infections effectively slow down the progression of infections and improve the quality of life for CF patients (3). Chronic airway infections are treated using suppressive antibiotic therapy in order to maintain lung function. Approved antibiotics for the inhalation treatment of respiratory infections in CF patients, including tobramycin, aztreonam, and colistimethate sodium. Tobramycin inhalation solutions (such as TOBI®, TIS®, Kitabis Pak®, and Bethkis®) and tobramycin inhalation powder (TOBI Podhaler™), are currently available for management of chronic *P. aeruginosa* infections (28). Nebulized monobactam aztreonam lysine inhalation solution (Cayston®) is a safe and efficacious formulation against chronic *P. aeruginosa* infections in CF patients (28). Clinical studies carried out to compare the efficacies of Cayston and TIS in CF patients demonstrated superiority of Cayston over TIS in improving lung function, reducing pulmonary exacerbations, and aiding patient weight gain (32–34). An open-label study of aztreonam lysine inhalation solution showed similar success rates in eradicating *P. aeruginosa* as those reported for other antibiotic regimens (35). Cayston is available in the United States, Canada, Switzerland, and the European Union (28). Typically patients age 7 and over alternate between 28-day treatments of tobramycin and aztreonam.

In Europe, colistimethate sodium, a prodrug that hydrolyzes in the lungs to its active form, colistin, a cyclic polypeptide antibiotic, is used as the last line of defense against multidrug resistant gram-negative organisms (28). Colistin has demonstrated very low resistance rates against *P. aeruginosa* compared to other antibiotics (36,37). It is administered intravenously or via inhalation (the European Union only) as the prodrug colistimethate sodium (CMS), which is less toxic and has fewer side effects than the non-prodrug form (38). It is not FDA approved for use via inhalation in the United States due to the death of a patient from overdosing on a premixed solution, which led to dosing with a high

bioactive concentration. CMS dry powder (Colobreathe DPI®) is well tolerated in adult and younger patients (28,39).

Limitations of current treatment strategies

In spite of significant improvements in the quality of life and median life span of CF patients, the ability to eradicate bacterial populations using current treatment strategies diminishes over time. This is attributed to various factors that initiate bacterial resistance, including poor patient compliance with burdensome treatment regimens, suboptimal drug deposition and dosing of antibiotics in the lungs, and the formation of biofilms.

The time, money, and health resources necessitated by a multipronged treatment regimen, which includes airway clearance and nutrient therapies in addition to therapeutic drug treatments, make the medical regimen burdensome. Poor patient compliance has been linked to the development of bacterial resistance. The poor taste of nebulized drugs during prolonged inhalation treatments, difficulties administering therapies to children, difficulties associated with cleaning and disinfecting drug delivery devices, and patient forgetfulness in administering drugs all increase the level of noncompliance with treatments (40,41).

Even when patients do complete treatment regimens, issues with administering drugs at high enough doses to completely eradicate bacterial populations still abound. *P. aeruginosa* infections in CF lungs start in the smaller airways and, as the infection progresses, move into the larger airways. As the exact progression of disease is difficult to ascertain, therapeutic treatments aim to target antibiotics throughout the airways (42). However, mucus plugs block bronchi and bronchioles, and inhibit the deposition of antibiotics in regions distal to the airway obstruction (42,43). This results in suboptimal dosing of antibiotics in certain regions of the lungs to below the minimum inhibitory concentration (MIC) required to inhibit infection progression. At sub-MIC concentrations, bacteria develop drug resistance. Larger drug doses that would be required to overcome this are not feasible due to systemic and organ toxicity (42,44).

P. aeruginosa isolates from CF airways display distinct properties from *P. aeruginosa* causing acute infections in other diseases, and the genotypes and phenotypes further evolve in late stages of infection (8,45). CF isolates of *P. aeruginosa* also display larger genomes than laboratory strains, suggesting the possibility of newly acquired genes during their adaptation and alteration to the present genes (46). Recent studies have reported high prevalence of antibiotic-resistant, biofilm-forming phenotypes of *P. aeruginosa* in CF airways (47). Bacteria embedded in biofilms display characteristics such as reduced metabolic activity, slow growth, loss of flagella, a higher rate of mutation, and an increase in the expression of efflux transporters on the cell membrane. These characteristics contribute to reduced bacterial susceptibility to antibiotics; thus, the persistence of chronic *P. aeruginosa* infections is largely due to biofilm growth (45). This results in the recurrence of infections, leading to progressive lung damage and severe deterioration in quality of life (48–50).

BACTERIAL BIOFILMS IN CF

Bacterial biofilms, colonies of bacteria that are attached to the airway surface and protected by a self-produced polymeric matrix, form and evolve in a series of stages (Figure 13.5). The first stage involves the attachment of planktonic (free-flowing) bacteria to a surface, such as the airway surface. Initial attachment is reversible, mediated by nonspecific van der Waals, Lewis acid-base, and electrostatic interactions (51–53), while factors such as high repulsive forces or nutrient availability weaken or deter bacterial attachment to the surface. *P. aeruginosa* biofilms have been found in the mucus layer overlaying the epithelial cells in CF airways (54–56). The sticky mucus surface and stunted mucociliary clearance in CF lungs provide an ideal environment for bacteria to attach and proliferate (stage 2). Attached bacteria then form microcolonies and undergo changes in gene expression and upregulation of factors that favor sessility. These changes trigger secretion of an extracellular polymeric substance (EPS) matrix that surrounds the colonies, leading to formation of young biofilms (stage 3). The EPS matrix is mainly composed of water and high molecular weight molecules such as polysaccharides, proteins, nucleic acids, lipids, and humic substances. Mucoid bacterial strains secrete alginate, an exopolysaccharide that confers bacterial biofilms with protection from antibiotics and immune responses (4,57). The matrix aids biofilm formation and stabilization, while protecting the embedded bacterial colonies against the host defense system and antimicrobials (58). These colonies and the surrounding matrix grow over time to form mature biofilms (stage 4). Nutrient and oxygen gradients develop within the matrix because of their consumption by biofilm bacteria. The bacteria develop biofilm-specific characteristics, such as presence of pili (used for attachment) rather than flagella (used for movement), reduction in metabolism in response to nutrient depletion, and upregulation of efflux receptors on cell membrane (52,58). These characteristics further contribute to reduced bacterial susceptibility to antibiotics (8,45). Within the biofilm, bacteria constantly sense environmental changes in the matrix, such as fluctuations in oxygen level, nutrient availability, and accumulation of toxins in the matrix. The bacteria can respond to favorable changes by dispersing out of the biofilm by degrading the matrix (stage 5). In doing so, they regain plankton-like characteristics to migrate to another surface for attachment, where they may initiate formation of new biofilms (52,58).

Antibiotic resistance in biofilms

The effectiveness of an antibiotic depends on its concentration at the site of infection. Subinhibitory antibiotic concentrations lead to development of resistance and aid in the development of biofilms (Figure 13.6) (60). Antibiotic resistance in bacterial biofilms can be broadly divided into two types: resistance by the bacterial cells and resistance by the biofilm matrix.

Bacterial cells can resist antibiotics by a variety of mechanisms. *Intrinsic resistances* are those resistances that are part of the bacterial genetic makeup. These lead to higher baseline antibiotic treatment doses required to eradicate the infection. An example of intrinsic resistance is the inherently lower outer membrane permeability of *P. aeruginosa*, which is 10–100 times less than that of other gram-negative bacterial species (49). *Adaptive resistances* are resistances that the bacteria develop in response to environmental stimuli, such as changes in

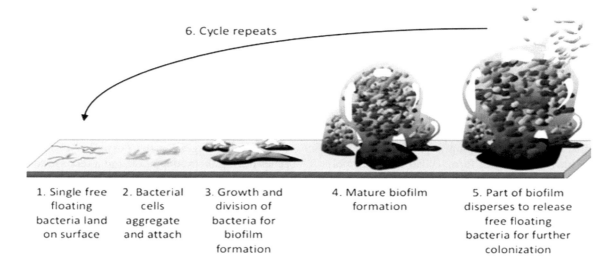

Figure 13.5 Stages involved in the formation, maturation, and propagation of biofilms. Stage 1, initial attachment; Stage 2, irreversible attachment; Stage 3, maturation I; Stage 4, maturation II; Stage 5, dispersion; Stage 6, formation of new colonies. (Adapted from Monroe, D., *PLoS Biol.*, 5, e307, 2007. This is an open-access article distributed under the terms of the Creative Commons Attribution License.)

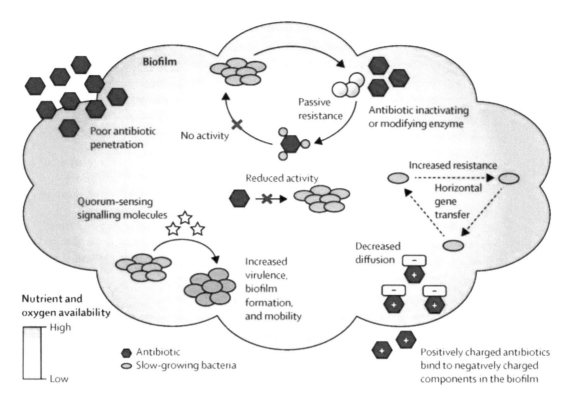

Figure 13.6 Factors affecting the susceptibility of biofilm bacteria to antibiotics. The permeability of antibiotics in the biofilm matrix is inhibited due to poor penetration and adsorption to various matrix components. Antibiotic-degrading enzymes such as β-lactamases break down the drug molecules in the matrix. Bacteria in the biofilm also display reduced metabolic activity in response to oxygen and nutrient depletion, resulting in reduced uptake of antibiotic molecules that manage to reach the bacterial cells. (Reprinted from *The Lancet*, 384, Sherrard, L.J. et al., Elborn, Antimicrobial resistance in the respiratory microbiota of people with cystic fibrosis, 703–713, 2014, with permission from Elsevier.)

nutrient levels and subinhibitory concentrations of antibiotics. Subinhibitory antibiotic concentrations trigger genetic changes in *P. aeruginosa* that allow the bacteria to withstand subsequent onslaughts of lethal antibiotic concentrations (49). For example, *P. aeruginosa* expresses efflux pumps such as MexAB-OprM and MexCD-OprJ on its cell membrane that assists in resistance against β-lactams and tetracyclines (61). *Acquired resistances* develop by acquisition of inheritable traits via transfer and sharing of antibiotic resistance genes between bacteria occupying the same environment. For example, *P. aeruginosa* are known to acquire plasmid-mediated extended spectrum β-lactamases from *Enterobacteriaceae*, which leads to inactivation of β-lactam antibiotics (48,49).

The biofilm matrix also plays an important role in protecting the embedded bacteria from antibiotics. The components of the biofilm matrix act as a physical barrier to antibiotics diffusing through the matrix. Negatively charged components of the matrix can adsorb positively charged antibiotics to further retard their diffusion. This ensures that the diffusing antibiotic does not achieve bactericidal concentrations near the organisms embedded in the matrix. The presence of antibiotic-degrading enzymes such as β-lactamase has also been observed in the matrix of *P. aeruginosa* biofilms (48).

As a result of these mechanisms, some bacterial cells within the biofilm survive after an antibiotic regimen. These cells, called persister cells, are often slow-growing or non-dividing cells. As the majority of available antibiotics target dividing cells, persisters cannot be eradicated until they undergo phenotypic changes resulting in plankton-like behavior. In the absence of antibiotics, persisters act as seeds for a new cycle of infection (49,50).

Biofilm busters: Novel strategies to eradicate bacterial biofilms

Various strategies to enhance the effectiveness of existing antimicrobial therapies against bacterial biofilms or to replace antibiotic therapies by providing better eradication of bacterial biofilms are currently being investigated. Some of the primary strategies under investigation are summarized in Table 13.1.

ANTIMICROBIAL PEPTIDES

Antimicrobial peptides (AMPs) are naturally occurring cationic components of the innate immune systems of most living organisms. Some AMPs display direct antimicrobial activity against gram-positive and gram-negative bacteria. AMPs have been investigated as an alternative to antibiotics

Table 13.1 Summary of biofilm busting strategies under *in vitro* and *in vivo* investigation

Strategy	Stage of testing	Mechanism of action	Advantages	References
Antimicrobial peptides	*In vivo*	Binds to bacterial membrane, rapid depolarization of cell and death; Inhibits synthesis of DNA and RNA	Naturally occurring; Broad-spectrum activity; Minimal toxicity; Low dose	(62–65)
Bacteriophage	*In vivo*	Replicate inside the host bacteria, increased phage density causes bacterial cell to burst	Minimal toxicity; Bacterial specificity; Low potential for resistance	(66–68)
Chelating agents	*In vitro*	Binds iron, a compound necessary for biofilm formation	Lower antibiotic dose required for eradication of infection	(69,70)
Dispersion compounds	*In vitro*	Entice bacteria to disperse out of biofilms using various stimuli, increasing their susceptibility to antibiotics	Minimal toxicity; Lowers antibiotic dose required for eradication of infection	(71–75)
Quorum sensing inhibitors	*In vivo*	Inhibit bacterial communication process important for biofilm formation	Lower antibiotic dose required for eradication of infection	(76–78)
Silver	*In vitro*	Binds to bacterial cell wall proteins, leading to cellular disintegration and death; Inhibits DNA replication	Broad spectrum; Minimal toxicity	(79–81)

due to their potency, minimal adverse effects in humans, and broad spectrum activity against bacteria (63,64). AMPs interact with anionic components of the bacterial membrane, leading to local disturbances in the membrane, rapid depolarization of the bacterial cell, and cell death. AMPs can also interact with bacterial DNA, RNA, and other cellular proteins or inhibit their synthesis (82).

Compared to traditional antibiotics, AMPs can reduce the concentration of a drug compound required for biofilm eradication by 4 to 500 times. LL-37, a major human host defense peptide, inhibited the formation of *in vitro* P. aeruginosa biofilms by 80% at subinhibitory concentrations of 16 µg/mL. LL-37 significantly reduced the initial bacterial attachment to a surface and downregulated important quorum-sensing systems necessary for biofilm communication and formation. This resulted in reduced thickness of *in vitro* biofilms by more than 50% from significant bacterial death at a low concentration (4 µg/mL) (62). Against clinical isolates obtained from CF patients, cathlecidin peptides derived from mammals inhibited formation of biofilms of P. aeruginosa and S. aureus at subinhibitory concentrations (63). Antibiotics and AMPs have displayed synergistic activity against P. aeruginosa biofilms, with an eightfold reduction in the minimum biofilm eradication concentration (MBEC) values of antibiotics (64). In rats, AMPs at low doses (10–15 µg) reduced bacterial load in lungs of CF rats by 94% compared to untreated rats (65). If the reduced dose required for complete biofilm eradication holds when tested in humans, several additional benefits would be conferred to patients, including reduced systemic toxicity, lower treatment costs, and improved patient compliance and patient outcomes.

BACTERIOPHAGE THERAPY

Bacteriophages (or phages) are viruses that infect bacteria, where they replicate to a high density and burst the bacterial cell (a process called amplification). Phage therapy represents a potential alterative treatment as antibiotic-resistant bacteria and biofilms do not present a challenge to phage (83). Pearl et al. (2008) demonstrated that phages remain alive within persister cells, then replicate when the persisters become active (66). Phages diffuse readily through biofilm matrices (67), expressing depolymerizing enzymes that degrade biofilm matrices and/or inducing the bacteria to express enzymes to further biofilm degradation (52,84). In mice with chronic P. aeruginosa infections, treatment with phages 24 or 48 hours post-infection resulted in complete clearance of P. aeruginosa from the lungs. After 6 days of infection, complete clearance was observed in 70% of the mice, with significant reduction in bacterial load in the remaining animals (68).

Phage therapy offers certain distinct advantages, such as low inherent toxicity, low potential for development of resistance, target specificity, minimal damage to normal flora, and antibiofilm activity (85). In spite of this, phage therapy has not made inroads as an antimicrobial therapy over concerns about the safety of phages and lack of financial investment by major pharmaceutical companies. Some phages (known as temperate phages) increase the pathogenicity of the target bacteria by modifying the organisms, which could lead to enhanced infections rather than eradication of the infections (86). Lack of financial investment has been primarily due to the high costs associated with phage characterization, such as full-genome sequencing and protein profiling, necessary for approval of the therapy. As bringing phage therapy to the market would require completing expensive, large-scale clinical trials in accordance with FDA guidelines, greater interest has remained focused on traditional antibiotic therapy (85,87).

CHELATING AGENTS

Iron is necessary for many bacterial physiologic functions such as bacterial metabolism, release of virulence factors, and regulation of gene expression (69). *P. aeruginosa* biofilms can form under both anaerobic and aerobic conditions regardless of iron levels; however, enhanced iron levels are required for formation of robust biofilms (88–91). As increased iron levels have been observed in the ASL of CF lungs, CF airways help promote substantial biofilm growth (69). Thus, a potential strategy to eliminate biofilms is starving bacteria of iron through the use of iron chelators. Iron chelation therapy has been approved by the FDA as an oral or parenteral therapy for the treatment of chronic iron overload due to blood transfusions (92).

Synthetic iron chelators, such as EDTA, and biological iron chelators, such as lactoferrin, have also been effective in destabilizing biofilm matrices. EDTA hindered biofilm formation and bacterial growth within *P. aeruginosa* biofilms *in vitro* (93). In contrast, the biological chelator lactoferrin significantly impaired biofilm formation but did not affect bacterial growth. Iron chelators have been also observed to inhibit the formation of robust biofilms. Mature biofilms of *P. aeruginosa* grown in the presence of the synthetic chelator 2,2′-dipyridyl (2DP) displayed a thin biofilm structure rather than the three-dimensional structure observed with untreated mature biofilms (70). The FDA-approved chelators, deferasirox (DSX) and deferoxamine (DFO), reduced mature biofilm biomass on airway epithelial cells by 42% and 99%, respectively, at clinically relevant concentrations. Chelating compounds also hold potential as an adjunct therapy to existing antibiotic therapy. Synergistic activity in reducing biofilm mass was demonstrated with tobramycin and DSX compared to tobramycin alone (69). While this strategy shows promise against biofilms *in vitro*, the safety and efficacy of these compounds in the lungs still remains to be demonstrated via *in vivo* studies.

DISPERSION COMPOUNDS

As part of the natural progression of biofilm maturation, bacteria disperse out of biofilms to colonize new sites in response to external stimuli such as nutrient availability; accumulation of toxic compounds in the matrix; pH changes; and external stressors such as salts, nitric oxide, and chelating agents (52,71,94–96). Once bacteria disperse from the biofilm, they display different phenotypic characteristics than those present in the biofilm, behaving more like free-swimming bacteria (97). As dispersed bacteria are more susceptible to antibiotics, if dispersion could be stimulated using dispersion compounds, bacterial eradication could be enhanced. Dispersion compounds are an

attractive co-therapy to be delivered with antibiotics as they can increase the antibiotic susceptibility of biofilm bacteria with minimal toxicity in patients.

Alginate is an important structural component of the matrix of mucoid bacterial biofilms, providing protection to bacteria is several ways. Alginate scavenges oxygen free radicals that are released by inflammatory cells as part of the immune response to infection, acts as a physicochemical barrier to phagocytic clearance, and blocks the diffusion of aminoglycoside antibiotics (tobramycin, gentamicin, and polymyxin B) (73,98–101). Alginate lyase is a glycoside hydrolase enzyme secreted by bacteria to degrade alginate, resulting in a structural breakdown of the biofilm and bacterial dispersion from biofilms (102). Treatment of cultured *P. aeruginosa* biofilms with the enzyme improved the diffusion of aminoglycoside antibiotics in the biofilm and enhanced pathogen killing (73). Further evidence of the potential benefit of matrix enzymes in dispersing biofilms and enhancing antimicrobial activity has been observed with clinical isolates of *P. aeruginosa*. Alipour et al. evaluated the antibacterial activity of aminoglycosides against mucoid and nonmucoid isolates of *P. aeruginosa*. Alginate lyase improved eradication of the mucoid clinical isolate 4 to 8 times when treated with aminoglycosides (74). Eradication of the nonmucoid clinical isolate was not affected by treatment with alginate lyase, proving the importance of the matrix in antibiotic resistance. Alkawash and coworkers showed that mucoid *P. aeruginosa* colonies incubated overnight with alginate lyase formed weaker biofilm structures. In addition, no bacterial growth was observed in biofilms treated with gentamicin and alginate lyase for 120 hours, while bacterial growth was observed in 13 out of 16 biofilms treated with only gentamicin (75). Therefore, enzymatic degradation of the biofilm matrix holds the potential both to prevent biofilm formation and to increase the susceptibility of biofilm bacteria to antimicrobial therapy.

Other dispersion strategies focus on altering the metabolic activity of bacteria within a biofilm. Bacterial biofilms display nutrient gradients in the EPS matrix, with nutrient availability progressively decreasing toward the interior of the matrix. In response to this low nutrient availability, bacteria embedded deep in the matrix exhibit low metabolic activity, reducing their susceptibility to antibiotics (52). The addition of a nutrient source to the biofilm environment could signal a favorable environmental change to the bacteria and induce dispersion. Bacteria can use various carbon sources such as succinate, citrate, and glutamate as nutrients. Sauer et al. (2004) investigated the effect of a sudden increase in carbon availability on *P. aeruginosa* biofilms. Bacterial dispersion, in the form of single cells exhibiting characteristics of free-flowing bacteria, was observed with the addition of nutrients. Biomass reductions of 72%–80% were observed (71). Sommerfield Ross and colleagues showed that co-delivery of nutrient dispersion compounds with common antibiotics led to synergistic eradication of *P. aeruginosa* biofilms *in vitro*. While all combinations displayed synergistic activity, citrate proved the most effective dispersion compound, leading to reductions in live bacterial population down to 3%–8%. They have further developed these combination treatments into dry powder aerosols, without loss of drug potency, to enable delivery of high doses of dispersion and antimicrobial compounds directly to the site of infection (72,103). The primary concern over dispersion therapy is the potential for dispersed bacteria to recolonize elsewhere in the lungs. Co-therapy with antimicrobials would produce locally high drug concentrations near the dispersed bacteria and could address this concern.

QUORUM SENSING INHIBITORS (QSIs)

Bacterial cells communicate and coordinate their behavior in response to stimuli by producing, secreting, and detecting signal molecules called autoinducers. This communication process, called quorum sensing (QS), allows bacteria to alter their gene expression with the accumulation of a minimal threshold concentration of autoinducers, resulting in behavioral changes (104). QS is closely linked to biofilm formation, playing a role in production of EPS matrix, virulence factors, and bacterial dispersion from biofilms. QSIs hinder biofilm formation by inhibiting the release of EPS and prevent the production of bacterial virulence factors (105,106). Several studies have quantified the effects of QSIs on *P. aeruginosa* biofilms.

Plants in the marine environment, such as seaweeds, have evolved to use secondary metabolites as protection against colonizing organisms. These compounds act as natural signal antagonists, targeting QSIs and inhibiting virulence factor expression in bacteria. Synthetic versions of these compounds have been tested for their ability to inhibit QS in *P. aeruginosa* biofilms, as well as in mice with pulmonary *P. aeruginosa* infections (76,107). Inhibition of QS through administration of furanones (10 μM C-30) increased the susceptibility of *in vitro P. aeruginosa* biofilms to antimicrobial therapy with 100 μg/mL tobramycin sulfate, compared to tobramycin alone. In mice, significant decreases in bacterial loads were observed. Other plant compounds such as 6-gingerol, a nonvolatile oil derived from ginger, have exhibited potency in inhibiting biofilm formation *in vitro* similar to that of C-30, as well as improved survival rates in mice infected with *P. aeruginosa* (108).

Yang et al. (2009) performed virtual screening of QSIs from a database of natural compounds and approved drugs (77). Salicylic acid, nifuroxazide, and chloroxazone were identified as QSI compounds that were active against *in vitro P. aeruginosa* biofilms. Biofilms treated with these compounds were thinner (biofilm biomass approximately 3 $\mu m^3/\mu m^2$) and less structured compared to untreated biofilms (biofilm biomass approximately 6.5 $\mu m^3/\mu m^2$), demonstrating the inability of the bacteria to produce or maintain biofilms in presence of QSIs. Flavanoids, including baicalin hydrate and cinnamaldehyde, have also shown promise as naturally derived QSIs (78). Both compounds enhanced the antimicrobial activity of tobramycin in young *P. aeruginosa* biofilms, by approximately 40%–60%. Furthermore, biacalin hydrate (2 mg/kg) has shown promise in mice infected with

Burkholderia cenocepacia lung infections administered in combination with tobramycin (30 mg/kg).

A large body of literature is developing around the discovery and use of QSIs against biofilms. Their ability to inhibit biofilm formation, coupled with minimal observed toxicity, makes QSIs one of the most promising strategies for busting biofilms in CF patients.

SILVER

Silver is an antimicrobial used in the treatment of chronic wounds and infected burns. Its antibacterial action is broad spectrum, and there are few reported cases of development of bacterial resistance to silver (79). Silver ions bind to bacterial proteins by electrostatic attraction, which leads to structural changes to the bacterial cell wall, cellular disintegration, and subsequent bacterial death. Even if silver does not kill the bacteria directly, the increased bacterial membrane permeability can enhance the antibacterial activity of antibiotics, as has been shown with *Escherichia coli in vitro* and *in vivo* (109). Silver ions further inhibit DNA replication in bacterial cells, expression of bacterial proteins, and bacterial electron transfer chain (52,110). Against *in vitro P. aeruginosa* biofilms, silver sulfadiazine (10 μg/mL) completely eradicated mature (4-day-old) biofilms, where high doses of tobramycin (380 μg/mL) had no effect (79). Similarly, biologically synthesized silver nanoparticles (100 nM) reduced 1-day-old biofilms by 95%–98% (80). In one case study, colloidal silver was given to a 12-year-old boy with CF for untreatable chronic lung infections. The patient, who was not responding well to nebulized antibiotic treatment, demonstrated a significant improvement in lung function (FEV1, from 24% to 60%) and overall quality of life after initiation of colloidal silver treatment. This allowed weaning the patient off inhaled antibiotics (81). While the toxicity of silver in humans is low, it will accumulate irreversibly in the body on ingestion, inhalation, or injection (111). With antimicrobial therapy, colloidal silver has been observed to interact with certain antibiotic treatments and decrease the effectiveness of these antibiotics (112). Colloidal silver is not recognized as safe or effective by the FDA and further *in vivo* and clinical studies would be necessary to prove the efficacy and safety of silver in human patients.

CONCLUSION

Antibiotic therapies have significantly improved the quality of life for CF patients and increased the median patient survival to almost 40 years. In spite of this progress, infections persist, leading to chronic lung infection and progressive lung damage. Bacterial survival strategies, such as biofilm formation, enable the organism to survive despite the aggressive use of antibiotics and an intense host immune response. Increased understanding of the factors that lead to bacterial persistence is enabling researchers to develop novel therapeutic approaches to combat these infections. Several strategies to bust biofilms by inhibiting their formation or disrupting their survival mechanisms are beginning to show success against *P. aeruginosa* in *in vitro* and *in vivo* studies. With further development, these strategies could prove efficacious in completely eliminating pathogenic bacteria in CF lungs.

REFERENCES

1. About Cystic Fibrosis: Cystic Fibrosis Foundation; [cited July 27, 2017]. Available from https://www.cff.org/What-is-CF/About-Cystic-Fibrosis/.

2. Pettit RS, Fellner C. CFTR modulators for the treatment of cystic fibrosis. *Pharmacy and Therapeutics*. 2014;39(7):500–511.

3. Flume PA, Van Devanter DR. State of progress in treating cystic fibrosis respiratory disease. *BMC Medicine*. 2012;10(1):88. doi:10.1186/1741-7015-10-88.

4. Lyczak JB, Cannon CL, Pier GB. Lung infections associated with cystic fibrosis. *Clinical Microbiology Reviews*. 2002;15(2):194–222. doi:10.1128/CMR.15.2.194-222.2002.

5. Mall MA, Hartl D. CFTR: Cystic fibrosis and beyond. *European Respiratory Journal*. 2014;44(4):1042–1054. doi:10.1183/09031936.00228013.

6. Stoltz DA, Meyerholz DK, Pezzulo AA, Ramachandran S, Rogan MP, Davis GJ, Hanfland RA et al. Cystic fibrosis pigs develop lung disease and exhibit defective bacterial eradication at birth. *Science Translational Medicine*. 2010;2(29):29ra31–29ra31. doi:10.1126/scitranslmed.3000928.

7. Esen M, Grassmé H, Riethmüller J, Riehle A, Fassbender K, Gulbins E. Invasion of human epithelial cells by *Pseudomonas aeruginosa* involves src-like tyrosine kinases p60Src and p59Fyn. *Infection Immunity*. 2001;69(1):281–287. doi:10.1128/IAI.69.1.281-287.2001.

8. Gibson RL, Burns JL, Ramsey BW. Pathophysiology and management of pulmonary infections in cystic fibrosis. *American Journal of Respiratory and Critical Care Medicine*. 2003;168(8):918–951. doi:10.1164/rccm.200304-505SO.

9. Chmiel JF, Davis PB. State of the art: Why do the lungs of patients with cystic fibrosis become infected and why can't they clear the infection? *Respiratory Research*. 2003;4(1):8.

10. Filkins LM, O'Toole GA. Cystic fibrosis lung infections: Polymicrobial, complex, and hard to treat. *PLoS Pathogens*. 2016;11(12):e1005258. doi:10.1371/journal.ppat.1005258.

11. Nixon GM, Armstrong DS, Carzino R, Carlin JB, Olinsky A, Robertson CF, Grimwood K. Clinical outcome after early *Pseudomonas aeruginosa* infection in cystic fibrosis. *The Journal of Pediatrics*. 2001;138(5):699–704. doi:10.1067/mpd.2001.112897.

12. Emerson J, Rosenfeld M, McNamara S, Ramsey B, Gibson RL. *Pseudomonas aeruginosa* and other predictors of mortality and morbidity in young children with cystic fibrosis. *Pediatric Pulmonology*. 2002;34(2):91–100. doi:10.1002/ppul.10127.

13. Firmida MC, Pereira RHV, Silva E, Marques EA, Lopes AJ. Clinical impact of *Achromobacter xylosoxidans* colonization/infection in patients with cystic fibrosis. *Brazilian Journal of Medical and Biological Research*. 2016;49(4):e5097. doi:10.1590/1414-431x20155097.

14. Waters V, Yau Y, Prasad S, Lu A, Atenafu E, Crandall I, Tom S et al. *Stenotrophomonas maltophilia* in cystic fibrosis. *American Journal of Respiratory and Critical Care Medicine*. 2011;183(5):635–640. doi:10.1164/rccm.201009-1392OC.

15. Horsley A, Jones AM, Lord R. Antibiotic treatment for *Burkholderia cepacia* complex in people with cystic fibrosis experiencing a pulmonary exacerbation. *Cochrane Database of Systematic Reviews*. 2016(1). doi:10.1002/14651858.CD009529.pub3.

16. Foundation CF. *Patient Registry Annual Data Report*. Bethesda, MD, 2015.

17. Isles A, Maclusky I, Corey M, Gold R, Prober C, Fleming P, Levison H. *Pseudomonas cepacia* infection in cystic fibrosis: An emerging problem. *The Journal of Pediatrics*. 1984;104(2):206–210. doi:10.1016/S0022-3476(84)80993-2.

18. Leitão JH, Sousa SA, Ferreira AS, Ramos CG, Silva IN, Moreira LM. Pathogenicity, virulence factors, and strategies to fight against *Burkholderia cepacia* complex pathogens and related species. *Applied Microbiology and Biotechnology*. 2010;87(1):31–40. doi:10.1007/s00253-010-2528-0.

19. Courtney JM, Dunbar KEA, McDowell A, Moore JE, Warke TJ, Stevenson M, Elborn JS. Clinical outcome of *Burkholderia cepacia* complex infection in cystic fibrosis adults. *Journal Cystic Fibrosis*. 2004;3(2):93–98. doi:10.1016/j.jcf.2004.01.005.

20. Lambiase A, Catania MR, del Pezzo M, Rossano F, Terlizzi V, Sepe A, Raia V. *Achromobacter xylosoxidans* respiratory tract infection in cystic fibrosis patients. *European Journal Clinical Microbiology Infectious Diseases*. 2011;30(8):973–980. doi:10.1007/s10096-011-1182-5.

21. Fraser A, Paul M, Almanasreh N, Tacconelli E, Frank U, Cauda R, Borok S et al. Benefit of appropriate empirical antibiotic treatment: Thirty-day mortality and duration of hospital stay. *The American Journal of Medicine*. 2006;119(11):970–976. doi:10.1016/j.amjmed.2006.03.034.

22. Kang C-I, Kim S-H, Park WB, Lee K-D, Kim H-B, Kim E-C, Oh M-d, Choe K-W. Bloodstream infections caused by antibiotic-resistant gram-negative bacilli: Risk factors for mortality and impact of inappropriate initial antimicrobial therapy on outcome. *Antimicrobial Agents and Chemotherapy*. 2005;49(2):760–766. doi:10.1128/AAC.49.2.760-766.2005.

23. Hirsch EB, Tam VH. Impact of multidrug-resistant *Pseudomonas aeruginosa* infection on patient outcomes. *Expert Review of Pharmacoeconomics & Outcomes Research*. 2010;10(4):441–451. doi:10.1586/erp.10.49.

24. Marshall B, Elbert A, Petren K, Rizvi S, Fink A, Ostrenga J, Sewall A, Loeffler D. Cystic Fibrosis Foundation Patient Registry 2015 Annual Data Report. Bethesda, MD: Cystic Fibrosis Foundation, 2016.

25. Hill UG, Floto RA, Haworth CS. Non-tuberculous mycobacteria in cystic fibrosis. *Journal of the Royal Society Medicine*. 2012;105(Suppl 2):S14–S8. doi:10.1258/jrsm.2012.12s003.

26. Cramer GW, Bosso JA, Maldonado WT, Guévremont C. The role of dornase alfa in the treatment of cystic fibrosis. *Annals of Pharmacotherapy*. 1996;30(6):656–661. doi:10.1177/106002809603000614.

27. Henke MO, Ratjen F. Mucolytics in cystic fibrosis. *Paediatric Respiratory Reviews*. 2007;8(1):24–29. doi:10.1016/j.prrv.2007.02.009.

28. Döring G, Flume P, Heijerman H, Elborn JS. Treatment of lung infection in patients with cystic fibrosis: Current and future strategies. *Journal of Cystic Fibrosis*. 2012;11(6):461–479. doi:10.1016/j.jcf.2012.10.004.

29. Mogayzel PJ, Naureckas ET, Robinson KA, Mueller G, Hadjiliadis D, Hoag JB, Lubsch L et al. Cystic fibrosis pulmonary guidelines. *American Journal of Respiratory and Critical Care Medicine*. 2013;187(7):680–689. doi:10.1164/rccm.201207-1160OE.

30. Tramper-Stranders GA, van der Ent CK, Molin S, Yang L, Hansen SK, Rau MH, Ciofu O et al. Initial *Pseudomonas aeruginosa* infection in patients with cystic fibrosis: Characteristics of eradicated and persistent isolates. *Clinical Microbiology and Infection*. 2012;18(6):567–574. doi:10.1111/j.1469-0691.2011.03627.x.

31. Chmiel JF, Konstan MW, Elborn JS. Antibiotic and anti-inflammatory therapies for cystic fibrosis. *Cold Spring Harbor Perspectives in Medicine*. 2013;3(10):a009779. doi:10.1101/cshperspect.a009779.

32. McCoy KS, Quittner AL, Oermann CM, Gibson RL, Retsch-Bogart GZ, Montgomery AB. Inhaled aztreonam lysine for chronic airway *pseudomonas aeruginosa* in cystic fibrosis. *American Journal of Respiratory and Critical Care Medicine*. 2008;178(9):921–928. doi:10.1164/rccm.200712-1804OC.

33. Retsch-Bogart GZ, Quittner AL, Gibson RL, Oermann CM, McCoy KS, Montgomery AB, Cooper PJ. Efficacy and safety of inhaled aztreonam lysine for airway Pseudomonas in cystic fibrosis. *Chest*. 2009;135(5):1223–1232. doi:10.1378/chest.08-1421.

34. Assael BM, Pressler T, Bilton D, Fayon M, Fischer R, Chiron R, LaRosa M et al. Inhaled aztreonam lysine vs. inhaled tobramycin in cystic fibrosis: A comparative efficacy trial. *Journal of Cystic Fibrosis*. 2013;12(2):130–140. doi:10.1016/j.jcf.2012.07.006.

35. Tiddens HA, De Boeck K, Clancy JP, Fayon M, Arets HGM, Bresnik M, Derchak A et al.. Open label study of inhaled aztreonam for Pseudomonas eradication in children with cystic fibrosis: The ALPINE study. *Journal of Cystic Fibrosis*. 2015;14(1):111–119. doi:10.1016/j.jcf.2014.06.003.

36. Pitt T, Sparrow M, Warner M, Stefanidou M. Survey of resistance of *Pseudomonas aeruginosa* from UK patients with cystic fibrosis to six commonly prescribed antimicrobial agents. *Thorax*. 2003;58(9):794–796. doi:10.1136/thorax.58.9.794.

37. Valenza G, Radike K, Schoen C, Horn S, Oesterlein A, Frosch M, Abele-Horn M, Hebestreit H. Resistance to tobramycin and colistin in isolates of *Pseudomonas aeruginosa* from chronically colonized patients with cystic fibrosis under antimicrobial treatment. *Scandinavian Journal of Infectious Diseases*. 2010;42(11–12):885–889. doi:10.3109/00365548.2010.509333.

38. Bergen PJ, Li J, Rayner CR, Nation RL. Colistin methanesulfonate is an inactive prodrug of colistin against *Pseudomonas aeruginosa*. *Antimicrobial Agents and Chemotherapy*. 2006;50(6):1953–1958. doi:10.1128/AAC.00035-06.

39. Koerner-Rettberg C, Ballmann M. Colistimethate sodium for the treatment of chronic pulmonary infection in cystic fibrosis: An evidence-based review of its place in therapy. *Core Evidence*. 2014;9:99–112. doi:10.2147/CE.S64980.

40. Greally P, Whitaker P, Peckham D. Challenges with current inhaled treatments for chronic *Pseudomonas aeruginosa* infection in patients with cystic fibrosis. *Current Medical Research and Opinion*. 2012;28(6):1059–1067. doi:10.1185/03007995.2012.674500.

41. Sawicki GS, Sellers DE, Robinson WM. High treatment burden in adults with cystic fibrosis: Challenges to disease self-management. *Journal of Cystic Fibrosis: Official Journal of the European Cystic Fibrosis Society*. 2009;8(2):91–96. doi:10.1016/j.jcf.2008.09.007.

42. Labiris NR, Dolovich MB. Pulmonary drug delivery. Part I: Physiological factors affecting therapeutic effectiveness of aerosolized medications. *British Journal of Clinical Pharmacology*. 2003;56(6):588–599. doi:10.1046/j.1365-2125.2003.01892.x.

43. Anderson PJ, Blanchard JD, Brain JD, Feldman HA, McNamara JJ, Heyder J. Effect of cystic fibrosis on inhaled aerosol boluses. *American Review of Respiratory Disease*. 1989;140(5):1317–1324. doi:10.1164/ajrccm/140.5.1317.

44. Touw DJ, Brimicombe RW, Hodson ME, Heijerman HG, Bakker W. Inhalation of antibiotics in cystic fibrosis. *European Respiratory Journal*. 1995;8(9):1594.

45. Gómez MI, Prince A. Opportunistic infections in lung disease: Pseudomonas infections in cystic fibrosis. *Current Opinion in Pharmacology*. 2007;7(3):244–251. doi:10.1016/j.coph.2006.12.005.

46. Spencer DH, Kas A, Smith EE, Raymond CK, Sims EH, Hastings M, Burns JL, Kaul R, Olson MV. Whole-genome sequence variation among multiple

isolates of *Pseudomonas aeruginosa*. *Journal of Bacteriology*. 2003;185(4):1316–1325. doi:10.1128/JB.185.4.1316-1325.2003.

47. Drenkard E, Ausubel FM. Pseudomonas biofilm formation and antibiotic resistance are linked to phenotypic variation. *Nature*. 2002;416(6882):740–743.

48. Sherrard LJ, Tunney MM, Elborn JS. Antimicrobial resistance in the respiratory microbiota of people with cystic fibrosis. *The Lancet*. 2014;384(9944):703–713. doi:10.1016/S0140-6736(14)61137-5.

49. Breidenstein EBM, de la Fuente-Núñez C, Hancock REW. *Pseudomonas aeruginosa*: All roads lead to resistance. *Trends in Microbiology*. 2011;19(8):419–426. doi:10.1016/j.tim.2011.04.005.

50. Lewis K. Persister cells and the riddle of biofilm survival. *Biochemistry (Moscow)*. 2005;70(2):267–274. doi:10.1007/s10541-005-0111-6.

51. Dunne WM. Bacterial adhesion: Seen any good biofilms lately? *Clinical Microbiology Reviews*. 2002;15(2):155–166. doi:10.1128/CMR.15.2.155-166.2002.

52. Kostakioti M, Hadjifrangiskou M, Hultgren SJ. Bacterial biofilms: Development, dispersal, and therapeutic strategies in the dawn of the postantibiotic era. *Cold Spring Harbor Perspectives in Medicine*. 2013;3(4):a010306/1-a/23. doi:10.1101/cshperspect.a010306.

53. Garrett TR, Bhakoo M, Zhang Z. Bacterial adhesion and biofilms on surfaces. *Progress in Natural Science*. 2008;18(9):1049–1056. doi:10.1016/j.pnsc.2008.04.001.

54. Moreau-Marquis S, Stanton BA, O'Toole GA. *Pseudomonas aeruginosa* biofilm formation in the cystic fibrosis airway. A short review. *Pulmonary Pharmacology & Therapeutics*. 2008;21(4):595–599. doi:10.1016/j.pupt.2007.12.001.

55. Worlitzsch D, Tarran R, Ulrich M, Schwab U, Cekici A, Meyer KC, Birrer P et al. Effects of reduced mucus oxygen concentration in airway Pseudomonas infections of cystic fibrosis patients. *The Journal of Clinical Investigation*. 2002;109(3):317–325. doi:10.1172/JCI13870.

56. Hassett DJ, Cuppoletti J, Trapnell B, Lymar SV, Rowe JJ, Sun Yoon S, Hilliard GM et al. Anaerobic metabolism and quorum sensing by *Pseudomonas aeruginosa* biofilms in chronically infected cystic fibrosis airways: Rethinking antibiotic treatment strategies and drug targets. *Advanced Drug Delivery Reviews*. 2002;54(11):1425–1443. doi:10.1016/S0169-409X(02)00152-7.

57. Leid JG, Willson CJ, Shirtliff ME, Hassett DJ, Parsek MR, Jeffers AK. The exopolysaccharide alginate protects *Pseudomonas aeruginosa* biofilm bacteria from IFN-γ-mediated macrophage killing. *The Journal of Immunology*. 2005;175(11):7512.

58. Masyuko RN, Lanni EJ, Driscoll CM, Shrout JD, Sweedler JV, Bohn PW. Spatial organization of *Pseudomonas aeruginosa* biofilms probed by combined matrix-assisted laser desorption ionization mass spectrometry and confocal Raman microscopy. *Analyst (Cambridge, UK)*. 2014;139(22):5700–5708. doi:10.1039/C4AN00435C.

59. Monroe D. Looking for chinks in the armor of bacterial biofilms. *PLoS Biology*. 2007;5(11):e307. doi:10.1371/journal.pbio.0050307.

60. Hoffman LR, D'Argenio DA, MacCoss MJ, Zhang Z, Jones RA, Miller SI. Aminoglycoside antibiotics induce bacterial biofilm formation. *Nature*. 2005;436(7054):1171–1175. http://www.nature.com/nature/journal/v436/n7054/suppinfo/nature03912_S1.html.

61. Gillis RJ, White KG, Choi K-H, Wagner VE, Schweizer HP, Iglewski BH. Molecular basis of azithromycin-resistant *Pseudomonas aeruginosa* biofilms. *Antimicrobial Agents and Chemotherapy*. 2005;49(9):3858–3867. doi:10.1128/AAC.49.9.3858-3867.2005.

62. Overhage J, Campisano A, Bains M, Torfs ECW, Rehm BHA, Hancock REW. Human host defense peptide LL-37 prevents bacterial biofilm formation. *Infection and Immunity*. 2008;76(9):4176–4182. doi:10.1128/IAI.00318-08.

63. Pompilio A, Scocchi M, Pomponio S, Guida F, Di Primio A, Fiscarelli E, Gennaro R, Di Bonaventura G. Antibacterial and anti-biofilm effects of cathelicidin peptides against pathogens isolated from cystic fibrosis patients. *Peptides*. 2011;32(9):1807–1814. doi:10.1016/j.peptides.2011.08.002.

64. Dosler S, Karaaslan E. Inhibition and destruction of *Pseudomonas aeruginosa* biofilms by antibiotics and antimicrobial peptides. *Peptides*. 2014;62:32–37. doi:10.1016/j.peptides.2014.09.021.

65. Zhang L, Parente J, Harris SM, Woods DE, Hancock REW, Falla TJ. Antimicrobial peptide therapeutics for cystic fibrosis. *Antimicrobial Agents and Chemotherapy*. 2005;49(7):2921–2927. doi:10.1128/AAC.49.7.2921-2927.2005.

66. Pearl S, Gabay C, Kishony R, Oppenheim A, Balaban NQ. Nongenetic individuality in the host–phage interaction. *PLoS Biology*. 2008;6(5):e120. doi:10.1371/journal.pbio.0060120.

67. Hanlon GW, Denyer SP, Olliff CJ, Ibrahim LJ. Reduction in exopolysaccharide viscosity as an aid to bacteriophage penetration through *Pseudomonas aeruginosa* biofilms. *Applied and Environmental Microbiology*. 2001;67(6):2746–2753. doi:10.1128/AEM.67.6.2746-2753.2001.

68. Waters EM, Neill DR, Kaman B, Sahota JS, Clokie MRJ, Winstanley C, Kadioglu A. Phage therapy is highly effective against chronic lung infections with *Pseudomonas aeruginosa*. *Thorax*. 2017.

69. Moreau-Marquis S, O'Toole GA, Stanton BA. Tobramycin and FDA-approved iron chelators eliminate *Pseudomonas aeruginosa* biofilms on cystic fibrosis cells. *American Journal Respiratory and Cell Molecular Biology*. 2009;41(3):305–313. doi:10.1165/rcmb.2008-0299OC.

70. O'May CY, Sanderson K, Roddam LF, Kirov SM, Reid DW. Iron-binding compounds impair *Pseudomonas aeruginosa* biofilm formation, especially under anaerobic conditions. *Journal of Medical Microbiology*. 2009;58(6):765–773. doi:10.1099/jmm.0.004416-0.

71. Sauer K, Cullen MC, Rickard AH, Zeef LAH, Davies DG, Gilbert P. Characterization of nutrient-induced dispersion in *Pseudomonas aeruginosa* PAO1 biofilm. *Journal Bacteriology*. 2004;186(21):7312–7326. doi:10.1128/JB.186.21.7312-7326.2004.

72. Sommerfeld Ross S, Fiegel J. Nutrient dispersion enhances conventional antibiotic activity against *Pseudomonas aeruginosa* biofilms. *International Journal Antimicrobial Agents*. 2012;40(2):177–181. doi:10.1016/j.ijantimicag.2012.04.015.

73. Hatch RA, Schiller NL. Alginate Lyase Promotes Diffusion of Aminoglycosides through the Extracellular Polysaccharide of Mucoid *Pseudomonas aeruginosa*. *Antimicrobial Agents and Chemotherapy*. 1998;42(4):974–977.

74. Alipour M, Suntres ZE, Omri A. Importance of DNase and alginate lyase for enhancing free and liposome encapsulated aminoglycoside activity against *Pseudomonas aeruginosa*. *Journal of Antimicrobial Chemotherapy*. 2009;64(2):317–325. doi:10.1093/jac/dkp165.

75. Alkawash MA, Soothill JS, Schiller NL. Alginate lyase enhances antibiotic killing of mucoid *Pseudomonas aeruginosa* in biofilms. *APMIS*. 2006;114(2):131–138. doi:10.1111/j.1600-0463.2006.apm_356.x.

76. Hentzer M, Wu H, Andersen JB, Riedel K, Rasmussen TB, Bagge N, Kumar N et al. Attenuation of *Pseudomonas aeruginosa* virulence by quorum sensing inhibitors. *The EMBO Journal*. 2003;22(15):3803–3815. doi:10.1093/emboj/cdg366.

77. Yang L, Rybtke MT, Jakobsen TH, Hentzer M, Bjarnsholt T, Givskov M, Tolker-Nielsen T. Computer-aided identification of recognized drugs as *Pseudomonas aeruginosa* quorum-sensing inhibitors. *Antimicrobial Agents and Chemotherapy*. 2009;53(6):2432–2443.

78. Brackman G, Cos P, Maes L, Nelis HJ, Coenye T. Quorum sensing inhibitors increase the susceptibility of bacterial biofilms to antibiotics in vitro and in vivo. *Antimicrobial Agents and Chemotherapy*. 2011;55(6):2655–2661.

79. Bjarnsholt T, Kirketerp-Moeller K, Kristiansen S, Phipps R, Nielsen AK, Jensen PO, Hoeiby N, Givskov M. Silver against *Pseudomonas aeruginosa* biofilms. *APMIS*. 2007;115(8):921–928. doi:10.1111/j.1600-0463.2007.apm_646.x.

80. Kalishwaralal K, BarathManiKanth S, Pandian SRK, Deepak V, Gurunathan S. Silver nanoparticles impede the biofilm formation by *Pseudomonas aeruginosa* and Staphylococcus epidermidis. *Colloids and Surfaces B: Biointerfaces*. 2010;79(2):340–344. doi:10.1016/j.colsurfb.2010.04.014.

81. Baral VR, Dewar AL, Connett GJ. Colloidal silver for lung disease in cystic fibrosis. *Journal of the Royal Society of Medicine*. 2008;101(Suppl 1):51–52. doi:10.1258/jrsm.2008.s18012.

82. Powers J-PS, Hancock REW. The relationship between peptide structure and antibacterial activity. *Peptides*. 2003;24(11):1681–1691. doi:10.1016/j.peptides.2003.08.023.

83. Alves DR, Perez-Esteban P, Kot W, Bean JE, Arnot T, Hansen LH, Enright MC, Jenkins ATA. A novel bacteriophage cocktail reduces and disperses *Pseudomonas aeruginosa* biofilms under static and flow conditions. *Microbial Biotechnology*. 2016;9(1):61–74. doi:10.1111/1751-7915.12316.

84. Harper DR, Parracho HMRT, Walker J, Sharp R, Hughes G, Werthén M, Lehman S, Morales S. Bacteriophages and biofilms. *Antibiotics*. 2014;3(3):270–284. doi:10.3390/antibiotics3030270.

85. Loc-Carrillo C, Abedon ST. Pros and cons of phage therapy. *Bacteriophage*. 2011;1(2):111–114. doi:10.4161/bact.1.2.14590.

86. Abedon ST, Kuhl SJ, Blasdel BG, Kutter EM. Phage treatment of human infections. *Bacteriophage*. 2011;1(2):66–85. doi:10.4161/bact.1.2.15845.

87. Kutateladze M, Adamia R. Bacteriophages as potential new therapeutics to replace or supplement antibiotics. *Trends in Biotechnology*. 2010;28(12):591–595. doi:10.1016/j.tibtech.2010.08.001.

88. Reid DW, Withers NJ, Francis L, Wilson JW, Kotsimbos TC. Iron deficiency in cystic fibrosis: Relationship to lung disease severity and chronic *Pseudomonas aeruginosa* infection. *Chest*. 2002;121(1):48–54. doi:10.1378/chest.121.1.48.

89. Reid DW, Kirov SM. Iron, *Pseudomonas aeruginosa* and cystic fibrosis. *Microbiology*. 2004;150(3):516. doi:10.1099/mic.0.26804-0.

90. Stites SW, Walters B, O'Brien-Ladner AR, Bailey K, Wesselius LJ. Increased iron and ferritin content of sputum from patients with cystic fibrosis or chronic bronchitis. *Chest*. 1998;114(3):814–819. doi:10.1378/chest.114.3.814.

91. Stites S, Plautz M, Bailey K, O'Brien-Ladner A, Wesselius L. Increased concentrations of iron and isoferritins in the lower respiratory tract of patients with stable cystic fibrosis. *American Journal of Respiratory and Critical Care Medicine*. 1999;160(3):796–801. doi:10.1164/ajrccm.160.3.9811018.

92. Vichinsky E, Onyekwere O, Porter J, Swerdlow P, Eckman J, Lane P, Files B et al. A randomised comparison of deferasirox versus

deferoxamine for the treatment of transfusional iron overload in sickle cell disease. *British Journal Haematology*. 2007;136(3):501–508. doi:10.1111/j.1365-2141.2006.06455.x.

93. Banin E, Brady KM, Greenberg EP. Chelator-induced dispersal and killing of *Pseudomonas aeruginosa* cells in a biofilm. *Applied and Environmental Microbiology*. 2006;72(3):2064–2069.

94. Gjermansen M, Ragas P, Sternberg C, Molin S, Tolker-Nielsen T. Characterization of starvation-induced dispersion in *Pseudomonas putida* biofilms. *Environmental Microbiology*. 2005;7(6):894–904. doi:10.1111/j.1462-2920.2005.00775.x.

95. Thormann KM, Saville RM, Shukla S, Spormann AM. Induction of rapid detachment in *Shewanella oneidensis* MR-1 biofilms. *Journal Bacteriology*. 2005;187(3):1014–1021.

96. Barraud N, Hassett DJ, Hwang S-H, Rice SA, Kjelleberg S, Webb JS. Involvement of nitric oxide in biofilm dispersal of *Pseudomonas aeruginosa*. *Journal Bacteriology*. 2006;188(21):7344–7353. doi:10.1128/JB.00779-06.

97. Sauer K, Camper AK, Ehrlich GD, Costerton JW, Davies DG. *Pseudomonas aeruginosa* displays multiple Phenotypes during development as a biofilm. *Journal of Bacteriology*. 2002;184(4):1140–1154. doi:10.1128/jb.184.4.1140-1154.2002.

98. Simpson JA, Smith SE, Dean RT. Scavenging by alginate of free radicals released by macrophages. *Free Radical Biology and Medicine*. 1989;6(4):347–353. doi:10.1016/0891-5849(89)90078-6.

99. Govan JR, Deretic V. Microbial pathogenesis in cystic fibrosis: Mucoid *Pseudomonas aeruginosa* and *Burkholderia cepacia*. *Microbiological Reviews*. 1996;60(3):539–574.

100. Ramsey DM, Wozniak DJ. Understanding the control of *Pseudomonas aeruginosa* alginate synthesis and the prospects for management of chronic infections in cystic fibrosis. *Molecular Microbiology*. 2005;56(2):309–322. doi:10.1111/j.1365-2958.2005.04552.x.

101. Lamppa JW, Griswold KE. Alginate lyase exhibits catalysis-independent biofilm dispersion and antibiotic synergy. *Antimicrobial Agents and Chemotherapy*. 2013;57(1):137–145. doi:10.1128/AAC.01789-12.

102. Fleming D, Rumbaugh KP. Approaches to dispersing medical biofilms. *Microorganisms*. 2017;5(2):15. doi:10.3390/microorganisms5020015.

103. Sommerfeld Ross S, Gharse S, Sanchez L, Fiegel J. Dry powder aerosols to co-deliver antibiotics and nutrient dispersion compounds for enhanced bacterial biofilm eradication. *International Journal Pharmaceutics*. 2017;531(1):14–23. doi:10.1016/j.ijpharm.2017.08.060.

104. Waters CM, Bassler BL. Quorum sensing: Cell-to-cell communication in bacteria. *Annual Review of Cell and Developmental Biology*. 2005;21(1):319–346. doi:10.1146/annurev.cellbio.21.012704.131001.

105. Nadell CD, Xavier JB, Levin SA, Foster KR. The evolution of quorum sensing in bacterial biofilms. *PLoS Biology*. 2008;6(1):e14. doi:10.1371/journal.pbio.0060014.

106. Rutherford ST, Bassler BL. Bacterial quorum sensing: Its role in virulence and possibilities for its control. *Cold Spring Harbor Perspectives in Medicine*. 2012;2(11):a012427.

107. Wu H, Song Z, Hentzer M, Andersen JB, Molin S, Givskov M, Høiby N. Synthetic furanones inhibit quorum-sensing and enhance bacterial clearance in *Pseudomonas aeruginosa* lung infection in mice. *Journal Antimicrobial Chemotherapy*. 2004;53(6):1054–1061. doi:10.1093/jac/dkh223.

108. Kim H-S, Lee S-H, Byun Y, Park H-D. 6-Gingerol reduces *Pseudomonas aeruginosa* biofilm formation and virulence via quorum sensing inhibition. *Scientific Reports*. 2015;5:8656. doi:10.1038/srep08656. https://www.nature.com/articles/srep08656#supplementary-information.

109. Morones-Ramirez JR, Winkler JA, Spina CS, Collins JJ. Silver enhances antibiotic activity against gram-negative bacteria. *Science Translational Medicine*. 2013;5(190):190ra81–ra81. doi:10.1126/scitranslmed.3006276.

110. Lansdown ABG. Silver I: Its antibacterial properties and mechanism of action. *Journal of Wound Care*. 2002;11(4):125–130. doi:10.12968/jowc.2002.11.4.26389.

111. Lansdown ABG. Silver in health care: Antimicrobial effects and safety in use. *Current Problems in Dermatology (Biofunctional Textiles and the Skin)*. 2006;33:17–34.

112. de Souza A, Mehta D, Leavitt RW. Bactericidal activity of combinations of Silver-Water Dispersion with 19 antibiotics against seven microbial strains. *Current Science*. 2006;91(7):926–929.

14

Current and future CFTR therapeutics

MARNE C. HAGEMEIJER, GIMANO D. AMATNGALIM, AND JEFFREY M. BEEKMAN

Cystic fibrosis respiratory disease	239	Making (anti)sense of the CFTR mutation	244
Lung disease pathophysiology	239	Correcting the F508del-CFTR folding defect	244
Airway epithelium host defense	240	Potentiating the open probability of the channel	245
CFTR dysfunctioning and CF lung disease	240	Potentiating corrected CFTR proteins	246
(Mal)functioning of the CFTR anion channel	241	Stabilizing CFTR protein synthesis	247
Structure and function of CFTR	241	The future of CFTR therapeutics	247
CFTR mutations and functional defects	241	F508del-CFTR restoration by small molecules	247
Approved and investigational CFTR-modulating compounds	242	Small molecule CFTR modulation beyond F508del-CFTR	248
Targeting nonsense mutations by read-through agents	242	Final conclusions	248
		Acknowledgments	248
Amplifying CFTR with class II defects	243	References	249

CYSTIC FIBROSIS RESPIRATORY DISEASE

Cystic fibrosis (CF) is a systemic disease that affects multiple organs (1) due to malfunctioning of the cystic fibrosis transmembrane conductance regulator (CFTR) protein (2). CF lung disease, however, is the main cause of morbidity and mortality of individuals with CF (3). It originates from an abnormal host defense mechanism in the lungs, leading to persistent colonization and recurrent infections of opportunistic respiratory pathogens (see Figure 14.1) (4).

Lung disease pathophysiology

Prior to the development of clinical symptoms in CF infants, microbial colonization with *Staphylococcus aureus* (*S. aureus*) already occurs in the lungs during the first month after birth (5). Although *S. aureus* is the main microbe observed in these infants, it is generally assumed that *Pseudomonas aeruginosa* (*P. aeruginosa*) is the major pathogen that contributes to CF lung disease progression later in life (6). It seems that epithelial remodeling and chronic

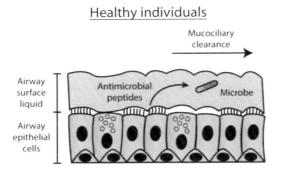
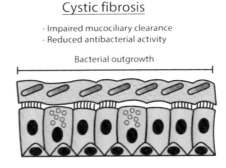

Figure 14.1 Impaired airway epithelial host defense in cystic fibrosis. In healthy individuals airway epithelial cells prevent microbial outgrowth via mucociliary clearance and antibacterial activity of antimicrobial proteins and peptides in the airway surface liquid (ASL) (left panel). CFTR dysfunction in subjects suffering from cystic fibrosis (CF) causes microbial outgrowth in the ASL due to ASL dehydration or enhanced mucus viscosity resulting in impaired mucociliary clearance, whereas acidification of the ASL impairs the activity of antimicrobial proteins and peptides (right panel).

inflammation alters the lung microenvironment in such a way that it favors persistent *P. aeruginosa* colonization (7). In addition, microbes such as *Burkholderia cepacia* are also observed upon disease progression with colonization of the nonmucoidal phenotype being associated with a more rapid lung function decline (8).

The presence of microbes in bronchoalveolar lavage (BAL) fluid correlates with inflammation in the lower airways in CF infants (9), suggesting that microbial colonization contributes to the onset of airway inflammation in CF. Indeed, it has been shown that microbial stimulation increases inflammatory responses in CF animal models and primary CF cell cultures (10,11), but it has also been proposed that CFTR dysfunction itself can cause these responses independent of microbial exposure (12). Airway inflammation in CF is characterized by excessive infiltrations of neutrophils and enhanced levels of associated biomarkers such as neutrophil elastase in BAL fluid (9). Degranulation and/or cell death of neutrophils leads to the release of cytotoxic mediators that can cause tissue damage (13). Therefore, it is assumed that enhanced neutrophil inflammation contributes to tissue injury and remodeling in CF lung disease, which is in agreement with the correlation between elastase activity in BAL fluid and epithelial remodeling in CF infants (14).

Taken together, CFTR dysfunction in the lungs causes an increased microbial burden that contributes to chronic airway inflammation and repetitive lung injury. This eventually results in irreversible tissue damage and remodeling with lung transplantation as the only and final solution (15).

Airway epithelium host defense

The prevailing general assumption is that impaired host defense due to CFTR malfunctioning in the airway epithelium is the primary cause of CF lung disease development (4). The airway epithelium lines the surface of the respiratory tract and includes the conductive airways and alveoli (16). The conductive airway epithelium consists of a pseudostratified layer of mature luminal ciliated and secretory epithelial cells that are essential in maintaining proper gas exchange in the alveoli by removing inhaled particles and microbes via mucociliary clearance (16,17). Gel-forming mucins (mucus) produced by secretory goblet cells and upper airway submucosal glands are secreted into the airway surface liquid (ASL), which captures and transports foreign substances via ciliary beating to the throat (17). The ASL also contains a mixture of antimicrobial factors that include lipids, reactive oxygen species, and numerous antimicrobial proteins and peptides (AMPs) that, together with submucosal glands and immune cells that produce antimicrobials, kill or inhibit inhaled microbes in the lungs (18). Mucociliary clearance and antimicrobial activity are both important contributors to the suppression of microbial outgrowth in the lungs, which are both affected in individuals with CF.

CFTR dysfunctioning and CF lung disease

CFTR functions as an anion channel that regulates ion and fluid homeostasis across various epithelia (2). In the airways, it is mainly expressed on ciliated cells and in serous cells located in submucosal glands (19). Several mechanisms have been proposed to explain how malfunctioning of CFTR in these cells can lead to impaired lung host defense and eventually into lung disease.

The dehydration hypothesis proposes that impaired CFTR-dependent chloride secretion on ciliated cells causes dehydration of ASL volume and impaired mucociliary transport, which seems to be due to an imbalance between CFTR-mediated chloride secretion and excessive sodium and fluid reabsorption by the epithelial sodium transporter channel (ENaC) (20). As a result, mucociliary clearance is impaired with the formation of mucus plugs that favor microbial colonization (7).

It has also been proposed that impaired antibacterial activity of AMPs contributes to increased microbial susceptibility. It has been demonstrated that antibacterial properties in CF patient-derived airway epithelial cells were reduced, which was not due to impaired expression levels of AMPs but due to altered physiological conditions of the ASL (21). This was also observed in CF newborn pigs (22), with this defect being present already after birth and might therefore be the underlying cause of the onset of CF lung disease (4). Several AMPs display pH-sensitive antibacterial properties (22), and it is assumed that reduced CFTR-mediated bicarbonate secretion impairs the ASL antibacterial activity, which allows for microbial outgrowth on epithelia (4,23). This process is normally regulated by the hydrogen potassium ATPase transporter H^+,K^+-ATPase ATP12A that prevents acidification of the ASL (22,23). pH reduction may also lead to impaired mucociliary clearance, due to increased mucus viscosity (24) or to ASL dehydration by abrogating ENaC inhibition of the pH-sensitive protein short palate lung and nasal epithelial clone 1 (SPLUNC1) (25).

The host defense properties of the submucosal glands are also affected by malfunctioning of CFTR (26). The submucosal glands are the primary source of AMPs in the upper airways (18), and an acidic pH at the surface epithelium might affect gland-produced AMP activity like lysozyme, lactoferrin, and LL-37 (22). Moreover, antibacterial function regulated by lactoperoxidase, secreted by submucosal glands, is also attenuated when CFTR function is dysregulated (27) and in CF pigs, secreted mucins from submucosal glands remain tethered to the cell surface (28).

Taken together, the CFTR anion channel has a central role in regulating airway epithelial defense. Current and future CFTR-modulating drugs may restore CFTR function, thereby reducing the microbial burden in CF patients and prevent further progression of respiratory disease symptoms.

(MAL)FUNCTIONING OF THE CFTR ANION CHANNEL

CF is the most prevalent life-threatening genetic disease in western countries and affects approximately 70,000 individuals worldwide. People with CF suffer from gastrointestinal and pulmonary complications due to malfunction of the CFTR epithelial anion channel and will eventually succumb from end-stage lung disease (see previous section). The median life expectancy of individuals with CF is around 35 years of age (29).

Structure and function of CFTR

The CFTR protein (also known as ABCC7) is a cAMP-dependent anion channel that regulates ion transport and fluid homeostasis across various epithelia (30). It is a member of the superfamily of ATP-binding cassette (ABC) transporter ATPases, with the 1480 amino acids of the protein encoding for different functional domains that include two membrane-spanning domains (MSDs), two cytoplasmic nucleotide-binding domains (NBDs), and a cytosolic regulatory (R) domain, which is unique for ABC transporters (2). A schematic representation of the CFTR protein and its corresponding topology are depicted in Figure 14.2.

The pore of the channel is formed by the two MSDs that each consist of six transmembrane (TM) domains (2). The ion conduction pathway has a narrow TM tunnel and a large cytoplasmic vestibule, with the inside being positively charged, which ensures selective transport of anions (chloride and bicarbonate) across the cellular membrane (31,32). Sodium is passively transported together with the chloride ions resulting in trans- and paracellular water transport, which ensures hydration of the luminal mucus layer together with correct regulation of the pH in the ASL (30).

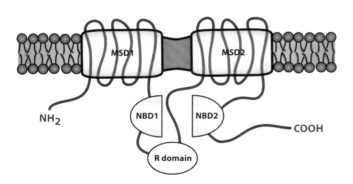

Figure 14.2 Schematic representation of the CFTR protein domain organization and topology. CFTR is an anion channel with two membrane-spanning domains (MSDs) that each consist of six transmembrane (TM) domains that form the pore of the channel. Opening and closing (gating) of the channel requires the consorted action of the regulatory (R) and nucleotide-binding domains (NBDs) as described in the section "Structure and function of CFTR."

Opening and closing of the ion channel (so-called *gating*) is regulated by an ATP-dependent gating cycle. Phosphorylation of the R domain by the cAMP-dependent protein kinase A (PKA) displaces the R domain, thereby allowing ATP to bind to the NBDs (33,34). NBD1 and NBD2 interact with each other and induce a conformational change in the MSDs that results in opening of the channel and ion transport (32). Hydrolysis of the NBD2-bound ATP results in loss of NBD heterodimers and conformational rearrangement of the protein, thereby closing the channel and preventing ion transport (35).

CFTR mutations and functional defects

The gene that encodes CFTR is located on chromosome 7 (7q31.2) (36,37). Until now, more than 2000 different mutations have been reported (38), of which approximately 90% are estimated to be CF disease-causing variants (39). The most common CFTR mutation present on at least one allele of 85% of people with CF is the deletion of a phenylalanine at position 508 (p.Phe508del, c.1521_1523delCTT, F508del). An additional 20 other variants occur at a frequency >0.1% in the CF population, but most of the remaining mutations, so-called orphan mutations, are rare due to their low incidence (38). Considerable progress in understanding the molecular and cellular mechanism of different CFTR mutations has resulted in a classification system according to the effect of a particular mutation on CFTR processing and functioning (40,41).

The majority of class I mutations are nonsense mutations that introduce premature termination codons and result in nonsense-mediated mRNA decay and nonfunctional CFTR protein synthesis. Severe splicing mutations in the consensus splice site sequence and frame-shift mutations also belong to this specific class. Class II mutations result in defective folding, processing, and trafficking of CFTR to the plasma membrane. F508del-CFTR is the most common class II mutation. When CFTR reaches the cell surface but is unable to properly perform channel regulation, i.e., opening and closing of the channel (*gating*), it is considered a class III mutation. Class IV mutants have reduced channel conductance activity, i.e., transport of chloride and bicarbonate ions through the obstructed pore. Defects resulting in decreased levels of CFTR due to aberrant or improper maturation of the protein belong to class V. Mutations leading to reduced stability of plasma membrane-localized CFTR due to increased endocytosis and/or decreased recycling of the protein belong to class VI. At the group level class I–III and VI mutations are considered to cause severe CF (no or limited residual CFTR function), whereas class IV and V mutations are associated with milder disease phenotypes (some residual CFTR function) (42). Although the classification system is useful to classify mutations, detailed analysis indicated that many mutations actually have mixed phenotypes, such as reported for F508del-CFTR, which exhibits features of class II, III, and VI (43).

The classification system of *CFTR* genotypes categorizes disease-causing mutations into different classes and allows for the development of mutation class-specific therapies that target similar functional protein defects. Current drug development programs aim to develop new CFTR-restoring therapies that target the underlying basic defect of the disease, especially the CFTR-F508del mutation as this is the most common CF-causing mutation in individuals with CF. For rare mutations, so-called theratyping efforts are undertaken to classify other mutational groups for therapeutic options. These efforts already resulted in the development of two existing CFTR modulators (which will be discussed in the next section). Despite this great achievement, the efficacy of these therapeutics has been variable between subjects and only reach half of the total CF population (44,45). Many individuals with a rare mutation on both alleles or in combination with F508del-CFTR on the other allele will not benefit from these drugs. As such, a clinical need for novel small molecule therapies that target a broad spectrum of CFTR mutations exists.

APPROVED AND INVESTIGATIONAL CFTR-MODULATING COMPOUNDS

In this section, we will give a concise overview of CFTR modulators that have passed the preclinical trial phase as reported by the Cystic Fibrosis Foundation (CFF) drug development pipeline and that act on the basic CFTR defect, for example, no gene-editing or bypass therapeutic approaches, see Figure 14.3 for an overview of approved and experimental CFTR-modulating approaches. Only those modulators of which sufficient literature is available, including publications and conference proceedings, will be discussed and include (i) existing modulators that are currently on the market, (ii) investigational modulators actively being tested in clinical trials, and (iii) modulator(s) that have been discontinued for clinical application.

Targeting nonsense mutations by read-through agents

Nonsense mutations (class I) in the *CFTR* gene generate premature termination codons in the mature messenger RNA (mRNA). Translation of such transcripts results in truncated nonfunctional CFTR proteins. A cellular quality control mechanism exists that recognizes these premature termination codons and degrades the aberrant mRNA via the translation-dependent nonsense-mediated mRNA decay (NMD) pathway. This pathway acts in a complex series of steps that involves (i) detection of the premature termination codon, (ii) tagging of the aberrant mRNA transcript, and (iii) exonucleolytic degradation of the target mRNA (46).

Restoration of abnormal protein synthesis due to premature termination codons can be achieved via a process known as *translational read-through*. Aminoglycosides, which are a class of antibiotics, have the capability to

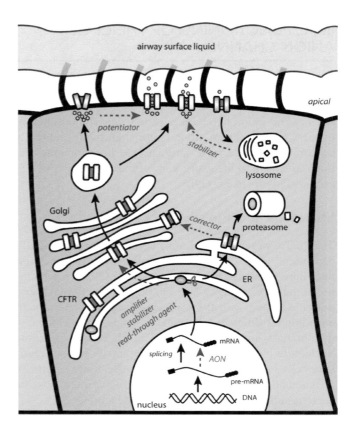

Figure 14.3 Overview of (aberrant) CFTR processing and functioning. Approved and experimental CFTR-modulating approaches are depicted in blue and are described in detail in the sections "Targeting nonsense mutations by read-through agents" through "Stabilizing CFTR protein synthesis."

promote nonsense suppression (47). Preclinical *in vitro* studies have demonstrated that geneticin (G-418) and gentamicin-induced read-through of CFTR stop codons is achievable (48,49) but that the clinical potential was limited due to difficult administration and toxicity of aminoglycosides to patients (50–52).

Ataluren (PTC124, Translarna™) is an oxadiazole of which the chemical structure is depicted in Figure 14.4. The drug is taken as an oral suspension and is metabolized by uridine diphosphate glucuronosyltransferase (UGT) enzymes in the liver into ataluren-O-1β-acyl glucuronide with (i) a tissue half-life of 2–6 hours, (ii) peak plasma levels being reached

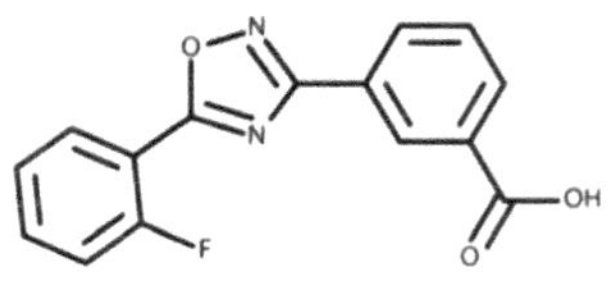

Ataluren
(read-through agent)

Figure 14.4 Chemical structure of the read-through agent Ataluren. (PTC124, Translarna™). (From Kim, S. et al., *Nucleic. Acids Res.*, 44, D1202–D1213, 2016.)

around 1.5 hours after administration, and (iii) 99.6% bound to plasma proteins (53). Ataluren was initially developed to treat Duchene muscular dystrophy (DMD) (54), for which it has been authorized in the European Union (53), but also seemed to be effective in clinical studies in individuals with CFTR premature termination mutations (55–57). The mechanism of action of Ataluren is not completely understood. It promotes translational read-through by stimulating insertion of near-cognate tRNAs at the premature termination codon with specific codon-anticodon preference for amino acid substitutions, for which direct binding to ribosomes seems to be required (58). The sequence surrounding the premature termination codon also seems to be important for this selection (59).

Administration of Ataluren is well tolerated in both adult (57) and pediatric CF subjects (56). Functional CFTR improvement measured by nasal potential difference (NPD) was observed in a phase II trial conducted in adult CF subjects with nonsense mutations who received Ataluren (55). Despite positive outcome results in earlier clinical trials, the primary endpoint (percent-predicted forced expiratory volume, [ppFEV$_1$]) in a phase 3 trial was not reached (60). Retrospective analysis of the patient population that was included in the trial revealed that chronic tobramycin inhalation (an aminoglycoside family member that binds to ribosomes) by trial participants might have negatively affected the efficacy of Ataluren in one of the studied subgroups. The inhibitory effect of tobramycin on the efficacy of Ataluren-mediated read-through was also observed in cell cultures (58). Ataluren-mediated nonsense suppression could not be detected in rectal organoids derived from CF subjects but limited G418-induced read-through activity was detected (61), which was in agreement with the reported phase 3 clinical trial results (60) and other studies (62–64). Clearly, preclinical (patient-specific) models that accurately predict CFTR modulator efficacy are desirable.

PTC Therapeutics Inc. decided to discontinue the clinical development of Ataluren for CF patients harboring nonsense mutations (65). Currently, no effective nonsense suppression therapy for people with CF is available and thus a need for the development of novel effective read-through agents that target this specific class of mutations exists, perhaps in combination with other approved and/or investigational CFTR modulator therapies.

Amplifying CFTR with class II defects

Existing small molecules available for clinical therapy (which will be described in "Correcting the F508del-CFTR folding defect" through "Potentiating corrected CFTR proteins") have demonstrated variable and modest benefits in lung function in homozygous F508del subjects but not in F508del compound heterozygous individuals (45,66). A possible explanation for this observation might be that these modulators do not have enough substrate, i.e. immature nonfunctional CFTR protein, to act upon and thus demonstrate any efficacy (67). Functional responses to

CFTR modulators in tissue cultures of subjects homozygous for F508del-CFTR are approximately twice as high compared to responses of tissue having only a single functional F508del allele, and thus support a hypothesis that a twofold increase of F508del expression might lead to therapeutically beneficial effects (68). Therefore, increasing the immature (nonfunctional) CFTR protein pool might be a potential approach to increase substrate availability for CFTR modulators.

Proteostasis Therapeutics Inc. initiated high-throughput screening efforts with the aim of identifying small molecules that would exhibit functional synergy with existing CFTR modulators. This approach resulted in the discovery of a novel class of CFTR modulators, which were termed *amplifiers* (67). Amplifiers increase the levels of immature CFTR protein but by themselves do not correct for the basic defect itself. Therefore, amplifiers require other CFTR modulators like *correctors* and *potentiators* (see "Correcting the F508del-CFTR folding defect" through "Potentiating corrected CFTR proteins") to restore CFTR function and as such might be promising candidates for future CFTR modulator combination therapies.

The identity of the investigational amplifiers in these high-throughput screens have not been disclosed by Proteostasis Therapeutics Inc., but **PTI-CH** represents this class of compounds (67), and **PTI-428** is the lead investigational oral amplifier. Not much data has been published with respect to the exact chemical structure of PTI-428 and its mechanism of action, but initial phase I clinical trial results have demonstrated safety and tolerability of PTI-428 in both CF and healthy individuals (69,70).

In human bronchial epithelial cells (HBECs), it was shown that amplifiers increased levels of immature F508del-CFTR more than the mature form (67). F508del-CFTR mRNA levels present at the ER were higher upon amplifier treatment, but to maintain this increase of CFTR, mRNA active translation was required (71). The first transmembrane domain (TM1) of CFTR acts as an inefficient signal sequence, which reduces effective membrane targeting for translation (72). *In silico* modeling of charged residues-to-alanine mutations residing in TM1, combined with *in vitro* experiments, demonstrated a lack of PTI-CH effectivity in these mutants (71). In the current model, PTI-428 and PTI-CH function by enhancing successful signal-sequence targeting of CFTR to the signal recognition particle (SRP), which in turn targets the ribosome-nascent chain complex to the translocon in the ER membranes for synthesis of the immature CFTR protein (69,71,73).

Preclinical studies have demonstrated that PTI-428 and/or PTI-CH increased CFTR function in CFTR model systems when combined with other CFTR modulators (67,74). These studies also demonstrated that amplifiers work across CFTR mutation classes (69). Recently, a proof-of-concept study demonstrated that PTI-CH was able to enhance ORKAMBI® (see "Potentiating corrected CFTR proteins") effectiveness in primary nasal cells for the p.Ile1234_Arg1239del (ΔI1234_R1239-CFTR) mutation, for which this drug was initially not registered (75). Read-through of p.Gly542X (c.1624G>T, G542X) in primary cell lines by co-treatment of the aminoglycoside G418 with PTI-428 resulted in enhanced read-through efficacy (73). Whether such treatment combinations are feasible with respect to the known toxicity of aminoglycosides needs to be investigated.

Making (anti)sense of the CFTR mutation

Development of small molecule therapies targeting F508-CFTR have mainly focused on the folding and processing defects of the protein (see "Correcting the F508del-CFTR folding defect"). Novel approaches using oligonucleotides that target the CFTR ribonucleic acid (RNA) for F508del-CFTR restoration are currently under investigation and will be discussed in this section.

Antisense oligonucleotides (AONs) are short complementary RNA molecules of approximately 15–30 nucleotides in size that base-pair specifically with their target RNA (76). Unmodified AONs are unstable and easily degraded by cellular endonucleases with poor pharmacokinetic properties (77). Various oligonucleotide chemistries can be applied to overcome these limitations, with several of these modified AONs already being used in clinical trials (78).

Zamecnik et al. demonstrated in 2004 that modified oligodeoxyribonucleotides can be used to restore CFTR-F508del function *in vitro* by a 33-mer oligonucleotide complex consisting of 2′-O-methyl (2′-OMe) RNA hybridized to an unmodified 11-mer RNA oligonucleotide duplex (79). This chemical modification at the ribose 2′ position renders oligonucleotides resistant against RNase-H nucleases (78). Using these AONs CFTR-mediated chloride transport in F508del-expressing cell lines was restored, and approximately 30% UGU mRNA insertion was detected without any genotypic changes. The specific mechanism of nucleotide insertion remains to be elucidated, but it was hypothesized that the AON complex hybridized and cleaved the mRNA followed by (i) a splicing event that inserted the AON into the target site or (ii) that the AON served as a template for individual nucleotide insertion (79).

Currently, ProQR Therapeutics has a lead candidate in development aimed at repairing the F508del-CFTR mRNA to restore channel function. **QR-010** is a single-stranded AON of 33 nucleotides with 2′-OMe sugar moieties and a phosphorothioate (PS) backbone complementary to the wild-type CFTR mRNA (80) with a similar sequence as published by Zamecnik et al. (79). The PS backbone–modified oligonucleotides renders the AONs nuclease-resistant, together with enhanced cellular uptake properties (78).

Preclinical *in vitro* data demonstrated that QR-010 is stable in sputum of CF subjects (approximately 48 hours) and that Cy5-tagged QR-010 was able to diffuse through CF-like mucus (5%–11% solids). In the presence of Pulmozyme®, fluticasone and salbutamol (inhalation therapies for CF patients), QR-010 remained stable (81). Improvement of CFTR activity in air-liquid interface (ALI) cultures of homozygous F508del primary bronchial epithelial cells could be detected after prolonged incubation with QR-010 by short-circuit current measurements in Ussing chambers when compared to nontreated cultures (82). Orotracheal dosing of nude mice with a single dose of QR-010 demonstrated that QR-010 localized to lung epithelial cells. *Ex vivo* analysis of sacrificed mice demonstrated a systemic absorption and distribution throughout multiple organs, including the lungs, and QR-010 did not accumulate in the liver and kidneys (83).

QR-010 is being developed as a regularly inhaled therapy for delivery to the lungs, which is quite a challenge as individuals with CF suffer from severe pulmonary complications that include viscous mucus and anti-inflammatory mediators as discussed in the section "Airway epithelium host defense." However, recent positive results of a phase Ib safety and tolerability trial in homozygous F508del-CFTR adult subjects demonstrated that inhaled administration of QR-010 was safe and well-tolerated, together with lung function improvements being reported (84). If this specific RNA inhalation therapy turns out to be successful, it will hold great promise to be applicable to all CFTR mutation classes in the future.

Correcting the F508del-CFTR folding defect

Numerous *CFTR* mutations, including F508del-CFTR, result in conformational defects and destabilization of the protein, and they do not pass the ER quality control (ERQC) machinery and are not targeted for ER-associated degradation (ERAD) via the ubiquitin-proteasome pathway (85). Depending on the severity of the mutation, low levels of protein might still reach the cell surface but will exhibit other structural defects. Restoration of these class II defects can be achieved by targeting the proteostasis network by using *amplifiers* or *stabilizers* as described in "Amplifying CFTR with class II defects" and "Stabilizing CFTR protein synthesis".

Another strategy to correct defective CFTR processing is by using pharmacological chaperones, called *correctors*, that bind to the misfolded CFTR protein. These correctors can be grouped according to their molecular targets. NBD1-MSD1 and NBD1-MSD2 are class I correctors, whereas class II correctors target NBD2. Chemical chaperones that stabilize the F508del-NBD1 defect belong to class III (86).

Lumacaftor (**VX-809**, Vertex Pharmaceuticals) is a CFTR *corrector* developed to restore the function of F508del-CFTR (see Figure 14.5a for the chemical structure). Lumacaftor has not been approved as monotherapy for individuals with the F508del-CFTR mutation but is available as combination therapy with a *potentiator* (ORKAMBI, see "Potentiating corrected CFTR proteins"). Lumacaftor absorption is increased twofold when taken orally with fat-containing foods with peak plasma levels 4 hours after intake and has a half-life of approximately 26 hours. It binds to plasma (99%),

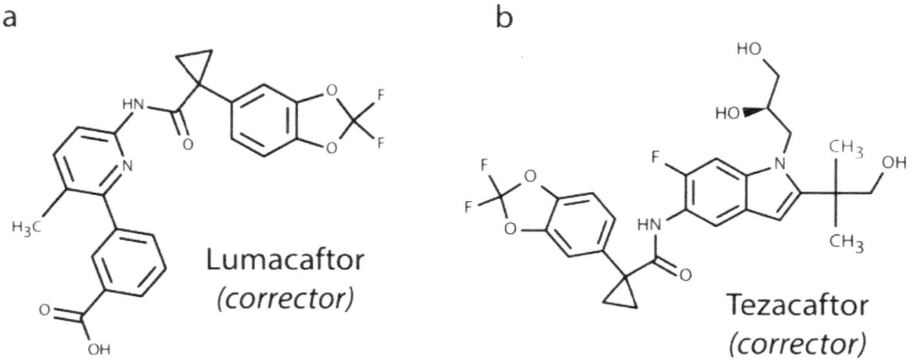

a

b

Lumacaftor
(corrector)

Tezacaftor
(corrector)

Figure 14.5 Chemical structures of the CFTR correctors (a) lumacaftor (VX-809) and (b) tezacaftor (VX-661). (From Kim, S. et al., *Nucleic. Acids Res.*, 44, D1202–D1213, 2016.)

is hardly metabolized, and is mainly (51%) excreted from the body in the feces (87).

It has been demonstrated that lumacaftor treatment of F508del-CFTR HBECs resulted in proper folding and chloride transport of the improperly processed CFTR in part of the treated cell cultures (88). Lumacaftor modulates the MSD1 structural conformation of F508del-CFTR (89) and binds directly to NBD1 to stabilize the protein (86,90). Indeed, a potential binding site of lumacaftor resides in MSD1 of the CFTR protein (91) that might be coupled to cytosolic loop (CL) 1 (92) or CL4 (90) upon lumacaftor binding. Lumacaftor also exhibits secondary activity by stabilizing partially rescued F508del-CFTR at the cell surface (93).

Lumacaftor monotherapy appears safe and well tolerated by people with CF harboring homozygous F508del-CFTR mutations. Modest improvement in sweat chloride concentration (SSC) in the lumacaftor-treated group was observed, but other biomarkers and clinical outcome parameters did not improve (94). To overcome the observed limited efficacy of lumacaftor monotherapy, it can be combined with CFTR potentiators to restore CFTR function at the cell surface (88). However, combination with the only clinical available *potentiator* ivacaftor resulted in a decrease of the therapeutic effect of lumacaftor (95,96), which will be discussed in more detail in "Potentiating the open probability of the channel" and "Potentiating corrected CFTR proteins."

Clearly, opportunities for the development of better corrector compounds exist. Indeed several pharmaceutical companies are developing novel CFTR correctors. **Tezacaftor (VX-661**, Vertex Pharmaceuticals) is a novel oral corrector compound that acts on F508del-CFTR and intended for combination therapy with ivacaftor. The chemical structure of tezacaftor is depicted in Figure 14.5b. Mono- or combination therapy of tezacaftor in F508del homozygous or F508del/G551D CF subjects demonstrated that tezacaftor does not induce CYP3A activity (which will be discussed in the next section) and was well absorbed, with steady-state levels of the drug detected after approximately 2 weeks (97). Recent phase III clinical trial results demonstrated that a combination therapy of tezacaftor and ivacaftor in CF subjects with a single copy or two copies of the 508del-CFTR mutation

resulted in a significant improvement in lung function (98). Galapagos NV together with AbbVie have various *correctors* and *potentiators* in their clinical portfolio. **GLPG2222 (GLPG2222/ABBV-2222)** is a promising type 1 (early) corrector currently in clinical development. The compound itself was well tolerated as an oral suspension in healthy volunteers and CF subjects with at least one F508del-CFTR allele and readily absorbed in the body, with a mean apparent elimination half-life of 12 hours and steady-state levels being obtained within 2 days. The pharmacokinetic data supports a once daily dosing regimen and, in contrast to lumacaftor but similar to tezacaftor, GLPG2222 does not induce CYP3A activation (99,100). Another corrector currently in clinical development is **FDL169** from Flatley Discovery Lab. When compared to lumacaftor, this compound demonstrated similar efficacy and potency in primary F508del-CFTR HBECs (101,102) but it was present at higher levels in the lungs of rats when compared to lumacaftor after treatment (102,103). In contrast to lumacaftor, FDL169 does not bind as much to human serum proteins, and CFTR corrected in CF-HBE cells by FDL169 were less affected by ivacaftor-induced decrease of CFTR correction (see "Potentiating the open probability of the channel") (102). Phase I clinical trials with FDL169 have been completed. Proteostasis Therapeutics has an investigational CFTR corrector called **PTI-801** in development. This compound is similar to FDL169 and can also prevent F508del-CFTR instability due to ivacaftor treatment and was able to complement other CFTR modulators in an *in vitro* setting (74).

Potentiating the open probability of the channel

CFTR mutations belonging to class III or class IV display gating or conductance defects, respectively. CFTR modulators called *potentiators* are small molecules that are able to increase the open probability of the activated CFTR channel and thereby increase chloride transport across the plasma membrane. Recently, the first clinically available CFTR potentiator entered the market and is now available for CF subjects with selected gating mutations. **Ivacaftor**

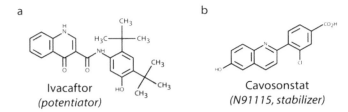

a   b

Ivacaftor
(potentiator)

Cavosonstat
(N91115, stabilizer)

Figure 14.6 Chemical structures of (a) the potentiator ivacaftor (KALYDECO®, VX-770) and (b) the stabilizer cavosonstat (N91115). The blue ellipses highlight the methyl (–CH₃) groups that are replaced by –DH₃ groups in the deuterium-substituted version of ivacaftor (CTP-656, d₉-ivacaftor). (From Kim, S. et al., *Nucleic. Acids Res.*, 44, D1202–D1213, 2016.)

(KALYDECO®, VX-770) was developed by Vertex Pharmaceuticals (the chemical structure is depicted in Figure 14.6a). Similar to lumacaftor, it has to be taken with fat-containing food because fat enhances absorption 2.5 to 4 times, with peak plasma levels obtained at 4 hours after administration and with 99% of it binding to plasma proteins. Ivacaftor has a half-life of 12 hours and is extensively metabolized, with approximately 88% of it being removed from the body via the feces (104).

The exact CFTR binding site of ivacaftor is still unknown but direct binding to the phosphorylated CFTR protein has been reported (105), with the transmembrane domains (TMDs) being suggested as possible binding site candidates (106). Ivacaftor stabilizes a posthydrolytic open state of CFTR and as a result stimulates decoupling of the gating and ATP hydrolysis cycle, resulting in an increased time period that the CFTR channel stays open (106). It is able to exert its function, as demonstrated in a reconstitution system with purified wild-type and mutant CFTR, via an ATP-independent mechanism (105). Indeed, it was reported that spontaneous opening of CFTR may occur without ATP and is coupled to NBD dimerization (107). *In vitro* studies, however, suggested that the effect of ivacaftor was due to an ATP-dependent increase of the opening rate and reduction of the closing rate of the channel (108). Clearly, more studies are required to elucidate ivacaftor's mode of action in more detail, which would be beneficial for future development of novel potentiator compounds.

Despite the lack of mechanistic insight, ivacaftor is available for a subgroup of the CF population. Clinical trials in subjects with at least one G551D allele demonstrated improvements in sweat chloride levels, nasal potential differences, and lung function (44,109,110). No clinical benefits were observed in homozygous F508del individuals treated with ivacaftor (111). Ivacaftor has been available for CF subject with ten gating mutations, including G551D-CFTR (44,109,112,113) and R117H-CFTR (114). Other studies have also demonstrated that ivacaftor was also effective for other missense mutations (68,115) and nonsense mutations (p.Trp1282X, c.3846G>A, W1282X) (116). Recently, the label has been extended with an additional 23 *CFTR* mutations (117).

Ivacaftor is a weak inhibitor of cytochrome P450, family 3, subfamily A (CYP3A) but it is also CYP3A-sensitive and is metabolized into two metabolites that circulate in human plasma: (i) hydroxymethyl ivacaftor (M1) and (ii) ivacaftor carboxylate (M6). The M1 metabolite is still pharmacologically active, albeit with less potency, whereas the M6 metabolite is not pharmacologically active (118). After metabolic conversion, 65% of ivacaftor is eliminated from the body in the feces as metabolites and around 23% as the parental drug (104).

A novel approach to improve pharmacokinetic properties of existing drugs is by a process known as selective precision deuterium substitution. This technique allows for creating more stable chemical bonds in a drug compound, which might result in potentially more favorable drug metabolism and pharmacokinetic properties without modifying the biological activity of the compound (119). Concert Pharmaceuticals Inc. developed an investigational deuterium-substituted version of ivacaftor termed **CTP-656 (d₉-ivacaftor**, see Figure 14.6a). CTP-656 has similar pharmacological properties as ivacaftor but is metabolically more stable *in vitro* and *in vivo*, with more of the parental drug being present in plasma than its less active metabolites (120,121). Clinical trial data of CTP-656 demonstrated that CTP-656 has an increased half-life of 40% *in vivo* compared to ivacaftor, which would allow for daily single dosing (121). Other companies are also developing novel experimental potentiators, which include **QBW251** of Novartis (122) and **PTI-808** of Proteostasis Therapeutics (74).

Potentiating corrected CFTR proteins

As described in "Correcting the F508del-CFTR folding defect," lumacaftor monotherapy in homozygous F508del subjects demonstrated moderate improvement in CFTR function (94). Pharmacologically corrected F508del-CFTR proteins localized at the plasma membrane demonstrate class III or class IV gating defects. Combination therapy of *corrector* and *potentiator* compounds might alleviate the gating and/or conductance defect present in corrected F508del-CFTR.

ORKAMBI (Vertex Pharmaceuticals) is a combination therapy of lumacaftor (*corrector*) and ivacaftor (*potentiator*) in tablet form for oral administration and contains 200 mg of lumacaftor and 125 mg of ivacaftor (87). It is the only approved and clinically available drug for people suffering from CF with homozygous F508del-CFTR mutations (45,66). A drawback of this *corrector-potentiator* combination is that lumacaftor is able to induce CYP3A enzymes to metabolize ivacaftor (but also other CYP3A substrates) in its less functional M1 and M6 metabolites (see the previous section). Co-administration of CYP3A inhibitors together with ORKAMBI, however, increases the concentration of available ivacaftor (87).

Co-treatment of F508del-CFTR cell cultures and organoids with ivacaftor and lumacaftor demonstrated that ivacaftor was able to restore channel gating and conductance of lumacaftor-corrected and plasma membrane–localized CFTR (68,88,108). Several clinical studies in which homozygous F508del-CFTR individuals were treated with ORKAMBI showed a modest but significant lung improvement (ppFEV$_1$) (45,66) that was not to the same extent, however, when compared to the observed G551D-CFTR lung improvement upon ivacaftor monotherapy (44,110). Recently, it has been published that ivacaftor negatively influences the therapeutic effects of lumacaftor, which might explain the observed limited efficacy of ORKAMBI. Chronic, but not acute, administration of ivacaftor resulted in a higher turnover rate of repaired F508del-CFTR with less protein stability and chloride secretion in F508del/F508del CF HBECs (95,96). Matthes et al. argued, however, that chronic ivacaftor exposure did not reduce CFTR functional restoration but that the limited efficacy of lumacaftor was responsible for the marginal effectiveness of ORKAMBI (123). Additional investigations are required to understand these drug–drug interactions in more detail in order to develop novel CFTR modulators that do not interfere with correction of F508del-CFTR.

Experimental studies demonstrated that in human R117H/F508del airway cells, ORKAMBI treatment restored CFTR activity more than in cells treated with ivacaftor monotherapy (124). Studies using intestinal organoids with various genotypes are ongoing to investigate whether ORKAMBI might be beneficial to the individuals from which these organoids were derived (68). Functional restoration of the F508del-CFTR allele by the current *corrector-potentiator* combination is moderate and variable between individuals. Novel combination therapies consisting of various (new) CFTR modulators are therefore required to enhance functional restoration for this specific mutation (see "The future of CFTR therapeutics").

Stabilizing CFTR protein synthesis

The proteostasis network includes cellular pathways that together maintain protein homeostasis by regulating protein synthesis, folding, trafficking, and degrading, and as such it is an attractive target for the development of therapeutic approaches (125). S-nitrosation (or S-nitrosylation) is a cellular post-translational modification by which nitric oxide (NO) is transferred to a protein thiol group and thereby regulates NO-mediated signaling pathways. The S-nitrosoglutathione reductase (GSNOR) alcohol dehydrogenase (ADH) enzyme is responsible for metabolizing S-nitrosoglutathione (GSNO), which is the main source of nitric oxide in cells, and as such regulates NO levels for protein S-nitrosation (126).

The amount of endogenous GSNO in the airways of people suffering from CF is low (127). Treatment of cell cultures with low (micromolar) doses of GSNO increased maturation, expression, and function of cell surface expressed wild-type and F508del-CFTR (128–131), with aerosolized GSNO treatment reported to be well tolerated in patients with CF (132). GSNO induces S-nitrosylation of the CFTR

co-chaperone heat shock protein 70/90 (HSP70/90) organizing protein (HOP), which results in less expression of HOP and decrease in ER-associated proteosomal degradation of CFTR, allowing it to fully mature and traffic to the cell surface (133). CFTR stability at the cell surface is also improved, thereby leading to prolonged CFTR activity (134). Increased expression of co-chaperone cysteine string protein (Csp) induced by GSNO seems to be necessary for the observed CFTR stabilization (135).

Nivalis Therapeutics (recently acquired by Alpine Immune Sciences) developed the orally bioavailable GSNOR inhibitor (GSNORi) **cavosonstat (N91115)**, which acts as a *stabilizer* compound developed to target the F508del-CFTR mutation (its chemical structure is depicted in Figure 14.6b). GSNOR is the primary catabolizing enzyme of GSNO on which N91115 exerts its inhibitory function (126), thereby increasing GSNO-mediated CFTR stabilization by the earlier described mechanism.

Oral administration of cavosonstat was safe and well tolerated in healthy volunteers (136) and homozygous F508del individuals (136,137). Clinical trial data indicated that cavosonstat by itself would not be suitable as monotherapy for individuals harboring the homozygous F508del mutation (136). However, in combination with *correctors* and/or *potentiators*, cavosonstat indeed demonstrated improved plasma membrane stability and CFTR activity *in vitro* (138,139), suggesting it to be a suitable candidate for combination therapies to target class II and class VI mutations. Due to results obtained in a phase II clinical trial, Nivalis Therapeutics decided to discontinue clinical development of cavosonstat (140), leaving an opportunity for other pharmaceutical companies to develop novel stabilizer compounds for CF.

THE FUTURE OF CFTR THERAPEUTICS

Current progress with small molecules targeting the defect(s) in the CFTR protein have led to impressive therapeutic benefits for individuals with CF and offer hope for the majority of them still awaiting effective treatment of their disease. The field is steadily moving forward to develop therapeutic strategies of the basic defect for most if not all CF patients.

F508del-CFTR restoration by small molecules

Small molecule rescue of CFTR has and will probably remain mainly focused on the F508del-CFTR mutation, with the aim of identifying compound combinations that can restore F508del-CFTR function beyond the threshold associated with disease. Recent phase 2 data of Vertex Pharmaceuticals appear highly promising in this context, reaching approximately 10% average lung function improvement in individuals having one F508del allele and a minimal residual disease mutation on the other allele upon triple combination treatments of two corrector and one potentiator compound (141).

Yet even these encouraging results do not fully normalize sweat chloride levels, illustrating that the efficacy of these novel generation modulators is still not sufficient to fully repair CFTR in all affected tissues. Optimal F508del-CFTR correction might involve new combination cocktails that target the primary folding defect in NBD1 as well as the various domain-domain assembly steps required for wild type conformation (86).

It has been highly encouraging to observe that within a decade or so, clinical trials have progressed from single to triple combination therapy for F508del-CFTR. The selection of compound combinations is becoming increasingly complex as efficacy, formulation, pharmacokinetic properties and drug–drug interactions need to be accounted for. With so many pharmaceutical companies now developing F508del modulators, another possibility may be that optimal F508del-CFTR restoration in in vitro models will be observed when drugs from different parties are combined. The clinical follow-up of such combinations may be highly challenging due to additional economical, organizational, and regulatory aspects.

It remains uncertain whether correction of F508del-CFTR by chemical chaperones alone may eventually reach sufficient CFTR function to prevent further progression of CF. Combinations of chemical chaperones with small molecules that target F508del using distinct modes of action such as amplifiers or RNA-targeting approaches may turn out to be essential. For now, the encouraging phase II data of triple combination therapy support the hope that efficacious F508del modulator therapies will become available in the coming decade for the approximately 85% of individuals with CF that have a single F508del allele.

Small molecule CFTR modulation beyond F508del-CFTR

The theratyping (or classification) of non-F508del mutations for CFTR modulators aims to ensure that others may benefit from drugs being developed that target F508del-CFTR. Recently, label extension of ivacaftor by the food and drug administration (FDA) was approved based on drug efficacy in heterologous cell systems expressing defined mutant CFTR cDNAs (117). This first example that a drug label is extended based on in vitro data alone shows that in vitro approaches can provide quick and cost-effective alternatives to enable access to safe drugs with a known mode-of-action. As such, these heterologous cell systems are valuable to select or deselect CFTR mutations for therapy, but they do not account for other individual genetic factors (within or outside the CFTR gene) that might modulate drug efficacy.

Patient-derived models from easy-to-access tissue may complement such heterologous models. CFTR modulator responses in intestinal organoids have been used to select individuals for treatment, and this living, in vitro biomarker shows correlation with other known biomarkers of CFTR function such as SCC and intestinal current measurements (ICMs) (68). Currently, a pilot study that

aims to demonstrate that intestinal organoids can be used to select the p.Ala455Glu (c.1364C>A, A455E) mutation for ORKAMBI treatment is almost completed. This study (i) was initiated based on efficacy data of ORKAMBI in organoids from three individuals with the A455E/F508del genotype and (ii) compared these responses with ORKAMBI efficacy in F508del/F508del organoids. Intestinal organoids, and potentially also airway cultures from the nasal cavity, may thus provide additional tools for the selection of CFTR mutations for therapy, even in a patient-specific manner.

The available CFTR modulators will not be efficacious for many premature stop codons, frameshifts, consensus splice-sites, and other difficult-to-treat missense mutations (e.g. p.Asn1303Lys (c.3909C>G, N1303K). For this group, mutation-specific therapies will be difficult to develop due to the low frequency of mutations and the costs associated with the development of such approaches. Potentially, CFTR mutation-specific approaches targeting CFTR mRNA may be further exploited as the defined molecular target requires nucleotide-pairing, which greatly limits the preclinical screening period for potential drug candidates. In this respect, compound series that were not developed for F508del-CFTR might also be redeveloped for other missense mutations (142). Other approaches that are currently being pursued actively are the development of more effective PTC read-through drugs, although these need to become significantly more efficacious than the currently known aminoglycosides. For a minority of subjects with CF, it is likely that CFTR mutation-independent approaches such as gene therapy need to be pursued to restore CFTR function in these individuals.

Final conclusions

In the last decade, treatment of CF has been revolutionized by the development of mutation-specific therapies that restore CFTR function. Currently, many pharmaceutical companies are developing small molecules with distinct modes of action that aim to restore or enhance function of the most dominant F508del-CFTR mutation that is present in the large majority of patients. The coming decade might bring a breakthrough for CF care when these treatments, or combinations thereof, can push F508del-CFTR function beyond the threshold of disease. However, therapeutic development for people not having F508del-CFTR will remain challenging, especially when subjects cannot benefit from the modulators being developed for F508del-CFTR. As such, the development of CFTR mutation-dependent and -independent approaches remains necessary when we aim to treat all individuals with CF.

ACKNOWLEDGMENTS

The authors would like to thank Domenique Zomer van Ommen and Eyleen de Poel for critically reading the manuscript and Florijn Dekkers for providing several of the figures that were adapted for this chapter.

REFERENCES

1. Elborn JS. Cystic fibrosis. *Lancet.* 2016;388(10059):2519–2531. doi:10.1016/S0140-6736(16)00576-6. PubMed PMID: 27140670.

2. Riordan JR. CFTR function and prospects for therapy. *Annu Rev Biochem.* 2008;77:701–726. doi:10.1146/annurev.biochem.75.103004.142532. PubMed PMID: 18304008.

3. Kerem E, Reisman J, Corey M, Canny GJ, Levison H. Prediction of mortality in patients with cystic fibrosis. *N Engl J Med.* 1992;326(18):1187–1191. doi:10.1056/NEJM199204303261804. PubMed PMID: 1285737.

4. Stoltz DA, Meyerholz DK, Welsh MJ. Origins of cystic fibrosis lung disease. *N Engl J Med.* 2015;372(4):351–362. doi:10.1056/NEJMra1300109. PubMed PMID: 25607428; PMCID: PMC4916857.

5. Sly PD, Brennan S, Gangell C, de Klerk N, Murray C, Mott L, Stick SM, Robinson PJ, Robertson CF, Ranganathan SC, Australian respiratory early surveillance team for cystic F. Lung disease at diagnosis in infants with cystic fibrosis detected by newborn screening. *Am J Respir Crit Care Med.* 2009;180(2):146–152. doi:10.1164/rccm.200901-0069OC. PubMed PMID: 19372250.

6. Koch C. Early infection and progression of cystic fibrosis lung disease. *Pediatr Pulmonol.* 2002;34(3):232–236. doi:10.1002/ppul.10135. PubMed PMID: 12203855.

7. Staudinger BJ, Muller JF, Halldorsson S, Boles B, Angermeyer A, Nguyen D, Rosen H et al. Conditions associated with the cystic fibrosis defect promote chronic Pseudomonas aeruginosa infection. *Am J Respir Crit Care Med.* 2014;189(7):812–824. doi:10.1164/rccm.201312-2142OC. PubMed PMID: 24467627; PMCID: PMC4225830.

8. Zlosnik JE, Costa PS, Brant R, Mori PY, Hird TJ, Fraenkel MC, Wilcox PG, Davidson AG, Speert DP. Mucoid and nonmucoid *burkholderia cepacia complex* bacteria in cystic fibrosis infections. *Am J Respir Crit Care Med.* 2011;183(1):67–72. doi:10.1164/rccm.201002-0203OC. PubMed PMID: 20709823.

9. Khan TZ, Wagener JS, Bost T, Martinez J, Accurso FJ, Riches DW. Early pulmonary inflammation in infants with cystic fibrosis. *Am J Respir Crit Care Med.* 1995;151(4):1075–1082. doi:10.1164/ajrccm.151.4.7697234. PubMed PMID: 7697234.

10. Becker MN, Sauer MS, Muhlebach MS, Hirsh AJ, Wu Q, Verghese MW, Randell SH. Cytokine secretion by cystic fibrosis airway epithelial cells. *Am J Respir Crit Care Med.* 2004;169(5):645–653. doi:10.1164/rccm.200207-765OC. PubMed PMID: 14670800.

11. Saadane A, Soltys J, Berger M. Acute Pseudomonas challenge in cystic fibrosis mice causes prolonged nuclear factor-kappa B activation, cytokine secretion, and persistent lung inflammation. *J Allergy Clin Immunol.* 2006;117(5):1163–1169. doi:10.1016/j.jaci.2006.01.052. PubMed PMID: 16675347.

12. Rubin BK. CFTR is a modulator of airway inflammation. *Am J Physiol Lung Cell Mol Physiol.* 2007;292(2):L381–L382. doi:10.1152/ajplung.00375.2006. PubMed PMID: 17012368.

13. Ralhan A, Laval J, Lelis F, Ballbach M, Grund C, Hector A, Hartl D. Current concepts and controversies in innate immunity of cystic fibrosis lung disease. *J Innate Immun.* 2016;8(6):531–540. doi:10.1159/000446840. PubMed PMID: 27362371.

14. Sly PD, Gangell CL, Chen L, Ware RS, Ranganathan S, Mott LS, Murray CP, Stick SM, Investigators AC. Risk factors for bronchiectasis in children with cystic fibrosis. *N Engl J Med.* 2013;368(21):1963–1970. doi:10.1056/NEJMoa1301725. PubMed PMID: 23692169.

15. Elborn JS, Bell SC, Madge SL, Burgel PR, Castellani C, Conway S, De Rijcke K et al. Report of the European Respiratory Society/European Cystic Fibrosis Society task force on the care of adults with cystic fibrosis. *Eur Respir J.* 2016;47(2):420–428. doi:10.1183/13993003.00592-2015. PubMed PMID: 26453627.

16. Crystal RG, Randell SH, Engelhardt JF, Voynow J, Sunday ME. Airway epithelial cells: Current concepts and challenges. *Proc Am Thorac Soc.* 2008;5(7):772–777. doi:10.1513/pats.200805-041HR. PubMed PMID: 18757316.

17. Knowles MR, Boucher RC. Mucus clearance as a primary innate defense mechanism for mammalian airways. *J Clin Invest.* 2002;109(5):571–577. doi:10.1172/JCI15217. PubMed PMID: 11877463; PMCID: PMC150901.

18. Ganz T. Antimicrobial polypeptides in host defense of the respiratory tract. *J Clin Invest.* 2002;109(6):693–697. doi:10.1172/JCI15218. PubMed PMID: 11901174; PMCID: PMC150915.

19. Kreda SM, Mall M, Mengos A, Rochelle L, Yankaskas J, Riordan JR, Boucher RC. Characterization of wild-type and deltaF508 cystic fibrosis transmembrane regulator in human respiratory epithelia. *Mol Biol Cell.* 2005;16(5):2154–21567. doi:10.1091/mbc. E04-11-1010. PubMed PMID: 15716351; PMCID: PMC1087225.

20. Boucher RC. Airway surface dehydration in cystic fibrosis: Pathogenesis and therapy. *Annu Rev Med.* 2007;58:157–170. doi:10.1146/annurev.med.58.071905.105316. PubMed PMID: 17217330.

21. Smith JJ, Travis SM, Greenberg EP, Welsh MJ. Cystic fibrosis airway epithelia fail to kill bacteria because of abnormal airway surface fluid. *Cell.* 1996;85(2):229–236. PubMed PMID: 8612275.

22. Pezzulo AA, Tang XX, Hoegger MJ, Abou Alaiwa MH, Ramachandran S, Moninger TO, Karp PH et al. Reduced airway surface pH impairs bacterial killing in the porcine cystic fibrosis lung. *Nature.* 2012;487(7405):109–113. doi:10.1038/nature11130. PubMed PMID: 22763554; PMCID: PMC3390761.

23. Shah VS, Meyerholz DK, Tang XX, Reznikov L, Abou Alaiwa M, Ernst SE, Karp PH et al. Airway acidification initiates host defense abnormalities in cystic fibrosis mice. *Science*. 2016;351(6272):503–507. doi:10.1126/science.aad5589. PubMed PMID: 26823428; PMCID: PMC4852973.

24. Tang XX, Ostedgaard LS, Hoegger MJ, Moninger TO, Karp PH, McMenimen JD, Choudhury B, Varki A, Stoltz DA, Welsh MJ. Acidic pH increases airway surface liquid viscosity in cystic fibrosis. *J Clin Invest*. 2016;126(3):879–891. doi:10.1172/JCI83922. PubMed PMID: 26808501; PMCID: PMC4767348.

25. Garland AL, Walton WG, Coakley RD, Tan CD, Gilmore RC, Hobbs CA, Tripathy A et al. Molecular basis for pH-dependent mucosal dehydration in cystic fibrosis airways. *Proc Natl Acad Sci U S A*. 2013;110(40):15973–15978. doi:10.1073/pnas.1311999110. PubMed PMID: 24043776; PMCID: PMC3791714.

26. Verkman AS, Song Y, Thiagarajah JR. Role of airway surface liquid and submucosal glands in cystic fibrosis lung disease. *Am J Physiol Cell Physiol*. 2003;284(1):C2–15. doi:10.1152/ajpcell.00417.2002. PubMed PMID: 12475759.

27. Conner GE, Wijkstrom-Frei C, Randell SH, Fernandez VE, Salathe M. The lactoperoxidase system links anion transport to host defense in cystic fibrosis. *FEBS Lett*. 2007;581(2):271–278. doi:10.1016/j.febslet.2006.12.025. PubMed PMID: 17204267; PMCID: PMC1851694.

28. Hoegger MJ, Fischer AJ, McMenimen JD, Ostedgaard LS, Tucker AJ, Awadalla MA, Moninger TO et al. Impaired mucus detachment disrupts mucociliary transport in a piglet model of cystic fibrosis. *Science*. 2014;345(6198):818–822. doi:10.1126/science.1255825. PubMed PMID: 25124441; PMCID: PMC4346163.

29. De Boeck K, Amaral MD. Progress in therapies for cystic fibrosis. *Lancet Respir Med*. 2016;4(8):662–674. doi:10.1016/S2213-2600(16)00023-0. PubMed PMID: 27053340.

30. Saint-Criq V, Gray MA. Role of CFTR in epithelial physiology. *Cell Mol Life Sci*. 2017;74(1):93–115. doi:10.1007/s00018-016-2391-y. PubMed PMID: 27714410; PMCID: PMC5209439.

31. Liu F, Zhang Z, Csanady L, Gadsby DC, Chen J. Molecular structure of the human CFTR Ion channel. *Cell*. 2017;169(1):85–95 e8. doi:10.1016/j.cell.2017.02.024. PubMed PMID: 28340353.

32. Zhang Z, Liu F, Chen J. Conformational changes of CFTR upon phosphorylation and ATP binding. *Cell*. 2017;170(3):483–91 e8. doi:10.1016/j.cell.2017.06.041. PubMed PMID: 28735752.

33. Gadsby DC, Nairn AC. Control of CFTR channel gating by phosphorylation and nucleotide hydrolysis. *Physiol Rev*. 1999;79(1 Suppl):S77–S107. PubMed PMID: 9922377.

34. Sheppard DN, Welsh MJ. Structure and function of the CFTR chloride channel. *Physiol Rev*. 1999;79(1 Suppl):S23–S45. PubMed PMID: 9922375.

35. Vergani P, Lockless SW, Nairn AC, Gadsby DC. CFTR channel opening by ATP-driven tight dimerization of its nucleotide-binding domains. *Nature*. 2005;433(7028):876–880. doi:10.1038/nature03313. PubMed PMID: 15729345; PMCID: PMC2756053.

36. Kerem B, Rommens JM, Buchanan JA, Markiewicz D, Cox TK, Chakravarti A, Buchwald M, Tsui LC. Identification of the cystic fibrosis gene: Genetic analysis. *Science*. 1989;245(4922):1073–1080. PubMed PMID: 2570460.

37. Zielenski J, Rozmahel R, Bozon D, Kerem B, Grzelczak Z, Riordan JR, Rommens J, Tsui LC. Genomic DNA sequence of the cystic fibrosis transmembrane conductance regulator (CFTR) gene. *Genomics*. 1991;10(1):214–228. PubMed PMID: 1710598.

38. Cystic Fibrosis Mutation Database (CFTR1); available at http://www.genet.sickkids.on.ca/app.

39. The Clinical and Functional TRanslation of CFTR (CFTR2); available at http://cftr2.org.

40. Haardt M, Benharouga M, Lechardeur D, Kartner N, Lukacs GL. C-terminal truncations destabilize the cystic fibrosis transmembrane conductance regulator without impairing its biogenesis. A novel class of mutation. *J Biol Chem*. 1999;274(31):21873–21877. PubMed PMID: 10419506.

41. Welsh MJ, Smith AE. Molecular mechanisms of CFTR chloride channel dysfunction in cystic fibrosis. *Cell*. 1993;73(7):1251–1254. PubMed PMID: 7686820.

42. Amaral MD. Novel personalized therapies for cystic fibrosis: Treating the basic defect in all patients. *J Intern Med*. 2015;277(2):155–166. doi:10.1111/joim.12314. PubMed PMID: 25266997.

43. Veit G, Avramescu RG, Chiang AN, Houck SA, Cai Z, Peters KW, Hong JS et al. From CFTR biology toward combinatorial pharmacotherapy: Expanded classification of cystic fibrosis mutations. *Mol Biol Cell*. 2016;27(3):424–433. doi:10.1091/mbc. E14-04-0935. PubMed PMID: 26823392; PMCID: PMC4751594.

44. Ramsey BW, Davies J, McElvaney NG, Tullis E, Bell SC, Drevinek P, Griese M et al. A CFTR potentiator in patients with cystic fibrosis and the G551D mutation. *N Engl J Med*. 2011;365(18):1663–1672. doi:10.1056/NEJMoa1105185. PubMed PMID: 22047557; PMCID: PMC3230303.

45. Wainwright CE, Elborn JS, Ramsey BW. Lumacaftor-Ivacaftor in patients with cystic fibrosis homozygous for Phe508del CFTR. *N Engl J Med*. 2015;373(18):1783–1784. doi:10.1056/NEJMc1510466. PubMed PMID: 26510034.

46. Popp MW, Maquat LE. Organizing principles of mammalian nonsense-mediated mRNA decay. *Annu Rev Genet*. 2013;47:139–165. doi:10.1146/annurev-genet-111212-133424. PubMed PMID: 24274751; PMCID: PMC4148824.

47. Hermann T. Aminoglycoside antibiotics: Old drugs and new therapeutic approaches. *Cell Mol Life Sci.* 2007;64(14):1841–18452. doi:10.1007/s00018-007-7034-x. PubMed PMID: 17447006.

48. Bedwell DM, Kaenjak A, Benos DJ, Bebok Z, Bubien JK, Hong J, Tousson A, Clancy JP, Sorscher EJ. Suppression of a CFTR premature stop mutation in a bronchial epithelial cell line. *Nat Med.* 1997;3(11):1280–1284. PubMed PMID: 9359706.

49. Howard M, Frizzell RA, Bedwell DM. Aminoglycoside antibiotics restore CFTR function by overcoming premature stop mutations. *Nat Med.* 1996;2(4):467–469. PubMed PMID: 8597960.

50. Clancy JP, Bebok Z, Ruiz F, King C, Jones J, Walker L, Greer H et al. Evidence that systemic gentamicin suppresses premature stop mutations in patients with cystic fibrosis. *Am J Respir Crit Care Med.* 2001;163(7):1683–1692. doi:10.1164/ajrccm.163.7.2004001. PubMed PMID: 11401894.

51. Sermet-Gaudelus I, Renouil M, Fajac A, Bidou L, Parbaille B, Pierrot S, Davy N et al. In vitro prediction of stop-codon suppression by intravenous gentamicin in patients with cystic fibrosis: A pilot study. *BMC Med.* 2007;5:5. doi:10.1186/1741-7015-5-5. PubMed PMID: 17394637; PMCID: PMC1852113.

52. Wilschanski M, Yahav Y, Yaacov Y, Blau H, Bentur L, Rivlin J, Aviram M et al. Gentamicin-induced correction of CFTR function in patients with cystic fibrosis and CFTR stop mutations. *N Engl J Med.* 2003;349(15):1433–1441. doi:10.1056/NEJMoa022170. PubMed PMID: 14534336.

53. Translarna : EPAR – Product Information. European Medicines Agency. First published: 04/09/2014. Last updated: 31/08/2018; available at https://www.ema.europa.eu/en/medicines/human/EPAR/translarna#overview-section.

54. Welch EM, Barton ER, Zhuo J, Tomizawa Y, Friesen WJ, Trifillis P, Paushkin S et al. PTC124 targets genetic disorders caused by nonsense mutations. *Nature.* 2007;447(7140):87–91. doi:10.1038/nature05756. PubMed PMID: 17450125.

55. Kerem E, Hirawat S, Armoni S, Yaakov Y, Shoseyov D, Cohen M, Nissim-Rafinia M et al. Effectiveness of PTC124 treatment of cystic fibrosis caused by nonsense mutations: A prospective phase II trial. *Lancet.* 2008;372(9640):719–727. doi:10.1016/S0140-6736(08)61168-X. PubMed PMID: 18722008.

56. Sermet-Gaudelus I, Boeck KD, Casimir GJ, Vermeulen F, Leal T, Mogenet A, Roussel D et al. Ataluren (PTC124) induces cystic fibrosis transmembrane conductance regulator protein expression and activity in children with nonsense mutation cystic fibrosis. *Am J Respir Crit Care Med.* 2010;182(10):1262–1272. doi:10.1164/rccm.201001-0137OC. PubMed PMID: 20622033.

57. Wilschanski M, Miller LL, Shoseyov D, Blau H, Rivlin J, Aviram M, Cohen M et al. Chronic ataluren (PTC124) treatment of nonsense mutation cystic fibrosis. *Eur Respir J.* 2011;38(1):59–69. doi:10.1183/09031936.00120910. PubMed PMID: 21233271.

58. Roy B, Friesen WJ, Tomizawa Y, Leszyk JD, Zhuo J, Johnson B, Dakka J et al. Ataluren stimulates ribosomal selection of near-cognate tRNAs to promote nonsense suppression. *Proc Natl Acad Sci U S A.* 2016;113(44):12508–125013. doi:10.1073/pnas.1605336113. PubMed PMID: 27702906; PMCID: PMC5098639.

59. Xue X, Mutyam V, Thakerar A, Mobley J, Bridges RJ, Rowe SM, Keeling KM, Bedwell DM. Identification of the amino acids inserted during suppression of CFTR nonsense mutations and determination of their functional consequences. *Hum Mol Genet.* 2017;26(16):3116–3129. doi:10.1093/hmg/ddx196. PubMed PMID: 28575328.

60. Kerem E, Konstan MW, De Boeck K, Accurso FJ, Sermet-Gaudelus I, Wilschanski M, Elborn JS et al. Cystic Fibrosis Ataluren Study G. Ataluren for the treatment of nonsense-mutation cystic fibrosis: A randomised, double-blind, placebo-controlled phase 3 trial. *Lancet Respir Med.* 2014;2(7):539–547. doi:10.1016/S2213-2600(14)70100-6. PubMed PMID: 24836205; PMCID: PMC4154311.

61. Zomer-van Ommen DD, Vijftigschild LA, Kruisselbrink E, Vonk AM, Dekkers JF, Janssens HM, de Winter-de Groot KM, van der Ent CK, Beekman JM. Limited premature termination codon suppression by read-through agents in cystic fibrosis intestinal organoids. *J Cyst Fibros.* 2016;15(2):158–162. doi:10.1016/j.jcf.2015.07.007. PubMed PMID: 26255232.

62. Auld DS, Lovell S, Thorne N, Lea WA, Maloney DJ, Shen M, Rai G et al. Molecular basis for the high-affinity binding and stabilization of firefly luciferase by PTC124. *Proc Natl Acad Sci U S A.* 2010;107(11):4878–4883. doi:10.1073/pnas.0909141107. PubMed PMID: 20194791; PMCID: PMC2841876.

63. Auld DS, Thorne N, Maguire WF, Inglese J. Mechanism of PTC124 activity in cell-based luciferase assays of nonsense codon suppression. *Proc Natl Acad Sci U S A.* 2009;106(9):3585–3590. doi:10.1073/pnas.0813345106. PubMed PMID: 19208811; PMCID: PMC2638738.

64. McElroy SP, Nomura T, Torrie LS, Warbrick E, Gartner U, Wood G, McLean WH. A lack of premature termination codon read-through efficacy of PTC124 (Ataluren) in a diverse array of reporter assays. *PLoS Biol.* 2013;11(6):e1001593. doi:10.1371/journal.pbio.1001593. PubMed PMID: 23824517.

65. PTC Therapeutics, Inc. PTC Therapeutics Announces Results from Pivotal Phase 3 Clinical Trial of Ataluren in Patients Living with Nonsense Mutation Cystic Fibrosis [Press release]. Retrieved from http://irptcbiocom/releasedetailcfm?ReleaseID=10154712017

66. Boyle MP, Bell SC, Konstan MW, McColley SA, Rowe SM, Rietschel E, Huang X, Waltz D, Patel NR, Rodman D, group VXs. A CFTR corrector (lumacaftor) and a CFTR potentiator (ivacaftor) for treatment of patients with cystic fibrosis who have a phe508del CFTR mutation: A phase 2 randomised controlled trial. *Lancet Respir Med.* 2014;2(7):527–538. doi:10.1016/S2213-2600(14)70132-8. PubMed PMID: 24973281.

67. Giuliano KA, Wachi S, Drew L, Dukovski D, Green O, Bastos C, Cullen MD et al. Use of a high-throughput phenotypic screening strategy to identify amplifiers, a novel pharmacological class of small molecules that exhibit functional synergy with potentiators and correctors. *SLAS Discov.* 2017:2472555217729790. doi:10.1177/2472555217729790. PubMed PMID: 28898585.

68. Dekkers JF, Berkers G, Kruisselbrink E, Vonk A, de Jonge HR, Janssens HM, Bronsveld I et al. Characterizing responses to CFTR-modulating drugs using rectal organoids derived from subjects with cystic fibrosis. *Sci Transl Med.* 2016;8(344):344ra84. doi:10.1126/scitranslmed.aad8278. PubMed PMID: 27334259.

69. Gilmartin G, Flume PA, Layish D, Mehdi N, Nasr S, Lee P-S, Wilson S, PTI-428–401. WS13.2 Phase 1 initial results evaluating novel CFTR amplifier PTI-428 in CF subjects. *40th European Cystic Fibrosis Conference. Journal of Cystic Fibrosis.* 2017:S23.

70. Mouded M, Layish D, Sawicki GS, Milla C, Flume PA, Tolle J, Vansaghi L et al. 187. Phase 1 initial results evaluating safety, tolerability, pk and biomarker data using PTI-428, a novel CFTR modulator, in patients with cystic fibrosis. *30th Annual North American Cystic Fibrosis Conference. Poster Session Abstracts. Pediatric Pulmonology.* 2016:S194–S485.

71. Dukovski D, Kombo DC, Villella A, Patel N, Cullen MD, Bastos CM, Aghamohammadzadeh S, Munoz B, Miller J. P112 Amplifiers co-translationally increase CFTR levels at the ER membrane by improving membrane targeting of CFTR. *14th ECFS Basic Science Conference; Portugal: Conference Programme & Abstract Book,* 2017; available at https://www.ecfs.eu/news/abstract-book-14th-ecfs-basic-science-conference

72. Lu Y, Xiong X, Helm A, Kimani K, Bragin A, Skach WR. Co- and posttranslational translocation mechanisms direct cystic fibrosis transmembrane conductance regulator N terminus transmembrane assembly. *J Biol Chem.* 1998;273(1):568–576. PubMed PMID: 9417117.

73. Tyler RE, Kim H, Dukovski D, Aghamohammadz S, Qiu D, Miller JP, Lee P-S, Munoz B. WS18.7 Amplifiers enhance the efficacy of small molecules to promote the translational read-through of CFTR nonsense mutations. *40th European Cystic Fibrosis Conference. Journal of Cystic Fibrosis.* 2017:S32.

74. Miller J, Drew L, Bastos C, Green O, Dukovski D, Villella A, Patel N et al. 39. Novel CFTR modulator combination of amplifier, corrector and potentiator provides advantages over two corrector-based combinations. *30th Annual North American Cystic Fibrosis Conference. Poster Session Abstracts. Pediatric Pulmonology.* 2016:S194–S485.

75. Molinski SV, Ahmadi S, Ip W, Ouyang H, Villella A, Miller JP, Lee PS et al. Orkambi(R) and amplifier co-therapy improves function from a rare CFTR mutation in gene-edited cells and patient tissue. *EMBO Mol Med.* 2017;9(9):1224–1243. doi:10.15252/emmm.201607137. PubMed PMID: 28667089; PMCID: PMC5582412.

76. Rigo F, Seth PP, Bennett CF. Antisense oligonucleotide-based therapies for diseases caused by pre-mRNA processing defects. *Adv Exp Med Biol.* 2014;825:303–352. doi:10.1007/978-1-4939-1221-6_9. PubMed PMID: 25201110.

77. Geary RS, Norris D, Yu R, Bennett CF. Pharmacokinetics, biodistribution and cell uptake of antisense oligonucleotides. *Adv Drug Deliv Rev.* 2015;87:46–51. doi:10.1016/j.addr.2015.01.008. PubMed PMID: 25666165.

78. Sharma VK, Sharma RK, Singh SK. Antisense oligonucleotides: Modifications and clinical trials. *Med Chem Commun.* 2014;5(10):1454–14571. doi:10.1039/C4MD00184B.

79. Zamecnik PC, Raychowdhury MK, Tabatadze DR, Cantiello HF. Reversal of cystic fibrosis phenotype in a cultured Delta 508 cystic fibrosis transmembrane conductance regulator cell line by oligonucleotide insertion. *P Natl Acad Sci USA.* 2004;101(21):8150–8155. doi:10.1073/pnas.0401933101. PubMed PMID: WOS:000221652000056.

80. Henig N, Beumer W, Anthonijsz H, Beka M, Panin N, Leal T, Matthee B, Ritsema T. QR-010, an RNA therapy, restores CFTR function in the saliva secretion assay. A37. It won't be long: Advances in adult cystic fibrosis. *American Thoracic Society 2015 International Conference Abstracts: American Journal of Respiratory and Critical Care Medicine.* 2015:A1449.

81. Brinks V, Lipinska K, Koppelaar M, Matthee B, Button B, Livraghi A, Henig N. QR-010 Penetrates the Mucus Barrier in Vitro and in Vivo. *11th Annual Meeting of the Oligonucleotide Therapeutics Society.* October 11–14, 2015. Leiden, the Netherlands: Poster available on website ProQR Therapeutics; 2015.

82. Swildens J, van Putten C, Potman M, Ritsema T. 241. QR-010, an antisense oligonucleotide, restores cftr function in δf508 cell cultures. *28th Annual North American Cystic Fibrosis Conference Poster Session Abstracts. Pediatric Pulmonology.* 2014:S216–S456.

83. Beumer W, Matthee B, Ritsema T. 216. QR-010 is taken up by airway epithelial cells showing systemic exposure after oro-tracheal dosing. *28th Annual North American Cystic Fibrosis Conference Poster Session Abstracts. Pediatric Pulmonology.* 2014:S216–S456.

84. ProQR Therapeutics NV. ProQR Announces Positive Top-Line Results from a Phase 1b Study of QR-010 in Subjects with Cystic Fibrosis [Press release]. Retrieved from http://irproqr-txcom/phoenixzhtml?c=253704&p=irol-newsArticle&ID=23026792017.

85. Farinha CM, Canato S. From the endoplasmic reticulum to the plasma membrane: Mechanisms of CFTR folding and trafficking. *Cell Mol Life Sci.* 2017;74(1):39–55. doi:10.1007/s00018-016-2387-7. PubMed PMID: 27699454.

86. Okiyoneda T, Veit G, Dekkers JF, Bagdany M, Soya N, Xu H, Roldan A, Verkman AS, Kurth M, Simon A, Hegedus T, Beekman JM, Lukacs GL. Mechanism-based corrector combination restores DeltaF508-CFTR folding and function. *Nat Chem Biol.* 2013;9(7):444–454. doi:10.1038/nchembio.1253. PubMed PMID: 23666117; PMCID: PMC3840170.

87. ORKAMBI® (lumacaftro/ivacaftor) [package insert]. Vertex Pharmaceuticals Incorporated; 2018; available at https://pi.vrtx.com/files/uspi_lumacaftor_ivacaftor.pdf.

88. Van Goor F, Hadida S, Grootenhuis PD, Burton B, Stack JH, Straley KS, Decker CJ et al. Correction of the F508del-CFTR protein processing defect in vitro by the investigational drug VX-809. *Proc Natl Acad Sci U S A.* 2011;108(46):18843–18848. doi:10.1073/pnas.1105787108. PubMed PMID: 21976485; PMCID: PMC3219147.

89. Ren HY, Grove DE, De La Rosa O, Houck SA, Sopha P, Van Goor F, Hoffman BJ, Cyr DM. VX-809 corrects folding defects in cystic fibrosis transmembrane conductance regulator protein through action on membrane-spanning domain 1. *Mol Biol Cell.* 2013;24(19):3016–30124. doi:10.1091/mbc. E13-05-0240. PubMed PMID: 23924900; PMCID: PMC3784376.

90. Hudson RP, Dawson JE, Chong PA, Yang Z, Millen L, Thomas PJ, Brouillette CG, Forman-Kay JD. Direct binding of the corrector VX-809 to human CFTR NBD1: Evidence of an allosteric coupling between the binding site and the NBD1:CL4 interface. *Mol Pharmacol.* 2017;92(2):124–135. doi:10.1124/mol.117.108373. PubMed PMID: 28546419.

91. Loo TW, Bartlett MC, Clarke DM. Corrector VX-809 stabilizes the first transmembrane domain of CFTR. *Biochem Pharmacol.* 2013;86(5):612–619. doi:10.1016/j.bcp.2013.06.028. PubMed PMID: 23835419.

92. Loo TW, Clarke DM. Corrector VX-809 promotes interactions between cytoplasmic loop one and the first nucleotide-binding domain of CFTR. *Biochem Pharmacol.* 2017;136:24–31. doi:10.1016/j.bcp.2017.03.020. PubMed PMID: 28366727.

93. Eckford PD, Ramjeesingh M, Molinski S, Pasyk S, Dekkers JF, Li C, Ahmadi S et al. VX-809 and related corrector compounds exhibit secondary activity stabilizing active F508del-CFTR after its partial rescue to the cell surface. *Chem Biol.* 2014;21(5):666–678. doi:10.1016/j.chembiol.2014.02.021. PubMed PMID: 24726831.

94. Clancy JP, Rowe SM, Accurso FJ, Aitken ML, Amin RS, Ashlock MA, Ballmann M et al. Results of a phase IIa study of VX-809, an investigational CFTR corrector compound, in subjects with cystic fibrosis homozygous for the F508del-CFTR mutation. *Thorax.* 2012;67(1):12–18. doi:10.1136/thoraxjnl-2011-200393. PubMed PMID: 21825083; PMCID: PMC3746507.

95. Cholon DM, Quinney NL, Fulcher ML, Esther CR, Jr., Das J, Dokholyan NV, Randell SH, Boucher RC, Gentzsch M. Potentiator ivacaftor abrogates pharmacological correction of DeltaF508 CFTR in cystic fibrosis. *Sci Transl Med.* 2014;6(246):246ra96. doi:10.1126/scitranslmed.3008680. PubMed PMID: 25101886; PMCID: PMC4272825.

96. Veit G, Avramescu RG, Perdomo D, Phuan PW, Bagdany M, Apaja PM, Borot F, Szollosi D, Wu YS, Finkbeiner WE, Hegedus T, Verkman AS, Lukacs GL. Some gating potentiators, including VX-770, diminish DeltaF508-CFTR functional expression. *Sci Transl Med.* 2014;6(246):246ra97. doi:10.1126/scitranslmed.3008889. PubMed PMID: 25101887; PMCID: PMC4467693.

97. Donaldson SH, Pilewski JM, Griese M, Cooke J, Viswanathan L, Tullis E, Davies JC, Lekstrom-Himes JA, Wang LT, Group VXS. Tezacaftor/Ivacaftor in Subjects with Cystic Fibrosis and F508del/F508del-CFTR or F508del/G551D-CFTR. *Am J Respir Crit Care Med.* 2017. doi:10.1164/rccm.201704-0717OC. PubMed PMID: 28930490.

98. Vertex Pharmaceuticals Inc. Two Phase 3 Studies of the Tezacaftor/Ivacaftor Combination Treatment Met Primary Endpoints with Statistically Significant Improvements in Lung Function (FEV1) in People with Cystic Fibrosis [Press release]. Retrieved from http://investorsvrtxcom/releasedetailcfm?releaseid=10191562017.

99. Van de Steen O, Namour F, Kanters D, Geller DE, de Kock H, Vanhoutte FP. 252. Safety, tolerability and pharmacokinetics of a novel CFTR corrector molecule GLPG2222 in healthy volunteers. *30th Annual North American Cystic Fibrosis Conference: Poster Session Abstracts. Pediatric Pulmonology.* 2016. s194–s485.

100. Van de Steen O, De Boeck K, Vermeulen F, Geller DE, De Kock H, Kanters D, Gesson C, Namour F. 58 Pharmacokinetics and safety of a novel CFTR corrector molecule GLPG2222 in subjects with cystic fibrosis (CF): Results from a phase Ib study. *40th European Cystic Fibrosis Conference. Journal of Cystic Fibrosis.* 2017:S79.

101. Patron T, Valdez R, Bhatt P, Deshpande A, Krouse M, Barsukov G, Handley K et al. 50. Discovery and development of novel δF508-cftr correctors. *27th Annual North American Cystic Fibrosis Conference: Poster Session Abstracts. Pediatric Pulmonology.* 2013: 207–453.

102. Zawistoski M, Sui J, Ordonez C, Mai V, Liu E, Li T, Kwok I et al. 32 Properties of a novel F508del-CFTR corrector FDL169. *39th European Cystic Fibrosis Conference. Journal of Cystic Fibrosis.* 2016: S59–S60.

103. Ferkany JW, Krouse ME, Kolodziej AF, Fitzpatrick R, Cole BM. 67. Lung partitioning of δF508-cftr correctors. *29th Annual North American Cystic Fibrosis Conference: Poster Session Abstracts. Pediatric Pulmonology,* 2015: S193–S453.

104. KALYDECO® (ivacaftor) [package insert]. Vertex Pharmaceuticals Incorporated; 2018; https://pi.vrtx.com/files/uspi_ivacaftor.pdf.

105. Eckford PD, Li C, Ramjeesingh M, Bear CE. Cystic fibrosis transmembrane conductance regulator (CFTR) potentiator VX-770 (ivacaftor) opens the defective channel gate of mutant CFTR in a phosphorylation-dependent but ATP-independent manner. *J Biol Chem.* 2012;287(44):36639–36649. doi:10.1074/jbc. M112.393637. PubMed PMID: 22942289; PMCID: PMC3481266.

106. Jih KY, Hwang TC. VX-770 potentiates CFTR function by promoting decoupling between the gating cycle and ATP hydrolysis cycle. *Proc Natl Acad Sci U S A.* 2013;110(11):4404–4409. doi:10.1073/pnas.1215982110. PubMed PMID: 23440202; PMCID: PMC3600496.

107. Mihalyi C, Torocsik B, Csanady L. Obligate coupling of CFTR pore opening to tight nucleotide-binding domain dimerization. *Elife.* 2016;5. doi:10.7554/eLife.18164. PubMed PMID: 27328319; PMCID: PMC4956468.

108. Kopeikin Z, Yuksek Z, Yang HY, Bompadre SG. Combined effects of VX-770 and VX-809 on several functional abnormalities of F508del-CFTR channels. *J Cyst Fibros.* 2014;13(5):508–514. doi:10.1016/j.jcf.2014.04.003. PubMed PMID: 24796242.

109. Accurso FJ, Rowe SM, Clancy JP, Boyle MP, Dunitz JM, Durie PR, Sagel SD et al. Effect of VX-770 in persons with cystic fibrosis and the G551D-CFTR mutation. *N Engl J Med.* 2010;363(21):1991–2003. doi:10.1056/NEJMoa0909825. PubMed PMID: 21083385; PMCID: PMC3148255.

110. Davies J, Sheridan H, Bell N, Cunningham S, Davis SD, Elborn JS, Milla CE, Starner TD, Weiner DJ, Lee PS, Ratjen F. Assessment of clinical response to ivacaftor with lung clearance index in cystic fibrosis patients with a G551D-CFTR mutation and preserved spirometry: A randomised controlled trial. *Lancet Respir Med.* 2013;1(8):630–638. doi:10.1016/S2213-2600(13)70182-6. PubMed PMID: 24461666.

111. Flume PA, Liou TG, Borowitz DS, Li H, Yen K, Ordonez CL, Geller DE, Group VXS. Ivacaftor in subjects with cystic fibrosis who are homozygous for the F508del-CFTR mutation. *Chest.* 2012;142(3):718–724. doi:10.1378/chest.11-2672. PubMed PMID: 22383668; PMCID: PMC3435140.

112. Davies JC, Cunningham S, Harris WT, Lapey A, Regelmann WE, Sawicki GS, Southern KW et al. Safety, pharmacokinetics, and pharmacodynamics of ivacaftor in patients aged 2–5 years with cystic fibrosis and a CFTR gating mutation (KIWI): An open-label, single-arm study. *Lancet Respir Med.* 2016;4(2):107–115. doi:10.1016/S2213-2600(15)00545-7. PubMed PMID: 26803277.

113. De Boeck K, Munck A, Walker S, Faro A, Hiatt P, Gilmartin G, Higgins M. Efficacy and safety of ivacaftor in patients with cystic fibrosis and a non-G551D gating mutation. *J Cyst Fibros.* 2014;13(6):674–680. doi:10.1016/j.jcf.2014.09.005. PubMed PMID: 25266159.

114. Moss RB, Flume PA, Elborn JS, Cooke J, Rowe SM, McColley SA, Rubenstein RC, Higgins M, Group VXS. Efficacy and safety of ivacaftor in patients with cystic fibrosis who have an Arg117His-CFTR mutation: A double-blind, randomised controlled trial. *Lancet Respir Med.* 2015;3(7):524–533. doi:10.1016/S2213-2600(15)00201-5. PubMed PMID: 26070913; PMCID: PMC4641035.

115. Van Goor F, Yu H, Burton B, Hoffman BJ. Effect of ivacaftor on CFTR forms with missense mutations associated with defects in protein processing or function. *J Cyst Fibros.* 2014;13(1):29–36. doi:10.1016/j.jcf.2013.06.008. PubMed PMID: 23891399.

116. Mutyam V, Libby EF, Peng N, Hadjiliadis D, Bonk M, Solomon GM, Rowe SM. Therapeutic benefit observed with the CFTR potentiator, ivacaftor, in a CF patient homozygous for the W1282X CFTR nonsense mutation. *J Cyst Fibros.* 2017;16(1):24–29. doi:10.1016/j.jcf.2016.09.005. PubMed PMID: 27707539; PMCID: PMC5241185.

117. Vertex Pharmaceuticals Inc. FDA Approves KALYDECO® (ivacaftor) for More Than 900 People Ages 2 and Older with Cystic Fibrosis Who Have Certain Residual Function Mutations [Press release]. Retrieved from http://investorsvrtxcom/releasedetailcfm?ReleaseID=10268642017.

118. Wainwright CE. Ivacaftor for patients with cystic fibrosis. *Expert Rev Respir Med.* 2014;8(5):533–538. doi:10.1586/17476348.2014.951333. PubMed PMID: 25148205.

119. Uttamsingh V, Gallegos R, Liu JF, Harbeson SL, Bridson GW, Cheng C, Wells DS, Graham PB, Zelle R, Tung R. Altering metabolic profiles of drugs by precision deuteration: Reducing mechanism-based inhibition of CYP2D6 by paroxetine. *J Pharmacol Exp Ther.* 2015;354(1):43–54. doi:10.1124/jpet.115.223768. PubMed PMID: 25943764.

120. Harbeson SL, Morgan AJ, Liu JF, Aslanian AM, Nguyen S, Bridson GW, Brummel CL et al. Altering metabolic profiles of drugs by precision deuteration 2: Discovery of a deuterated analog of ivacaftor with differentiated pharmacokinetics for clinical development. *J Pharmacol Exp Ther.* 2017;362(2):359–367. doi:10.1124/jpet.117.241497. PubMed PMID: 28611092.

121. Uttamsineh V, Pilja L, Grotbeck B, Brummei CL, Uddin N, Harbeson SL, Braman V, Cassella J. WS13.6 CTP-656 tablet confirmed superiority of pharmacokinetic profile relative to Kalydeco® in Phase I clinical studies. 39th *European Cystic Fibrosis Conference. Journal of Cystic Fibrosis.* 2016;15:S22.

122. Kazani S, Alcantara J, Debonnett L, Doucet J, Jones I, Kulmatycki K, Machineni S et al. QBW251 is a safe and efficacious CFTR potentiator for patients with cystic Fibrosis. A51. Bronchiectasis: Clinical and epidemiologic studies. *American Thoracic Society 2016 International Conference Abstracts: American Journal of Respiratory and Critical Care Medicine* 2016:A7789–A.

123. Matthes E, Goepp J, Carlile GW, Luo Y, Dejgaard K, Billet A, Robert R, Thomas DY, Hanrahan JW. Low free drug concentration prevents inhibition of F508del CFTR functional expression by the potentiator VX-770 (ivacaftor). *Br J Pharmacol.* 2016;173(3):459–470. doi:10.1111/bph.13365. PubMed PMID: 26492939; PMCID: PMC4728415.

124. Gentzsch M, Ren HY, Houck SA, Quinney NL, Cholon DM, Sopha P, Chaudhry IG et al. Restoration of R117H CFTR folding and function in human airway cells through combination treatment with VX-809 and VX-770. *Am J Physiol Lung Cell Mol Physiol.* 2016;311(3):L550–L559. doi:10.1152/ajplung.00186.2016. PubMed PMID: 27402691; PMCID: PMC5142211.

125. Balch WE, Morimoto RI, Dillin A, Kelly JW. Adapting proteostasis for disease intervention. *Science.* 2008;319(5865):916–919. doi:10.1126/science.1141448. PubMed PMID: 18276881.

126. Barnett SD, Buxton ILO. The role of S-nitrosoglutathione reductase (GSNOR) in human disease and therapy. *Crit Rev Biochem Mol Biol.* 2017;52(3):340–354. doi:10.1080/10409238.2017.1304353. PubMed PMID: 28393572; PMCID: PMC5597050.

127. Grasemann H, Gaston B, Fang K, Paul K, Ratjen F. Decreased levels of nitrosothiols in the lower airways of patients with cystic fibrosis and normal pulmonary function. *J Pediatr.* 1999;135(6):770–772. PubMed PMID: 10586185.

128. Andersson C, Gaston B, Roomans GM. S-Nitrosoglutathione induces functional DeltaF508-CFTR in airway epithelial cells. *Biochem Biophys Res Commun.* 2002;297(3):552–557. PubMed PMID: 12270130.

129. Chen L, Patel RP, Teng X, Bosworth CA, Lancaster JR, Jr., Matalon S. Mechanisms of cystic fibrosis transmembrane conductance regulator activation by S-nitrosoglutathione. *J Biol Chem.* 2006;281(14):9190–9199. doi:10.1074/jbc.M513231200. PubMed PMID: 16421103.

130. Howard M, Fischer H, Roux J, Santos BC, Gullans SR, Yancey PH, Welch WJ. Mammalian osmolytes and S-nitrosoglutathione promote Delta F508 cystic fibrosis transmembrane conductance regulator (CFTR) protein maturation and function. *J Biol Chem.* 2003;278(37):35159–351567. doi:10.1074/jbc.M301924200. PubMed PMID: 12837761.

131. Zaman K, McPherson M, Vaughan J, Hunt J, Mendes F, Gaston B, Palmer LA. S-nitrosoglutathione increases cystic fibrosis transmembrane regulator maturation. *Biochem Biophys Res Commun.* 2001;284(1):65–70. doi:10.1006/bbrc.2001.4935. PubMed PMID: 11374871.

132. Snyder AH, McPherson ME, Hunt JF, Johnson M, Stamler JS, Gaston B. Acute effects of aerosolized S-nitrosoglutathione in cystic fibrosis. *Am J Respir Crit Care Med.* 2002;165(7):922–926. doi:10.1164/ajrccm.165.7.2105032. PubMed PMID: 11934715.

133. Marozkina NV, Yemen S, Borowitz M, Liu L, Plapp M, Sun F, Islam R et al. Hsp 70/Hsp 90 organizing protein as a nitrosylation target in cystic fibrosis therapy. *Proc Natl Acad Sci U S A.* 2010;107(25):11393–11398. doi:10.1073/pnas.0909128107. PubMed PMID: 20534503; PMCID: PMC2895117.

134. Zaman K, Bennett D, Fraser-Butler M, Greenberg Z, Getsy P, Sattar A, Smith L et al. S-Nitrosothiols increases cystic fibrosis transmembrane regulator expression and maturation in the cell surface. *Biochem Biophys Res Commun.* 2014;443(4):1257–1262. doi:10.1016/j.bbrc.2013.12.130. PubMed PMID: 24393850; PMCID: PMC3974270.

135. Zaman K, Carraro S, Doherty J, Henderson EM, Lendermon E, Liu L, Verghese G et al. S-nitrosylating agents: A novel class of compounds that increase cystic fibrosis transmembrane conductance regulator expression and maturation in epithelial cells. *Mol Pharmacol.* 2006;70(4):1435–1442. doi:10.1124/mol.106.023242. PubMed PMID: 16857740.

136. Donaldson SH, Solomon GM, Zeitlin PL, Flume PA, Casey A, McCoy K, Zemanick ET et al. Pharmacokinetics and safety of cavosonstat (N91115) in healthy and cystic fibrosis adults homozygous for F508DEL-CFTR. *J Cyst Fibros*. 2017;16(3):371–379. doi:10.1016/j.jcf.2017.01.009. PubMed PMID: 28209466.

137. Donaldson SH. 270. Safety and pharmacokinetics of n91115 in patients with cystic fibrosis homozygous for the f508del-cftr mutation. *29th Annual North American Cystic Fibrosis Conference: Poster Session Abstracts. Pediatric Pulmonology*. 2015:S193–S453.

138. Angers RC, Mutka S, Bove PF, Gabriel SE. 74. Pharmacological correction and acute inhibition of gsnor results in improved in vitro CFTR function. *28th Annual North American Cystic Fibrosis Conference: Poster Session Abstracts. Pediatric Pulmonology*. 2014:S216–S456.

139. Bove PF, Look KM, Mehra NK, Veit G, Lukacs GL, Gabriel S. 283. Enhanced CFTR modulation with s-nitrosoglutathione reductase inhibitor in addition to CFTR corrector and potentiator. *30th Annual North American Cystic Fibrosis Conference: Poster Session Abstracts. Pediatric Pulmonol*. 2016:S194–S485.

140. Nivalis Therapeutics Inc. and Alpine Immune Sciences Inc. Nivalis Therapeutics and Alpine Immune Sciences Agree to Combine [Press release]. Retrieved from https://wwwalpineimmunesciencescom/alpine-nivalis-combination/2017.

141. Vertex Pharmaceuticals Inc. Vertex Announces Positive Phase 1 & Phase 2 Data from Three Different Triple Combination Regimens in People with Cystic Fibrosis Who Have One F508del Mutation and One Minimal Function Mutation (F508del/Min) [Press release]. Retrieved from http://investorsvrtxcom/releasedetailcfm?ReleaseID=10335592017.

142. Dekkers JF, Gogorza Gondra RA, Kruisselbrink E, Vonk AM, Janssens HM, de Winter-de Groot KM, van der Ent CK, Beekman JM. Optimal correction of distinct CFTR folding mutants in rectal cystic fibrosis organoids. *Eur Respir J*. 2016;48(2):451–458. doi:10.1183/13993003.01192-2015. PubMed PMID: 27103391.

143. Kim S, Thiessen PA, Bolton EE, Chen J, Fu G, Gindulyte A, Han L et al. PubChem substance and compound databases. *Nucleic Acids Res*. 2016;44(D1):D1202–D1213. doi:10.1093/nar/gkv951. PubMed PMID: 26400175; PMCID: PMC4702940.

15

Innate and adaptive barrier properties of airway mucus

ALISON SCHAEFER AND SAMUEL K. LAI

Introduction	257	Mucus clearance	263
The mucus barrier	257	Ciliary-mediated clearance	263
Composition and characteristics	257	Cough-driven clearance	263
Mucin properties and structure	258	Mucus in disease	263
Mucins into mucus	259	Cystic fibrosis	263
Nonmucin components	259	Asthma	264
Innate barrier properties of airway mucus	259	Immune cells and adaptive immune responses in the lung	264
Steric obstruction by the mucin mesh	259	Anatomy of immune response	264
Adhesive interactions with mucins	259	Immunomodulation in the lung	265
Adaptive barrier properties of AM	261	Conclusion	266
IgA in airway mucus	261	Acknowledgments	266
IgG in airway mucus	261	References	266
Antibody-mediated trapping	262		

INTRODUCTION

Over 8000 liters of air enter the lungs every day, passing through the continually branching airways and arriving at the nearly 100 m^2 surface area of the alveoli. Extremely thin type I epithelial cells line the alveoli, which together with the alveolar capillaries present a diffusion distance of less than one micrometer (1,2). It is at this interface that the most essential function of the lungs occurs: oxygen is transported into and carbon dioxide is removed from the bloodstream. This large, thin surface make the lungs not only highly efficient at gas exchange but also a desirable target for drug delivery, as evident by the rapid onset of the effects of inhaled nicotine experienced by smokers (3). In addition to oxygen, inhaled air carries with it foreign matter ranging from dust and soot to bacteria and viruses, reaching up to 100 billion particles over the course of the day (1). Naturally, the lungs have developed an array of sophisticated defense mechanisms designed to trap particulate matter and neutralize pathogens before they reach the alveolar cells. This includes the mucus barrier, which not only can physically obstruct pathogens from reaching the underlying cells but also acts as the first battleground for the innate and adaptive immune system. Drug carriers delivered to the airways must quickly penetrate mucus in order to provide effective and sustained drug delivery.

THE MUCUS BARRIER

Composition and characteristics

The respiratory tract consists of distinct components, including the nose, nasal passages, larynx, and pharynx of the upper respiratory system; and the trachea, bronchi, bronchioles, and alveoli of the lower tract. From the bronchioles to the nose, the airway epithelium is covered by airway mucus (AM), a highly viscoelastic gel layer between 5–50 μm thick overlaying a periciliary liquid layer (Figure 15.1) (4–6). Its major function is to trap foreign particles deposited in the airways, which are then quickly purged from the lung by natural mucocilliary clearance mechanisms, followed by eventual sterilization by the acidic and degradative environments of the stomach (7). AM is composed almost entirely of water, with solids typically representing less than 3% of

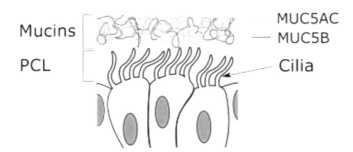

Figure 15.1 Mucus coats the airway epithelium. A viscoelastic mucus layer lays on top of a periciliary liquid layer in which cilia can beat in a coordinated fashion to facilitate continuous mucus clearance.

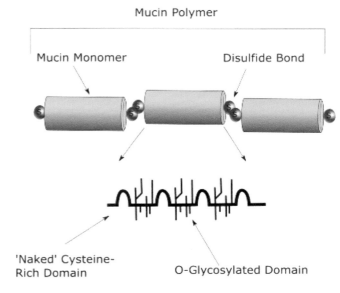

Figure 15.2 Structure of mucins. Mucin monomers are joined together by disulfide bonds. Monomers are composed of O-glycosylated regions interspersed with "naked" unglycosylated, cysteine-rich domains.

mucus by weight (8). The solid component is made of lipids, salts, cell debris, and various proteins. Mucin represents the most abundant protein in AM, serving as the key structural component of the dense matrix in mucus. Mucin is essential to maintaining the hydration and rheological properties of AM, as well as aiding in the retention and function of host-defense proteins.

Mucin properties and structure

Mucins are a family of high molecular weight, intricate, O-linked glycoproteins that are generally divided into two categories. The first group are monomeric, cell-tethered mucins found almost exclusively at the cell surface, whereas the other group are secreted oligomers that can undergo extensive end-linking and entanglement to form the mucus gel. Mucins isolated from the airways are typically organized as linear polymers composed of a variable number of monomers linked together by disulfide bonds (Figure 15.2) (9,10). These structural elements of AM can range in mass from 2–50 MDa, and in length from 0.5–10 µm, depending on the extent of polymerization (11–13).

Mucins are polyanionic, due to the extensive glycosylation (more than 70% carbohydrate by weight) of the mucin backbone. The glycans are concentrated into regions that are rich in proline, threonine, and serine. Mucins possess a diverse array of O-linked glycans, often sialyated or sulfated, with a limited number of N-glycans (14,15). The extensive glycosylation results in a stiff "bottle-brush" conformation for mucins, and contributes to ion binding, water retention, and pathogen binding (14).

The glycosylated regions of mucins are separated by "naked" protein that lack sites for glycosylation (16–19). These domains are typically 110 amino acids long and rich in cysteine (19). These regions result in globular, folded structures that are stabilized by disulfide bonds (Figure 15.2) (19,20). These hydrophobic domains adsorb a significant amount of lipids and other hydrophobic proteins. Low-affinity bonds between these lipids and overlapping mucins, together with entanglement of mucins, contribute to the bulk viscoelasticity of the mucus gel (21).

Mucin-secreting cells achieve an impressive metabolic feat: the cellular machinery must assemble and transport a large polypeptide at least 1 MDa in size through the endoplasmic reticulum to the Golgi, while keeping sugar acceptor sites accessible to the Golgi enzymes to enable O-glycosylation to take place (22). Cells must also polymerize and tightly package mucins into secretory granules. Upon exocytosis, they can expand by over 500 times in only 50 milliseconds (10). In studies of MUC5AC, a common mucin in AM, the process of synthesis and secretion took two hours to complete (23). Expansion after secretion is controlled by a Donnan potential based on the exchange of Ca^{2+} ions shielding mucins with Na^+ ions from the extracellular space, with the degree of expansion affecting the rheology of the mucus (24,25).

While there are many known mucins, AM largely contains MUC5AC produced by goblet cells in the surface epithelium, and MUC5B produced by cells of the submucosal glands (Figure 15.3) (7,15,26,27). MUC2 has also been detected in small quantities, estimated at 0.2%–2.5% of total mucins by weight (28–33). MUC5B is present in both high- and low-charge glycoforms, produced by distinct cell populations, with the low charge glycoform being the more abundant (31,34). MUC5AC tends to have a lower mass per unit length compared to MUC5B, suggesting the incorporation of smaller O-glycan side chains. It also remains in a stiffer, more open conformation compared to MUC5B, which exhibits a more compact structure (35). Submucosal glands are associated with both sympathetic and parasympathetic nerves, while goblet cells are not associated with either. Different regulatory mechanisms mean that the mucin composition of AM can change in response to changing environmental conditions (36,37).

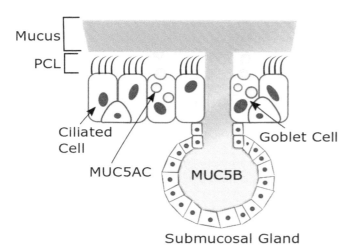

Figure 15.3 Goblet cells at the epithelial surface produce predominately MUC5AC and only small amounts of MUC5B, whereas submucosal glands produce most of the MUC5B.

MUC5AC and MUC5B play different roles in mucosal defense. MUC5AC has been indicated in preventing growth of certain bacteria (38,39). However, in studies comparing MUC5AC and MUC5B knockout mice, MUC5B$^{-/-}$ mice had much lower survival rates compared to MUC5AC$^{-/-}$ mice due to higher bacterial burden in the lungs as well as impaired mucociliary clearance, which was measured by assessing clearance of fluorescent microspheres from the nose and lungs. This suggests MUC5B to be critical to microbial control and clearance in ways that MUC5AC is not (40). Additionally, MUC5AC may potentially play a detrimental role under specific conditions. For example, MUC5AC$^{-/-}$ mice sustained significantly less tissue damage after exposure to a ventilator compared to wild-type mice (41), and increased MUC5AC production is associated with remodeling of the airways in asthma (42). MUC5AC is also frequently induced as a result of allergic inflammation, and MUC5AC$^{-/-}$ mice experience reduced mucus plugging even in the presence of ongoing inflammation (43). The protective role of MUC5B means that therapeutics aimed at mucin reduction may need to be carefully selected in order to preserve critical host defenses.

Mucins into mucus

As discussed above, secreted mucins form end-links with other mucin molecules to create large macromolecules that span microns. In turn, those mucin oligomers can undergo extensive entanglement with each other to form a viscoelastic gel network that supports the different functions of mucus (15). Reversible, noncovalent, calcium-ion-dependent crosslinking of adjacent polymers also contribute to the network formation, particularly through modulation of the organization of MUC5B molecules (44). The naked protein domains along mucins can also interact with the same domains on other mucin molecules, thereby binding mucins

together into large cable-like structures (45). The hydration of the dense mucin matrix is dictated by the glycan side chains that are capable of binding hundreds of times their weight in water. The availability of water and other ions in the extracellular environment can greatly affect the viscoelastic properties and clearance of the gel (4,46,47).

Nonmucin components

Although mucins are the primary building block of mucus, mucus is home to a diverse array of other molecules. There are over 250 other proteins found in sputum, as well as other components such as lipids and cell debris (44,48). In particular, AM is a reservoir of host defense molecules such as antibodies, lactoferrins, lysozyme, macrophages, and cytokines. Mucus provides an extracellular environment for these molecules to function, resulting in antimicrobial, antiprotease, and antioxidant properties (49).

INNATE BARRIER PROPERTIES OF AIRWAY MUCUS

Steric obstruction by the mucin mesh

At the most basic level, mucus limits the free Brownian diffusion of particles by steric obstruction through the dense network of mucins. Particles that are larger than the pore size of the mucin mesh are naturally slowed or stopped entirely. Only particles substantially smaller than the mesh pores and that do not adhesively interact with mucins (see the section called "Adhesive interactions with mucins" below) can undergo rapid diffusion in the low viscosity aqueous environment of the interstitial fluid between the mesh elements and penetrate through the mucus barrier to reach the underlying airway epithelium. The pores in healthy AM are estimated to be 100–200 nanometers in size (50,51). The size-dependent diffusion of nanoparticles is best illustrated by studies using muco-inert PEGylated beads (Figure 15.4) (50,52). The pore size in many lung diseases is even more restricted and may vary substantially from patient to patient. As a result, inhaled therapies with particles significantly larger than 100nm are unlikely to quickly penetrate the AM (53).

Adhesive interactions with mucins

In addition to physical obstruction, mucins can directly capture particles through adhesive interactions with mucins. For instance, the dense array of glycans extending from the protein backbone offers an abundance of carboxylic acid and hydroxyl groups, which in turn can form electrostatic interactions with cationic entities as well as undergo hydrogen bonding (54). For example, nonviral gene vectors are frequently formulated with cationic polymers and lipids in order to condense DNA into nanoparticles, typically yielding a net positive surface charge. The movement of these cationic DNA-loaded particles are strongly hindered in

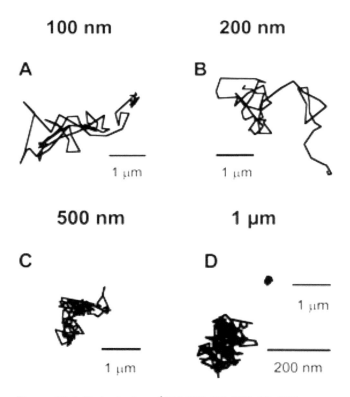

100 nm

A

200 nm

B

500 nm

C

1 µm

D

Figure 15.4 Trajectories of **(A)** 100, **(B)** 200, **(C)** 500 nm, and **(D)** 1 µm PEGylated beads in human cervico-vaginal mucus. Smaller particles are able to diffuse farther than larger ones over this timescale. (Reproduced from Lai, S.K., *PLoS One*, 4, e4294, 2009.)

mucus, thereby precluding effective delivery to the underlying epithelium (55–58).

Similarly, the periodic hydrophobic domains allow mucins to capture hydrophobic particles. For instance, hydrophobic amine-modified polystyrene nanoparticles with near-neutral surface charges are immobilized in cystic fibrosis sputum (51). Lipid-based nanoparticles are another example that exhibit poor mucus penetration due to hydrophobic interactions with mucins unless hydrophobic-hydrophilic surface properties are carefully tuned (59). The diffusion of nanoparticles with surface carboxylic acid groups that yield a negative surface charge are also strongly hindered in different mucus secretions, likely due to adhesive interactions with hydrophobic regions of the mucin fiber, and/or hydrogen bonds with mucin glycans (50,60–62). Dense PEGylation can shield the charged or hydrophobic core from these interactions and has been used to improve distribution, penetration, and retention of particles in the airways for enhancing drug delivery (Figure 15.5) (51,56,58,63).

Mucus can also form specific adhesive interactions with incoming particles. Many viruses, for example, enter the cell by binding to specific sugars on the cell surface. A mucin may display the same sugar, thus binding the virus before it ever reaches a cell (64). One example may be adeno-associated virus (AAV), often used as a vector by inhaled gene therapies. Many AAV serotypes specifically bind cell-associated glycans such as heparan sulfate or α 2,3/2,6-linked sialic acids. AAV serotypes 1, 2, and 5 all

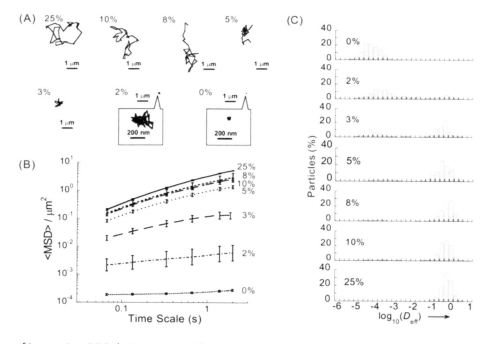

Figure 15.5 Effect of increasing PEGylation on particle transport in mucus. **(A)** Representative trajectories over 3 seconds. Particles with PEGylation above 5% are able to move largely unhindered. **(B)** Ensemble-averaged geometric mean square displacement (<MSD>) as a function of time scale for different PEGylated particles. **(C)** Distribution of the log of individual particle effective diffusivities at a 1-second time scale. (Reprinted with permission from Xu, Q. et al., *ACS Nano*, 9, 9217–9227, 2015. Copyright 2015 American Chemical Society.)

appear to strongly associate to mucins (65). In the case of AAV2, mutations that eliminate binding to heparan sulfate increased its mobility in mucus twofold (53). Mucolytics that can partially break down the mucus gel have also been used to enhance the diffusion of AAV and other virus vectors through mucus (53,66,67).

ADAPTIVE BARRIER PROPERTIES OF AM

Immunoglobulins in AM play a major role in defense against foreign pathogens and enter the lung through multiple mechanisms. At the gas-exchange surface of the alveoli, the barrier to the blood is thin and a fraction of immunoglobulins in the blood can enter via passive transudation (68). Along the conducting airways, plasma cells associated with local lymphoid tissue can secrete immunoglobulins (69).

IgA in airway mucus

IgA is frequently associated with mucosal protection, and abundant quantities are found in AM secretions. Dimeric IgA (dIgA) is produced by plasma cells in the lamina propria and includes two IgA molecules linked by a J-chain protein (Figure 15.6). The dIgA is then bound by secretory component (SC), a protein found in the plasma membrane on the basolateral surfaces of a subpopulation of mucosal epithelial cells. This dIgA-SC complex on the plasma membrane is then transcytosed and released at the luminal surface as secretory IgA (sIgA) (70,71). While almost 90% of IgA in the blood exits in monomeric (mIgA) form, roughly half of IgA is found in the dimeric form as (sIgA) (72,73). In the lung, IgA has two subclasses, IgA1 and IgA2. IgA2 represents at most 20% of total serum IgA, but it represents 30% of lung IgA (74); these differences reflect considerable local production of IgA in the lung.

sIgA has four binding sites, giving it greater crosslinking capacity. Both secretory component and the higher presence of IgA2 contribute to a greater resistance of the antibody against bacterial degradation (75–77). sIgA contributes to

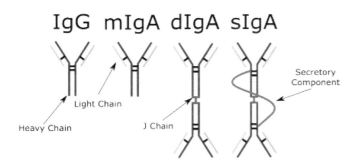

IgG mIgA dIgA sIgA

Heavy Chain · Light Chain · J Chain · Secretory Component

Figure 15.6 Schematic illustrating the structures of IgG and IgA antibodies. IgG and monomeric IgA (mIgA) are y-shaped proteins composed of two heavy and two light chains. Dimeric IgA (dIgA) consists of two IgA monomers joined by a J-chain protein. Secretory IgA (sIgA), the most present in mucus, consists of dIgA linked to secretory component.

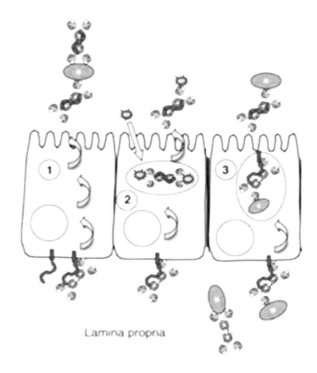

Lamina propria

Figure 15.7 sIgA and dIgA facilitate immune defense (1) in the lumen, (2) the epithelium, and (3) the lamina propria. (Reproduced from Corthésy, B., *Front. Immunol.*, 4, 85, 2013.)

antigen neutralization at all three levels of the mucosal tissues: the lumen, the epithelium, and the lamina propria. In the lumen, sIgA can agglutinate bacteria into aggregates that are too large to penetrate through the pores of mucus to inhibit adherence of bacteria at the epithelial surface, a process frequently referred to as immune exclusion. sIgA can also directly neutralize viruses both in the mucus layer and intraepithelially. dIgA can also bind antigen in the lamina propia, and the immune complex is then cleared to the lumen via binding with pIgR and subsequent endocytosis (Figure 15.7) (78–81). FcαRI, an IgA Fc receptor present on myeloid immune cells, can bind to IgA-opsonized pathogens, resulting in a proinflammatory immune response.

IgG in airway mucus

Abundant quantities of IgG are also found in AM. All four subtypes of IgG have been found in the lung, with IgG3 and IgG4 being produced locally in relatively greater amounts than IgG1 and IgG2 (82). Plasma cells producing IgG are located in the bronchial mucosa (83,84). Similar to IgA, IgG can bind to critical epitopes on the viral surface and neutralize the virus directly. In addition, IgG can facilitate other effector functions, such as complement activation, opsonization, and antibody-dependent cellular cytotoxicity (ADCC). IgG can interact with lung-specific surfactant protein A (SP-A), which modulates some of these functions. IgG-opsonized pathogens bound by SP-A exhibit enhanced phagocytosis (85). SP-A can also inhibit complement activation, and complement activity in bronchoalveolar lavage fluid is reduced compared to serum, even at similar levels of detectable complement protein (86,87). Alveolar macrophages mediate ADCC in the lung (88): approximately 25% of alveolar macrophages can bind IgG3, approximately 10% bind IgG4, with little binding IgG1 or IgG2 (89).

Antibody-mediated trapping

In addition to the aforementioned classical immune defense mechanisms, antibodies can also reinforce the diffusional barrier of mucus by acting as third-party crosslinkers that crosslink the pathogens to the mucin mesh. This unique mechanism of mucosal antibody function was long overlooked because the affinity of individual antibody molecules to mucins was thought to be far too weak to facilitate effective crosslinking. Indeed, the diffusion coefficient of IgG and IgA antibodies in human mucus was only slowed approximately 10% compared to the rate in water, indicating that any bond between antibodies and mucins is exceedingly transient (seconds or less) and readily broken up by thermal excitation (90). Nevertheless, multiple antibodies can bind the same virus or bacteria, and the array of bound antibody on any individual pathogen/antibody complex can form multivalent interactions with the mucin mesh, sufficient to trap individual pathogens with near permanent avidity. This concept was first illustrated with herpes simplex virus (HSV), where both exogenous and endogenous HSV-specific antibodies mediated effective trapping of HSV in human cervico-vaginal mucus and protected against vaginal HSV transmission in mice (Figure 15.8) (91), most likely by excluding access to the underlying epithelium. Extension of this concept to AM was recently illustrated with influenza virus, whose mobility were directly correlated with endogenous influenza-binding antibodies in AM, even for influenza virus-like particles (VLPs) that lack the ability to bind sialic acids on mucins (92).

The interactions between antibodies and mucins appear to be mediated by specific N-glycans on the Fc-domain of the antibodies; removal of either the Fc or the N-glycans markedly abrogated the trapping potency (91). There is likely a Goldilocks zone for the affinity between individual antibody molecules and mucins (93): if the affinity is too weak, many antibody molecules must be bound to an individual pathogen to generate sufficient avidity to trap, whereas if the affinity is too strong, antibodies would lose their ability to undergo rapid diffusion in mucus and quickly accumulate on the pathogen surface. The ability of antibodies to interact with mucins effectively transforms mucus, despite its relatively static and well-conserved biochemistry, into a potent adhesive barrier against a diverse array of pathogens (93).

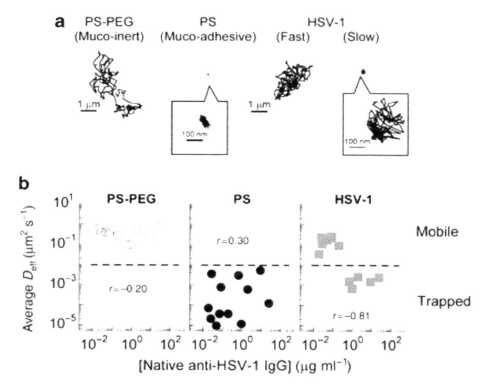

Figure 15.8 Herpes simplex virus serotype 1 (HSV-1) is immobilized in human cervicovaginal mucus (CVM) samples with high levels of endogenous anti-HSV-1 IgG but mobile in samples with low levels of endogenous anti-HSV-1 IgG. (a) Representative 20s traces of HSV-1 and control particles with effective diffusivity (D_{eff}) at a timescale τ of 1s. Control particles include muco-inert (polyethylene glycol (PEG)-coated polystyrene (PS); PS-PEG) which are freely diffusive in CVM and muco-adhesive (uncoated; PS) beads which are trapped in CVM. (b) Geometric average D_{eff} (τ = 1 s) for PS-PEG, PS, and HSV-1 in individual CVM samples from unique donors. Dashed lines represent the D_{eff} cutoff below which particles are immobile. (Reproduced from Wang, Y.Y. et al., *Mucosal Immunol.*, 7, 1036–1044, 2014.)

Antibodies, particularly multimeric IgM and sIgA, may crosslink multiple pathogens together to create an aggregate that is much too large to penetrate through the pores of mucus, a process known as agglutination. Agglutination is distinct from trapping of individual pathogens via antibody-mucin crosslinking. Since individual pathogens must first collide with each other before becoming agglutinated, agglutination is likely less effective against pathogens transmitted at relatively lower titers (94). Indeed, in a recent study comparing the muco-trapping potency of IgG and IgM, no agglutination was observed with both antibodies against modest doses of nanoparticles (95).

Antibody-mediated trapping in mucus may pose a challenge to drug and gene carriers. A significant fraction of the population harbors antibodies against many of the AAV vectors used in gene therapies. For instance, antibodies against AAV1, 2, 5, 6, and 7 have been found in the airways of individuals both with and without lung disease (96–98). Similarly, anti-PEG antibodies may also impede the diffusion of PEG-coated nanoparticles that otherwise can readily penetrate mucus. Detectable quantities of anti-PEG antibodies were found in approximately 72% of serum specimens from the general population, with a small number possessing high titers in excess of 1 µg/ml (99). Numerous studies have also shown that systemic administration of PEGylated therapeutic can induce high titers of circulating anti-PEG antibodies (100–104). Systemic antibodies can enter mucus through passive transudation or FcRn-mediated transcytosis (105); for example, antigen-specific monoclonal antibodies have been found in the genital secretions of mice and macaques after the antibodies were delivered systemically (106–108). We have recently shown that the presence of PEG-binding antibodies in mucus resulted in extensive trapping of PEGylated nanoparticles, with the fraction of mobile particles reduced from 95% in control mucus specimens to 34% and 7% with anti-PEG IgG and IgM, respectively (95). This in turn limited the flux of particles reaching the epithelium. The presence of anti-PEG antibodies in AM may impede the diffusion and alter the biodistribution of PEGylated drug carriers delivered to the airways, but this remains to be investigated.

MUCUS CLEARANCE

Ciliary-mediated clearance

A hallmark of AM is its continuous clearance from the airways. The primary route of mucus clearance is through ciliary beating, pushing the mucus up the respiratory tract and out of the trachea, which is then swallowed and sterilized by the acidic gastric environment (4,64). The top mucus layer (10–50 µm) rests atop a 7–10 µm thick perciliary liquid layer (PCL), about the size of an extended cilia. Cilia beat normally at a rate between 8 and 15 Hz (109). Each stroke of coordinated beating facilitates the transport of the mucus layer. During clearance, the stroke of the cilia engages the bottom side of the mucus layer, pushing the layer unidirectionally. Frictional forces between the mucus and the PCL cause the PCL to be dragged along with the mucus layer, at very similar velocities (4).

The rate of mucus transport varies locally along the proximal and distal regions of the respiratory tract, getting slower near the periphery. Actual clearance time of deposited particulates is affected by the overall pattern of deposition, the size of particles, and the disease state of the lungs. Particles deposited in the lungs can be cleared in as little as 15 minutes, with generally all but the smallest being cleared in 24 hours (110,111). This means that therapeutics delivered to the respiratory tract must quickly penetrate through the mucus if they are to reach the underlying epithelium at time scales faster than natural mucus clearance.

Although mucociliary clearance represents a key mechanism that helps limit microbial proliferation, it is likely insufficient on its own. For example, some bacteria can double in as little as 20 minutes, meaning that bacterial loads could overwhelm the rate of mucus clearance under specific circumstances. Antimicrobial factors such as lactoferrin, lysozyme, and secretory leukoproteinase inhibitor generally help limit bacterial growth sufficiently to allow for clearance (112). Nevertheless, the innate antimicrobial defense alone is also inadequate: decline in mucus clearance rates can result in heavy bacterial loads and has serious implications for overall health (113).

Cough-driven clearance

The lungs have another important means of clearing mucus: coughing. Coughing is independent of the actions of cilia and can efficiently transport mucus even in diseases where the cilia have been rendered nonfunctional. However, its effectiveness is still dependent on several properties of AM. Increased mucus viscosity results in reduced ability to clear via cough (114). The presence of PCL is also vital, since the lubricating function facilitates the movement of mucus along the epithelium—an absence or reduction in the PCL results in interactions between mobile mucins in the top layer, and the cell-tethered mucins below (4,115). These interactions prevent cough clearance in addition to mucocilliary clearance (4,116).

MUCUS IN DISEASE

Mucus dysfunction can be observed in virtually all inflammatory airway diseases, such as cystic fibrosis and asthma (Figure 15.9). Mucus in disease conditions often exhibits higher viscoelasticity than secretions from healthy persons (7,117), making the barrier even more difficult to penetrate and also making it more difficult to clear by natural mucociliary mechanisms.

Cystic fibrosis

Cystic fibrosis (CF) is the result of a mutation in the cystic fibrosis transmembrane regulator (CFTR) (118,119). The main consequence of CFTR mutation is dehydration of the

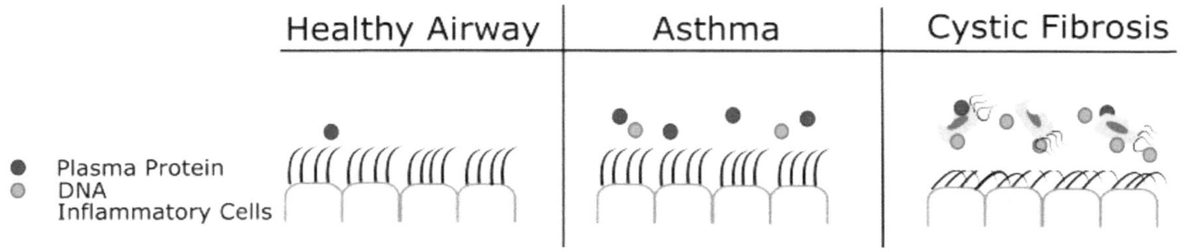

Healthy Airway | Asthma | Cystic Fibrosis

- Plasma Protein
- DNA
  Inflammatory Cells

Figure 15.9 Contrasting mucus properties in disease. Asthma exhibits increased mucus production as a result of goblet cell hyperplasia, and higher levels of plasma proteins prevent breakdown of mucus leading to plugs. Cystic fibrosis is characterized elevated levels of DNA, actin, and inflammatory cells. The collapse of PCL impairs clearance, which causes mucus buildup and results in bacterial colonization.

mucus (116,120,121). The height of the PCL is reduced, which compromises the ability of cilia to beat. Additionally, the reduced PCL is less effective at protecting the cell surfaces from the mucus above. The gel layer can now interact with the glycan side chains of the cell-tethered mucins below, essentially fastening the mucus to the cell surface and preventing cough clearance (4). Lack of clearance contributes to bacterial colonization as mucus continues to secrete, forming a thicker mucus layer and mucus plugs. The thicker layer and increased oxygen consumption by CF epithelia create steep oxygen gradients that provide an anaerobic environment ideal for colonization by *P. aeruginosa* (122).

There are other changes to the mucus besides dehydration. MUC5A and the low-charge glycoform of MUC5B are hypersecreted compared to healthy mucus (123). Inflammatory responses lead to a build-up of cellular debris, making the mucus of CF patients replete with neutrophils, DNA, and actin (124–126). The combination of greater amounts of biomacromolecules with dehydration results in a much more viscous mucus layer and a tighter mesh, where pore size can be less than 100 nm (53). The increase in DNA concentration also increases the negative charge, possibly leading to increased adhesivity (64).

Asthma

Though characterization and treatment of asthma is often focused on relieving hyperinflammatory responses and bronchoconstriction, mucus dysfunction has been recognized as central to airway obstruction in severe asthma (127,128). Mucus is hypersecreted by an increased number of goblet cells, which results in a thicker and more difficult to clear mucus barrier. The obstructive effects of smooth muscle contraction are thus exacerbated by the thickened mucus layer in the airway (129). In addition, the ratio of mucins is skewed compared to normal airways, with MUC5A levels persistently elevated in asthmatic lungs (Figure 15.10) (42,130). There is an increased concentration of plasma proteins in the mucus, which reduces mucin degradation by proteases (131), contributing to mucus plugging.

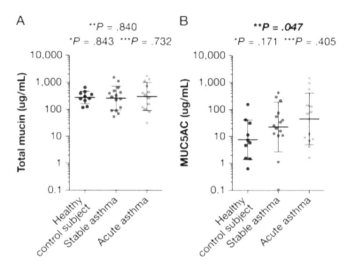

Figure 15.10 Mucin quantification by means of Western blotting on sputum samples from children with stable asthma, children with acute asthma, and healthy control subjects. **(a)** Total mucin content and **(b)** MUC5AC content. (Adapted from Welsh, K.G. et al., *Chest*, 152, 771–779, 2017.)

IMMUNE CELLS AND ADAPTIVE IMMUNE RESPONSES IN THE LUNG

Anatomy of immune response

The upper and lower respiratory tracts tend to be exposed to different types of environmental stimuli and pathogens. In addition to mucus coatings, they are also protected by the immune system in slightly different ways. In the upper respiratory tract. Immune responses are guided by the superficial and deep cervical lymph nodes, as well as other lymphoid tissues such as the tonsils and adenoids. The lower respiratory tract, on the other hand, is guided by the mediastinal and hilar lymph nodes in addition to the bronchus-associated lymphoid tissues (BALT) (132).

Not surprisingly, the dominant immunoglobulins also differ between the upper and lower respiratory tracts. B-cell responses in the lymphoid tissues of the upper tract tend to favor IgA over IgG, while the opposite is true in the lower tract (133,134). This may be a consequence of their local environments. IgA can be actively transported across the thick, pseudostratified epithelia in the upper tract, whereas IgG can more easily enter from the alveolar capillaries in the deep lung (133,135). Exogenously administered antibodies have shown that IgA is ineffective at preventing infection in the deep lung but excellent at reducing nasal viral shedding, while the opposite was true of IgG (133).

The deep lung also has an additional means to eliminate foreign particles, namely, alveolar macrophages. The abundant macrophages, with 5–7 macrophages per alveolus (136) readily phagocytose nearly all particulate matter deposited into the deep lung (137). Once phagocytosed, the macrophages are cleared either via the lymphatic system or up the mucociliary clearance escalator (138). The efficiency of macrophage phagocytosis depends on both the size and shape of the particulate. They appear to preferentially uptake particles 3–6 μm in size (139), as well as particles with low aspect-to-volume ratios (i.e., spheres over elongated disks) (Figure 15.11) (140,141).

In the airways, when infectious pathogens breach the mucus barrier and reach the underlying epithelium, the epithelial cells initiate a cascade of classical immune responses through common triggers such as pattern recognition receptors (PRRs) and toll-like receptors (TLRs) (142–144). The upregulation of interferons will then trigger inflammation and adaptive immune cell recruitment and differentiation (145).

In the deep lung, both alveolar macrophages and dendritic cells can contribute cytokine and chemokine secretion that either maintains or escalates the immune response (146). PRR ligation and cytokine signaling both contribute to the maturation of dendritic cells, which in turn aid the induction of adaptive immune response via antigen presentation (147,148). Mature dendritic cells then migrate to the draining lymph nodes where they activate naïve T-cells (149). This results in three different possible outcomes for T-cells: a T-helper 1 (Th1) response, a T-helper 2 (Th2) response, or regulatory T (Treg) cells. Th1 response is typical in response to viruses or bacteria, and Th2 is typical following contact with extracellular parasites or allergens (150). Treg response is the most common response during homeostasis.

T-cells are found intraepithelially and in the lamina propria. Most of the epithelial T-cells are CD8 cells, while CD4+ T-cells are typical of the lamina propria (150). Many studies have found that T-cell proliferation can be influenced by nanoparticles, making them a potential therapeutic target (147,151–154). CD4+ T-cells aid in B cells differentiation into antibody-secreting plasma cells and memory B-cells following antigen recognition. In turn, the secreted high-affinity antibodies can facilitate trapping of pathogens in mucus, facilitate direct neutralization of virus, or activate other effector functions such as complement activation or opsonization. Once antigen is cleared, some plasma cells differentiate into a long-lived variety, helping to prime responses to future exposure (150).

Immunomodulation in the lung

The immune system in the lung must mount the most potent responses against foreign entities while minimizing the possibility of causing loss of function. Indeed, the

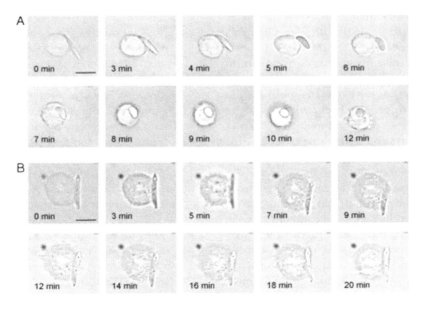

Figure 15.11 Shape-dependent uptake by macrophages. (A) Uptake of PLGA particles by macrophage after a shapeshift from rods to spheres. (B) Failure to uptake in the absence of shape switch. (Reproduced from Yoo, J.W. and Mitragotri, S., *PNAS*, 107, 11205–11210, 2010.)

lungs are constantly exposed to foreign matter, and if the lungs were not able to tightly regulate the local immune responses, the result would be an immunopathological state of constant damaging inflammation. One such immunoregulatory mechanisms is the upregulation of indoleamine 2,3-dioxygenase (IDO) expression in resident lung cells following exposure to TLR ligands. The IDO enzyme persists for several days in the lung and regulates T-cell activation. It can inhibit Th1- and Th2-mediated lung inflammation by preventing trafficking of T-cells to the lung and killing those cells that do enter. Such IDO-mediated repression in response to TLR activation is not seen in otherwise sterile organs, such as the spleen (155).

T-cells themselves play an integral role in balancing tissue damage versus pathogen clearance. Effector CD8+ T-cells increase production of IL-10 at inflamed sites, which, via negative feedback mechanisms, can reduce adaptive immune responses (156). T-cells also promote inhibitory receptors like PD-1 after an antigen is cleared, which in turn suppresses effector functions through rapid reduction in B and T-cells via apoptosis (157). Specialized Treg cells also work to prevent immunopathology. Following infection, activated Treg cells have been found to accumulate in the lung and suppress antigen-specific CD8+ T-cells (158). Recruitment of Treg cells to the lung has also been shown to reduce vaccine-enhanced disease following some vaccinations, such as FI-RSV, while recruitment of other T-cells may worsen it (159).

The lung has a series of additional measures that can aid in control of immune response. MUC1, a cell-tethered mucin on airway epithelial cells, is upregulated during bacterial infection of the airways (160). Reduction of MUC1 amplified inflammation during *in vitro* models of RSV infection indicates that MUC1 plays a role in regulating lung inflammation (161). Other mechanisms include heightened expression of CD200 (OX-2) membrane glycoprotein by alveolar macrophages, and reduced expression of pattern recognition receptors such as TLRs (155,162,163). In addition, the lung works to rapidly restore epithelial integrity postinfection. For example, innate lymphoid cells that generate proinflammatory cytokines work to remodel the airways and repair lung tissue postinfection (163).

Various studies have looked into how the properties of drug-loaded particles interact with the immune system in the lung. Size dictates where an inhaled particle may deposit within the lung and what cells may uptake it. For example, dendritic cells preferentially internalize particles approximately 20–50 nm in diameter, and few particles outside that range are found in lymphatic drainage (137). Positively charged particles seem to increase uptake among almost all of the antigen-presenting cells present in the lungs, but they may also increase the burden of antigen-specific T-cells (164,165). These findings indicate that the precise physiochemical properties of inhaled particles could be used to tune downstream immune responses in the respiratory

system. Understanding the ways that particle design can influence pulmonary immune response or prevent inflammatory responses is critical to developing effective inhalable therapeutics.

CONCLUSION

Drug delivery to the lung is essential for treatment of a variety of pulmonary indications, but effective delivery must overcome a multitude of barriers. In the airways, the mucus secretions coupled with rapid mucocilliary clearance can effectively trap and remove inhaled foreign particulates, thereby preventing access for a drug or preventing sustained drug delivery to the underlying cells. In the deep lung, the abundance of macrophages and immune cells also serve to readily eliminate foreign particles. In addition, lung diseases are often characterized by enhanced mucosal barrier properties as well as active immune responses, creating an even more challenging barrier to delivery. Thus, drug delivery systems to the lung must be carefully engineered to overcome these various physiological barriers to achieve effective therapy.

ACKNOWLEDGMENTS

Financial support was provided by the National Science Foundation CAREER Award (DMR-1151477, S.K.L.), the David and Lucile Packard Foundation (2013–39274), National Institutes of Health (R21EB017938, S.K.L.), and the NC TraCS Institute.

REFERENCES

1. Janssen WJ, Stefanski AL, Bochner BS, Evans CM. Control of lung defense by mucins and macrophages: Ancient defense mechanisms with modern functions. *European Respiratory Journal* 2016;48(4):1201–1214. doi:10.1183/13993003.00120-2015.

2. Ruge CA, Kirch J, Lehr C-M. Pulmonary drug delivery: From generating aerosols to overcoming biological barriers—therapeutic possibilities and technological challenges. *The Lancet Respiratory Medicine* 2013;1(5):402–413. doi:10.1016/S2213-2600(13)70072-9.

3. Benowitz NL, Hukkanen J, Jacob P. Nicotine chemistry, metabolism, kinetics and biomarkers. *Handbook of Experimental Pharmacology* 2009(192):29–60. doi:10.1007/978-3-540-69248-5_2.

4. Knowles MR, Boucher RC. Mucus clearance as a primary innate defense mechanism for mammalian airways. *J Clin Invest.* 2002;109(5):571–577. doi:10.1172/JCI15217.

5. Tarran R, Button B, Boucher RC. Regulation of normal and cystic fibrosis airway surface liquid volume by phasic shear stress. *Annual Review of Physiology* 2006;68(1):543–561. doi:10.1146/annurev.physiol.68.072304.112754.

6. Widdicombe JG. Airway liquid: A barrier to drug diffusion? *European Respiratory Journal* 1997;10(10):2194–2197.

7. Fahy JV, Dickey BF. Airway mucus function and dysfunction. *The New England Journal of Medicine 2010*; 363(23):2233–2247. doi:10.1056/NEJMra0910061.

8. Hill DB, Vasquez PA, Mellnik J, McKinley SA, Vose A, Mu F, Henderson AG et al. A biophysical basis for mucus solids concentration as a candidate biomarker for airways disease. *PLOS ONE 2014*;9(2):e87681. doi:10.1371/journal.pone.0087681.

9. Carlstedt I, Lindgren H, Sheehan JK. The macromolecular structure of human cervical-mucus glycoproteins. Studies on fragments obtained after reduction of disulphide bridges and after subsequent trypsin digestion. *Biochemical Journal 1983*;213(2):427–435.

10. Cone RA. Barrier properties of mucus. *Advanced Drug Delivery Reviews 2009*;61(2):75–85. doi:10.1016/j.addr.2008.09.008.

11. Thornton DJ, Davies JR, Kraayenbrink M, Richardson PS, Sheehan JK, Carlstedt I. Mucus glycoproteins from "normal" human tracheobronchial secretion. *Biochemical Journal 1990*;265(1):179–186.

12. Thornton DJ, Sheehan JK, Lindgren H, Carlstedt I. Mucus glycoproteins from cystic fibrotic sputum. Macromolecular properties and structural "architecture." *Biochemical Journal 1991*;276(Pt 3):667–675.

13. Davies JR, Hovenberg HW, Lindén CJ, Howard R, Richardson PS, Sheehan JK, Carlstedt I. Mucins in airway secretions from healthy and chronic bronchitic subjects. *Biochemical Journal 1996*;313(Pt 2):431–439.

14. Lamblin G, Degroote S, Perini J-M, Delmotte P, Scharfman A, Davril M, Lo-Guidice J-M. et al. Human airway mucin glycosylation: A combinatory of carbohydrate determinants which vary in cystic fibrosis. *Glycoconjugate Journal 2001*;18(9):661–684. doi:10.1023/A:1020867221861.

15. Thornton DJ, Rousseau K, McGuckin MA. Structure and function of the polymeric mucins in airways mucus. *Annual Review of Physiology 2008*;70(1):459–486. doi:10.1146/annurev.physiol.70.113006.100702.

16. Desseyn J-L, Guyonnet-Dupérat V, Porchet N, Aubert J-P, Laine A. Human mucin gene MUC5B, the 10.7-kb large central exon encodes various alternate subdomains resulting in a super-repeat structural evidence for a 11p15.5 gene family. *Journal of Biological Chemistry 1997*;272(6):3168–3178. doi:10.1074/jbc.272.6.3168.

17. Escande F, Aubert JP, Porchet N, Buisine MP. Human mucin gene MUC5AC: Organization of its 5'-region and central repetitive region. *Biochemical Journal 2001*;358(Pt 3):763–772.

18. Toribara NW, Gum JR, Culhane PJ, Lagace RE, Hicks JW, Petersen GM, Kim YS. MUC-2 human small intestinal mucin gene structure. Repeated arrays and polymorphism. *Journal of Clinical Investigation 1991*; 88(3):1005–1013.

19. Johansson MEV, Ambort D, Pelaseyed T, Schütte A, Gustafsson JK, Ermund A, Subramani DB. et al. Composition and functional role of the mucus layers in the intestine. *Cellular and Molecular Life Sciences 2011*;68(22):3635. doi:10.1007/s00018-011-0822-3.

20. Escande F, Porchet N, Aubert J-P, Buisine M-P. The mouse Muc5b mucin gene: CDNA and genomic structures, chromosomal localization and expression. *Biochemical Journal 2002*;363(Pt 3):589–598.

21. Murty VLN, Sarosiek J, Slomiany A, Slomiany BL. Effect of lipids and proteins on the viscosity of gastric mucus glycoprotein. *Biochemical and Biophysical Research Communications 1984*;121(2):521–529. doi:10.1016/0006-291X(84)90213-4.

22. Hang HC, Bertozzi CR. The chemistry and biology of mucin-type O-linked glycosylation. *Bioorganic & Medicinal Chemistry 2005*;13(17):5021–5034. doi:10.1016/j.bmc.2005.04.085.

23. Sheehan JK, Kirkham S, Howard M, Woodman P, Kutay S, Brazeau C, Buckley J, Thornton DJ. Identification of molecular intermediates in the assembly pathway of the MUC5AC mucin. *Journal of Biological Chemistry 2004*;279(15):15698–15705. doi:10.1074/jbc. M313241200.

24. Tam PY, Verdugo P. Control of mucus hydration as a Donnan equilibrium process. *Nature 1981*;292(5821):340–342. doi:10.1038/292340a0.

25. Verdugo P. Mucin exocytosis. *The American Review of Respiratory Disease 1991*;144(3_pt_2):S33–S37. doi:10.1164/ajrccm/144.3_pt_2.S33.

26. Chen Y, Zhao YH, Di Y-P, Wu R. Characterization of human mucin 5B gene expression in airway epithelium and the genomic clone of the amino-terminal and 5'-flanking region. *American Journal of Respiratory Cell and Molecular Biology 2001*;25(5):542–553. doi:10.1165/ajrcmb.25.5.4298.

27. Rose MC, Voynow JA. Respiratory tract mucin genes and mucin glycoproteins in health and disease. *Physiological Reviews 2006*;86(1):245–278. doi:10.1152/physrev.00010.2005.

28. Kirkham S, Sheehan JK, Knight D, Richardson PS, Thornton DJ. Heterogeneity of airways mucus: Variations in the amounts and glycoforms of the major oligomeric mucins MUC5AC and MUC5B. *Biochemical Journal 2002*;361(Pt 3):537–546.

29. Sheehan JK, Howard M, Richardson PS, Longwill T, Thornton DJ. Physical characterization of a low-charge glycoform of the MUC5B mucin comprising the gel-phase of an asthmatic respiratory mucous plug. *Biochemical Journal 1999*;338(Pt 2):507–513.

30. Thornton DJ, Carlstedt I, Howard M, Devine PL, Price MR, Sheehan JK. Respiratory mucins: Identification of core proteins and glycoforms. *Biochemical Journal 1996*;316(Pt 3):967–975.

31. Thornton DJ, Howard M, Khan N, Sheehan JK. Identification of two glycoforms of the MUC5B mucin in human respiratory mucus evidence for a cysteine-rich sequence repeated within the molecule. *Journal of Biological Chemistry* 1997;272(14):9561–9566. doi:10.1074/jbc.272.14.9561.

32. Davies JR, Svitacheva N, Lannefors L, Kornfält R, Carlstedt I. Identification of MUC5B, MUC5AC and small amounts of MUC2 mucins in cystic fibrosis airway secretions. *Biochemical Journal* 1999;344(Pt 2):321–330.

33. Hovenberg HW, Davies JR, Herrmann A, Lindén C-J, Carlstedt I. MUC5AC, but not MUC2, is a prominent mucin in respiratory secretions. *Glycoconjugate Journal* 1996;13(5):839–847. doi:10.1007/BF00702348.

34. Buisine M-P, Devisme L, Copin M-C, Durand-Réville M, Gosselin B, Aubert J-P, Porchet N. Developmental mucin gene expression in the human respiratory tract. *American Journal of Respiratory Cell and Molecular Biology* 1999;20(2):209–218. doi:10.1165/ajrcmb.20.2.3259.

35. Thornton DJ, Sheehan JK. From mucins to mucus. *Proceedings of the American Thoracic Society* 2004;1(1):54–61. doi:10.1513/pats.2306016.

36. Davis CW. *Goblet Cells: Physiology and Pharmacology. Airway Mucus: Basic Mechanisms and Clinical Perspectives.* Boston, MA; Basel, Switzerland: Birkhauser, 1997, pp. 149–177.

37. Fung DC, Rogers DF. *Airway Submucosal Glands: Physiology and Pharmacology. Airway Mucus: Basic Mechanisms and Clinical Perspectives.* Boston, MA; Basel, Switzerland: Birkhasuer, 1997, pp. 170–210.

38. Kawakubo M, Ito Y, Okimura Y, Kobayashi M, Sakura K, Kasama S, Fukuda MN, Fukuda M, Katsuyama T, Nakayama J. Natural antibiotic function of a human gastric mucin against helicobacter pylori infection. *Science* 2004;305(5686):1003–1006. doi:10.1126/science.1099250.

39. Lindén S, Nordman H, Hedenbro J, Hurtig M, Borén T, Carlstedt I. Strain- and blood group-dependent binding of Helicobacter pylori to human gastric MUC5AC glycoforms. *Gastroenterology* 2002;123(6):1923–1930. doi:10.1053/gast.2002.37076.

40. Roy MG, Livraghi-Butrico A, Fletcher AA, McElwee MM, Evans SE, Boerner RM, Alexander SN, et al. Muc5b is required for airway defense. *Nature* 2014;505(7483):412–416. doi:10.1038/nature12807.

41. Koeppen M, McNamee EN, Brodsky KS, Aherne CM, Faigle M, Downey GP, Colgan SP, Evans CM, Schwartz DA, Eltzschig HK. Detrimental role of the airway mucin Muc5ac during ventilator-induced lung injury. *Mucosal Immunology* 2013;6(4):762–775. doi:10.1038/mi.2012.114.

42. Ordoñez CL, Khashayar R, Wong HH, Ferrando R, Wu R, Hyde DM, Hotchkiss JA, et al. Mild and moderate asthma is associated with airway goblet cell hyperplasia and abnormalities in mucin gene expression. *American Journal of Respiratory and Critical Care Medicine* 2001;163(2):517–523. doi:10.1164/ajrccm.163.2.2004039.

43. Evans CM, Raclawska DS, Ttofali F, Liptzin DR, Fletcher AA, Harper DN, McGing MA, et al. The polymeric mucin Muc5ac is required for allergic airway hyperreactivity. *Nature Communications* 2015;6:6281. doi:10.1038/ncomms7281.

44. Raynal BDE, Hardingham TE, Sheehan JK, Thornton DJ. Calcium-dependent protein interactions in MUC5B provide reversible cross-links in salivary mucus. *Journal of Biological Chemistry* 2003;278(31):28703–28710. doi:10.1074/jbc. M304632200.

45. Lai SK, Wang Y-Y, Hida K, Cone R, Hanes J. Nanoparticles reveal that human cervicovaginal mucus is riddled with pores larger than viruses. *Proceedings of the National Academy of Sciences of the United States of America* 2010;107(2):598–603. doi:10.1073/pnas.0911748107.

46. Boucher RC. New concepts of the pathogenesis of cystic fibrosis lung disease. *European Respiratory Journal* 2004;23(1):146–158. doi:10.11 83/09031936.03.00057003.

47. Wills PJ, Hall RL, Chan W, Cole PJ. Sodium chloride increases the ciliary transportability of cystic fibrosis and bronchiectasis sputum on the mucus-depleted bovine trachea. *Journal of Clinical Investigation* 1997;99(1):9–13.

48. Nicholas B, Skipp P, Mould R, Rennard S, Davies DE, O'Connor CD, Djukanović R. Shotgun proteomic analysis of human-induced sputum. *Proteomics* 2006;6(15):4390–4401. doi:10.1002/pmic.200600011.

49. Ali M, Lillehoj EP, Park Y, Kyo Y, Kim KC. Analysis of the proteome of human airway epithelial secretions. *Proteome Science* 2011;9:4. doi:10.1186/1477-5956-9-4.

50. Schuster BS, Suk JS, Woodworth GF, Hanes J. Nanoparticle diffusion in respiratory mucus from humans without lung disease. *Biomaterials* 2013;34(13):3439–3446. doi:10.1016/j.biomaterials.2013.01.064.

51. Suk JS, Lai SK, Wang Y-Y, Ensign LM, Zeitlin PL, Boyle MP, Hanes J. The penetration of fresh undiluted sputum expectorated by cystic fibrosis patients by non-adhesive polymer nanoparticles. *Biomaterials* 2009;30(13):2591–2597. doi:10.1016/j.biomaterials.2008.12.076.

52. Lai SK, Wang Y-Y, Cone R, Wirtz D, Hanes J. Altering mucus rheology to "Solidify" human mucus at the nanoscale. *PLoS One* 2009;4(1):e4294.doi:10.1371/journal.pone.0004294.

53. Schuster BS, Kim AJ, Kays JC, Kanzawa MM, Guggino WB, Boyle MP, Rowe SM, Muzyczka N, Suk JS, Hanes J. Overcoming the cystic fibrosis sputum barrier to leading adeno-associated virus gene therapy vectors. *Molecular Therapy 2014*;22(8):1484–1493. doi:10.1038/mt.2014.89.

54. Lieleg O, Vladescu I, Ribbeck K. Characterization of particle translocation through mucin hydrogels. *Biophysical Journal 2010*;98(9):1782–1789. doi:10.1016/j.bpj.2010.01.012.

55. Sanders NN, De Smedt SC, Demeester J. Mobility and stability of gene complexes in biogels. *Journal of Controlled Release 2003*;87(1):117–129. doi:10.1016/S0168-3659(02)00355-3.

56. Suk JS, Kim AJ, Trehan K, Schneider CS, Cebotaru L, Woodward OM, Boylan NJ, Boyle MP, Lai SK, Guggino WB, Hanes J. Lung gene therapy with highly compacted DNA nanoparticles that overcome the mucus barrier. *Journal of Controlled Release 2014*;178:8–17. doi:10.1016/j.jconrel.2014.01.007.

57. Kim AJ, Boylan NJ, Suk JS, Hwangbo M, Yu T, Schuster BS, Cebotaru L. et al. Use of single-site-functionalized PEG dendrons To prepare gene vectors that penetrate human mucus barriers. *Angewandte Chemie International Edition 2013*;52(14):3985–3988. doi:10.1002/anie.201208556.

58. Mastorakos P, da Silva AL, Chisholm J, Song E, Choi WK, Boyle MP, Morales MM, Hanes J, Suk JS. Highly compacted biodegradable DNA nanoparticles capable of overcoming the mucus barrier for inhaled lung gene therapy. *Proceedings of the National Academy of Sciences of the United States of America 2015*;112(28):8720–8725. doi:10.1073/pnas.1502281112.

59. Wu L, Liu M, Shan W, Cui Y, Zhang Z, Huang Y. Lipid nanovehicles with adjustable surface properties for overcoming multiple barriers simultaneously in oral administration. *International Journal of Pharmaceutics 2017*;520(1):216–227. doi:10.1016/j.ijpharm.2017.02.015.

60. Sanders NN, De Smedt SC, Van Rompaey E, Simoens P, De Baets F. Demeester journal cystic fibrosis sputum. *American Journal of Respiratory and Critical Care Medicine 2000*;162(5):1905–1911. doi:10.1164/ajrccm.162.5.9909009.

61. Lai SK, O'Hanlon DE, Harrold S, Man ST, Wang Y-Y, Cone R, Hanes J. Rapid transport of large polymeric nanoparticles in fresh undiluted human mucus. *Proceedings of the National Academy of Sciences of the United States of America 2007*;104(5):1482–1487. doi:10.1073/pnas.0608611104.

62. Braeckmans K, Peeters L, Sanders NN, De Smedt SC, Demeester J. Three-Dimensional fluorescence recovery after photobleaching with the confocal scanning laser microscope. *Biophysical Journal 2003*;85(4):2240–2252.

63. Xu Q, Ensign LM, Boylan NJ, Schön A, Gong X, Yang J-C, Lamb NW. et al. Impact of surface polyethylene glycol (PEG) density on biodegradable nanoparticle transport in mucus ex vivo and distribution in vivo. *ACS Nano 2015*;9(9):9217–9227. doi:10.1021/acsnano.5b03876.

64. Duncan GA, Jung J, Hanes J, Suk JS. The mucus barrier to inhaled gene therapy. *Molecular Therapy 2016*;24(12):2043–2053. doi:10.1038/mt.2016.182.

65. Hida K, Lai SK, Suk JS, Won SY, Boyle MP, Hanes J. Common gene therapy viral vectors do not efficiently penetrate sputum from cystic fibrosis patients. *PLoS One 2011*;6(5):e19919. doi:10.1371/journal.pone.0019919.

66. Araújo F, Martins C, Azevedo C, Sarmento B. Chemical modification of drug molecules as strategy to reduce interactions with mucus. *Advanced Drug Delivery Reviews 2017*. doi:10.1016/j.addr.2017.09.020.

67. Suk JS, Boylan NJ, Trehan K, Tang BC, Schneider CS, Lin J-MG, Boyle MP et al. N-acetylcysteine enhances cystic fibrosis sputum penetration and airway gene transfer by highly compacted DNA nanoparticles. *Molecular Therapy 2011*;19(11):1981–1989. doi:10.1038/mt.2011.160.

68. Reynolds HY. Immunoglobulin G and its function in the human respiratory tract*. *Mayo Clinic Proceedings 1988*;63(2):161–174. doi:10.1016/S0025-6196(12)64949-0.

69. Burnett D. Immunoglobulins in the lung. *Thorax 1986*;41(5):337–344.

70. Goodman MR, Link DW, Brown WR, Nakane PK. Ultrastructural evidence of transport of secretory IgA across bronchial epithelium. *The American Review of Respiratory Disease 1981*;123(1):115–119. doi:10.1164/arrd.1981.123.1.115.

71. Mostov KE, Blobel G. A transmembrane precursor of secretory component. The receptor for transcellular transport of polymeric immunoglobulins. *Journal of Biological Chemistry 1982*;257 (19):11816–11821.

72. Newkirk MM, Klein MH, Katz A, Fisher MM, Underdown BJ. Estimation of polymeric IgA in human serum: An assay based on binding of radiolabeled human secretory component with applications in the study of IgA nephropathy, IgA monoclonal gammopathy, and liver disease. *The Journal of Immunology 1983*;130(3):1176–1181.

73. Stockley RA, Afford SC, Burnett D. Assessment of 7S and 11S immunoglobulin a in sputum. *The American Review of Respiratory Disease 1980*;122(6):959–964. doi:10.1164/arrd.1980.122.6.959.

74. Delacroix DL, Dive C, Rambaud JC, Vaerman JP. IgA subclasses in various secretions and in serum. *Immunology 1982*;47(2):383–385.

75. Kornfeld SJ, Plaut AG. Secretory immunity and the bacterial IgA proteases. *Reviews of Infectious Diseases* 1981;3(3):521–534.

76. Longet S, Miled S, Lötscher M, Miescher SM, Zuercher AW, Corthésy B. Human plasma-derived polymeric IgA and IgM antibodies associate with secretory component to yield biologically active secretory-like antibodies. *Journal of Biological Chemistry* 2013;288(6):4085–4094. doi:10.1074/jbc.M112.410811.

77. Marcotte H, Lavoie MC. Oral microbial ecology and the role of salivary immunoglobulin A. *Microbiology and Molecular Biology Reviews* 1998;62(1):71–109.

78. Mazanec MB, Nedrud JG, Kaetzel CS, Lamm ME. A three-tiered view of the role of IgA in mucosal defense. *Immunology Today* 1993;14(9):430–435. doi:10.1016/0167-5699(93)90245-G.

79. Kim S-H, Jang Y-S. The development of mucosal vaccines for both mucosal and systemic immune induction and the roles played by adjuvants. *Clinical and Experimental Vaccine Research* 2017;6(1):15–21. doi:10.7774/cevr.2017.6.1.15.

80. Corthésy B. Multi-faceted functions of secretory IgA at mucosal surfaces. *Frontiers in Immunology* 2013;4:85. doi:10.3389/fimmu.2013.00185.

81. Bakema JE, Egmond Mv. The human immunoglobulin A Fc receptor FcαRI: A multifaceted regulator of mucosal immunity. *Mucosal Immunology* 2011;4(6):mi201136. doi:10.1038/mi.2011.36.

82. Merrill WW, Naegel GP, Olchowski JJ, Reynolds HY. Immunoglobulin G subclass proteins in serum and lavage fluid of normal subjects. *The American Review of Respiratory Disease* 1985;131(4):584–587. doi:10.1164/arrd.1985.131.4.584.

83. Soutar CA. Distribution of plasma cells and other cells containing immunoglobulin in the respiratory tract in chronic bronchitis. *Thorax* 1977;32(4):387–396.

84. Nijhuis-Heddes JM, Lindeman J, Otto AJ, Snieders MW, Kievit-Tyson PA, Dijkman JH. Distribution of immunoglobulin-containing cells in the bronchial mucosa of patients with chronic respiratory disease. *European Journal of Respiratory Diseases* 1982;63(3):249–256.

85. Lin PM, Wright JR. Surfactant protein A binds to IgG and enhances phagocytosis of IgG-opsonized erythrocytes. *AJP: Lung Cellular and Molecular Physiology* 2006;291(6):L1199–L206. doi:10.1152/ajplung.00188.2006.

86. Watford WT, Ghio AJ, Wright JR. Complement-mediated host defense in the lung. *American Journal of Physiology—Lung Cellular and Molecular Physiology* 2000;279(5):L790–L798.

87. Watford WT, Wright JR, Hester CG, Jiang H, Frank MM. Surfactant protein a regulates complement activation. *The Journal of Immunology* 2001;167(11):6593–600. doi:10.4049/jimmunol.167.11.6593.

88. Garagiola DM, Huard TK, LoBuglio AF. Comparison of monocyte and alveolar macrophage antibody-dependent cellular cytotoxicity and Fc-receptor activity. *Cellular Immunology* 1981;64(2):359–370. doi:10.1016/0008-8749(81)90487-1.

89. Naegel GP, Young KR, Reynolds HY. Receptors for human IgG subclasses on human alveolar macrophages. *The American Review of Respiratory Disease* 1984;129(3):413–418. doi:10.1164/arrd.1984.129.3.413.

90. Olmsted SS, Padgett JL, Yudin AI, Whaley KJ, Moench TR, Cone RA. Diffusion of macromolecules and virus-like particles in human cervical mucus. *Biophysical Journal* 2001;81(4):1930–1937.

91. Wang Y-Y, Kannan A, Nunn KL, Murphy MA, Subramani DB, Moench T, Cone R, Lai SK. IgG in cervicovaginal mucus traps HSV and prevents vaginal herpes infections. *Mucosal Immunology* 2014;7(5):1036–1044. doi:10.1038/mi.2013.120.

92. Wang Y-Y, Harit D, Subramani DB, Arora H, Kumar PA, Lai SK. Influenza-binding antibodies immobilise influenza viruses in fresh human airway mucus. *European Respiratory Journal* 2017;49(1):1601709. doi:10.1183/13993003.01709-2016.

93. Newby J, Schiller JL, Wessler T, Edelstein J, Forest MG, Lai SK. A blueprint for robust crosslinking of mobile species in biogels with weakly adhesive molecular anchors. *Nature Communications* 2017;8. doi:10.1038/s41467-017-00739-6.

94. Chen A, McKinley SA, Shi F, Wang S, Mucha PJ, Harit D, Forest MG, Lai SK. Modeling of virion collisions in cervicovaginal mucus reveals limits on agglutination as the protective mechanism of secretory immunoglobulin A. *PLoS One* 2015;10(7). doi:10.1371/journal.pone.0131351.

95. Henry CE, Wang Y-Y, Yang Q, Hoang T, Chattopadhyay S, Hoen T, Ensign LM, et al. Anti-PEG antibodies alter the mobility and biodistribution of densely PEGylated nanoparticles in mucus. *Acta Biomater* 2016;43:61–70. doi:10.1016/j.actbio.2016.07.019.

96. Chirmule N, Propert KJ, Magosin SA, Qian Y, Qian R, Wilson JM. Immune responses to adenovirus and adeno-associated virus in humans. *Gene Therapy* 1999;6(9):3300994. doi:10.1038/sj.gt.3300994.

97. Calcedo R, Vandenberghe LH, Gao G, Lin J, Wilson JM. Worldwide epidemiology of neutralizing antibodies to adeno-associated viruses. *The Journal of Infectious Diseases* 2009;199(3):381–390. doi:10.1086/595830.

98. Halbert CL, Miller AD, McNamara S, Emerson J, Gibson RL, Ramsey B, Aitken ML. Prevalence of neutralizing antibodies against adeno-associated virus (AAV) types 2, 5, and 6 in cystic fibrosis and normal populations: Implications for gene therapy using AAV vectors. *Human Gene Therapy* 2006;17(4):440–447. doi:10.1089/hum.2006.17.440.

99. Yang Q, Lai SK. Anti-PEG immunity: Emergence, characteristics, and unaddressed questions. *Wiley Interdisciplinary Reviews: Nanomedicine and Nanobiotechnology* 2015;7(5):655–677. doi:10.1002/wnan.1339.

100. Cheng T-L, Wu P-Y, Wu M-F, Chern J-W, Roffler SR. Accelerated clearance of polyethylene glycol-modified proteins by anti-polyethylene glycol IgM. *Bioconjugate Chemistry* 1999;10(3):520–528. doi:10.1021/bc980143z.

101. Zhang C, Fan K, Ma X, Wei D. Impact of large aggregated uricases and PEG Diol on accelerated blood clearance of PEGylated canine uricase. *PLoS One* 2012;7(6):e39659. doi:10.1371/journal.pone.0039659.

102. Shimizu T, Ichihara M, Yoshioka Y, Ishida T, Nakagawa S, Kiwada H. Intravenous administration of polyethylene glycol-coated (PEGylated) proteins and PEGylated adenovirus elicits an anti-PEG immunoglobulin M response. *Biological and Pharmaceutical Bulletin* 2012;35(8):1336–1342.

103. Zhao Y, Wang L, Yan M, Ma Y, Zang G, She Z, Deng Y. Repeated injection of PEGylated solid lipid nanoparticles induces accelerated blood clearance in mice and beagles. *International Journal of Nanomedicine* 2012;7:2891–2900. doi:10.2147/IJN.S30943.

104. Ichihara M, Shimizu T, Imoto A, Hashiguchi Y, Uehara Y, Ishida T, Kiwada H. Anti-PEG IgM response against PEGylated liposomes in mice and rats. *Pharmaceutics* 2010;3(1):1–11. doi:10.3390/pharmaceutics3010001.

105. Li Z, Palaniyandi S, Zeng R, Tuo W, Roopenian DC, Zhu X. Transfer of IgG in the female genital tract by MHC class I-related neonatal Fc receptor (FcRn) confers protective immunity to vaginal infection. *Proceedings of the National Academy of Sciences of the United States of America* 2011;108(11):4388–4393. doi:10.1073/pnas.1012861108.

106. Mascola JR, Stiegler G, VanCott TC, Katinger H, Carpenter CB, Hanson CE, Beary H. et al. Protection of macaques against vaginal transmission of a pathogenic HIV-1/SIV chimeric virus by passive infusion of neutralizing antibodies. *Nature Medicine* 2000;6(2):nm0200_207. doi:10.1038/72318.

107. Deruaz M, Moldt B, Le KM, Power KA, Vrbanac VD, Tanno S, Ghebremichael MS. et al. Protection of humanized mice from repeated intravaginal HIV challenge by passive immunization: A model for studying the efficacy of neutralizing antibodies in vivo. *The Journal of Infectious Diseases* 2016;214(4):612–616. doi:10.1093/infdis/jiw203.

108. Hessell AJ, Rakasz EG, Poignard P, Hangartner L, Landucci G, Forthal DN, Koff WC, Watkins DI, Burton DR. Broadly neutralizing human anti-HIV antibody 2G12 Is effective in protection against mucosal SHIV challenge even at low serum neutralizing titers. *PLoS Pathogens* 2009;5(5):e1000433. doi:10.1371/journal.ppat.1000433.

109. Tarran R. Regulation of airway surface liquid volume and mucus transport by active ion transport. *Proceedings of the American Thoracic Society* 2004;1(1):42–46. doi:10.1513/pats.2306014.

110. Donaldson SH, Corcoran TE, Laube BL, Bennett WD. Mucociliary clearance as an outcome measure for cystic fibrosis clinical research. *Proceedings of the American Thoracic Society* 2007;4(4):399–405. doi:10.1513/pats.200703-042BR.

111. Todoroff J, Vanbever R. Fate of nanomedicines in the lungs. *Current Opinion in Colloid & Interface Science* 2011;16(3):246–254. doi:10.1016/j.cocis.2011.03.001.

112. Ganz T. Antimicrobial polypeptides in host defense of the respiratory tract. *Journal of Clinical Investigation* 2002;109(6):693–697. doi:10.1172/JCI15218.

113. Cole AM, Dewan P, Ganz T. Innate antimicrobial activity of nasal secretions. *Infection and Immunity* 1999;67(7):3267–3275.

114. Zahm JM, King M, Duvivier C, Pierrot D, Girod S, Puchelle E. Role of simulated repetitive coughing in mucus clearance. *European Respiratory Journal* 1991;4(3):311–315.

115. Matsui H, Grubb BR, Tarran R, Randell SH, Gatzy JT, Davis CW, Boucher RC. Evidence for periciliary liquid layer depletion, not abnormal ion composition, in the pathogenesis of cystic fibrosis airways disease. *Cell* 1998;95(7):1005–1015.

116. Boucher RC. Cystic fibrosis: A disease of vulnerability to airway surface dehydration. *Trends in Molecular Medicine* 2007;13(6):231–40. doi:10.1016/j.molmed.2007.05.001.

117. Tang XX, Ostedgaard LS, Hoegger MJ, Moninger TO, Karp PH, McMenimen JD, Choudhury B, Varki A, Stoltz DA, Welsh MJ. Acidic pH increases airway surface liquid viscosity in cystic fibrosis. *Journal of Clinical Investigation* 126(3):879–891. doi:10.1172/JCI83922.

118. Collawn JF, Matalon S. CFTR and lung homeostasis. *American Journal of Physiology—Lung Cellular and Molecular Physiology* 2014;307(12):L917–L923. doi:10.1152/ajplung.00326.2014.

119. Gadsby DC, Vergani P, Csanády L. The ABC protein turned chloride channel whose failure causes cystic fibrosis. *Nature* 2006;440(7083):477–483. doi:10.1038/nature04712.

120. Rowe SM, Miller S, Sorscher EJ. Mechanisms of disease: Cystic fibrosis. *The New England Journal of Medicine* 2005;352(19):1992–2001.

121. Davis PB. Cystic fibrosis since 1938. *American Journal of Respiratory and Critical Care Medicine* 2006;173(5):475–482.

122. Worlitzsch D, Tarran R, Ulrich M, Schwab U, Cekici A, Meyer KC, Birrer P et al. Effects of reduced mucus oxygen concentration in airway Pseudomonas infections of cystic fibrosis patients. *Journal of Clinical Investigation* 2002;109(3):317–325. doi:10.1172/JCI13870.

123. Henke MO, John G, Germann M, Lindemann H, Rubin BK. MUC5AC and MUC5B mucins increase in cystic fibrosis airway secretions during pulmonary exacerbation. *American Journal of Respiratory and Critical Care Medicine* 2007;175(8):816–821. doi:10.1164/rccm.200607-1011OC.

124. Hubeau C, Lorenzato M, Couetil JP, Hubert D, Dusser D, Puchelle E, Gaillard D. Quantitative analysis of inflammatory cells infiltrating the cystic fibrosis airway mucosa. *Clinical and Experimental Immunology* 2001;124(1):69–76. doi:10.1046/j.1365-2249.2001.01456.x.

125. Potter JL, Spector S, Matthews LW, Lemm J. Studies on pulmonary secretions. *The American Review of Respiratory Disease* 1969;99(6):909–916. doi:10.1164/arrd.1969.99.6.909.

126. Perks B, Shute JK. DNA and Actin Bind and Inhibit Interleukin-8 Function in cystic fibrosis sputa. *American Journal of Respiratory and Critical Care Medicine* 2000;162(5):1767–1772. doi:10.1164/ajrccm.162.5.9908107.

127. Evans CM, Kim K, Tuvim MJ, Dickey BF. Mucus hypersecretion in asthma: Causes and effects. *Current Opinion in Pulmonary Medicine* 2009;15(1):4–11. doi:10.1097/MCP.0b013e32831da8d3.

128. Morcillo EJ, Cortijo J. Mucus and MUC in asthma. *Current Opinion in Pulmonary Medicine* 2006;12(1):1–6.

129. Bergeron C, Al-Ramli W, Hamid Q. Remodeling in asthma. *Proceedings of the American Thoracic Society* 2009;6(3):301–305. doi:10.1513/pats.200808-089RM.

130. Welsh KG, Rousseau K, Fisher G, Bonser LR, Bradding P, Brightling CE, Thornton DJ, Gaillard EA. MUC5AC and a glycosylated variant of MUC5B alter mucin composition in children with acute asthma. *Chest* 2017;152(4):771–779. doi:10.1016/j.chest.2017.07.001.

131. Innes AL, Carrington SD, Thornton DJ, Kirkham S, Rousseau K, Dougherty RH, Raymond WW, Caughey GH, Muller SJ, Fahy JV. Ex vivo sputum analysis reveals impairment of protease-dependent mucus degradation by plasma proteins in acute asthma. *American Journal of Respiratory and Critical Care Medicine* 2009;180(3):203–210. doi:10.1164/rccm.200807-1056OC.

132. Allie SR, Randall TD. Pulmonary immunity to viruses. *Clinical Science* 2017;131(14):1737–1762. doi:10.1042/CS20160259.

133. Renegar KB, Small PA, Boykins LG, Wright PF. Role of IgA versus IgG in the control of influenza viral infection in the murine respiratory tract. *The Journal of Immunology* 2004;173(3):1978–1986. doi:10.4049/jimmunol.173.3.1978.

134. Tamura S, Tanimoto T, Kurata T. Mechanisms of broad cross-protection provided by influenza virus infection and their application to vaccines. *Japanese Journal of Infectious Diseases* 2005;58(4):195.

135. Johansen F-E, Kaetzel C. Regulation of the polymeric immunoglobulin receptor and IgA transport: New advances in environmental factors that stimulate pIgR expression and its role in mucosal immunity. *Mucosal Immunology* 2011;4(6):598–602. doi:10.1038/mi.2011.37.

136. Labiris NR, Dolovich MB. Pulmonary drug delivery. Part I: Physiological factors affecting therapeutic effectiveness of aerosolized medications. *British Journal of Clinical Pharmacology* 2003;56(6):588–599. doi:10.1046/j.1365-2125.2003.01892.x.

137. Blank F, Stumbles PA, Seydoux E, Holt PG, Fink A, Rothen-Rutishauser B, Strickland DH, von Garnier C. Size-dependent uptake of particles by pulmonary antigen-presenting cell populations and trafficking to regional lymph nodes. *American Journal of Respiratory Cell and Molecular Biology* 2013;49(1):67–77. doi:10.1165/rcmb.2012-0387OC.

138. Folkesson HG, Matthay MA, Westrom BR, Kim KJ, Karlsson BW, Hastings RH. Alveolar epithelial clearance of protein. *Journal of Applied Physiology* 1996;80(5):1431–1445.

139. Hirota K, Hasegawa T, Hinata H, Ito F, Inagawa H, Kochi C, Soma G-I, Makino K, Terada H. Optimum conditions for efficient phagocytosis of rifampicin-loaded PLGA microspheres by alveolar macrophages. *Journal of Controlled Release* 2007;119(1):69–76. doi:10.1016/j.jconrel.2007.01.013.

140. Patel B, Gupta N, Ahsan F. Particle engineering to enhance or lessen particle uptake by alveolar macrophages and to influence the therapeutic outcome. *European Journal of Pharmaceutics and Biopharmaceutics* 2015;89:163–174. doi:10.1016/j.ejpb.2014.12.001.

141. Yoo J-W, Mitragotri S. Polymer particles that switch shape in response to a stimulus. *PNAS* 2010;107(25):11205–11210. doi:10.1073/pnas.1000346107.

142. Cleaver JO, You D, Michaud DR, Pruneda FAG, Juarez MML, Zhang J, Weill PM. et al. Lung epithelial cells are essential effectors of inducible resistance to pneumonia. *Mucosal Immunology* 2014;7(1):78–88. doi:10.1038/mi.2013.26.

143. Barlow PG, Findlay EG, Currie SM, Davidson DJ. Antiviral potential of cathelicidins. *Future Microbiology* 2014;9(1):55–73. doi:10.2217/fmb.13.135.

144. Vareille M, Kieninger E, Edwards MR, Regamey N. The airway epithelium: Soldier in the fight against respiratory viruses. *Clinical Microbiology Reviews* 2011;24(1):210–229. doi:10.1128/CMR.00014-10.

145. Yoo J-K, Kim TS, Hufford MM, Braciale TJ. Viral infection of the lung: Host response and sequelae. *Clinical and Experimental Immunology* 2013;132(6). doi:10.1016/j.jaci.2013.06.006.

146. Guilliams M, Lambrecht BN, Hammad H. Division of labor between lung dendritic cells and macrophages in the defense against pulmonary infections. *Mucosal Immunology* 2013;6(3):464–473. doi:10.1038/mi.2013.14.

147. Legge KL, Braciale TJ. Lymph node dendritic cells control CD8+ T cell responses through regulated fasL expression. *Immunity* 2005;23(6):649–659. doi:10.1016/j.immuni.2005.11.006.

148. Legge KL, Braciale TJ. Accelerated migration of respiratory dendritic cells to the regional lymph nodes is limited to the early phase of pulmonary infection. *Immunity* 2003;18(2):265–277. doi:10.1016/S1074-7613(03)00023-2.

149. Vermaelen K, Pauwels R. Pulmonary Dendritic Cells. *American Journal of Respiratory and Critical Care Medicine* 2005;172(5):530–551. doi:10.1164/rccm.200410-1384SO.

150. Blank F, Fytianos K, Seydoux E, Rodriguez-Lorenzo L, Petri-Fink A, von Garnier C, Rothen-Rutishauser B. Interaction of biomedical nanoparticles with the pulmonary immune system. *Journal of Nanobiotechnology* 2017;15. doi:10.1186/s12951-016-0242-5.

151. Nembrini C, Stano A, Dane KY, Ballester M, Vlies AJvd, Marsland BJ, Swartz MA, Hubbell JA. Nanoparticle conjugation of antigen enhances cytotoxic T-cell responses in pulmonary vaccination. *PNAS* 2011;108(44):E989–E997. doi:10.1073/pnas.1104264108.

152. Frick SU, Bacher N, Baier G, Mailänder V, Landfester K, Steinbrink K. Functionalized polystyrene nanoparticles trigger human dendritic cell maturation resulting in enhanced CD4+ T cell activation. *Macromolecular Bioscience* 2012;12(12):1637–1647. doi:10.1002/mabi.201200223.

153. Blank F, Gerber P, Rothen-Rutishauser B, Sakulkhu U, Salaklang J, Peyer KD, Gehr P. et al. Biomedical nanoparticles modulate specific CD4+ T cell stimulation by inhibition of antigen processing in dendritic cells. *Nanotoxicology* 2011;5(4):606–621. doi:10.3109/17435390.2010.541293.

154. Hardy CL, LeMasurier JS, Belz GT, Scalzo-Inguanti K, Yao J, Xiang SD, Kanellakis P, Bobik A, Strickland DH, Rolland JM, O'Hehir RE, Plebanski M. Inert 50 nm polystyrene nanoparticles that modify pulmonary dendritic cell function and inhibit allergic airway inflammation. *The Journal of Immunology* 2012;188(3):1431–1441. doi:10.4049/jimmunol.1100156.

155. Raz E. Organ-specific regulation of innate immunity. *Nature Immunology* 2007;8(1):3–4. doi:10.1038/ni0107-3.

156. Sun J, Madan R, Karp CL, Braciale TJ. Effector T cells control lung inflammation during acute influenza virus infection by producing IL-10. *Nature Medicine* 2009;15(3):277–284. doi:10.1038/nm.1929.

157. Chiu C, Openshaw PJ. Antiviral B cell and T cell immunity in the lungs. *Nature Immunology* 2015;16(1):18–26. doi:10.1038/ni.3056.

158. Loebbermann J, Thornton H, Durant L, Sparwasser T, Webster KE, Sprent J, Culley FJ, Johansson C, Openshaw PJ. Regulatory T cells expressing granzyme B play a critical role in controlling lung inflammation during acute viral infection. *Mucosal Immunology* 2012;5(2):161–172. doi:10.1038/mi.2011.62.

159. Loebbermann J, Durant L, Thornton H, Johansson C, Openshaw PJ. Defective immunoregulation in RSV vaccine-augmented viral lung disease restored by selective chemoattraction of regulatory T cells. *Proceedings of the National Academy of Sciences of the United States of America* 2013;110(8):2987–2992. doi:10.1073/pnas.1217580110.

160. Umehara T, Kato K, Park YS, Lillehoj EP, Kawauchi H, Kim KC. Prevention of lung injury by Muc1 mucin in a mouse model of repetitive pseudomonas aeruginosa infection. *Inflammation Research* 2012;61(9):1013–1020. doi:10.1007/s00011-012-0494-y.

161. Li Y, Dinwiddie DL, Harrod KS, Jiang Y, Kim KC. Anti-inflammatory effect of MUC1 during respiratory syncytial virus infection of lung epithelial cells in vitro. *American Journal of Physiology—Lung Cellular and Molecular Physiology* 2010;298(4):L558–L563. doi:10.1152/ajplung.00225.2009.

162. Snelgrove RJ, Goulding J, Didierlaurent AM, Lyonga D, Vekaria S, Edwards L, Gwyer E, Sedgwick JD, Barclay AN, Hussell T. A critical function for CD200 in lung immune homeostasis and the severity of influenza infection. *Nature Immunology* 2008;9(9):1074–1083. doi:10.1038/ni.1637.

163. Monticelli LA, Sonnenberg GF, Abt MC, Alenghat T, Ziegler CGK, Doering TA, Angelosanto JM. et al. Innate lymphoid cells promote lung-tissue homeostasis after infection with influenza virus. *Nature Immunology 2011*;12(11):1045–1054. doi:10.1038/ni.2131.

164. Fromen CA, Rahhal TB, Robbins GR, Kai MP, Shen TW, Luft JC, DeSimone JM. Nanoparticle surface charge impacts distribution, uptake and lymph node trafficking by pulmonary antigen-presenting cells. *Nanomedicine 2016*;12(3):677–687. doi:10.1016/j.nano.2015.11.002.

165. Rodriguez-Lorenzo L, Fytianos K, Blank F, von Garnier C, Rothen-Rutishauser B, Petri-Fink A. Fluorescence-encoded gold nanoparticles: Library design and modulation of cellular uptake into dendritic cells. *Small 2014*;10(7):1341–1350. doi:10.1002/smll.201302889.

16

Nontuberculous mycobacteria

M. GHADIRI, P.M. YOUNG, AND D. TRAINI

Introduction	275		Microbiologic laboratory diagnosis	277
Pulmonary NTM disease	276		Treatment of pulmonary NTM disease	277
Epidemiology and prevalence	276		Antibiotic therapy	277
Classification of NTM species in lung disease	276		Inhaled antibiotics	278
Slow growers	276		Devices used for inhaled antibiotics	279
Fast growers	276		Surgery	279
The pathogenesis of NTM infections in human lung	276		Limitations of treatments in NTM lung disease	279
Predisposing factors	276		Drug resistance of nontuberculous mycobacteria	279
Chronic lung diseases	276		Drug toxicity and side effects	280
Age	276		Drug–drug interaction	280
Sex	277		Drug discovery pipeline for NTM	280
Race	277		Clinical studies of NTM treatment	281
Immunocompromised patients	277		Conclusion	281
Diagnosis of NTM lung disease	277		References	284
Clinical and radiographic criteria	277			

INTRODUCTION

Mycobacterium (*M.*) has more than 190 well-characterized species (1), some are pathogens for humans, like *M. tuberculosis* and *M. leprae,* while others are normally environmental *Mycobacterium* and poorly pathogenic for humans. They can, however, be responsible for opportunistic diseases. The term *nontuberculous mycobacteria (NTM)* generally refers to mycobacteria other than *M. tuberculosis* and *M. leprae.* NTM are ubiquitous organisms commonly isolated from environments such as drinking water, natural water, and soil (2). The NTMs are a diverse group of organisms with a broad spectrum of virulence and potential for causing disease in humans. Host factors, such as genetic susceptibility, immune defects, and structural lung disease, as well as environmental factors, including humidity, altitude, and shower systems, may also influence the development of NTM lung diseases (3,4). Among the diverse range of NTMs, *M. avium* complex (MAC), *M. abscessus* (MAB), and *M. kansasii* are

the most commonly encountered and important etiologic organisms (5). NTMs are aerobic, nonmotile organisms that appear positive with acid-fast alcohol staining. They are known for their lipid-rich, hydrophobic cell wall, which is substantially thicker than that of most other bacteria. The structure of the cell wall makes mycobacteria impermeable to hydrophilic nutrients and resistant to heavy metals, disinfectants, and antibiotics (6), contributing to forming resistant biofilms to disinfectants and antibiotic therapy (7).

Human diseases related to NTM infection are classified into four distinct clinical syndromes: chronic pulmonary disease (8), lymphadenitis (9), cutaneous disease (10), and disseminated disease (11), with pulmonary infections being the most frequent (12). The lung can easily be affected by inhalation of aerosolized mycobacteria and is by far the most frequent site of human mycobacteriosis. In this chapter, pulmonary NTM infection will be addressed; the chapter will focus mainly on epidemiology, pathogenesis, diagnosis, and treatment strategies.

PULMONARY NTM DISEASE

Epidemiology and prevalence

The incidence and prevalence of NTM lung diseases are increasing worldwide, and they can affect both immunocompetent and *immunocompromised* individuals (13). Capturing accurate data to estimate pulmonary NTM incidence and prevalence is challenging because pulmonary NTM is not reportable to public health authorities, although increasingly, incidence and prevalence of NTM lung disease has started to be reported in many countries, including western countries such as the United States (14), Canada (15), Australia (16), and the United Kingdom (17), as well as Asian countries like Iran (18), Korea (19), Japan (20), and Taiwan (21).

Classification of NTM species in lung disease

NTM can be divided into two groups based on their rate of growth on solid culture medium, rapid and slow growers, and their pigment color, with growth rate having more clinically important consequences then colony pigmentation. Slow growers are most often responsible for pulmonary and lymphonodal diseases (22), whereas rapid growers usually affect skin, bones, and joints (23). However, in some cases, rapid growers can also cause pulmonary infection (24).

SLOW GROWERS

Slow growers take 7 days or more to grow and have been classified by their pigment color: photochromogens if the pigment is only generated on exposure to light; scotochromogens if the pigment is produced in the absence of light; and non-photochromogens if they are not strongly pigmented. Slow-growing species are mainly responsible for pulmonary infection (25,26), but they can cause other diseases as well. Among the slowly growing mycobacteria, the most clinically relevant species in pulmonary diseases are members of *MAC*, *M. kansasii*, *M. malmoense*, and *M. xenopi*.

FAST GROWERS

Fast growers grow in less than 7 days, still slower than most other bacteria (27). They have a propensity to produce skin and soft-tissue infections; however, they can cause pulmonary infection as well. The most clinically relevant species include *M. abscessus*, *M. fortuitum*, and *M. chelonae* (24). *M. abscessus* is the most pathogenic and most likely to produce pulmonary disease, causing approximately 80% of lung disease (28).

The pathogenesis of NTM infections in human lung

Among all NTM species, about 91 different species (29) were isolated from the clinical pulmonary samples. These isolated species have the potential to cause community-acquired and healthcare-associated infections. Infection is believed to occur from the environment; person-to-person spread happens rarely, although evidence for this type of transmission has been reported for cystic fibrosis (CF) patients infected with *M. abscessus* complex (30). Inhalation appears to be the primary transmission route of NTM causing pulmonary disease (31). This usually occurs in artificial water environments such as hot tubs and showers, but it may involve garden soil and house dust (32). NTM have been isolated from natural water environments in which aerosolization increases the concentration of NTM in the air (33). Mycobacteria may aerosolize more readily than other bacteria as they have highly hydrophobic cell walls (34). Probably both environmental exposure and host susceptibility are required for the establishment of pulmonary NTM.

Infection begins when the mycobacterium enters the lungs via inhalation, reaches the alveolar space, and enters the resident alveolar macrophages. If alveolar macrophages fail to eliminate the bacteria, it invades the lung interstitial tissue, either by the bacteria directly infecting the alveolar epithelium or by the migration of the infected alveolar macrophages to the lung parenchyma (35). The infected macrophage produces cytokine signals (e.g., interleukin 12) that recruit and stimulate lymphocytes to make the immune response to help kill the invading mycobacteria. In the lung, this event leads to the formation of granuloma (35). Then the bacteria replicate within the growing granuloma, leading to the expansion and rupture of the granuloma and release of mycobacterium. When an expanding granuloma meets an airway, it fuses with its structure to form a cavity. Released content of the granuloma to the luminal side of the cavity contains both intracellular and extracellular bacteria, which later can show in the sputum (36).

Predisposing factors

CHRONIC LUNG DISEASES

In a substantial number of cases, prior lung infection as well as chronic obstructive pulmonary disease (COPD) (37) and genetic diseases such as CF (30), Alpha-1 antitrypsin deficiency (38), hyper immunoglobulin E syndrome (39), and primary ciliary dyskinesia (PCD) (40) are considered as main predisposing factors for pulmonary NTM infection. However, it is still not completely clear why some people get infected and some do not. Patients with severe COPD are predisposed to NTM lung infections, which can be attributed to the weight loss due to increased breathing rate, decreased oral intake, and catabolic effects of inflammatory cytokines. Thereby, low body mass index (BMI) in these individuals may also contribute to pulmonary NTM disease (22).

AGE

Older people are more susceptible to NTM infection (41), suggesting that low systemic immunity in the elderly is causing NTM infection. Indeed, Umrao et al. showed that the annual prevalence of pulmonary NTM among adults 65 years or older significantly increased by 8.2% per year (42).

SEX

Women are 1.4 times more likely to get pulmonary NTM infection than men (43). Caucasian women in particular are more vulnerable to NTM infection (44). The observation that NTM lung infections are more common in slender, older women without any overt immune defects suggests that abnormal expression of adipokines, sex hormones, and TGF-beta may play an important role in their susceptibility (44). Leptin deficiency has also been suggested as a reason for the higher susceptibility of women to NTM infections (45).

RACE

Relative to white individuals, Asian/Pacific Islander individuals have been shown to be twice as likely to get NTM, whereas black individuals are half as likely (46,47).

IMMUNOCOMPROMISED PATIENTS

Patients who are severely immunosuppressed due to genetic disorders in the cellular immune system or treatment with immunosuppressive drugs more frequently present with NTM disease (48). Illnesses which feature immune dysregulation, such as autoimmune disorders like Sjogren's disease (49) or rheumatoid arthritis (50), and HIV infection (51) may also increase NTM.

DIAGNOSIS OF NTM LUNG DISEASE

Diagnosis of NTM lung disease requires the clinician to integrate clinical, radiographic, and microbiological data. Symptomatic patients with compatible radiographic findings should meet the microbiological criteria in order to establish a diagnosis of NTM lung disease. According to the American Thoracic Society/Infectious Diseases Society of America (ATS/IDSA) statement, two clinical criteria and one microbiological criterion need to be fulfilled to confirm the diagnosis (52).

Clinical and radiographic criteria

The clinical and radiographic criteria include (1) pulmonary symptoms (chronic cough, often with purulent sputum and sometimes haemoptysis) and systemic symptoms (malaise, fatigue, and weight loss); (2) chest radiograph to check nodular or cavity opacities; and (3) in the absence of cavitation, a high-resolution computed tomography (HRCT) to show a multifocal bronchiectasis with multiple small nodules needs to be performed. All clinical criteria need to be fulfilled for NTM diagnosis.

Microbiologic laboratory diagnosis

The isolation of NTM remains a clinical dilemma, since it exists naturally in the environment, and therefore isolation of NTM from nonsterile respiratory specimens does not mean they cause lung disease. According to ATS/IDSA (52),

for accurate microbiologic diagnosis of NTM, one out of three main criteria should be positive. These three criteria are (1) positive growth obtained from at least two separate sputum samples; (2) positive culture obtained from at least one bronchial wash or lavage; or (3) transbronchial or other lung biopsy with mycobacterial histopathological features and a positive growth for NTM, or biopsy showing mycobacterial histopathological features and a positive NTM growth with sputum or bronchial wash.

However, in cases where patients who are suspected of having NTM lung disease but do not meet the diagnostic criteria, these patients will need to be followed up until a firm diagnosis is proven. A diagnosis of NTM lung disease does not necessitate the immediate initiation of treatment. Treatment should be based on potential risks and benefits of therapy for each patient, taking into consideration age, comorbidities, and disease type.

TREATMENT OF PULMONARY NTM DISEASE

The treatment of NTM infections remains challenging due to the need for multiple antibiotic treatments for prolonged periods of time, which causes multiple drug side effects and drug–drug interactions (53), and the intrinsic problem associate with antibiotic resistance. Once treatment commences, the goal of curative therapy in NTM lung disease is 12 months of culture negativity. In some cases, surgery is needed to remove infected areas of the lung, although incidence of this procedure is rare.

Antibiotic therapy

Treatment for NTM species causing pulmonary diseases includes multiple antibiotic therapy, for example, combining clarithromycin, azithromycin, rifampin, and ethambutol, depending on the severity of disease and type of NTM. However, specific to each species, there are different therapeutic regimens, as discussed below in detail and summarized in Table 16.1.

Generally, for most slow-growing NTM, the recommended regimen consists of rifampicin (or rifabutin), ethambutol, and a macrolide antibiotic given for 18–24 months; in severe disease conditions, amikacin or streptomycin can be added to the regimen in the initial 3–6 months. For the rapid-growing species, regimens are primarily based on *in vitro* drug susceptibility test results.

1. **Treatment of pulmonary MAC disease.** MAC is the most common cause of NTM infections and may cause pulmonary or disseminated disease (54). Treatment of pulmonary NTM caused by MAC is usually 2 or 3 antibiotics for at least 12 months (55). First-line drugs include macrolides (clarithromycin or azithromycin), ethambutol, and rifamycins (rifampin, rifabutin). Adjuvant therapeutics are aminoglycosides,

Table 16.1 Treatment regimens for common pulmonary NTMs

Species	Treatment	Duration of treatment	Other treatments
MAC	Clarithromycin or azithromycin, rifampin or rifabutin, and ethambutol	1 year until the culture is negative	Aerosolized amikacin, Bedaquiline, Surgery
M. kansasii	Isoniazid, rifampin, and ethambutol	1 year until the culture is negative	Clarithromycin, Moxifloxacin, Surgery
M. xenopi	Rifampicin, isoniazid, clarithromycin and ethambutol, streptomycin (initial 3–6 months)	1 year until the culture is negative	
M. malmoense	Rifampicin, isoniazid, and ethambutol, quinolone and macrolide	1 year until the culture is negative	
M. abscessus	Intensive phase: Amikacin, cefoxitin (or imipenem) for 2–4 months, Azithromycin or clarithromycin Continuation phase: Azithromycin or clarithromycin + inhaled amikacin, clofazimine	1 year until the culture is negative	Tigecycline, Linezolid, Bedaquiline

such as streptomycin and amikacin, even aerosolized amikacin (56); fluoroquinolones (levofloxacin, moxifloxacin); and clofazimine, due to their poor outcome compared with macrolide-containing regimens. Linezolid and ketolides also have demonstrated good *in vitro* activity against MAC and other mycobacteria (57).

2. **Treatment of pulmonary *M. kansasii* disease and other slow growers.** *M. kansasii* is known to be highly pathogenic and is rarely isolated from humans in the absence of disease (58). However, *M. kansasii* is more susceptible to treatment than any other NTM. The key to successful therapy of *M. kansasii* lung disease is the presence of rifampin in a multidrug regimen (58). The current ATS recommendation for treatment of lung disease caused by *M. kansasii* is the regimen of isoniazid, rifampin, and ethambutol given daily for 18 months (52). Patients with *M. kansasii* pulmonary infection should be closely monitored with routine clinical examinations and regular sputum for smears test and cultures for mycobacteria during the treatment period. A high-dose regimen of isoniazid, rifampicin, and ethambutol is used to treat slow-growing mycobacteria. When rifampicin is resistant, ethambutol and isoniazide and sulfamethoxazole plus amikacin or streptomycin is used as the replacement therapy (59). Patients should be treated until the culture is negative for 1 year.

3. **Treatment of pulmonary *M. Abscessus* disease and other rapid growers.** *M. abscessus* is the third most frequently isolated NTM pathogen in pulmonary disease in the United States (60), isolated four times more frequently than the other rapid growers combined. *M. abscessus* has acquired the reputation of being the most infectious and drug-resistant member of the rapid growers (61). There are no drug regimens of proven or predictable efficacy for treatment of *M. abscessus* lung disease (62). For rapid growers, treatment regimens are based on *in vitro* drug susceptibility test results, with the goal of improving clinical outcomes and not complete eradication of the infection. It has been shown that multidrug regimens that include clarithromycin may cause symptomatic improvement and disease deterioration (63). Surgery of localized disease areas in addition to multidrug clarithromycin-based therapy offers the best chance for better outcomes.

INHALED ANTIBIOTICS

Use of inhaled antibiotics is increasing worldwide due to the benefits they offer: high drug concentrations at the site of infection (64), low systemic toxicity (65), and reduced systemic absorption (66). In the United States, inhaled antibiotics are used in up to 10% of patients with NTM infections (67). Current marketed inhaled antibiotics include aztreonam for inhalation solution (Cayston), tobramycin inhalation solution (such as TOBI®, Bethkis®, Kitabis Pak®), tobramycin inhalation powder (TOBI® Podhaler™) and colistimethate powder for reconstitution for nebulization (Colistin®), ciprofloxacin dry powder and liposomal ciprofloxacin for jet nebulizer (Pulmaquin™), levofloxacin solution (Aeroquin®), colistimethate powder for reconstitution (Colomycin®, Colobreathe®), vancomycin dry powder (AeroVanc™), and amphotericin B dry powder (ABIP). Additionally, injectable formulations of antibiotics such as gentamicin, tobramycin, amikacin, ceftazidime, and amphotericin are currently nebulized off label in non-CF bronchiectasis, drug-resistant pulmonary NTM infection (68).

Inhaled amikacin (Arikace, Insmed) has been granted qualified infectious disease product designation by the FDA (69). It is being assessed as a treatment for lung infections caused by NTM in CF patients. In patients with treatment-refractory pulmonary nontuberculous mycobacterial infection, the addition of inhaled amikacin was associated with microbiologic and/or symptomatic improvement (70). Although amikacin has been demonstrated to have high activity against NTM infection, its narrow toxicity index and the need for parenteral administration limit its application. Inhaled amikacin still has systemic toxicity like ototoxicity and nephrotoxicity, as shown in the clinical trials (71), which resulted in formulation of inhaled liposomal amikacin to further decrease systemic toxicity and increase its efficacy (72). It has been shown that the addition of aerosolized liposomal amikacin to standard oral antibiotic therapy for NTM infection improved the efficacy and decreased systemic toxicity (66). Encapsulation of amikacin in the liposomes also permits sustained release of high concentrations of the drug, which translates into less frequent administration and decreased systemic toxicity (65). Therefore, inhaled amikacin can reduce the amount of the drug given and decrease the number of administrations.

Inhaled liposomal amikacin *in vivo* has demonstrated similar effectiveness to almost 25% higher total dose of parenterally administered amikacin at reducing *M. avium* in the lungs (60). It achieved bactericidal levels at the site of infection without causing systemic toxicity.

DEVICES USED FOR INHALED ANTIBIOTICS

Inhaled antibiotics for the treatment of pulmonary infections are more challenging than other inhaled formulations, often due to the prolonged administration time and high dose of treatments. Nebulizers and dry powder inhalers (DPIs) are the common devices utilized for delivering antibiotics, although in NTM infection nebulizers are most commonly used (71). The type of nebulizer used for this purpose is critical to the efficiency of inhalation and deposition of the drug in the lung (72). Although traditional jet-nebulizers are still in use, new generations of nebulizers have been manufactured with better efficiency. These new nebulizers are faster and more efficient; therefore the administration time has been improved. This will result in increased patient adherence to therapy.

Two examples of these new technologies used to deliver antibiotics in NTM infection are:

1. Vibrating mesh technology (VMT) driven by piezoelectric actuators (73). Droplets generated are similar in size to the mesh aperture (usually about 2.5 μm), thus reducing heterodispersion compared with traditional nebulizers. They are also portable devices, as they can be hand-held and battery-powered. An example of this nebulizer is the eFlow (Pari Medical, UK). Tobi, Arikace®, Cayston, and Aeroquin formulation are nebulized with eFlow and eFlow Rapid nebulizers equipped with VMT technology (73).

2. Adaptive aerosol delivery (AAD) (74). This new technology only delivers medication on inhalation during the individual's breathing cycle. Devices that utilize AAD technology deliver a specific predetermined drug dose and use reduced volumes of drug because they are not continuous flow devices delivering drug throughout the inspiratory and expiratory cycle (i.e., they reduce drug wastage during exhalation). The Ineb device combines two technologies of VMT and AAD. It is used to deliver colistimethate sodium formulation to CF patients with pulmonary NTM infection (75).

Although nebulized antibiotics have been available for more than 30 years, intensive research has also focused on particle engineering for inhaled delivery of antibiotics using DPIs. Advances over the past decade in particle engineering technology have resulted in the development of antibiotic formulations delivered by DPIs (64). Current DPI formulations available in the market are tobramycin (TOBI Podhaler, Novartis Pharmaceuticals) (64,76), colistin (Colobreathe) (77), ciprofloxacin (Podhaler, Byer) (78) and amphotericin B (Podhaler, Novartis) (79). Inhaled tobramycin is delivered with a portable, capsule-based inhaler that does not require an external power source. In addition, the device is breath-actuated with low airflow resistance, and its delivery is independent of the patient's peak inspiratory flow rate, thus reducing variability in drug delivery (80). Ciprofloxacin DPI is also being evaluated for its ability to inhibit bronchiectasis exacerbation or reduce frequency of pulmonary attacks (78).

Inhaled antibiotics require high doses of drug, on the order of milligrams (i.e., Tip TOBI = 112 mg), which means patients must inhale multiple drug-containing capsules when taking their daily dose of antibiotics. Challenges facing device loading and multiple inhalation maneuvers cause lack of patients adherence, which can further result in incomplete antibiotic therapy and higher risk of re-infection for patients. Recently, Pharmaxis Limited (http://www.pharmaxis.com.au) has developed a multi-breath DPI device, the Orbital DPI®, designed to deliver high doses of dry powder antibiotics directly into the respiratory tract from a disposable, single-dose device (81,82). The use of this revolutionary device could change the way therapies requiring high payload of drug are delivered to patients.

Surgery

Pulmonary NTM infection in some patients may require surgical excision of focal pulmonary nodules (83). Lobectomy is recommended only for patients with extensive lung infection who have not responded to antibiotics in the past (83). Although surgery is considered a treatment option, it is not often used by clinicians.

Limitations of treatments in NTM lung disease

Current systemic therapy for NTM infection is limited by poor clinical response rates due to multidrug resistance, drug toxicities, and drug–drug interactions.

DRUG RESISTANCE OF NONTUBERCULOUS MYCOBACTERIA

Infections due to the NTM pathogens are difficult to treat because these mycobacteria are intrinsically resistant not only to the classical antimycobacterial drugs but also to most of the antibiotics currently available (84). Intrinsic antibiotic resistant mechanisms include slow growth, the presence of a thick impermeable cell wall (which acts as a physical size exclusion and a chemical-hydrophobic barrier), drug export systems (efflux pumps), and genetic polymorphism of targeted genes (antibiotic-modifying/inactivating enzymes) (53,85).

Some species of NTM have been shown to form biofilms, which is another successful survival strategy for these pathogens that enhances resistance to disinfectants and antimicrobial agents (86). Due to the drug resistance of NTM pathogens, a drug susceptibility test needs to be performed on the isolated species before the start of treatment (87).

DRUG TOXICITY AND SIDE EFFECTS

Many of the antibiotics for NTM infection have undesirable side effects (56). However, mild side effects can be tolerated by patients for short time periods, but it is difficult to tolerate daily nausea and vomiting for prolonged treatment periods (12–24 months). For example, amikacin is an effective drug against most NTM species, but daily or intermittent use of systemic amikacin can have undesirable adverse effects, such as ototoxicity and nephrotoxicity (76). Gastrointestinal side effects with oral antibiotics are also common. Due to severe gastrointestinal disturbances, the use of macrolides may require dose adjustment. Renal function testing is also needed, especially for aminoglycosides. Rifampin, macrolides, imipenem, or tigecycline can cause drug-induced hepatotoxicity; therefore, liver function needs to be monitored regularly (88).

DRUG–DRUG INTERACTION

Multidrug therapy for NTM infection results in inevitable drug interactions (41). Therefore, clinicians should consider drug–drug interactions following concomitant therapies, especially in elderly patients. Drug interaction may result in increased toxicity of drugs, often leading to reduced peak serum levels, which could partially explain the higher toxicity of concomitant therapies as well as poor outcomes of currently recommended treatment regimens. For example, simultaneous use of rifampin can decrease peak serum levels for macrolides and moxifloxacin (89). Clarithromycin is both a substrate for and an inhibitor of cytochrome P 3A enzymes, whereas azithromycin is not (90). Thus, azithromycin is often preferred in order to avoid drug interactions, including interactions with rifamycin. Conclusively, the medication list of patients with NTM lung disease should be reviewed before starting antimicrobial therapy, and potential drug–drug interactions should be monitored.

Drug discovery pipeline for NTM

To meet the challenges for successful NTM therapy, new drugs are needed and existing drugs must be preserved. In addition, it is necessary to improve our understanding of intrinsic and acquired drug resistance in these pathogens. Given the diversity of drug resistance mechanisms in NTM pathogens, such understanding will be achieved only through direct genomic, molecular, and clinical investigation of the various NTM diseases.

The following novel compounds have been proposed as effective agents against NTM infection and are depicted in Figure 16.1.

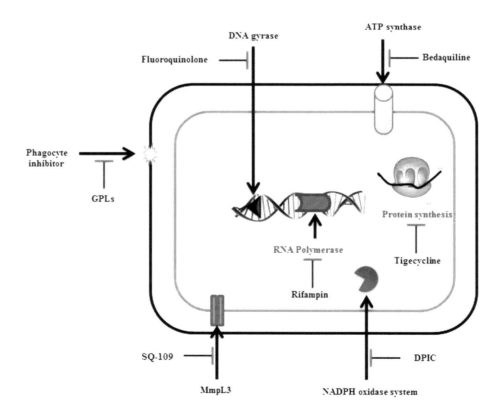

Figure 16.1 Various targets of currently utilized drugs and novel targets against NTM.

1. Diphenyleneiodonium chloride (DPIC) is an NADPH/NADH oxidase inhibitor. Singh et al. demonstrated that DPIC has a concentration-dependent bactericidal activity against *M. fortuitum* in a murine neutropenic infection model (91). DPIC caused a significant reduction in bacterial load in kidney and spleen. The reduction in bacterial count is comparable to amikacin at a 100-fold lower concentration. DPIC has not been tested on pulmonary NTM infection.

2. Surface-exposed mycobacterial glycopeptidolipids (GLPs), or GLP extracted by mechanical treatment from the outermost cell layer of the nonpathogenic *M. smegmatis*, specifically and dose dependently inhibits the phagocytosis of both *M. smegmatis* and the opportunistic pathogen *M. kansasii*. GLP is an efficient competitor of the interaction between macrophages and mycobacteria and, as such, has been tested as a novel drug for anti-NTM infections (92). GLP is the outermost molecule of the mycobacteria. The occurrence of a high amount of GLPs on the surface of mycobacteria leads to lower invasion abilities and lower internalization by macrophages.

3. Thiopeptide antibiotics are highly modified sulfur-rich peptides of ribosomal origin. They exhibit a dual mode of action against intracellular pathogens (like NTM) by affecting both host and microbe (93). They not only have innate antibacterial activity but also have been found to possess a wide range of biological properties, including anticancer (94), antiplasmodial (95), and immunosuppressive (96). Tigecycline is a member of this family and has been tested on NTM infections. A large clinical trial using tigecycline-containing regimens resulted in improvement in >60% of patients with *M. abscessus* and *M. chelonae* infections, including those with underlying CF, despite failure of prior antibiotic therapy (97). Adding tigecycline to clarithromycin regimen against *M. avium* improved clarithromycin activity and prevented clarithromycin resistance (98). Tigecycline is the first in the glycylcycline class of protein synthesis inhibitors that have been approved by the FDA since 2005 and possess antimicrobial activity against NTM (85).

4. Bedaquiline (BDQ) is the first approved antibiotic for the treatment of multidrug-resistant tuberculosis (MDR-TB) in 40 years (99). It was discovered and developed by Johnson & Johnson (100). It has been used off label for treatment of lung disease caused by MAC (101,102), targeting the ATP synthase of mycobacteria. *In vitro* activity of BDQ against rapidly growing NTM has also been confirmed (100). In the study by Aguilar et al., *in vitro* activity of BDQ against 18 rapidly growing NTM was assessed by evaluating the minimal inhibitory concentration (MIC) and minimal bactericidal concentration (MBC) against these specious. Preliminary promising results from this study demonstrated that BDQ exhibited a strong inhibitory effect against most NTM tested; however, for some NTM strains, the MBC was significantly higher than the MIC.

5. Gallium (Ga) compounds exhibit potent growth-inhibitory capacity against the ATCC strain and antibiotic-resistant clinical isolates of *M. abscessus* (103). Ga is an attractive "Trojan horse" metabolic inhibitor since it can both compete with Fe (Iron) for acquisition and inhibit Fe-dependent enzymes if it is substituted for Fe in their active sites. It is known that Fe is essential for the growth of most microorganisms, including *M. abscessus* (104).

6. DNA gyrase inhibitors (fluoroquinolones belong to this group) inhibit the supercoiling action of DNA gyrase (105). A new generation of this group (DC-159a) has been developed by Daiichi Sankyo (Japan) and has been shown to have an excellent activity against *M. tuberculosis*, and *M. kansasii* (106).

7. Dinitrobenzamide (107) and indolcarboxamides (108) are cell wall biosynthesis inhibitors primarily discovered for the treatment of tropical diseases, later have demonstrated anti-mycobacterial potency against both slow-growing and fast-growing mycobacterial species. The molecular target of these compounds is trehalose monomycolate transporter MmpL3, which is essential for mycobacterial cell wall biosynthesis. SQ-190 targets MmpL3, a membrane transporter of trehalose monomycolate involved in mycolic acid donation to the cell wall core of mycobacteria (109).

CLINICAL STUDIES OF NTM TREATMENT

So far, a review of the NIH clinical trials database showed only 15 randomized trials for the treatment of NTM pulmonary disease (either completed or currently recruiting), which were summarized in Table 16.2. With this limited number of clinical trials, it is vital that more studies examining the efficacy and safety of antibiotics regimens in treating NTM lung disease are developed and funded. Furthermore, robust multicenter trials, although costlier to conduct, would provide the patient numbers needed to conduct rigorous and adequately powered clinical trials in patients with NTM infections.

CONCLUSION

There are many challenges facing NTM infection, which represent one of the major threats to human health worldwide. These challenges can be classified as diagnostic limitations, challenges in therapeutic options, and management of disease due to microbial resistance and difficulties in development of new drugs. Delay in disease diagnosis, which varies by preexisting underlying lung diseases, requires a focus on more clinically relevant species, such as *M. avium* complex and *M. abscessus*, because there are more than 160 species of NTM and the treatment of these infections varies. Meanwhile, with advanced molecular methods, species-specific environmental niches of NTMs should be also isolated and investigated for better treatment strategies.

The lack of therapeutic options and regimens for pulmonary NTM infections makes the treatment of NTM infections even harder. Present treatment options are limited, lengthy,

Table 16.2 Summary of recent clinical trials for pulmonary NTM

Study title	Status	Intervention	Conditions	Objectives	Identifier
Clarithromycin for the Treatment of Infections Caused by NTM	Completed (2017)	Oral clarithromycin	Nontuberculous Mycobacteria; Mycobacterium avium Complex	Open Study of Clarithromycin for the Treatment of Infections Caused by Nontuberculous Mycobacteria (NTM)	NCT00600769
Interleukin-12 in the Treatment of Severe NTM Infections	Completed (2003)	Interleukin-12	Atypical Mycobacterium Infection	Safety and Effectiveness of a Interleukin-12 in Fighting Severe Infectious with NTM	NCT00001911
Arikayce for NTM	Completed (2015)	Liposomal amikacin for inhalation (LAI)	Mycobacterium Infections, Nontuberculous	Efficacy of Liposomal Amikacin for Inhalation (Arikayce®) in Patients with Recalcitrant Nontuberculous Mycobacterial Lung Disease	NCT01315236
Linezolid for Treatment of NTM	Not yet recruiting	Oral tablet of linezolid	Nontuberculous Mycobacterial Diseases	Efficacy and Tolerability of Linezolid for Treatment of NTM Disease	NCT03220074
Study to Evaluate Efficacy of LAI When Added to Multi-Drug Regimen Compared to Multi-Drug Regimen Alone	Active but not recruiting	Liposomal amikacin for inhalation	Mycobacterium Infections, Nontuberculous	Efficacy of Liposomal Amikacin for Inhalation (LAI) in Adult Patients with Pulmonary NTM Caused by Mycobacterium avium Complex (MAC) That Are Refractory to Treatment	NCT02344004
Effectiveness of Rifabutin in the Treatment of Mycobacterium avium Complex	Completed (2017)	Rifabutin	Nontuberculous Mycobacterial Infections	Clinical Efficacy of Rifabutin in the Treatment of Serious and Life-Threatening Infections Due to Mycobacterium avium Complex	NCT03164291
Treatment of Non-Tuberculous Mycobacterial Infections with Interferon Gamma	Completed (2008)	Interferon gamma	Nontuberculous Mycobacterial Infections	Treatment of Non-Tuberculous Mycobacterial Infections with Interferon Gamma	NCT00001318
Liposomal Amikacin for Inhalation (LAI) in the Treatment of Mycobacterium abscessus Lung Disease	Recruiting	LAI plus multidrug regimens	Mycobacterium Infections, Nontuberculous; Mycobacteria, Atypical	Efficacy, Safety and Tolerability of Liposomal Amikacin for Inhalation (LAI) Once Daily in the Treatment of Mycobacterium abscessus Lung Disease	NCT03038178

(Continued)

Table 16.2 (Continued) Summary of recent clinical trials for pulmonary NTM

Study title	Status	Intervention	Conditions	Objectives	Identifier
Sildenafil for Pulmonary NTM Infection	Completed (2015)	Sildenafil	Nontuberculous Mycobacterial Infections	To Study the Effect of Sildenafil on CBF and NO levels in People with PNTM Infection	NCT01853540
Treatment of Mycobacterium xenopi Pulmonary Infection	Recruiting	Clarithromycin; moxifloxacin	Atypical; Mycobacterium, Pulmonary, Tuberculous	Efficacy of Clarithromycin or Moxifloxacin Containing Regimen in 6 Months Sputum Conversion of Mycobacterium xenopi	NCT01298336
Clofazimine in the Treatment of Pulmonary Mycobacterium avium Complex (MAC)	Recruiting	Clofazimine	Mycobacterium avium Complex	Phase 2 Study of Clofazimine for the Treatment of Pulmonary Mycobacterium avium Disease	NCT02968212
Clarithromycin Versus Azithromycin in the Treatment of Mycobacterium avium Complex (MAC) Lung Infections	Not yet recruiting	Clarithromycin azithromycin rifampicin, ethambutol	Mycobacterium avium Complex	Clarithromycin versus Azithromycin in the Treatment of Mycobacterium avium Complex (MAC) Lung Infections	NCT03236987

expensive, and time consuming, with drug regimens associated with significant failure and side effects. Moreover, due to the microbial resistance, and variable treatment responses based on the NTM species, urgent novel therapeutic options are required, as are more prospective clinical studies to define suitable drug regimens for different NTM species, since many of the novel drugs being developed for treating tuberculosis mycobacteria do not exhibit any antimicrobial activity against NTM. The lack of standard animal models mimicking NTM human disease and pathology also add to this problem. Clearly, further work in the area of diagnosis, treatment, and drug development is warranted; however, for the time being, continued attention to at risk populations and strict patient adherence to the updated international treatment guidelines remain the main key to control pulmonary NTM disease.

REFERENCES

1. King HC, Khera-Butler T, James P, Oakley BB, Erenso G, Aseffa A, Knight R, Wellington EM, Courtenay O. Environmental reservoirs of pathogenic mycobacteria across the Ethiopian biogeographical landscape. *Plos One* 2017;12(3). doi:10.1371/journal.pone.0173811. PubMed PMID: WOS:000399102200025.

2. Cook JL. Nontuberculous mycobacteria: Opportunistic environmental pathogens for predisposed hosts. *Brit Med Bull 2010*;96(1):45–59. doi:10.1093/bmb/ldq035. PubMed PMID: WOS:000284637600004.

3. Floto RA, Haworth CS. The growing threat of nontuberculous mycobacteria in CF. *J Cyst Fibros*. 2015;14(1):1–2. doi:10.1016/j.jcf.2014.12.002. PubMed PMID: 25487786.

4. Jordao Junior CM, Lopes FC, David S, Farache Filho A, Leite CQ. Detection of nontuberculous mycobacteria from water buffalo raw milk in Brazil. *Food Microbiol*. 2009;26(6):658–661. doi:10.1016/j.fm.2009.04.005. PubMed PMID: 19527843.

5. Johnson MM, Odell JA. Nontuberculous mycobacterial pulmonary infections. *J Thorac Dis*. 2014;6(3):210–220. Epub 2014/03/14. doi:10.3978/j.issn.2072-1439.2013.12.24. PubMed PMID: 24624285; PMCID: PMC3949190.

6. Shahraki AH, Heidarieh P, Bostanabad SZ, Khosravi AD, Hashemzadeh M, Khandan S, Biranvand M, Schraufnagel DE, Mirsaeidi M. "Multidrug-resistant tuberculosis" may be nontuberculous mycobacteria. *Eur J Intern Med*. 2015;26(4):279–284. doi:10.1016/j.ejim.2015.03.001. PubMed PMID: WOS:000353549900019.

7. Aung TT, Yam JKH, Lin SM, Salleh SM, Givskov M, Liu SP, Lwin NC, Yang L, Beuerman RW. Biofilms of pathogenic nontuberculous mycobacteria targeted by new therapeutic approaches. *Antimicrob Agents Ch*. 2016;60(1):24–35. doi:10.1128/Aac.01509-15. PubMed PMID: WOS:000369154600004.

8. Kurahara Y, Tachibana K, Tsuyuguchi K, Suzuki K. Mixed pulmonary infection with three types of nontuberculous mycobacteria. *Internal Med*. 2013;52(4):507–510. doi:10.2169/internalmedicine.52.8907. PubMed PMID: WOS:000318244500017.

9. Losurdo G, Castagnola E, Cristina E, Tasso L, Toma P, Buffa P, Giacchino R. Cervical lymphadenitis caused by nontuberculous mycobacteria in immunocompetent children: Clinical and therapeutic experience. *Head Neck-J Sci Spec*. 1998;20(3):245–249. doi:10.1002/(Sici)1097-0347(199805)20:3 < 245::Aid-Hed10 > 3.0.Co;2-J. PubMed PMID: WOS:000073097500010.

10. Bartralot R, Pujol RM, Garcia-Patos V, Sitjas D, Martin-Casabona N, Coll P, Alomar A, Castells A. Cutaneous infections due to nontuberculous mycobacteria: Histopathological review of 28 cases. Comparative study between lesions observed in immunosuppressed patients and normal hosts. *J Cutan Pathol*. 2000;27(3):124–129. doi:10.1034/j.1600-0560.2000.027003124.x. PubMed PMID: WOS:000085540200006.

11. Gimenez-Sanchez F, Cobos-Carrascosa E, Sanchez-Forte M, Martinez-Lirola M, Lopez-Ruzafa E, Galera-Martinez R, Del Rosal-Babes T, Martinez-Gallo M. Different penetrance of disseminated infections caused by nontuberculous Mycobacteria in mendelian susceptibility to mycobacteria disease associated with a novel mutation. *Pediatr Infect Dis J*. 2014;33(3):328–330. doi:10.1097/Inf.0000000000000099. PubMed PMID: WOS:000331699000031.

12. van Ingen J, Boeree MJ, Dekhuijzen PN, van Soolingen D. Environmental sources of rapid growing nontuberculous mycobacteria causing disease in humans. *Clin Microbiol Infect*. 2009;15(10):888–893. doi:10.1111/j.1469-0691.2009.03013.x. PubMed PMID: 19845700.

13. Wei MC, Banaei N, Yakrus MA, Stoll T, Gutierrez KM, Agarwal R. Nontuberculous mycobacteria infections in immunocompromised patients single institution experience. *J Pediat Hematol Onc*. 2009;31(8):556–560. PubMed PMID: WOS:000268815000006.

14. Plongla R, Preece CL, Perry JD, Gilligan PH. Evaluation of RGM medium for isolation of nontuberculous mycobacteria from respiratory samples from patients with cystic fibrosis in the United States. *J Clin Microbiol*. 2017;55(5):1469–1477. doi:10.1128/JCM.02423-16. PubMed PMID: 28228494.

15. Pham-Huy A, Robinson JL, Tapiero B, Bernard C, Daniel S, Dobson S, Dery P, Le Saux N, Embree J, Valiquette L, Quach C. Current trends in nontuberculous mycobacteria infections in Canadian children: A pediatric investigators collaborative network on

infections in Canada (PICNIC) study. *Paed Child Healt-Can.* 2010;15(5):276–282. PubMed PMID: WOS:000278701200010.

16. Thomson R, Donnan E, Konstantinos A. Notification of nontuberculous mycobacteria: An Australian perspective. *Ann Am Thorac Soc.* 2017;14(3):318–323. doi:10.1513/AnnalsATS.201612-994OI. PubMed PMID: WOS:000397430100006.

17. Rolin SA, Sharma S, Myers JD. Prevalence and clinical significance of nontuberculous mycobacteria isolated in Cornwall, United Kingdom. *Am J Resp Crit Care.* 2011;183. PubMed PMID: WOS:000208770302690.

18. Heidarieh P, Mirsaeidi M, Hashemzadeh M, Feizabadi MM, Bostanabad SZ, Nobar MG, Shahraki AH. In vitro antimicrobial susceptibility of nontuberculous mycobacteria in Iran. *Microb Drug Resist.* 2016;22(2):172–178. doi:10.1089/mdr.2015.0134. PubMed PMID: WOS:000371872100012.

19. Koh WJ, Kwon OJ, Jeon K, Kim TS, Lee KS, Park YK, Bai GH. Clinical significance of nontuberculous mycobacteria isolated from respiratory specimens in Korea. *Chest 2006*;129(2):341–348. doi:DOI 10.1378/chest.129.2.341. PubMed PMID: WOS:000235646100021.

20. Yamanashi K, Marumo S, Fukui M, Huang CL. Nontuberculous mycobacteria infection and prognosis after surgery of lung cancer: A retrospective study. *Thorac Cardiovasc Surg.* 2016. doi:10.1055/s-0036-1584883. PubMed PMID: 27380380.

21. Lai CC, Tan CK, Chou CH, Hsu HL, Liao CH, Huang YT, Yang PC, Luh KT, Hsueh PR. Increasing incidence of nontuberculous mycobacteria, Taiwan, 2000–2008. *Emerg Infect Dis.* 2010;16(2):294–296. doi:10.3201/eid1602.090675. PubMed PMID: WOS:000274400300018.

22. Somoskovi A, Salfinger M. Nontuberculous mycobacteria in respiratory infections advances in diagnosis and identification. *Clin Lab Med.* 2014;34(2):271-+. doi:10.1016/j.cll.2014.03.001. PubMed PMID: WOS:000337643300006.

23. van Ingen J, Boeree MJ, Dekhuijzen PNR, van Soolingen D. Environmental sources of rapid growing nontuberculous mycobacteria causing disease in humans. *Clin Microbiol Infec.* 2009;15(10):888–893. doi:10.1111/j.1469-0691.2009.03013.x. PubMed PMID: WOS:000270958300002.

24. Han XY, De I, Jacobson KL. Rapidly growing mycobacteria: Clinical and microbiologic studies of 115 cases. *Am J Clin Pathol.* 2007;128(4):612–621. Epub 2007/09/19. doi:10.1309/1kb2gkyt1bueylb5. PubMed PMID: 17875513.

25. Koh WJ. Nontuberculous mycobacteria: Overview. *Microbiol Spectr.* 2017;5(1). doi:10.1128/microbiolspec. TNMI7-0024-2016. PubMed PMID: WOS:000397274600023.

26. Suomalainen S, Koukila-Kahkola P, Brander E, Katila ML, Piilonen A, Paulin L, Mattson K. Pulmonary infection caused by an unusual, slowly growing nontuberculous mycobacterium. *J Clin Microbiol.* 2001;39(7):2668–2671. doi:10.1128/Jcm.39.7.2668-2671.2001. PubMed PMID: WOS:000169586400050.

27. Kim EK, Shim TS, Kim DS. Clinical manifestations of pulmonary infection due to rapidly growing nontuberculous mycobacteria. *Chest 2003*;124(4):115s-116s. PubMed PMID: WOS:000186070400144.

28. Lee MR, Sheng WH, Hung CC, Yu CJ, Lee LN, Hsueh PR. *Mycobacterium abscessus* complex infections in humans. *Emerg Infect Dis.* 2015;21(9):1638–1646. doi:10.3201/eid2109.141634. PubMed PMID: WOS:000359894000024.

29. Hoefsloot W, van Ingen J, Andrejak C, Angeby K, Bauriaud R, Bemer P, Beylis N et al. Nontuberculous mycobacteria network European trials G. The geographic diversity of nontuberculous Mycobacteria isolated from pulmonary samples: An NTM-NET collaborative study. *Eur Respir J.* 2013;42(6):1604–1613. doi:10.1183/09031936.00149212. PubMed PMID: 23598956.

30. Bryant JM, Grogono DM, Greaves D, Foweraker J, Roddick I, Inns T, Reacher M et al. Whole-genome sequencing to identify transmission of *Mycobacterium abscessus* between patients with cystic fibrosis: A retrospective cohort study. *Lancet* (London, England). 2013;381(9877):1551–1560. Epub 2013/04/02. doi:10.1016/s0140-6736(13)60632-7. PubMed PMID: 23541540; PMCID: PMC3664974.

31. D'Antonio S, Rogliani P, Paone G, Altieri A, Alma MG, Cazzola M, Puxeddu E. An unusual outbreak of nontuberculous mycobacteria in hospital respiratory wards: Association with nontuberculous mycobacterial colonization of hospital water supply network. *Int J Mycobact.* 2016;5(2):244–247. doi:10.1016/j.ijmyco.2016.04.001. PubMed PMID: WOS:000376688000022.

32. Falkinham JO. Surrounded by mycobacteria: nontuberculous mycobacteria in the human environment. *J Appl Microbiol.* 2009;107(2):356–367. doi:10.1111/j.1365-2672.2009.04161.x. PubMed PMID: WOS:000267882800002.

33. Falkinham JO. Nontuberculous mycobacteria from household plumbing of patients with nontuberculous mycobacteria disease. *Emerg Infect Dis.* 2011;17(3):419–424. doi:10.3201/eid1703.101510. PubMed PMID: WOS:000288147000012.

34. Niederweis M, Danilchanka O, Huff J, Hoffmann C, Engelhardt H. Mycobacterial outer membranes: in search of proteins. *Trends Microbiol.* 2010;18(3):109–116. doi:10.1016/j.tim.2009.12.005. PubMed PMID: WOS:000276135500002.

35. Helguera-Repetto AC, Chacon-Salinas R, Cerna-Cortes JF, Rivera-Gutierrez S, Ortiz-Navarrete V, Estrada-Garcia I, Gonzalez-y-Merchand JA. Differential macrophage response to

slow- and fast-growing pathogenic mycobacteria. *Biomed Res Int.* 2014. doi:10.1155/2014/916521. PubMed PMID: WOS:000336586200001.

36. Holland SM. Host defense against nontuberculous mycobacterial infections. *Semin Respir Infect.* 1996;11(4):217–230. Epub 1996/12/01. PubMed PMID: 8976576.

37. Hoefsloot W, van Ingen J, Magis-Escurra C, Reijers MH, van Soolingen D, Dekhuijzen RP, Boeree MJ. Prevalence of nontuberculous mycobacteria in COPD patients with exacerbations. *J Infect.* 2013;66(6):542–545. doi:10.1016/j.jinf.2012.12.011. PubMed PMID: 23298891.

38. Chan ED, Kaminska AM, Gill W, Chmura K, Feldman NE, Bai X, Floyd CM, Fulton KE, Huitt GA, Strand MJ, Iseman MD, Shapiro L. Alpha-1-antitrypsin (AAT) anomalies are associated with lung disease due to rapidly growing mycobacteria and AAT inhibits *Mycobacterium abscessus* infection of macrophages. *Scand J Infect Dis.* 2007;39(8):690–696. Epub 2007/07/27. doi:10.1080/00365540701225744. PubMed PMID: 17654345.

39. Melia E, Freeman AF, Shea YR, Hsu AP, Holland SM, Olivier KN. Pulmonary nontuberculous mycobacterial infections in hyper-IgE syndrome. *J Allergy Clin Immunol.* 2009;124(3):617–618. doi:10.1016/j.jaci.2009.07.007. PubMed PMID: PMC2740750.

40. Noone PG, Leigh MW, Sannuti A, Minnix SL, Carson JL, Hazucha M, Zariwala MA, Knowles MR. Primary ciliary dyskinesia: Diagnostic and phenotypic features. *Am J Respir Crit Care Med.* 2004;169(4):459–467. Epub 2003/12/06. doi:10.1164/rccm.200303-365OC. PubMed PMID: 14656747.

41. Mirsaeidi M, Farshidpour M, Ebrahimi G, Aliberti S, Falkinham JO. Management of nontuberculous mycobacterial infection in the elderly. *Eur J Intern Med.* 2014;25(4):356–363. doi:10.1016/j.ejim.2014.03.008. PubMed PMID: PMC4067452.

42. Umrao J, Singh D, Zia A, Saxena S, Sarsaiya S, Singh S, Khatoon J, Dhole TN. Prevalence and species spectrum of both pulmonary and extrapulmonary nontuberculous mycobacteria isolates at a tertiary care center. *Int J Mycobact.* 2016;5(3):288–293. doi:10.1016/j.ijmyco.2016.06.008. PubMed PMID: WOS:000390941700008.

43. Mirsaeidi M, Sadikot RT. Gender susceptibility to mycobacterial infections in patients with non-CF bronchiectasis. *Int J Mycobact.* 2015;4(2):92–96. doi:10.1016/j.ijmyco.2015.05.002. PubMed PMID: WOS:000372919300002.

44. Chan ED, Iseman MD. Slender, older women appear to be more susceptible to nontuberculous mycobacterial lung disease. *Gender Med.* 2010;7(1):5–18. doi:10.1016/j.genm.2010.01.005. PubMed PMID: WOS:000275475600003.

45. Kartalija M, Ovrutsky AR, Bryan CL, Pott GB, Fantuzzi G, Thomas J, Strand MJ, et al., Patients with nontuberculous mycobacterial lung disease exhibit unique body and immune phenotypes. *Am J Resp Crit Care.* 2013;187(2):197–205. doi:10.1164/rccm.201206-1035OC. PubMed PMID: PMC5446199.

46. Honda JR, Williams D, Hasan NA, Epperson E, Reynolds PR, Davidson RM, Bankowski MJ, et al., Prevalence of environmental nontuberculous mycobacteria in the Hawaiian Islands: Absence of mycobacterium avium and predominance of mycobacterium chimaera from household biofilms and respiratory samples. *Am J Resp Crit Care.* 2015;191. PubMed PMID: WOS:000377582807080.

47. Thomas BS, Okamoto K. Role of race/ethnicity in pulmonary nontuberculous Mycobacterial disease. *Emerg Infect Dis.* 2015;21(3):544–545. doi:10.3201/eid2103.141369. PubMed PMID: PMC4344281.

48. Henkle E, Winthrop KL. Nontuberculous mycobacteria infections in immunosuppressed hosts. *Clin Chest Med.* 2015;36(1):91–99. doi:10.1016/j.ccm.2014.11.002. PubMed PMID: WOS:000350612700010.

49. Uji M, Matsushita H, Watanabe T, Suzumura T, Yamada M. [A case of primary Sjogren's syndrome presenting with middle lobe syndrome complicated by nontuberculous mycobacteriosis]. Nihon Kokyuki Gakkai zasshi. *The Journal of the Japanese Respiratory Society.* 2008;46(1):55–59. Epub 2008/02/12. PubMed PMID: 18260312.

50. Faulk TI, Hill EM, Griffith ME, Battafarano DF, Morris MJ. Rheumatoid arthritis and tracheal chondritis complicated by pulmonary nontuberculous mycobacteria infection. *Jcr-J Clin Rheumatol.* 2013;19(6):353–355. doi:10.1097/RHU.0b013e31829cf5ce. PubMed PMID: WOS:000330461800012.

51. Marinho A, Fernandes G, Carvalho T, Pinheiro D, Gomes I. Nontuberculous mycobacteria in non-AIDS patients. *Rev Port Pneumol.* 2008;14(3):323–337. PubMed PMID: WOS:000256984100001.

52. Griffith DE, Aksamit T, Brown-Elliott BA, Catanzaro A, Daley C, Gordin F, Holland SM, et al., An official ATS/IDSA statement: Diagnosis, treatment, and prevention of nontuberculous mycobacterial diseases. *Am J Respir Crit Care Med.* 2007;175(4):367–416. Epub 2007/02/06. doi:10.1164/rccm.200604-571ST. PubMed PMID: 17277290.

53. Brown-Elliott BA, Nash KA, Wallace RJ. Antimicrobial susceptibility testing, drug resistance mechanisms, and therapy of infections with nontuberculous mycobacteria. *Clin Microbiol Rev.* 2012;25(4):721. doi:10.1128/Cmr.000055-12. PubMed PMID: WOS:000309528200009.

54. Kirschner RA, Parker BC, Falkinham JO. Epidemiology of infection by nontuberculous mycobacteria: Mycobacterium-Avium,

Mycobacterium-Intracellulare, and Mycobacterium-Scrofulaceum in acid, brown-water swamps of the southeastern United States and their association with environmental variables. *Am Rev Respir Dis.* 1992;145(2):271–275. PubMed PMID: WOS:A1992HC99800007.

55. van Ingen J, Kuijper EJ. Drug susceptibility testing of nontuberculous mycobacteria. *Future Microbiol.* 2014;9(9):1095–1110. doi:10.2217/Fmb.14.60. PubMed PMID: WOS:000344177500008.

56. Davis KK, Kao PN, Jacobs SS, Ruoss SJ. Aerosolized amikacin for treatment of pulmonary Mycobacterium aviuminfections: An observational case series. *BMC Pulm Med.* 2007;7(1):2. doi:10.1186/1471-2466-7-2.

57. Berlin GW, Yatabe JAH, Lau WK, Patnaik M, Shaffer BS, Cruz PM. Antimycobacterial activity of Linezolid against selected nontuberculous species of Mycobacterium. *Clin Infect Dis.* 2001;33(7):1186. PubMed PMID: WOS:000171226900598.

58. Griffith DE. Management of disease due to *Mycobacterium kansasii*. *Clin Chest Med.* 2002;23(3):613–621, vi. Epub 2002/10/10. PubMed PMID: 12370997.

59. Tsukatani T, Suenaga H, Shiga M, Ikegami T, Ishiyama M, Ezoe T, Matsumoto K. Rapid susceptibility testing for slowly growing nontuberculous mycobacteria using a colorimetric microbial viability assay based on the reduction of water-soluble tetrazolium WST-1. *Eur J Clin Microbiol.* 2015;34(10):1965–1973. doi:10.1007/s10096-015-2438-2. PubMed PMID: WOS:000361071400006.

60. Adjemian J, Frankland TB, Daida YG, Honda JR, Olivier KN, Zelazny A, Honda S, Prevots DR. Epidemiology of nontuberculous mycobacterial lung disease and tuberculosis, Hawaii, USA. *Emerg Infect Dis.* 2017;23(3):439–447. doi:10.3201/eid2303.161827. PubMed PMID: WOS:000394830900008.

61. Petrini B. *Mycobacterium abscessus*: An emerging rapid-growing potential pathogen. *Apmis.* 2006;114(5):319–328. doi:10.1111/j.1600-0463.2006.apm_390.x.

62. Jeon K, Kwon OJ, Lee NY, Kim BJ, Kook YH, Lee SH. Antibiotic treatment of *Mycobacterium abscessus* lung disease: A retrospective analysis of 65 patients. *Am J Respir Crit Care Med.* 2009;180. doi:10.1164/rccm.200905-0704OC.

63. Nessar R, Cambau E, Reyrat JM, Murray A, Gicquel B. *Mycobacterium abscessus*: A new antibiotic nightmare. *J Antimicrob Chemoth.* 2012;67(4):810–818. doi:10.1093/jac/dkr578.

64. Hoppentocht M, Hagedoorn P, Frijlink HW, de Boer AH. Formulation of dry powder tobramycin for the twincer (Tm) high dose, disposable inhaler. *J Aerosol Med Pulm D.* 2013;26(4):A237–A238. PubMed PMID: WOS:000322439800004.

65. Biller JA, Eagle G, McGinnis JP, Micioni L, Daley CL, Winthrop KL, Ruoss SJ, et al., Efficacy of liposomal amikacin for inhalation (LAI) in achieving nontuberculous mycobacteria (NTM) culture negativity in patients whose lung infection is refractory to guideline-based therapy. *Am J Resp Crit Care.* 2015;191. PubMed PMID: WOS:000377582808530.

66. Rose SJ, Neville ME, Gupta R, Bermudez LE. Delivery of aerosolized Liposomal amikacin as a novel approach for the treatment of nontuberculous mycobacteria in an experimental model of pulmonary infection. *Plos One.* 2014;9(9):e108703. doi:10.1371/journal.pone.0108703. PubMed PMID: WOS:000345745400107.

67. Aksamit TR, O'Donnell AE, Barker A, Olivier KN, Winthrop KL, Daniels MLA, Johnson M, et al., Adult patients with bronchiectasis. *Chest.* 2017;151(5):982–992. doi:10.1016/j.chest.2016.10.055.

68. Martin AR, Finlay WH. Nebulizers for drug delivery to the lungs. *Expert Opin Drug Deliv.* 2015;12(6):889–900. doi:10.1517/17425247.2015.995087.

69. Winthrop KL, Eagle G, McGinnis JP, Micioni L, Daley CL, Ruoss SJ, Addrizzo-Harris DJ, et al., Subgroup analyses of baseline demographics and efficacy in patients with refractory nontuberculous mycobacteria (NTM) lung infection treated with liposomal amikacin for inhalation (LAI). *Am J Resp Crit Care.* 2015;191. PubMed PMID: WOS:000377582808529.

70. Daglian D, Lau S, Eagle G, McGinnis J, Micioni L, Addrizzo-Harris D. Case report of a patient with treatment-refractory nontuberculous mycobacteria (NTM) lung infection treated with once daily (QD) liposomal amikacin for inhalation (LAI). *Chest.* 2015;148(4). doi:10.1378/chest.2265301. PubMed PMID: WOS:000366134400158.

71. Quon BS, Goss CH, Ramsey BW. Inhaled antibiotics for lower airway infections. *Ann Am Thorac Soc.* 2014;11(3):425–434. doi:10.1513/AnnalsATS.201311-395FR. PubMed PMID: PMC4028738.

72. Bassetti M, Luyt CE, Nicolau DP, Pugin J. Characteristics of an ideal nebulized antibiotic for the treatment of pneumonia in the intubated patient. *Ann Intensive Care.* 2016;6. doi:10.1186/s13613-016-0140-x. PubMed PMID: WOS:000374329800002.

73. Coates AL, Denk O, Leung K, Ribeiro N, Chan J, Green M, Martin S, Charron M, Edwardes M, Keller M. Higher tobramycin concentration and vibrating mesh technology can shorten antibiotic treatment time in cystic fibrosis. *Pediatr Pulm.* 2011;46(4):401–408. doi:10.1002/ppul.21376. PubMed PMID: WOS:000288463400010.

74. Denyer J, Dyche T. The adaptive aerosol delivery (AAD) technology: Past, present, and future. *J Aerosol Med Pulm D.* 2010;23:S1–S10. doi:10.1089/jamp.2009.0791. PubMed PMID: WOS:000276413100002.

75. Mullinger, B. Inhalation therapy can be improved in CF patients by controlling the breathing pattern during inspiration. *J Cyst Fibros* 2004;3:S65

76. Wee WB, Tavernini S, Martin AR, Amirav I, Majaesic C, Finlay WH. Dry powder inhaler delivery of tobramycin in in vitro models of tracheostomized children. *J Aerosol Med Pulm D.* 2017;30(1):64−+. doi:10.1089/jamp.2016.1309. PubMed PMID: WOS:000392880300006.

77. Westerman EM, De Boer AH, Le Brun PP, Touw DJ, Roldaan AC, Frijlink HW, Heijerman HG. Dry powder inhalation of colistin in cystic fibrosis patients: A single dose pilot study. *J Cyst Fibros.* 2007;6(4):284–292. Epub 2006/12/23. doi:10.1016/j.jcf.2006.10.010. PubMed PMID: 17185047.

78. Dorkin HL, Staab D, Operschall E, Alder J, Criollo M. Ciprofloxacin DPI: A randomised, placebo-controlled, phase IIb efficacy and safety study on cystic fibrosis. *BMJ Open Respiratory Research.* 2015;2(1):e000100.

79. Shah SP, Misra A. Development of liposomal amphotericin B dry powder inhaler formulation. *Drug Deliv.* 2004;11(4):247–253. doi:10.1080/10717540490467375. PubMed PMID: WOS:000223065900004.

80. Zhu B, Padronia M, Colombo G, Phillips G, Crapper J, Young PM, Traini D. The development of a single-use, capsule-free multi-breath tobramycin dry powder inhaler for the treatment of cystic fibrosis. *Int J Pharmaceut.* 2016;514(2):392–398. doi:10.1016/j.ijpharm.2016.04.009. PubMed PMID: WOS:000387778600008.

81. Zhu B, Young PM, Ong HX, Crapper J, Flodin C, Qiao EL, Phillips G, Traini D. Tuning aerosol performance using the multibreath orbital (R) dry powder inhaler device: Controlling delivery parameters and aerosol performance via modification of puck orifice geometry. *J Pharm Sci-Us.* 2015;104(7):2169–2176. doi:10.1002/jps.24458. PubMed PMID: WOS:000356705500007.

82. Young PM, Crapper J, Philips G, Sharma K, Chan HK, Traini D. Overcoming dose limitations using the orbital((R)) multi-breath dry powder inhaler. *J Aerosol Med Pulm D.* 2014;27(2):138–147. doi:10.1089/jamp.2013.1080. PubMed PMID: WOS:000333405700009.

83. Koh WJ, Kim YH, Kwon OJ, Choi YS, Kim K, Shim YM, Kim J. Surgical treatment of pulmonary diseases due to nontuberculous mycobacteria. *J Korean Med Sci.* 2008;23(3):397–401. doi:10.3346/jkms.2008.23.3.397. PubMed PMID: WOS:000257442300007.

84. van Ingen J, Boeree MJ, van Soolingen D, Mouton JW. Resistance mechanisms and drug susceptibility testing of nontuberculousm Mycobacteria. *Drug resist update.* 2012;15(3):149–161. doi:10.1016/j.drup.2012.04.001. PubMed PMID: WOS:000307417100002.

85. Zhang ZY, Sun ZQ, Wang ZL, Wen ZL, Sun QW, Zhu ZQ, Song YZ, et al., Complete genome sequence of a novel clinical isolate, the nontuberculous mycobacterium strain JDM601. *J Bacteriol.* 2011;193(16):4300–4301. doi:10.1128/Jb.05291-11. PubMed PMID: WOS:000293222600048.

86. Aung TT, Yam JK, Lin S, Salleh SM, Givskov M, Liu S, Lwin NC, Yang L, Beuerman RW. Biofilms of pathogenic nontuberculous mycobacteria targeted by new therapeutic approaches. *Antimicrob Agents Chemother.* 2015;60(1):24–35. doi:10.1128/AAC.01509-15. PubMed PMID: 26459903; PMCID: PMC4704195.

87. Li G, Pang H, Guo Q, Huang M, Tan Y, Li C, Wei J, Xia Y, Jiang Y, Zhao X, Liu H, Zhao LL, Liu Z, Xu D, Wan K. Antimicrobial susceptibility and MIC distribution of 41 drugs against clinical isolates from China and reference strains of nontuberculous mycobacteria. *Int J Antimicrob Agents.* 2017;49(3):364–374. doi:10.1016/j.ijantimicag.2016.10.024. PubMed PMID: 28131606.

88. Egelund EF, Fennelly KP, Peloquin CA. Medications and monitoring in nontuberculous mycobacteria infections. *Clin Chest Med.* 2015;36(1):55–66. doi:10.1016/j.ccm.2014.11.001. PubMed PMID: WOS:000350612700007.

89. Huang L, Liu J, Yu X, Shi L, Liu J, Xiao H, Huang Y. Drug–drug interactions between moxifloxacin and rifampicin based on pharmacokinetics in vivo in rats. *Biomedical Chromatography: BMC.* 2016;30(10):1591–1598. Epub 2016/03/31. doi:10.1002/bmc.3726. PubMed PMID: 27028459.

90. Westphal JF. Macrolide-induced clinically relevant drug interactions with cytochrome P-450A (CYP) 3A4: An update focused on clarithromycin, azithromycin and dirithromycin. *Br J Clin Pharmacol.* 2000;50(4):285–295. doi:10.1046/j.1365-2125.2000.00261.x. PubMed PMID: PMC2015000.

91. Singh AK, Thakare R, Karaulia P, Das S, Soni I, Pandey M, Pandey AK, Chopra S, Dasgupta A. Biological evaluation of diphenyleneiodonium chloride (DPIC) as a potential drug candidate for treatment of nontuberculous Mycobacterial infections. *J Antimicrob Chemoth.* 2017;72(11):3117–3121.

92. Villeneuve C, Etienne G, Abadie V, Montrozier H, Bordier C, Laval F, Daffe M, Maridonneau-Parini I, Astarie-Dequeker C. Surface-exposed glycopeptidolipids of Mycobacterium smegmatis specifically inhibit the phagocytosis of mycobacteria by human macrophages: identification of a novel family of glycopeptidolipids. *J Biol Chem.* 2003;278(51):51291–51300. doi:10.1074/jbc. M306554200. PubMed PMID: WOS:000187206300056.

93. Zheng QF, Wang QL, Wang SF, Wu JQ, Gao Q, Liu W. Thiopeptide Antibiotics exhibit a dual mode of action against intracellular pathogens by affecting both host and microbe. *Chem Biol.* 2015;22(8):1002–1007. doi:10.1016/j.chembiol.2015.06.019. PubMed PMID: WOS:000361879200006.

94. Nicolaou KC, Zak M, Rahimipour S, Estrada AA, Lee SH, O'Brate A, Giannakakou P, Ghadiri MR. Discovery of a biologically active thiostrepton fragment. *J Am Chem Soc.* 2005;127(43):15042–15044. Epub 2005/10/27. doi:10.1021/ja0552803. PubMed PMID: 16248640.

95. Schoof S, Pradel G, Aminake MN, Ellinger B, Baumann S, Potowski M, Najajreh Y, Kirschner M, Arndt HD. Antiplasmodial thiostrepton derivatives: Proteasome inhibitors with a dual mode of action. *Angewandte Chemie* (International ed in English). 2010;49(19):3317–3321. Epub 2010/04/02. doi:10.1002/anie.200906988. PubMed PMID: 20358566.

96. Ueno M, Furukawa S, Abe F, Ushioda M, Fujine K, Johki S, Hatori H, Ueda H. Suppressive effect of antibiotic siomycin on antibody production. *J. Antibiot.* 2004;57(9):590–596. Epub 2004/12/08. PubMed PMID: 15580960.

97. Wallace RJ, Dukart G, Brown-Elliott BA, Griffith DE, Scerpella EG, Marshall B. Clinical experience in 52 patients with tigecycline-containing regimens for salvage treatment of *Mycobacterium abscessus* and Mycobacterium chelonae infections. *J Antimicrob Chemoth.* 2014;69(7):1945–1953. doi:10.1093/jac/dku062. PubMed PMID: PMC4054987.

98. Bax HI, Bakker-Woudenberg IAJM, ten Kate MT, Verbon A, de Steenwinkel JEM. Tigecycline potentiates clarithromycin activity against Mycobacterium avium in vitro. *Antimicrob Agents Ch.* 2016;60(4):2577–2579. doi:10.1128/Aac.02864-15. PubMed PMID: WOS:000376496100084.

99. Mahajan R. Bedaquiline: First FDA-approved tuberculosis drug in 40 years. *Int J Appl Basic Med Res.* 2013;3(1):1–2. doi:10.4103/2229-516X.112228. PubMed PMID: PMC3678673.

100. Aguilar-Ayala DA, Cnockaert M, Andre E, Andries K, Gonzalez YMJA, Vandamme P, Palomino JC, Martin A. In vitro activity of bedaquiline against rapidly growing nontuberculous mycobacteria. *J Med Microbiol.* 2017;66(8):1140–1143. Epub 2017/07/28. doi:10.1099/jmm.0.000537. PubMed PMID: 28749330.

101. Yadav S, Rawal G, Baxi M. Bedaquiline: a novel antitubercular agent for the treatment of multidrug-resistant tuberculosis. *J Clin Diagn Res.* 2016;10(8):Fm1–Fm2. doi:10.7860/Jcdr/2016/19052.8286. PubMed PMID: WOS:000397978800043.

102. Philley JV, Wallace RJ, Jr., Benwill JL, Taskar V, Brown-Elliott BA, Thakkar F, Aksamit TR, Griffith DE. Preliminary results of bedaquiline as salvage therapy for patients with nontuberculous Mycobacterial lung disease. *Chest.* 2015;148(2):499–506. Epub 2015/02/13. doi:10.1378/chest.14-2764. PubMed PMID: 25675393; PMCID: PMC4694173.

103. Abdalla MY, Switzer BL, Goss CH, Aitken ML, Singh PK, Britigan BE. Gallium compounds exhibit potential as new therapeutic agents against *Mycobacterium abscessus. Antimicrob Agents Ch.* 2015;59(8):4826–4834. doi:10.1128/AAC.00331-15. PubMed PMID: PMC4505262.

104. De Voss JJ, Rutter K, Schroeder BG, Barry CE. Iron acquisition and metabolism by mycobacteria. *J Bacteriol.* 1999;181(15):4443–4451. PubMed PMID: WOS:000081706100001.

105. Hooper DC, Jacoby GA. Topoisomerase inhibitors: Fluoroquinolone mechanisms of action and resistance. *Csh Perspect Med.* 2016;6(9):a025320. doi:10.1101/cshperspect.a025320. PubMed PMID: WOS:000388317500006.

106. Sekiguchi J, Disratthakit A, Maeda S, Doi N. Characteristic resistance mechanism of mycobacterium tuberculosis to DC-159a, a new respiratory quinolone. *Antimicrob Agents Ch.* 2011;55(8):3958–3960. doi:10.1128/Aac.00417-10. PubMed PMID: WOS:000292733800044.

107. Batt SM, Jabeen T, Bhowruth V, Quill L, Lund PA, Eggeling L, Alderwick LJ, Futterer K, Besra GS. Structural basis of inhibition of mycobacterium tuberculosis DprE1 by benzothiazinone inhibitors. *P Natl Acad Sci USA.* 2012;109(28):11354–11359. doi:10.1073/pnas.1205735109. PubMed PMID: WOS:000306642100066.

108. Kozikowski AP, Onajole OK, Stec J, et al., Targeting mycolic acid transport by indole-2-carboxamides for the treatment of *Mycobacterium abscessus* infections. *J Med Chem.* 2017;60(13):5876–5888. doi:10.1021/acs.jmedchem.7b00582. PubMed PMID: WOS:000405764900041.

109. Tahlan K, Wilson R, Kastrinsky DB, et al., SQ109 targets MmpL3, a membrane transporter of trehalose monomycolate involved in mycolic acid donation to the cell wall core of mycobacterium tuberculosis. *Antimicrob Agents Chemother.* 2012;56(4):1797–1809. Epub 2012/01/19. doi:10.1128/aac.05708-11. PubMed PMID: 22252828; PMCID: PMC3318387.

17

Inhalational therapies for non-cystic fibrosis bronchiectasis

ASHVINI DAMODARAN, DUSTIN R. FRAIDENBURG, AND ISRAEL RUBINSTEIN

Introduction	291
Influence of bronchiectasis pathophysiology on aerosol deposition	292
Aerosolized medications in the treatment of non-CF bronchiectasis	293
Acute exacerbations	293
Eradication therapy	294
Long-term inhaled antibiotic therapy	294
Aminoglycosides	295
Colistin	295
Fluoroquinolones	295
Bronchodilator and inhaled corticosteroid therapy	296
Inhaled bronchodilators	296
Inhaled corticosteroids	296
Mucoactive agents	296
Expectorant agents	296
Mucokinetic agents	296
Mucoregulators	297
Conclusion	297
References	297

INTRODUCTION

Clinical bronchiectasis is defined as chronic bronchial sepsis in the setting of irreversibly damaged and dilated bronchi. Bronchiectasis has an extensive list of etiologies that includes cystic fibrosis (CF), congenital defects, aspiration injury, severe pneumonia, immune deficiency, asthma, allergic bronchopulmonary aspergillosis, and primary bronchiolar disorders, among others (Table 17.1). CF is the most common inherited form of bronchiectasis worldwide and much research has identified both the unique pathophysiology as well as distinct therapies, both systemic and inhaled. The cystic fibrosis and inhaled therapies are discussed in Chapter 13 separately, and this chapter will focus on the etiologies that make up non–CF bronchiectasis, which share both clinical and pathogenic features.

The pathogenesis of bronchiectasis is described by Cole's vicious cycle model: an inflammatory response to a pulmonary infection leads to partial destruction of the airways, which results in mucus stasis and hence chronic infection and inflammation. The primary goal of therapy is to disrupt this cycle of inflammation, mucus stasis, and chronic infection (1). In adults, *Haemophilus influenzae* is the most common colonizer, followed by *Pseudomonas aeruginosa*, and bacterial colonization has been linked to higher rates of exacerbations and hospitalizations, poorer lung function, and diminished quality of life (2–4). Treatment options for management of bronchiectasis have been studied extensively in the CF population; whereas the research done on bronchiectasis due to other causes is limited. As a result, justification of many of the clinical practices on the non-CF bronchiectasis population put forth by the British Thoracic Society (BTS) and the European Respiratory Society (ERS) are derived mostly from either expert opinion or extrapolated from studies done on the CF population, with some exceptions. This chapter will focus on the role of aerosolized medications in the treatment of non-CF bronchiectasis. It will specifically discuss the impact the pathophysiology of this disease has on aerosol deposition as well as antimicrobial and adjunctive aerosolized medications for treating acute exacerbations and ameliorating chronic symptoms related to this disease.

Table 17.1 Causes of bronchiectasis

Cystic fibrosis (CF)
Ciliary dysfunction
    Primary ciliary dyskinesia
    Congenital bronchiectasis
Aspiration
    Foreign body aspiration
    Gastric aspiration
Inhalation of smoke or other noxious gases
Infections
    Previous severe lower respiratory tract infections
    Mycobacterial infections
Immune deficiencies
    Primary antibody deficiency syndromes
        Common variable immunodeficiency syndrome
        X-linked agammaglobulinemia
        IgA deficiency
    Secondary immunodeficiency syndromes
Asthma
Allergic bronchopulmonary aspergillosis
Autoimmune diseases
    Rheumatoid arthritis
    Systemic sclerosis
    Systemic lupus erythematosus
    Ankylosing spondylitis
Connective tissue diseases
    Marfan's disease
    Ehlers-Danlos syndrome
    Mounier-Kuhn syndrome (tracheobronchomegaly)
    Relapsing polychondritis
    Williams-Campbell syndrome (cartilage deficiency)
Inflammatory bowel diseases
    Crohn's disease
    Ulcerative colitis
    Celiac disease
Alpha-1 antitrypsin deficiency
Yellow nail syndrome
Young's syndrome

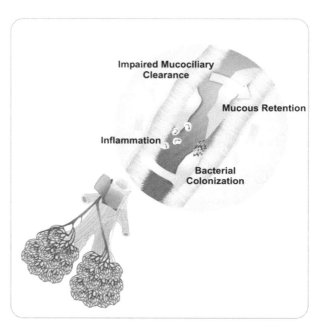

Figure 17.1 The pathogenesis of bronchiectasis. The pathogenic model proposed by Cole et al. (5) depicts an inciting event causing an inflammatory response which leads to structural damage to the airways and impaired mucociliary clearance. This milieu favors retained mucous and creates an environment that predisposes to bacterial colonization which then promotes sustained inflammation, thus creating a vicious cycle leading to the disease state.

INFLUENCE OF BRONCHIECTASIS PATHOPHYSIOLOGY ON AEROSOL DEPOSITION

The development of bronchiectasis involves a series of events that lead to what we know as the "vicious cycle" in the development of bronchiectasis (Figure 17.1). In this schema, inflammation induces a response from the host, causing destruction of the airway tissue, which in turn contributes to impaired defenses and mucous clearance that leads to bacterial colonization and further bronchial inflammation (5). These pathologic features of the bronchiectasis have important implications in aerosol delivery and deposition in the diseased lung.

Both the aerosol particle size and inspiratory flow rate are important factors in delivery and distribution of any inhaled therapy (6). Particles that are less than or equal to 1 μm may be eliminated during exhalation, resulting in less

lung deposition; particles that are greater than 5 μm are deposited predominately in the oropharynx, never reaching the airways (7). The presence of bronchiectasis is often associated with airflow limitations due to increased mucous secretion, chronic inflammation, and airway hyperreactivity. The presence of airflow obstruction has a significant impact on the deposition of aerosol particles in the lung (8,9). The optimal particle size for airway deposition in those with severe airflow obstruction may be somewhat larger than in a normal host (8). Despite this, subjects with CF and airflow obstruction have shown increased aerosol deposition, based on decreased exhaled concentrations, which is thought to relate to impairment in expiratory flow and volume (9). The distribution of these aerosols seems to be less uniform and favor the large, central airways in these subjects with bronchiectasis (9,10). Therefore, in the diseased lung, the areas that are most severely affected may receive the least amount of aerosol deposition (11). The high variability of aerosol deposition in the lung of CF patients can be improved by controlling the breathing pattern of these patients to target a minute ventilation of 12–5 L/min during nebulization (12). The high variability of aerosol delivery and deposition based on particle size and flow rate highlights the importance of controlled breathing and careful formulation of inhaled aerosols.

Aerosol drug absorption and clearance are also important considerations related to the effect of any therapeutic agent. Mucociliary clearance is an important part of the innate immunity providing a defense against bacteria and other foreign material in the bronchi. This mechanism indiscriminately clears particles from the lung and has been shown to transport mucus containing drug upward at a speed of 20 cm/h, clearing 80% of undissolved particles within 24 hours (13). This mechanism is impaired in bronchiectasis as a result of both increased mucous production and abnormal ciliary function (5,14). This impaired mucociliary clearance is shown to decrease the clearance of aerosolized drugs from the central airways, and aerosolized particles are predominately eliminated through coughing (15). Mucous plugs in the bronchi and bronchioles may prevent deposition to the small airways, which are often the site of chronic infection and thus may limit the effect of inhaled antimicrobial agents (9). Pseudomonas aeruginosa, the most common identified bacterial colonizer in bronchiectasis, also has host defenses that include formation of mucoid biofilms that may protect from penetration of aerosolized therapies. Absorption of aerosolized therapies can also be affected by the pathologic features of bronchiectasis. Increased mucous production can be thought to create a barrier to systemic absorption of aerosolized agents, while airway inflammation and epithelial injury is shown to impair barrier function and increase permeability (16).

The pathophysiologic features of bronchiectasis can have dramatic effects on aerosol delivery and deposition.

Development of inhaled therapies must take into account the impact of chronic airflow obstruction, uneven distribution of ventilation, impaired mucociliary clearance, and abnormal absorption on drug delivery.

AEROSOLIZED MEDICATIONS IN THE TREATMENT OF NON-CF BRONCHIECTASIS

Inhalation therapy is capable of directly targeting the airways, creating a higher and more sustained local tissue concentration and thereby increasing the therapeutic index, improving efficacy, minimizing toxicities, and decreasing the time of onset for the administered drug. As described above, many factors are related to aerosol particle engineering, drug delivery, and pathogenic features of bronchiectasis that can affect the overall efficacy of inhaled therapies. Despite this, it is clear that these inhaled therapies can be used either alone or as an adjunct to conventional systemic treatment in order to maximize the benefit to the patient (Table 17.2).

Acute exacerbations

An acute exacerbation of bronchiectasis is generally characterized as deterioration of respiratory symptoms related to the underlying bronchiectasis over several days. However,

Table 17.2 Inhaled therapies for management of stable bronchiectasis

Therapeutic goal	Indication for treatment	Available inhaled therapies
Eradicate P. aeruginosa	• Consider eradication therapy in those patients with new P. aeruginosa colonization (2 positive cultures at least 3 months apart) • Inhaled antibiotic therapy in combination with systemic therapy in patients who failed initial treatment with oral or IV antibiotic or who are at high risk of failure	Aminoglycosides (tobramycin gentamycin, and amikacin) Colistin Fluoroquinolones
Minimize bacterial burden	• Consider long-term antibiotic therapy for patients with >/= 3 exacerbations per year • Consider inhaled antibiotics for patients who have failed standard therapy or in patients at high risk of failure due to multidrug resistance	Aminoglycosides (tobramycin gentamycin, and amikacin) Colistin Fluoroquinolones
Address airway obstruction	Early use of bronchodilators recommended in symptomatic patients only	β_2 agonists Anticholinergics Inhaled corticosteroids (for those with moderate to severe airways obstruction)
Facilitate airway clearance	Consider after failing standard airway clearance strategies *Recombinant human DNAse contraidicated in non-CF bronchiectasis	Expectorants Hypertonic saline Mannitol Mucokinetics Terbutaline β_2 agonists Mucoregulator/Mucolytic Bromhexine Erdosteine

until recently, there have been no strict diagnostic criteria for an acute exacerbation of bronchiectasis, making the existing clinical studies difficult to compare. The classic symptoms and signs of an acute exacerbation include increases in cough severity and frequency; increased sputum volume and purulence; wheezing; worsening dyspnea; and, in severe cases, hypoxemia (Table 17.3). Other symptoms and signs may include hemoptysis, worsening spirometry results, and radiographic changes (17,18). In 2017, BTS formally defined an acute exacerbation of bronchiectasis as "a person with bronchiectasis with a deterioration in three or more of the following key symptoms for at least 48 h: cough; sputum volume and/or consistency; sputum purulence, breathlessness and/or exercise tolerance; fatigue and/or malaise; haemoptysis AND a clinician determines that a change in bronchiectasis treatment is required" (19). It is important to distinguish these symptoms from the chronic but stable daily symptoms and signs that many of these patients suffer, including mucopurulent cough and persistently positive sputum cultures for respiratory pathogens, as antibiotic therapy is not mandated in many of such patients. The current BTS guidelines recommend first empirically treating patients with an oral antibiotic and then narrowing therapy to treat the culprit organisms cultured in the sputum. Beta-lactam treatment is preferred because the most common organism is *H. influenza*, but ciprofloxacin or another quinolone should be given if *P. aeruginosa* is a concern (20). ERS guidelines recommend treatment duration of at least 14 days, regardless of which antibiotic regimen is chosen (21). There are very few studies that examine the use of inhaled antibiotics in these patients, and the results from these studies are mixed. A study examining the use of inhaled carbenicillin plus oral probenecid for 7–17 days found that 12 of the 15 subjects with severe acute exacerbations secondary to *P. aeruginosa* who had failed therapy with up to four courses of antibiotics had showed mild to significant clinical improvement as well as eradication of *P. aeruginosa* in their sputum at 2 months (22). A larger, double-blind randomized control trial involving 53 subjects analyzed the addition of inhaled tobramycin to oral ciprofloxacin to treat acute exacerbations, again secondary to *P. aeruginosa*. This study found that after 21 days of therapy, there was no statistically significant difference in clinical improvement between the two groups. The study did find that the percentage of

patients with negative sputum cultures at the end of the study was higher in the experimental arm compared to the placebo arm, but again this difference was not statistically significant in this small study group (23). Based on the limited evidence, inhaled antimicrobial therapy is often employed in combination with systemic antimicrobial agents after failure of an initial regimen or in the presence of multidrug resistant pathogens in which there is a concern for failure of systemic antimicrobial treatment.

Eradication therapy

Due to impaired mucociliary function and compromised innate antimicrobial mechanisms, patients with bronchiectasis are particularly prone to bacterial colonization (Table 17.4). The majority of these patients are eventually colonized with common upper respiratory bacteria such as *H. influenza*, *S. pneumoniae*, and *M. catarrhalis*, but some are colonized with the opportunistic bacterium *P. aeruginosa* (24,25). *P. aeruginosa* poses unique treatment difficulties due to its ability to form protective biofilms, thus sheltering it from innate immune defenses and barricading it away from systemic antibiotics (26). Moreover, chronic infection with *P. aeruginosa* has been associated with poorer mortality outcomes, increased hospitalization rates, increased exacerbation frequency, and worsening lung function (27). It is currently recommended that eradication of *P. aeruginosa* be attempted on patients with a new diagnosis of bacterial colonization (i.e., at least two sputum cultures positive for *P. aeruginosa* at least 3 months apart). This recommendation does not yet extend to those patients who have had known colonization for many years (21). It is based largely on two recent studies, one retrospective and one prospective, that examined the efficacy of systemic antibiotics plus nebulized antibiotics for patients with *P. aeruginosa* chronic infection. Both studies found that eradication therapy was associated with fewer exacerbations and lower hospitalization rates (28,29). Treatment of chronic colonization with other bacterial species to eradicate them from the sputum is not currently recommended.

Long-term inhaled antibiotic therapy

The goals of long-term therapy in this patient population are to (1) control chronic symptoms, (2) prevent exacerbations, and (3) preserve lung function (20). A number of

Table 17.3 Common symptoms seen in bronchiectasis exacerbations

Increased cough
Increased wheezing
Increased sputum production
Increased sputum purulence
Worsening dyspnea
Hemoptysis
Chest pain
Hemoptysis

Table 17.4 Most common organisms associated with bronchiectasis exacerbations

Streptococcus pneumoniae
Haemophilus influenza
Moraxella catarrhalis
Methicillin-sensitive *Staphylococcus aureus*
Methicillin-resistant *Staphylococcus aureus*
Coliforms (Klebsiella, Enterobacter)
Pseudomonas aeruginosa

studies have shown that long-term antibiotic use can help decrease the frequency and duration of lower respiratory illnesses, as well as improve functional status and quality of life, decrease bacterial burden, and suppress ongoing inflammation (24,30,31). Current guidelines recommend considering long-term antibiotic therapy in those patients who have either three or more exacerbations per year that require antibiotic therapy, or those who suffer from severe symptoms at baseline. The choice of antibiotic should be based on sensitivities determined from sputum cultures. Oral antibiotics should be attempted first, but inhaled antibiotics can be considered if oral therapy fails (20,21). The first-line therapy for chronic inhaled antibiotic use in this population is inhaled aminoglycosides administered as a cycle of 28 days of therapy followed by a 28-day inhaled drug holiday. The evidence supporting this practice stems from literature from the CF population (32). In adults, a number of studies have investigated the use of long-term nebulized antibiotics, the caveat to all of these studies being that there are no high-powered randomized placebo-controlled trials investigating the efficacy of nebulized antibiotics in the long-term management of non-CF bronchiectasis.

AMINOGLYCOSIDES

Aminoglycosides are a class of bactericidal antibiotics that were first isolated from *Streptomyces* and *Micromonospora*. The primary mechanism of action is disrupting protein synthesis through irreversible inhibition of the 30S ribosomal subunit, and have activity primarily against gram-negative bacilli. Though their use declined after the development of beta lactams, aminoglycosides are still often used for severe gram-negative infections and *P. aeruginosa* in particular. The serious side effects of nephrotoxicity, ototoxicity, and neurotoxicity of aminoglycosides is the primary reason why its use has declined compared to beta lactams, which are seen to have a more favorable side effect profile. Aminoglycosides have multiple possible routes of administration, with tobramycin being the most common nebulized agent in the class (33).

To date, one of the more extensively studied antibiotics for the long-term treatment of non-CF bronchiectasis is nebulized tobramycin in patients chronically infected with *P. aeruginosa*. Inhaled tobramycin has been shown to decrease bacterial load and symptom severity, but it has been associated with higher rates of intolerance due to bronchospasms and has not been shown to improve lung function (34–36). Inhaled gentamicin has also been shown to be effective in reducing bacterial load and symptoms without affecting pulmonary function (37). These agents remain the most commonly utilized class of inhaled antimicrobials in non-CF bronchiectasis.

COLISTIN

Developed in the 1940s, colistin is a polymyxin antibiotic and is one of the oldest antibiotics in use. Its use declined significantly after other antibiotic classes were discovered,

but it has experienced a recent rise in popularity due to the increase of drug-resistant bacteria and the dearth of novel antibiotics on the market. Colistin is a bactericidal antibiotic that acts by disrupting the cellular membrane through binding of lipopolysaccharide (LPS), and it is also known to neutralize endotoxins. It acts in a concentration-dependent manner mostly against aerobic gram-negative bacilli, but its use has been especially of interest against multidrug-resistant bacteria, namely, *P. aeruginosa*, *Acinetobacter baumanni*, *Klebsiella pneumoniae*, and *Stenotrophomonas maltophilia*. The two forms of colistin available are colistin sulfate and its prodrug, colisthimetate sodium. The drug's nephrotoxic effects are the most common side effect seen, though it has also been known to cause neurotoxicity, bronchospasm, and hypersensitivity pneumonitis (38). In its nebulized form, colistin has been shown to reduce exacerbations with good adherence to therapy, improve lung function and quality of life, reduce sputum volume and bacterial load, and generally be well tolerated (39–41).

FLUOROQUINOLONES

Fluoroquinolones are a class of synthetic broad-spectrum bactericidal antimicrobial agents that act by inhibiting DNA gyrase and topoisomerase IV (42). Originally developed to treat urinary tract infections, these drugs now have a diverse array of clinical indications that include bacterial prostatitis and sexually transmitted infections, in addition to infections involving the gastrointestinal system, skin, bone, joints, and respiratory tract (43). In the respiratory tract, fluoroquinolones are active against many organisms, notably *P. aeruginosa*, *H. influenza*, *Legionella pneumophila*, and mycobacterial infections (44). There are a number of recently completed and ongoing clinical trials examining the use of ciprofloxacin in this population. The ORBIT-2 trial was a phase II, multicenter, randomized, double-blind placebo-controlled trial that studied the use of nebulized dual-release liposomal ciprofloxacin in 42 subjects with ciprofloxacin-sensitive *P. aeruginosa*. Those subjects treated with nebulized ciprofloxacin had a delayed time to first pulmonary exacerbation, decreased bacterial density in their sputum, and similar incidence of systemic adverse events compared to placebo (31). This has now been followed up with two phase III clinical trials, RESPIRE 1 showed a significantly longer time to first exacerbation and decreased frequency of exacerbations in patients from Europe, North and South America, Australia and Japan who were treated with a 14-day course of inhaled ciprofloxacin (45). RESPIRE 2 failed to show a significant benefit with a 14-day course of inhaled ciprofloxacin (46). Both trials also showed a trend to benefit in patients treated with a 28-day course of inhaled ciprofloxacin though this did not reach statistical significance. An FDA advisory committee has therefore not recommended approval of ciprofloxacin dry powder inhalation for the treatment of non-CF bronchiectasis.

Bronchodilator and inhaled corticosteroid therapy

Bronchiectasis is not considered an indication for bronchodilator and/or inhaled corticosteroid (ICS) therapy. In general, ICS therapy is limited to those patients who have evidence of airflow obstruction on pulmonary function testing, while β_2-agonists therapy can be considered in certain patients who are severely symptomatic (20,21).

INHALED BRONCHODILATORS

Inhaled β_2-adrenergic agonists and anticholinergics improve dyspnea by reducing bronchoconstriction. β_2-agonists have the added benefit of promoting ciliary beating to facilitate mucus clearance, and anticholinergics decrease mucus production by inhibiting glandular secretion (47–49). The use of these agents has been studied extensively in the asthma and COPD population, but not as much in the non-CF bronchiectasis patient population. There is one small study that illustrated an improvement in lung function after bronchodilator use, but, to date, there are no randomized control trials investigating the use of bronchodilators in this population (50,51). Nevertheless, the ERS suggests considering the use of long-acting bronchodilators when patients are severely dyspneic. Bronchodilators should also be considered prior to inhaled antibiotic and mucolytic administration, as well as before physiotherapy, to increase medication deposition and activity tolerance, respectively (21).

INHALED CORTICOSTEROIDS

Like inhaled bronchodilators, ICSs have a role in the management of asthma and COPD. Their potential role in management of non-CF bronchiectasis has been of interest, particularly because of the importance of airway inflammation in the pathophysiology of the disease. However, the evidence showing meaningful clinical benefit is minimal. ICS use has been associated with reduced leukocyte density and other inflammatory markers in sputum without an effect on bacterial density (52). It has also been shown to decrease sputum volume and increase quality-of-life measures, but not significantly improve lung function or frequency of exacerbations (53–55). Therefore, current recommendations advocate not routinely using ICS medications in non-CF bronchiectasis patients (21).

Mucoactive agents

Promoting airway clearance of mucus is one of the primary objectives of bronchiectasis management. Mucoactive agents in conjunction with chest physiotherapy are particularly essential for those patients with chronic productive cough or mucus plugging as seen on high-resolution computed tomography (HRCT) imaging because it decreases the frequency of coughing by augmenting mucociliary clearance (20). The mucoactive agents used in non-CF bronchiectasis can be divided into expectorants, mucokinetic agents, and mucoregulators (Figure 17.2) (56).

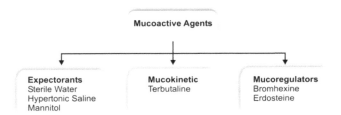

Figure 17.2 Mucoactive aerosols as therapy for bronchiectasis. The three categories of mucoactive agents in the therapeutic arsenal for treatment of bronchiectasis include expectorants, mucokinetics, and mucoregulators. Expectorants decrease sputum osmolality improving clearance. The mucokinetic agent terbutaline improves ciliary function to impact mucous clearance while mucoregulators affect sputum production and viscosity. These agents are often used in combination to improve mucous clearance and improve both symptoms and quality of life for patients with bronchiectasis.

EXPECTORANT AGENTS

Expectorant agents include sterile water, normal saline, hypertonic saline, and mannitol. Long-term use of humidified air with sterile water has been demonstrated to be a cost-effective way to reduce frequency and duration of exacerbations, increase forced expiratory volume in one second (FEV1) and forced vital capacity (FVC), and improve quality-of-life scores (57,58). Nebulized saline formulations improve ciliary clearance of sputum by decreasing sputum osmolality in bovine trachea models and can help increase the expectorated amount of sputum during chest physiotherapy (59,60). Hypertonic saline in particular has also been associated with immunomodulating effects, with one study showing a reduction of IL-8 concentrations in the sputum of CF patients (61). Clinically, the use of normal saline and hypertonic saline has been shown to improve quality of life, healthcare utilization rates, lung function, and changes in bacterial colonization, although the data on the superiority of one over the other are mixed (62,63). Mannitol is another osmotic agent that has been shown to improve mucus clearance in a dose-dependent fashion (64,65). In a 52-week, double-blind, randomized control trial involving 485 subjects from 84 centers worldwide, inhaled mannitol 400 mg twice daily was compared to a control of inhaled mannitol 50 mg twice daily (previously shown to not have significant clinical benefit). There was no significant difference in exacerbation rates, lung function, and sputum weight between the two groups, but the treatment group did show significantly longer time to exacerbation and more improvement in quality-of-life measures compared to the control group (66).

MUCOKINETIC AGENTS

β_2-adrenergic agonists, as described above, are thought primarily to affect bronchoconstriction and the airflow limitation identified in severe forms of bronchiectasis, yet these agents also have an important impact on mucociliary clearance. Terbutaline can help improve sputum production when administered before chest physiotherapy (60), and its β_2-adrenergic properties have the added benefit of improving sputum clearance by inducing bronchodilation and stimulating ciliary beat frequency by increasing intracellular cAMP levels (67,68). This is shown to be a class effect in preclinical models with agents such as albuterol, salmeterol, and salbutamol, all shown to improve ciliary beat frequency (48,69), yet the clinical effects with respect to mucokinetic action in non-CF bronchiectasis patients is not known.

MUCOREGULATORS

Agents that affect the structure or secretion of mucous glycoproteins include mucolytic, secretolytic, and proteolytic enzymes. Many oral agents have been explored and used to varying degrees in the treatment of non-CF bronchiectasis, including glucocorticoids and macrolide antibiotics, but they will not be discussed in this chapter. Of the inhaled mucolytics available, only bromhexine and erdosteine have been shown to have clinical benefit (70). In one study, bromhexine use increased ease of expectoration and decreased sputum production and cough severity, but did not significantly change lung function compared to placebo (71). Similarly, in a small pilot study comparing erdosteine plus chest physiotherapy versus physiotherapy alone, the treatment group exhibited improvement in sputum purulence and small but statistically significant improvements in lung function when compared to the control group (72).

There is an extensive body of evidence highlighting the benefits of recombinant human DNase (rhDNase) therapy in the CF population. These studies have shown rhDNase is a fairly well-tolerated and cost-effective way to improve lung function, and may also improve quality of life and decrease frequency of exacerbations (73–75). The benefit stems from the rhDNase reducing the viscosity of the sputum by degrading the DNA released from neutrophils, thereby easing sputum clearance independent of chest physical therapy (76,77). However, similar investigations into the utility of rhDNase in non-CF bronchiectasis have failed to show similar benefit in this population and may even cause harm; therefore, they are contraindicated in these patients (20,70). A double-blind, randomized, placebo-controlled and multicenter study involving 349 adult patients with stable idiopathic bronchiectasis investigated the use of twice-daily administration 2.5 mg of aerosolized rhDNase over 24 weeks compared to placebo. The rhDNase group had a statistically significant decline in FEV1 and FVC in addition to increased hospitalization rate and antibiotic use. The rhDNase subjects also had a higher rate of exacerbations, though that difference was not statistically significant (78). The different effect of rhDNase in non-CF bronchiectasis may be due to the lower level of DNA in the sputum compared to CF sputum as well as the regional involvement of CF compared to non-CF bronchiectasis (79).

CONCLUSION

Non-CF bronchiectasis includes numerous entities that share common clinical and pathologic features characterized by bronchial inflammation with structural damage, impaired mucociliary clearance, bacterial colonization, and recurrent infection. Inhalational therapies are now a mainstay in the treatment of this disease as they are seen to have direct activity at the site of injury, producing high concentration of drug and pharmacologic activity while minimizing systemic effects and adverse outcomes. Inhaled antimicrobial agents are often used either alone or in combination with systemic agents in severe infections or those that have not responded to oral antimicrobials alone. These inhaled antimicrobials are shown to create high drug concentrations at the site of infection and in many studies have shown improved antibacterial activity and clinical outcomes. Inhaled bronchodilators and ICS therapy can have effects on quality of life in select patients, but routine use is not recommended and there is both limited evidence and mixed results regarding the beneficial effects of these agents. Agents that are routinely considered as inhalational therapies are the mucoactive agents, including expectorants, mucokinetics, and mucoregulators. These agents are employed to facilitate mucous clearance through cough and ciliary function and can be used as a single agent or in combination. There are many different inhalational therapies that, together with systemic therapies, create a dynamic therapeutic arsenal to fight this morbid condition. The nature of bronchiectasis being such a diverse entity requires that these therapies be individualized and that the evidence be used accordingly within populations to give the best chance of improved length and quality of life.

REFERENCES

1. McShane PJ, Naureckas ET, Tino G, Strek ME. Non-cystic fibrosis bronchiectasis. *American Journal of Respiratory and Critical Care Medicine*. 2013;188(6):647–656. doi:10.1164/rccm.201303-0411CI. PubMed PMID: 23898922.

2. Davies G, Wells AU, Doffman S, Watanabe S, Wilson R. The effect of *Pseudomonas aeruginosa* on pulmonary function in patients with bronchiectasis. *The European Respiratory Journal*. 2006;28(5):974–979. doi:10.1183/09031936.06.00074605. PubMed PMID: 16899482.

3. King PT, Holdsworth SR, Freezer NJ, Villanueva E, Holmes PW. Microbiologic follow-up study in adult bronchiectasis. *Respiratory Medicine*. 2007;101(8):1633–1638. doi:10.1016/j.rmed.2007.03.009. PubMed PMID: 17467966.

4. Wilson CB, Jones PW, O'Leary CJ, Hansell DM, Cole PJ, Wilson R. Effect of sputum bacteriology on the quality of life of patients with bronchiectasis. *The European Respiratory Journal*. 1997;10(8):1754–1760. PubMed PMID: 9272915.

5. Cole PJ. Inflammation: A two-edged sword--the model of bronchiectasis. *European Journal of Respiratory Diseases Supplement*. 1986;147:6–15. PubMed PMID: 3533593.

6. Laube BL, Jashnani R, Dalby RN, Zeitlin PL. Targeting aerosol deposition in patients with cystic fibrosis: Effects of alterations in particle size and inspiratory flow rate. *Chest*. 2000;118(4):1069–1076. PubMed PMID: 11035679.

7. Kuhn RJ. Pharmaceutical considerations in aerosol drug delivery. *Pharmacotherapy*. 2002;22(3 Pt 2):80S-5S. PubMed PMID: 11898885.

8. Zanen P, Go LT, Lammers JW. Optimal particle size for beta 2 agonist and anticholinergic aerosols in patients with severe airflow obstruction. *Thorax*. 1996;51(10):977–980. PubMed PMID: 8977595; PubMed Central PMCID: PMC472643.

9. Anderson PJ, Blanchard JD, Brain JD, Feldman HA, McNamara JJ, Heyder J. Effect of cystic fibrosis on inhaled aerosol boluses. *The American Review of Respiratory Disease*. 1989;140(5):1317–1324. doi:10.1164/ajrccm/140.5.1317. PubMed PMID: 2817594.

10. Smaldone GC, Messina MS. Flow limitation, cough, and patterns of aerosol deposition in humans. *Journal of Applied Physiology*. 1985;59(2):515–520. doi:10.1152/jappl.1985.59.2.515. PubMed PMID: 4030604.

11. Lourenco RV, Loddenkemper R, Carton RW. Patterns of distribution and clearance of aerosols in patients with bronchiectasis. *The American Review of Respiratory Disease*. 1972;106(6):857–866. doi:10.1164/arrd.1972.106.6.857. PubMed PMID: 4641221.

12. Ilowite JS, Gorvoy JD, Smaldone GC. Quantitative deposition of aerosolized gentamicin in cystic fibrosis. *The American Review of Respiratory Disease*. 1987;136(6):1445–1449. doi:10.1164/ajrccm/136.6.1445. PubMed PMID: 3688646.

13. Backman P, Adelmann H, Petersson G, Jones CB. Advances in inhaled technologies: Understanding the therapeutic challenge, predicting clinical performance, and designing the optimal inhaled product. *Clinical Pharmacology and Therapeutics*. 2014;95(5):509–520. doi:10.1038/clpt.2014.27. PubMed PMID: 24503626.

14. Rossman CM, Lee RM, Forrest JB, Newhouse MT. Nasal ciliary ultrastructure and function in patients with primary ciliary dyskinesia compared with that in normal subjects and in subjects with various respiratory diseases. *The American Review of Respiratory Disease*. 1984;129(1):161–167. doi:10.1164/arrd.1984.129.1.161. PubMed PMID: 6703474.

15. Isawa T, Teshima T, Hirano T, Anazawa Y, Miki M, Konno K et al. Mucociliary clearance and transport in bronchiectasis: Global and regional assessment.

Journal of Nuclear Medicine: Official Publication, Society of Nuclear Medicine. 1990;31(5):543–548. PubMed PMID: 2341890.

16. Olson N, Greul AK, Hristova M, Bove PF, Kasahara DI, van der Vliet A. Nitric oxide and airway epithelial barrier function: Regulation of tight junction proteins and epithelial permeability. *Archives of Biochemistry and Biophysics*. 2009;484(2):205–213. doi:10.1016/j.abb.2008.11.027. PubMed PMID: 19100237; PubMed Central PMCID: PMC2753865.

17. Brill SE, Patel AR, Singh R, Mackay AJ, Brown JS, Hurst JR. Lung function, symptoms and inflammation during exacerbations of non-cystic fibrosis bronchiectasis: A prospective observational cohort study. *Respiratory Research*. 2015;16:16. doi:10.1186/s12931-015-0167-9. PubMed PMID: 25849856; PubMed Central PMCID: PMC4324878.

18. Chang AB, Bilton D. Exacerbations in cystic fibrosis: 4—non-cystic fibrosis bronchiectasis. *Thorax*. 2008;63(3):269–276. doi:10.1136/thx.2006.060913. PubMed PMID: 18308962.

19. Hill AT, Haworth CS, Aliberti S, Barker A, Blasi F, Boersma W et al. Pulmonary exacerbation in adults with bronchiectasis: A consensus definition for clinical research. *The European Respiratory Journal*. 2017;49(6). doi:10.1183/13993003.00051-2017. PubMed PMID: 28596426.

20. Pasteur MC, Bilton D, Hill AT. British thoracic society bronchiectasis non CFGG. British thoracic society guideline for non-CF bronchiectasis. *Thorax*. 2010;65 Suppl 1:i1–58. doi:10.1136/thx.2010.136119. PubMed PMID: 20627931.

21. Polverino E, Goeminne PC, McDonnell MJ, Aliberti S, Marshall SE, Loebinger MR et al. European respiratory society guidelines for the management of adult bronchiectasis. *The European Respiratory Journal*. 2017;50(3). doi:10.1183/13993003.00629-2017. PubMed PMID: 28889110.

22. Pines A, Raafat H, Siddiqui GM, Greenfield JS. Treatment of severe pseudomonas infections of the bronchi. *British Medical Journal*. 1970;1(5697):663–665. PubMed PMID: 4986284; PubMed Central PMCID: PMC1700575.

23. Bilton D, Henig N, Morrissey B, Gotfried M. Addition of inhaled tobramycin to ciprofloxacin for acute exacerbations of *Pseudomonas aeruginosa* infection in adult bronchiectasis. *Chest*. 2006;130(5):1503–1510. doi:10.1378/chest.130.5.1503. PubMed PMID: 17099030.

24. Chalmers JD, Smith MP, McHugh BJ, Doherty C, Govan JR, Hill AT. Short- and long-term antibiotic treatment reduces airway and systemic inflammation in non-cystic fibrosis bronchiectasis. *American Journal of Respiratory and Critical Care Medicine*. 2012;186(7):657–665. doi:10.1164/rccm.201203-0487OC. PubMed PMID: 22744718.

25. Whitters D, Stockley R. Immunity and bacterial colonisation in bronchiectasis. *Thorax.* 2012;67(11):1006–1013. doi:10.1136/thoraxjnl-2011-200206. PubMed PMID: 21933944.

26. Chalmers JD, Hill AT. Mechanisms of immune dysfunction and bacterial persistence in non-cystic fibrosis bronchiectasis. *Molecular Immunology.* 2013;55(1):27–34. doi:10.1016/j.molimm.2012.09.011. PubMed PMID: 23088941.

27. Finch S, McDonnell MJ, Abo-Leyah H, Aliberti S, Chalmers JD. A comprehensive analysis of the impact of *Pseudomonas aeruginosa* colonization on prognosis in adult bronchiectasis. *Annals of the American Thoracic Society.* 2015;12(11):1602–1611. doi:10.1513/AnnalsATS.201506-333OC. PubMed PMID: 26356317.

28. Orriols R, Hernando R, Ferrer A, Terradas S, Montoro B. Eradication therapy against *Pseudomonas aeruginosa* in non-cystic fibrosis bronchiectasis. *Respiration: International Review of Thoracic Diseases.* 2015;90(4):299–305. doi:10.1159/000438490. PubMed PMID: 26340658.

29. White L, Mirrani G, Grover M, Rollason J, Malin A, Suntharalingam J. Outcomes of *Pseudomonas* eradication therapy in patients with non-cystic fibrosis bronchiectasis. *Respiratory Medicine.* 2012;106(3):356–360. doi:10.1016/j.rmed.2011.11.018. PubMed PMID: 22204744.

30. Altenburg J, de Graaff CS, Stienstra Y, Sloos JH, van Haren EH, Koppers RJ et al. Effect of azithromycin maintenance treatment on infectious exacerbations among patients with non-cystic fibrosis bronchiectasis: The BAT randomized controlled trial. *JAMA.* 2013;309(12):1251–1259. doi:10.1001/jama.2013.1937. PubMed PMID: 23532241.

31. Serisier DJ, Bilton D, De Soyza A, Thompson PJ, Kolbe J, Greville HW et al. Inhaled, dual release liposomal ciprofloxacin in non-cystic fibrosis bronchiectasis (ORBIT-2): A randomised, double-blind, placebo-controlled trial. *Thorax.* 2013;68(9):812–817. doi:10.1136/thoraxjnl-2013-203207. PubMed PMID: 23681906; PubMed Central PMCID: PMC4770250.

32. Ramsey BW, Pepe MS, Quan JM, Otto KL, Montgomery AB, Williams-Warren J et al. Intermittent administration of inhaled tobramycin in patients with cystic fibrosis. Cystic Fibrosis Inhaled Tobramycin Study Group. *The New England Journal of Medicine.* 1999;340(1):23–30. doi:10.1056/NEJM199901073400104. PubMed PMID: 9878641.

33. Avent ML, Rogers BA, Cheng AC, Paterson DL. Current use of aminoglycosides: Indications, pharmacokinetics and monitoring for toxicity. *Internal Medicine Journal.* 2011;41(6):441–449. doi:10.1111/j.1445-5994.2011.02452.x. PubMed PMID: 21309997.

34. Barker AF, Couch L, Fiel SB, Gotfried MH, Ilowite J, Meyer KC et al. Tobramycin solution for inhalation reduces sputum *Pseudomonas aeruginosa* density in bronchiectasis. *American Journal of Respiratory and Critical Care Medicine.* 2000;162(2 Pt 1):481–485. doi:10.1164/ajrccm.162.2.9910086. PubMed PMID: 10934074.

35. Couch LA. Treatment with tobramycin solution for inhalation in bronchiectasis patients with *Pseudomonas aeruginosa.* *Chest.* 2001;120(3 Suppl):114S-7S. PubMed PMID: 11555565.

36. Scheinberg P, Shore E. A pilot study of the safety and efficacy of tobramycin solution for inhalation in patients with severe bronchiectasis. *Chest.* 2005;127(4):1420–1426. doi:10.1378/chest.127.4.1420. PubMed PMID: 15821224.

37. Murray MP, Govan JR, Doherty CJ, Simpson AJ, Wilkinson TS, Chalmers JD et al. A randomized controlled trial of nebulized gentamicin in non-cystic fibrosis bronchiectasis. *American Journal of Respiratory and Critical Care Medicine.* 2011;183(4):491–499. doi:10.1164/rccm.201005-0756OC. PubMed PMID: 20870753.

38. Yahav D, Farbman L, Leibovici L, Paul M. Colistin: New lessons on an old antibiotic. *Clinical Microbiology and Infection: The Official Publication of the European Society of Clinical Microbiology and Infectious Diseases.* 2012;18(1):18–29. doi:10.1111/j.1469-0691.2011.03734.x. PubMed PMID: 22168320.

39. Dhar R, Anwar GA, Bourke SC, Doherty L, Middleton P, Ward C et al. Efficacy of nebulised colomycin in patients with non-cystic fibrosis bronchiectasis colonised with *Pseudomonas aeruginosa.* *Thorax.* 2010;65(6):553. doi:10.1136/thx.2008.112284. PubMed PMID: 20522858.

40. Haworth CS, Foweraker JE, Wilkinson P, Kenyon RF, Bilton D. Inhaled colistin in patients with bronchiectasis and chronic *Pseudomonas aeruginosa* infection. *American Journal of Respiratory and Critical Care Medicine.* 2014;189(8):975–982. doi:10.1164/rccm.201312-2208OC. PubMed PMID: 24625200; PubMed Central PMCID: PMC4098097.

41. Steinfort DP, Steinfort C. Effect of long-term nebulized colistin on lung function and quality of life in patients with chronic bronchial sepsis. *Internal Medicine Journal.* 2007;37(7):495–498. doi:10.1111/j.1445-5994.2007.01404.x. PubMed PMID: 17547727.

42. Cheng G, Hao H, Dai M, Liu Z, Yuan Z. Antibacterial action of quinolones: From target to network. *European Journal of Medicinal Chemistry.* 2013;66:555–562. doi:10.1016/j.ejmech.2013.01.057. PubMed PMID: 23528390.

43. Hooper DC, Wolfson JS. Fluoroquinolone antimicrobial agents. *The New England Journal of Medicine.* 1991;324(6):384–394. doi:10.1056/NEJM199102073240606. PubMed PMID: 1987461.

44. Appelbaum PC, Hunter PA. The fluoroquinolone antibacterials: Past, present and future perspectives. *International Journal of Antimicrobial Agents.* 2000;16(1):5–15. PubMed PMID: 11185413.

45. De Soyza A, Asamit T, Bandel TJ, Criollo M, Elborn JS, Operschall E et al. RESPIRE 1: A phase III placebo-controlled randomised trial of ciprofloxacin dry powder for inhalation in non-cystic fibrosis bronchiectasis. *European Respiratory Journal.* 2018;51(1):1702052. doi:10.1183/13993003.02052-2017. PubMed PMID: 29371383.

46. Aksamit T, De Soyza A, Bandel TJ, Criollo M, Elborn JS, Operschall E et al. RESPIRE 2: A phase III placebo-controlled randomised trial of ciprofloxacin dry powder for inhalation in non-cystic fibrosis bronchiectasis. *European Respiratory Journal.* 2018;51(1):1702053. doi:10.1183/13993003.02053-2017. PubMed PMID: 29371384.

47. Cazzola M, Page CP, Rogliani P, Matera MG. Beta2-agonist therapy in lung disease. *American Journal of Respiratory and Critical Care Medicine.* 2013;187(7):690–696. doi:10.1164/rccm.201209-1739PP. PubMed PMID: 23348973.

48. Devalia JL, Sapsford RJ, Rusznak C, Toumbis MJ, Davies RJ. The effects of salmeterol and salbutamol on ciliary beat frequency of cultured human bronchial epithelial cells, in vitro. *Pulmonary Pharmacology.* 1992;5(4):257–263. PubMed PMID: 1362105.

49. Moulton BC, Fryer AD. Muscarinic receptor antagonists, from folklore to pharmacology: Finding drugs that actually work in asthma and COPD. *British Journal of Pharmacology.* 2011;163(1):44–52. doi:10.1111/j.1476-5381.2010.01190.x. PubMed PMID: 21198547; PubMed Central PMCID: PMC3085867.

50. Hassan JA, Saadiah S, Roslan H, Zainudin BM. Bronchodilator response to inhaled beta-2 agonist and anticholinergic drugs in patients with bronchiectasis. *Respirology.* 1999;4(4):423–426. PubMed PMID: 10612580.

51. Lasserson T, Holt K, Evans D, Greenstone M. Anticholinergic therapy for bronchiectasis. *The Cochrane Database of Systematic Reviews.* 2001(4):CD002163. doi:10.1002/14651858.CD002163. PubMed PMID: 11687147.

52. Tsang KW, Ho PL, Lam WK, Ip MS, Chan KN, Ho CS et al. Inhaled fluticasone reduces sputum inflammatory indices in severe bronchiectasis. *American Journal of Respiratory and Critical Care Medicine.* 1998;158(3):723–727. doi:10.1164/ajrccm.158.3.9710090. PubMed PMID: 9730996.

53. Elborn JS, Johnston B, Allen F, Clarke J, McGarry J, Varghese G. Inhaled steroids in patients with bronchiectasis. *Respiratory Medicine.* 1992;86(2):121–124. PubMed PMID: 1615177.

54. Martinez-Garcia MA, Perpina-Tordera M, Roman-Sanchez P, Soler-Cataluna JJ. Quality-of-life determinants in patients with clinically stable bronchiectasis. *Chest.* 2005;128(2):739–745. doi:10.1378/chest.128.2.739. PubMed PMID: 16100162.

55. Tsang KW, Tan KC, Ho PL, Ooi GC, Ho JC, Mak J et al. Inhaled fluticasone in bronchiectasis: A 12 month study. *Thorax.* 2005;60(3):239–243. doi:10.1136/thx.2002.003236. PubMed PMID: 15741443; PubMed Central PMCID: PMC1747352.

56. Balsamo R, Lanata L, Egan CG. Mucoactive drugs. *European Respiratory Review: An Official Journal of the European Respiratory Society.* 2010;19(116):127–133. doi:10.1183/09059180.00003510. PubMed PMID: 20956181.

57. Milne RJ, Hockey H, Rea H. Long-term air humidification therapy is cost-effective for patients with moderate or severe chronic obstructive pulmonary disease or bronchiectasis. *Value in Health: The Journal of the International Society for Pharmacoeconomics and Outcomes Research.* 2014;17(4):320–327. doi:10.1016/j.jval.2014.01.007. PubMed PMID: 24968990.

58. Rea H, McAuley S, Jayaram L, Garrett J, Hockey H, Storey L et al. The clinical utility of long-term humidification therapy in chronic airway disease. *Respiratory Medicine.* 2010;104(4):525–533. doi:10.1016/j.rmed.2009.12.016. PubMed PMID: 20144858.

59. Shibuya Y, Wills PJ, Cole PJ. Effect of osmolality on mucociliary transportability and rheology of cystic fibrosis and bronchiectasis sputum. *Respirology.* 2003;8(2):181–185. PubMed PMID: 12753533.

60. Sutton PP, Gemmell HG, Innes N, Davidson J, Smith FW, Legge JS et al. Use of nebulised saline and nebulised terbutaline as an adjunct to chest physiotherapy. *Thorax.* 1988;43(1):57–60. PubMed PMID: 3353875; PubMed Central PMCID: PMC461097.

61. Reeves EP, Williamson M, O'Neill SJ, Greally P, McElvaney NG. Nebulized hypertonic saline decreases IL-8 in sputum of patients with cystic fibrosis. *American Journal of Respiratory and Critical Care Medicine.* 2011;183(11):1517–1523. doi:10.1164/rccm.201101-0072OC. PubMed PMID: 21330456.

62. Kellett F, Robert NM. Nebulised 7% hypertonic saline improves lung function and quality of life in bronchiectasis. *Respiratory Medicine.* 2011;105(12):1831–1835. doi:10.1016/j.rmed.2011.07.019. PubMed PMID: 22018993.

63. Nicolson CH, Stirling RG, Borg BM, Button BM, Wilson JW, Holland AE. The long term effect of inhaled hypertonic saline 6% in non-cystic fibrosis bronchiectasis. *Respiratory Medicine.* 2012;106(5):661–667. doi:10.1016/j.rmed.2011.12.021. PubMed PMID: 22349069.

64. Daviskas E, Anderson SD, Eberl S, Chan HK, Bautovich G. Inhalation of dry powder mannitol improves clearance of mucus in patients with bronchiectasis. *American Journal of Respiratory and Critical Care Medicine.* 1999;159(6):1843–1848. doi:10.1164/ajrccm.159.6.9809074. PubMed PMID: 10351929.

65. Daviskas E, Anderson SD, Eberl S, Young IH. Effect of increasing doses of mannitol on mucus clearance in patients with bronchiectasis. *The European Respiratory Journal.* 2008;31(4):765–772. doi:10.1183/09031936.00119707. PubMed PMID: 18057051.

66. Bilton D, Tino G, Barker AF, Chambers DC, De Soyza A, Dupont LJ et al. Inhaled mannitol for non-cystic fibrosis bronchiectasis: A randomised, controlled trial. *Thorax.* 2014;69(12):1073–1079. doi:10.1136/thoraxjnl-2014-205587. PubMed PMID: 25246664.

67. Salathe M. Effects of beta-agonists on airway epithelial cells. *The Journal of Allergy and Clinical Immunology.* 2002;110(6 Suppl):S275–S281. PubMed PMID: 12464936.

68. Shiima-Kinoshita C, Min KY, Hanafusa T, Mori H, Nakahari T. Beta 2-adrenergic regulation of ciliary beat frequency in rat bronchiolar epithelium: Potentiation by isosmotic cell shrinkage. *The Journal of Physiology.* 2004;554(Pt 2):403–416. doi:10.1113/jphysiol.2003.056481. PubMed PMID: 14594991; PubMed Central PMCID: PMC1664781.

69. Frohock JI, Wijkstrom-Frei C, Salathe M. Effects of albuterol enantiomers on ciliary beat frequency in ovine tracheal epithelial cells. *Journal of Applied Physiology.* 2002;92(6):2396–2402. doi:10.1152/japplphysiol.00755.2001. PubMed PMID: 12015353.

70. Wilkinson M, Sugumar K, Milan SJ, Hart A, Crockett A, Crossingham I. Mucolytics for bronchiectasis. *The Cochrane Database of Systematic Reviews.* 2014(5):CD001289. doi:10.1002/14651858.CD001289.pub2. PubMed PMID: 24789119.

71. Olivieri D, Ciaccia A, Marangio E, Marsico S, Todisco T, Del Vita M. Role of bromhexine in exacerbations of bronchiectasis. Double-blind randomized multicenter study versus placebo. *Respiration: International Review of Thoracic Diseases.* 1991;58(3–4):117–121. PubMed PMID: 1745841.

72. Crisafulli E, Coletti O, Costi S, Zanasi E, Lorenzi C, Lucic S et al. Effectiveness of erdosteine in elderly patients with bronchiectasis and hypersecretion: A 15-day, prospective, parallel, open-label, pilot study. *Clinical Therapeutics.* 2007;29(9):2001–2009. doi:10.1016/j.clinthera.2007.09.003. PubMed PMID: 18035199.

73. Fuchs HJ, Borowitz DS, Christiansen DH, Morris EM, Nash ML, Ramsey BW et al. Effect of aerosolized recombinant human DNase on exacerbations of respiratory symptoms and on pulmonary function in patients with cystic fibrosis. The Pulmozyme Study Group. *The New England Journal of Medicine.* 1994;331(10):637–642. doi:10.1056/NEJM199409083311003. PubMed PMID: 7503821.

74. Harms HK, Matouk E, Tournier G, von der Hardt H, Weller PH, Romano L et al. Multicenter, open-label study of recombinant human DNase in cystic fibrosis patients with moderate lung disease. DNase International Study Group. *Pediatric Pulmonology.* 1998;26(3):155–161. PubMed PMID: 9773909.

75. Yang C, Chilvers M, Montgomery M, Nolan SJ. Dornase alfa for cystic fibrosis. *The Cochrane Database of Systematic Reviews.* 2016;4:CD001127. doi:10.1002/14651858.CD001127.pub3. PubMed PMID: 27043279.

76. Laube BL, Auci RM, Shields DE, Christiansen DH, Lucas MK, Fuchs HJ et al. Effect of rhDNase on airflow obstruction and mucociliary clearance in cystic fibrosis. *American Journal of Respiratory and Critical Care Medicine.* 1996;153(2):752–760. doi:10.1164/ajrccm.153.2.8564129. PubMed PMID: 8564129.

77. Shak S, Capon DJ, Hellmiss R, Marsters SA, Baker CL. Recombinant human DNase I reduces the viscosity of cystic fibrosis sputum. *Proceedings of the National Academy of Sciences of the United States of America.* 1990;87(23):9188–9192. PubMed PMID: 2251263; PubMed Central PMCID: PMC55129.

78. O'Donnell AE, Barker AF, Ilowite JS, Fick RB. Treatment of idiopathic bronchiectasis with aerosolized recombinant human DNase I. rhDNase Study Group. *Chest.* 1998;113(5):1329–1334. PubMed PMID: 9596315.

79. Wills PJ, Wodehouse T, Corkery K, Mallon K, Wilson R, Cole PJ. Short-term recombinant human DNase in bronchiectasis. Effect on clinical state and in vitro sputum transportability. *American Journal of Respiratory and Critical Care Medicine.* 1996;154(2 Pt 1):413–417. doi:10.1164/ajrccm.154.2.8756815. PubMed PMID: 8756815.

18

Pulmonary fibrosis

PRIYA MURALIDHARAN, DON HAYES, Jr., AND HEIDI M. MANSOUR

Introduction	303	Pulmonary fibrosis models	306
Idiopathic pulmonary fibrosis	303	Inhaled therapies for IPF	306
Cystic fibrosis and pulmonary fibrosis	304	Future of IPF research	308
Pharmacological interventions	304	References	310

INTRODUCTION

Chronic respiratory diseases dramatically affect quality of life for patients, particularly because they limit their physical ability to perform simple activities of daily living, even limiting their ability to walk. Respiratory diseases can be identified as obstructive or restrictive diseases. Obstructive diseases are often associated with airway limitation due to narrowed, damaged, or diseased airways. It affects the person's ability to exhale air normally. Inhalation is not generally affected; however, the breathing rate is affected since the exhalation rate can't keep up with the inhalation rate. As a result, the patient is often left with a feeling of incomplete breathing or, in other words, feeling "out of breath." A classic example of obstructive disease is a chronic obstructive pulmonary disease (COPD); other diseases include asthma, bronchiectasis, and cystic fibrosis (CF). In restrictive respiratory diseases, on the other hand, the patient can inhale and exhale at the same rate, but the lungs can't expand fully, which can be due to scarring or weak muscles or stiffness of the chest wall or damaged nerves, and so on. Examples of restrictive diseases include interstitial lung diseases (idiopathic pulmonary fibrosis [IPF]) and sarcoidosis.

In general, fibrosis is excess deposition of connective tissues that can lead to scarring and thickening of the affected tissues. Fibrosis is intended to be the body's response to an injury or damage, but when exaggerated, it leads to a pathological condition that can eventually obliterate the structure and function of the underlying organ. Fibrosis occurs in many parts of the body, such as the lungs (pulmonary fibrosis), liver (cirrhosis), heart (cardiac fibrosis), kidney (renal fibrosis), and so on.

As is evident from the name, *pulmonary fibrosis* is scarring of the lungs, categorized as chronic fibrosing interstitial lung disease (ILD). It is characterized by an excessive accumulation of scar tissue in the alveolar walls, thereby making gaseous exchange difficult, and hence reducing oxygen delivery into the circulation. Figure 18.1 is a schematic representation of the alveolar region in pulmonary fibrosis. The changes to the interstitial space can be noted in the figure. This difficulty in gas exchange is manifested as shortness of breath or trouble in breathing, particularly during walking and/or exercising (conditions where the body has excess oxygen demand).

Pulmonary fibrosis can have the following causes:

- Occupational exposure to, for example, silica, beryllium
- Toxicity of drugs such as methotrexate, amiodarone, nitrofurantoin
- Connective tissue disease like scleroderma
- Idiopathic with unknown etiology

IDIOPATHIC PULMONARY FIBROSIS

Idiopathic pulmonary fibrosis (IPF) is the most common and fatal form of pulmonary fibrosis. Its prevalence in the United States is estimated to be 42.7 per 100,000 persons on a broad definition (1). IPF is defined as "a specific form of chronic, progressive fibrosing interstitial pneumonia of unknown cause, occurring primarily in older adults, limited to the lungs and associated with the histopathological and/or radiologic pattern of usual interstitial pneumonia (UIP)" (2). It is a subclass of ILD with unknown etiology.

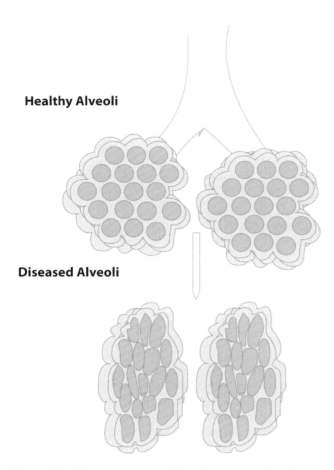

Healthy Alveoli

Diseased Alveoli

Figure 18.1 Representation of the changes in alveolar region during pulmonary fibrosis.

The incidence of IPF increases with age, with definitive diagnosis possible between the ages of 60 and 70 years. The global prevalence and incidence of IPF are unclear; however, it has been reported that the prevalence of IPF is increasing worldwide (3,4). This is mainly because it is difficult to diagnose IPF: the symptoms overlap with other chronic lung diseases such as emphysema. Therefore, in 2011, the American Thoracic Society (ATS), in collaboration with the European Respiratory Society (ERS), the Japanese Respiratory Society (JRS), and the Latin American Thoracic Association (ALAT), developed an evidence-based guideline for diagnosis and management of IPF. It requires three characteristics for a diagnosis of IPF: (1) exclusion of other known causes of interstitial lung disease (for example, hazardous exposure, connective tissue disease, drug toxicity), (2) the presence of UIP pattern on high-resolution computed tomography (HRCT), and (3) surgical lung biopsy pattern (2).

CYSTIC FIBROSIS AND PULMONARY FIBROSIS

It is important to understand the difference between the two main fibrotic diseases occurring in the lungs, which are pulmonary fibrosis (PF) and cystic fibrosis (CF). As previously

mentioned, PF is a progressive scarring of lungs localized to one organ (lungs), while CF is a progressive genetic disease affecting many exocrine secretory glands of the body, including the pancreas, lungs, liver, intestine, and reproductive system. CF is caused by mutation of the genes responsible for the production of a protein called cystic fibrosis transmembrane conductance regulator (CFTR). Defective CTFR gene results in thick and sticky mucus. When mucus in the airway is affected, it leads to poor mucociliary clearance, and the patient is susceptible to repeated lung infections. On the other hand, the progression of the scar tissue in PF leads to the impaired gas exchange, diminished lung function, limited physical ability to perform exercise, poor quality of life, and ultimately death. It is reported that the survival rate of IPF is worse than some cancers (5). CF is an inherited disease that can be diagnosed at any age depending on the severity of the symptoms; symptoms usually do not show up until the teen years or early adulthood. In contrast, PF is primarily a disease seen mostly in patients older than 50 years. No ethnic specificity has been identified for PF, while northern European Caucasians are identified to be at higher risk of inheriting CF. Medical advances in the treatment and care of CF have improved the quality of life for CF patients. Specifically, lung transplant can extend the life of patients and encourage them to do things that they enjoy, such as exercising (6,7). Transplant improves quality of life and potentially extends the life of some patients with CF; however, other organs in the body remain affected by CF and thus patients require chronic care for the duration of their lives. It is important to weigh the benefits against the risks of having a lung transplant since it is a physical, emotional, and financially challenging process (8–10).

PHARMACOLOGICAL INTERVENTIONS

Despite the etiology of IPF remaining elusive, inflammation, oxidative stress, and coagulation disturbances have been explored for their involvement in IPF (11). Unfortunately, there is no panacea for IPF, but clinical treatment includes pharmacological intervention, symptom relief, and co-morbidity management (12). Figure 18.2 identifies the different treatment modalities for IPF management as recognized by ATS. When these therapies fail to stabilize lung function, the patient is considered for single or bilateral lung transplantation. If the patient is deemed an appropriate lung transplant candidate, the wait time for a matching donor can be lengthy, hence emphasizing the need for a cure. Until recently, there was no therapies specifically marketed to treat IPF. Two drugs—pirfenidone (Esbriet®) and nintedanib (Ofev®)—were the first FDA-approved drugs for IPF treatment. Both the drugs received US FDA approval in 2014 following successful results from the ASCEND and INPULSIS clinical trials. Pirfenidone and nintedanib both slow the progression of the disease in mild to moderate IPF. Pirfenidone was approved in Japan in 2008, Europe in 2011, and in the United States in 2014. That same year, nintedanib also received approval for IPF treatment in the

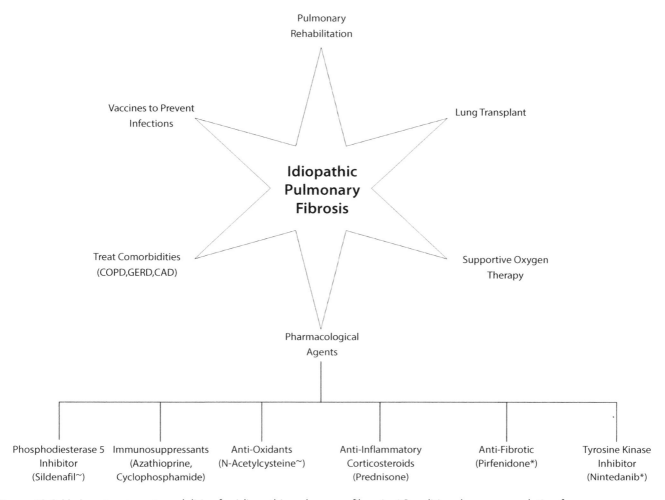

Figure 18.2 Various treatment modalities for idiopathic pulmonary fibrosis. *Conditional recommendation for use; ~conditional recommendation against use (reference ATS documents from 2011 and 2015). Conditional recommendations are not to be used in the majority of patients with IPF but can be used in minority of patient populations.

United States (13). This was seen as the first anticipatory step toward advancement in treating IPF, a devastating chronic respiratory disease. Both medications only slow disease progression, so a lack of curative drugs (14) is a motivating force behind drug development for this disease.

Other pharmacological interventions commonly used in treating patients with IPF include corticosteroids (prednisone), immunosuppressants (azathioprine, cyclophosphamide), anti–gastroesophageal reflux (GER) treatment, and phosphodiesterase 5 inhibitor (sildenafil) if pulmonary hypertension is a comorbidity to stabilize the patient's clinical stability or improve quality of life. Most of these drugs are small-molecule compounds. Figure 18.3 shows the structure and properties of the drug compounds used in IPF treatment. In 2015, the ATS/ERS/JPS/ALAT committee updated the evidence-based clinical practice guideline with the new recommended drug treatment for IPF.

Among the currently available drugs, pirfenidone is an antifibrotic with anti-inflammatory properties, which inhibits the synthesis of growth factors responsible for fibrogenesis. The therapeutic dose given orally is a high dose of 801 mg three times daily. This has been shown to have some gastrointestinal (GI) side effects, including nausea, abdominal pain, dyspepsia, and diarrhea in addition to photosensitivity and rash (14). Nintedanib is a tyrosine kinase receptor inhibitor targeting growth factors that eventually attenuates fibrosis development (15). It is given as 150 mg capsules twice daily orally. Nintedanib is also known to cause GI side effects such as diarrhea, nausea, abdominal pain, and vomiting and liver enzyme elevation. Although nintedanib received a conditional recommendation for its clinical use, the other tyrosine kinase receptor inhibitor imatinib was not recommended for IPF treatment. The committee has strongly recommended against the use of imatinib due to the high cost incurred and the lack of effective benefit from the clinical trial involving 119 patients (16). The use of corticosteroids is also limited due to the reduced clinical benefit. It is recommended only for acute disease exacerbations (15). Anti-GER therapies such as proton pump inhibitors or histamine 2 blocker receptor antagonists are commonly prescribed for IPF patients since GER is commonly seen in IPF patients.

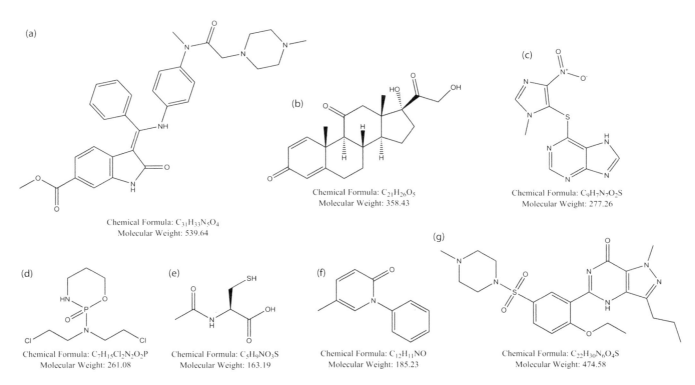

Figure 18.3 Chemical structures (ChemDraw 14.0, CambridgeSoft, Cambridge, MA) of drugs used in treating idiopathic pulmonary fibrosis (IPF). **(a)** Nintedanib, **(b)** prednisone, **(c)** azathioprine, **(d)** cyclophosphamide, **(e)** N-acetylcysteine, **(f)** pirfenidone, **(g)** sildenafil.

PULMONARY FIBROSIS MODELS

There is a need for advanced *in vitro* models and animal models to better mimic the human conditions in fibrosis because they serve as a screening tool for preclinical testing of novel drug compounds. Hence, a better representation of the human conditions is of paramount importance. This section of the chapter briefly introduces the various *in vitro* cell culture and *in vivo* animal models that are commonly used in PF research. There are two-dimensional (2D), 2.5-dimensional (2.5D), and three-dimensional (3D) *in vitro* cell culture models as described by Sundarakrishnan et al. (17). A 2D model is used to test the effect of the drug compound on an individual cell line, while 2.5D and 3D models consider the neighboring cells too. Two-dimensional culture models have stiff substrates that grow single type cell lines such as the tissue culture plate and glass substrates; 2.5D models are intermediate between the other two types and allow cell adhesion in the X-Y plane, similar to 2D models while permitting epithelial maturation that is possible only in 3D models. Three-dimensional *in vitro* models depict the microenvironment of the lung by allowing cell-cell and cell-matrix interaction (17). A relevant aspect of 2.5D and 3D culture models in PF is the ability to mimic the air-liquid interface of the lungs. Hence, there is some promise for future development of suitable *in vitro* cell-tissue culture models to depict PF. On the other hand, it has been very difficult to replicate all the features of PF in an animal model. Nonetheless, some commonly used *in vivo* animal models are used to replicate PF by either (1) instillation of compounds such as bleomycin, fluorescein thiocyanate (FITC), silica, vanadium, asbestos; (2) overexpression of cytokines such as TGF-β, TGF-α, IL-13, TNF-α, and IL-1β; or (3) using aged mice since fibrosis is an age-related disease (18,19). In any case, for novel therapies to be successful, it is important to develop and improve the tools used to study them for the diseases. In fact, ATS has recommended the use of 3D *in vitro* models with animal models to compliment findings from both studies (17).

INHALED THERAPIES FOR IPF

Although there is no inhaled drug therapy recommended for IPF, there is mounting interest in this route of administration. The oral administration of three tablets of pirfenidone given three times a day has known to cause adverse effects. Hence, a pulmonary delivery of the pirfenidone directly to the lungs can decrease the associated adverse events. Some investigations have been conducted in developing an aerosol formulation of pirfenidone. This section of the chapter discusses the details of the preclinical study of aerosol formulations targeted to treat PF. The investigation of inhalation route of administration for PF is still in its infancy; many of these aerosol formulations are entering clinical trials in humans. Nevertheless, the results of these studies are very promising to pursue the inhaled aerosol route of administration in the future.

A multicenter, randomized clinical trial conducted in Japan evaluated the efficacy of inhaled N-acetylcysteine (NAC) therapy (20); 352.4 mg of NAC dissolved in 4 mL saline was nebulized twice daily using Ne-U22, Omron vibrating mesh technology. The device generated aerosol with a particle size distribution between 1 and 8 μm and a mass median aerodynamic diameter of 5 μm. The inhaled NAC demonstrated positive results in some patients (20). However, the use of NAC monotherapy is not recommended by the ATS/ERS/JRS/ALAT in the recent clinical guidelines due to lack of significant benefit on mortality. Also, the use of a three-drug combination containing NAC, azathioprine, and prednisone is not recommended due to an increase in mortality and no significant difference in forced vital capacity (FVC) and lung diffusion capacity (DL_{CO}) (21,22).

Another study that developed lipid nanoparticles containing prostaglandin E and siRNA in the size range of 400 nm (23). When these particles were nebulized (inhalation aerosol) into bleomycin mice model for three weeks, it decreased the fibrotic tissue in lungs by 3.8 times and increased the survival rate. This cocktail containing gene therapy was found to downregulate five different transforming growth factors (TGFs) and connective tissue growth factors (CTGFs) that play a key role in fibrosis (23).

A clinical study of inhaled interferon-γ (IFN-γ) (Actimmune, InterMune, Brisbane, California) using I-neb vibrating mesh nebulizer showed a high local concentration of IFN-γ in the lungs (24). The treatment lasted for 80 weeks with no systemic side effects. The *in vivo* lung deposition using I-neb was found to be 65% of the original dose with 12.5% oropharyngeal deposition (24). This study has shown the possibility to effectively aerosolize IFN-γ to the lungs without losing its protein activity. It was also determined that the MMAD of the aerosolized particles generated using I-neb was 1.7 μm. This is the ideal particle size range to target the lower airways. A meta-analysis has shown that inhaled IFN-γ significantly improved the diffusion capacity of the lungs and attributes the failure of previous IFN-γ treatment to the parenteral route of administration (25).

An *in vivo* rodent study was conducted to test pirfenidone inhalation aerosol efficacy compared to oral administration (26). This study employed an ultrasonic nebulizer to deliver pirfenidone for 14 days. The oral dose delivered to the rats was 200 mg/kg.day, while a dose of 20 mg/kg.day was administered by inhalation. Not much difference between the oral and the inhalation route was observed when comparing histopathology, oxidative stress, proinflammatory and fibrotic gene expression. It was certain that 10 times lesser dose was able to achieve similar results via inhalation. However, it was uncertain if any fraction of the drug got into the systemic circulation to cause an adverse effect. Nonetheless, the study showed that the inhalation route can dramatically reduce the dose of pirfenidone administered (26). Particle-engineered pirfenidone powder was made by spray drying with L-leucine to form particles with a mean diameter of 1.75 μm (27). The aqueous spray-dried particles were seen to possess a corrugated surface, which is highly desirable for dry powder inhaler formulation to reduce the interparticular interactions. During the *in vitro* aerosol dispersion study using inertial impactor, the results indicated that about approximately 60% of the drug deposition was in impactor stages ≤ 3.45 μm. This is a significant amount of drug deposition in the given size range, which would mean that the aerosol formulation possesses the capability to reach the lower regions of the airways, where IPF is predominantly seen. This study also showed that an aerosol formulation of pirfenidone has less systemic absorption from the lungs, which leads to decreased adverse effect (27). The jet milling process made another powder formulation of pirfenidone. The micronized (milled) drug was blended with lactose to formulate an inhalable powder (28). The particle size distribution of the drug was micronized with a mean diameter of 7 μm. However, when the aerosol dispersion was tested using an Andersen cascade impactor, it was determined that 23% of the particles were fine particles (≤5.8 μm) and about approximately 56% of the blended particles was not respirable, which accounted for device retention and losses. Another interesting observation made in this study was that the inhalation route of administration of pirfenidone reduced the phototoxic side effect seen when given orally (28). From the above two studies, it can be inferred that the effective dose administered through inhalation aerosol was much lower than the oral dose; hence this formulation can invite better patient compliance compared to oral dose regimen of pirfenidone.

Pirfenidone is a low potent drug with minimal lung levels when administered orally. The high, 801 mg three-times-daily dose is because of the very high dose required to achieve sufficient level of the drug in the lung tissue when administered orally. On the other hand, an inhaled dose means higher concentrations of the drug locally in the lung tissue, which can in turn increase the duration of drug efficacy. Hence, an aqueous-buffered formulation of pirfenidone using co-solvents and salts has shown to be effective in increasing the C_{max} in lung tissue and plasma following nebulization compared to oral delivery. This systematic study reported in U.S. Patent US20120192861A1 describes several liquid formulations of pirfenidone that are suitable for aerosolization using different nebulizer devices (29). Pirfenidone is highly water soluble. The liquid formulation of pirfenidone in this study was comprised of co-solvents (ethanol, propylene glycol, glycerol) 1%–40%, surfactant (polysorbate 80 or cetyl-pyridium bromide), taste masking/sweetening agents (saccharine), buffers (phosphate, citrate) and salts (sodium chloride or magnesium chloride) to adjust tonicity for inhalation. The concentration of pirfenidone in these liquid formulations varied from 0.1 mg/mL to 60 mg/mL, with various combinations of co-solvents, surfactant, and other components. For example, the formulations used in pharmacokinetic (PK) analysis of aerosolized pirfenidone in rat contained 12.5 mg/mL pirfenidone in ethanol and propylene glycol at a 1:2 ratio, and a 5 mM phosphate buffer to maintain pH of 6.5 by QSing with water to a final volume of 30 mL. The aerosolization efficiency of a similar liquid formulation was studied using three different nebulizer devices, namely, Philips I-neb® AAD, PARI eFlow®, and Aerogen Aeroneb®. The liquid aerosol that was generated possessed characteristics suitable for a pulmonary delivery with a geometric standard deviation (emitted droplet size distribution) of 1.0–2.5 μm, volumetric mean diameter of 1–5 μm, mass median aerodynamic diameter (MMAD) of 1–5 μm, fine particle fraction (FPF % $\leq$ 5 μm) at least 30%. The PK rodent study showed that the local concentrations of pirfenidone in the lung was higher when administered as an aerosol by 80%–120% when compared to oral delivery. Based on this result and allometric scaling, it is possible to deliver 0.1 mg–360 mg of pirfenidone in 20 minutes to human lungs with an MMAD of 1–5 μm (29).

A preliminary study showed a formulation development of dry powder inhaler of tilorone using Easyhaler® and Twister™ dry powder inhaler devices. This study found an emitted dose of 2.95–4.77 mg of tilorone and fine particle fraction ($\leq$ 5 μm) of 22%–30% was achievable. This result was comparable to similarly aerosolized formulations of pirfenidone and nintedanib (30). The potential effect of tilorone in restoring impaired bone morphogenetic protein (BMP) signaling in the lungs was studied in a silica-induced fibrosis mice model (31). This compound must be further studied in vitro and in vivo to elucidate its mechanistic approach in PF.

Alpha-1 antitrypsin deficiency (AATD) is a commonly overlooked cause of lung disease (32). Inhaled alpha-1 antitrypsin (AAT) that is derived from human plasma has completed clinical trials phase 2 for the treatment of CF. Nebulized AAT solution at a concentration of 250 mg/10 mL 0.9% saline solution was aerosolized using a CR-60 high flow compressor and Ventstream nebulizer to study its effect in bronchiectasis patients with chronic bronchial infection. Kamada has developed this inhaled AAT formulation with potential use in AATD, CF, and bronchiectasis. Several clinical trials have shown the safety of this formulation in CF patients.

FUTURE OF IPF RESEARCH

Lack of a curative or preventive therapy in IPF and only a few treatments that slow disease progress necessitate an enormous demand for further research directed at preventing or reversing PF or halting the progression even more compared to the limited options available now (33). Given the prevalence and incidence of PF in the United States, European countries, and Asia, ATS has identified the need to form a global lung fibrosis initiative (33). Such an effort will help in gathering information regarding associated risk factors, and a common registry to collect epidemiological data, cross-reference patient's symptoms, and unify global diagnosis of PF. A collaborative effort with different countries on investigational research can identify potential new drugs.

Cellular and molecular mechanisms involvement of NADPH oxidase isoform 4 (Nox4), which is a key source of reactive oxygen species (ROS) in IPF, is a new avenue of research. Investigational compounds targeting this pathway might be useful in treating fibrotic disorders (34–38). Regenerative medicine using stem cell therapy has shown promising results in the early stage of development, including a clinical trial assessing the safety of stem cell infusion (39–41). Table 18.1 lists drug inventions currently in clinical trials to treat IPF. Aerodone™ solution is the inhaled pirfenidone, which is delivered via Pari eFlow nebulizer system. It was developed by Avalyn Pharma and has entered a clinical trial in healthy volunteers in Australia. It is worth noting that some marketed drugs are entering clinical trials as inhalation aerosol to treat IPF. The future of IPF therapy will include a targeted local drug delivery to the lung, which will reduce adverse effects. As the therapeutic profile for IPF expands, treatment regimens will likely include multiple drug combinations that target different mechanisms of the disease such as antifibrotic, anti-inflammatory, and antioxidant (12,14).

A recent study identified that thyroid hormone (TH) inhibits lung fibrosis in mice models. The antifibrotic effect of T_3 (3,5,3′-triiodothyronine) molecule was studied by aerosolizing it in bleomycin-induced mice. The fibrosis reduction effect of aerosolized T_3 was comparable to orally administered pirfenidone and nintedanib. There was no effect on the systemic levels of the T_3, suggesting a more targeted local delivery to the airways. This effect of TH was due to attenuation of mitochondrial dysfunction in pulmonary epithelial cells. TH was capable of reversing bleomycin-induced mitochondrial derangement in vivo and in vitro by induction of mitochondrial biogenesis and mitophagy. In the future, the exploration of biologics for IPF should be considered and may become relevant in humans (42).

Table 18.1 List of recent clinical trials with drug inventions in treating pulmonary fibrosis

	Drug/compound investigated	Phase	NCT number	Class of drug	Route of administration
1	Aerosol interferon alpha	Phase 1	NCT00563212	Immunotherapy	Inhalation
2	Inhaled pirfenidone[b]	Phase 1	ACTRN12617001501336[b]	Antifibrotic	Inhalation Inhalation
3	Dasatinib, quercetin	Phase 1	NCT02874989	Tyrosine kinase inhibitor, antioxidant	N/A
4	Rituximab, methylprednisone	Phase 1|2	NCT01266317	Monoclonal antibody, corticosteroid	IV
5	FG-3019	Phase 2	NCT01890265	N/A	IV infusion
6	Lebrikizumab, pirfenidone	Phase 2	NCT01872689	Monoclonal antibody, antifibrotic	SC
7	Tipelukast	Phase 2	NCT02503657	Anti-inflammatory	Oral
8	KD025	Phase 2	NCT02688647	N/A	Oral
9	GBT440	Phase 2	NCT02846324	N/A	Oral
10	Rituximab	Phase 2	NCT01969409	N/A	IV
11	CC-90001	Phase 2	NCT03142191	N/A	Oral
12	Nintedanib, sildenafil	Phase 3	NCT02802345	Tyrosine kinase inhibitor/ phosphodiesterase 5 inhibitor	Oral
13	Tralokinumab	Phase 2	NCT01629667	Anti–IL-13 monoclonal antibody	IV
14[a]	Pirfenidone, vismodegib	Phase 1	NCT02648048	Antifibrotic/ hedgehog pathway inhibitors	Oral
15[a]	GS-6624	Phase 1	NCT01362231	N/A	IV
16[a]	GC10088	Phase 1	NCT00125385	N/A	IV
17[a]	Zileuton	Phase 2	NCT00262405	Leukotriene synthesis inhibitor	N/A
18[a]	Gefapixant (AF-219, MK-7264)	Phase 2	NCT02477709, NCT02502097	Analgesic	Oral
19[a]	SAR156597	Phase 2	NCT02345070, NCT01529853	N/A	SC
20[a]	QAX576	Phase 2	NCT00532233	N/A	N/A
21[a]	BMS-986020	Phase 2	NCT01766817	N/A	Oral
22[a]	BG00011	Phase 2	NCT01371305	N/A	SC
23[a]	Beclomethasone/ formoterol[c]	Phase 2	NCT02048644	Anti-inflammatory/ bronchodilator	Inhalation
24[a]	CNTO 888	Phase 2	NCT00786201	N/A	IV infusion
24[a]	Sildenafil, losartan	Phase 2|3	NCT00981747	Phosphodiesterase 5 inhibitor/angiotensin II receptor antagonist	Oral
25[a]	Bosentan	Phase 3	NCT00391443	Endothelin receptor antagonist	N/A
26[a]	Sildenafil citrate	Phase 3	NCT00517933	Phosphodiesterase 5 inhibitor	Oral

Sources: Australia NZCTR. Australia New Zealand Clinical Trials Registry [March 7, 2018]. Available from http://www.anzctr.org.au/; Elsevier. Elsevier; [March 7, 2018]. Available from www.embase.com; European MA. European Medicines Agency; [March 7, 2018]. Available from https://www.clinicaltrialsregister.eu/; Springer I. Springer International; [March 7, 2018]. Available from http://adisinsight.springer.com/; US NLoM. US National Library of Medicine; [March 7, 2018]. Available from www.clinicaltrials.gov.

[a] Study completed.
[b] Global study conducted in Australia/New Zealand.
[c] Global study conducted in United Kingdom.
IV: intravenous, N/A: not available, SC: subcutaneous.

REFERENCES

1. Raghu G, Chen SY, Hou Q, Yeh WS, Collard HR. Incidence and prevalence of idiopathic pulmonary fibrosis in US adults 18–64 years old. *Eur Respir J.* 2016;48(1):179–186. doi:10.1183/13993003.01653-2015.

2. Raghu G, Collard HR, Egan JJ, Martinez FJ, Behr J, Brown KK, Colby TV, et al. An official ATS/ERS/JRS/ALAT statement: Idiopathic pulmonary fibrosis: Evidence-based guidelines for diagnosis and management. *Am J Respir Crit Care Med.* 2011;183(6):788–824. doi:10.1164/rccm.2009-040GL.

3. Hutchinson J, Fogarty A, Hubbard R, McKeever T. Global incidence and mortality of idiopathic pulmonary fibrosis: A systematic review. *Eur Respir J.* 2015;46(3):795–806. doi:10.1183/09031936.00185114.

4. Ley B, Collard HR. Epidemiology of idiopathic pulmonary fibrosis. *Clin Epidemiol.* 2013;5:483–492. doi:10.2147/CLEP.S54815.

5. Flaherty KR, Travis WD, Colby TV, Toews GB, Kazerooni EA, Gross BH, Jain A, Strawderman RL, Flint A, Lynch JP, Martinez FJ. Histopathologic variability in usual and nonspecific interstitial pneumonias. *Am J Resp Crit Care.* 2001;164(9):1722–1727. doi:10.1164/ajrccm.164.9.2103074.

6. Hayes D, Jr., Tumin D, Daniels CJ, McCoy KS, Mansour HM, Tobias JD, Kirkby SE. Pulmonary artery pressure and benefit of lung transplantation in adult cystic fibrosis patients. *Ann Thorac Surg.* 2016;101(3):1104–1109. doi:10.1016/j.athoracsur.2015.09.086.

7. Hayes D, Jr., Kopp BT, Kirkby SE, Reynolds SD, Mansour HM, Tobias JD, Tumin D. Impact of donor arterial partial pressure of oxygen on outcomes after lung transplantation in adult cystic fibrosis recipients. *Lung.* 2016;194(4):547–553. doi:10.1007/s00408-016-9902-3.

8. Hayes D, Jr., Auletta JJ, Whitson BA, Black SM, Kirkby S, Tobias JD, Mansour HM. Human leukocyte antigen mismatching and survival after lung transplantation in adult and pediatric patients with cystic fibrosis. *J Thorac Cardiov Sur.* 2016;151(2):549–557. doi:10.1016/j.jtcvs.2015.08.022.

9. Hayes D, Jr., Kirkby S, Whitson BA, Black SM, Sheikh SI, Tobias JD, Mansour HM, Kopp BT. Mortality risk and pulmonary function in adults with cystic fibrosis at time of wait listing for lung transplantation. *Ann Thorac Surg.* 2015;100(2):474–479. doi:10.1016/j.athoracsur.2015.04.022.

10. Hayes D, Jr, Kopp BT, Tobias JD, Woodley FW, Mansour HM, Tumin D, Kirkby SE. Survival in patients with advanced non-cystic fibrosis bronchiectasis versus cystic fibrosis on the waitlist for lung transplantation. *Lung.* 2015;193(6):933–938. doi:10.1007/s00408-015-9811-x.

11. Todd NW, Luzina IG, Atamas SP. Molecular and cellular mechanisms of pulmonary fibrosis. *Fibrosis Tissue Rep.* 2012;5(1):11. doi:10.1186/1755-1536-5-11.

12. Raghu G, Richeldi L. Current approaches to the management of idiopathic pulmonary fibrosis. *Resp Med.* 2017;129:24–30. doi:10.1016/j.rmed.2017.05.017.

13. Robalo-Cordeiro C, Campos P, Carvalho L, Borba A, Clemente S, Freitas S, Furtado S, et al. Idiopathic pulmonary fibrosis in the era of antifibrotic therapy: Searching for new opportunities grounded in evidence. *Rev Port Pneumol.* 2017. doi:10.1016/j.rppnen.2017.05.005.

14. Sathiyamoorthy G, Sehgal S, Ashton RW. Pirfenidone and Nintedanib for Treatment of Idiopathic Pulmonary Fibrosis. *South Med J.* 2017;110(6):393–398. doi:10.14423/SMJ.0000000000000655.

15. Xaubet A, Molina-Molina M, Acosta O, Bollo E, Castillo D, Fernandez-Fabrellas E, Rodriguez-Portal JA, et al. Guidelines for the medical treatment of idiopathic pulmonary fibrosis. *Arch Bronconeumol.* 2017;53(5):263–269. doi:10.1016/j.arbres.2016.12.011.

16. Daniels CE, Lasky JA, Limper AH, Mieras K, Gabor E, Schroeder DR, Imatinib IPFSI. Imatinib treatment for idiopathic pulmonary fibrosis: Randomized placebo-controlled trial results. *Am J Respir Crit Care Med.* 2010;181(6):604–610. doi:10.1164/rccm.200906-0964OC.

17. Sundarakrishnan A, Chen Y, Black LD, Aldridge BB, Kaplan DL. Engineered cell and tissue models of pulmonary fibrosis. *Adv Drug Deliv Rev.* 2017. doi:10.1016/j.addr.2017.12.013.

18. B BM, Lawson WE, Oury TD, Sisson TH, Raghavendran K, Hogaboam CM. Animal models of fibrotic lung disease. *Am J Respir Cell Mol Biol.* 2013;49(2):167–179. doi:10.1165/rcmb.2013-0094TR.

19. Tashiro J, Rubio GA, Limper AH, Williams K, Elliot SJ, Ninou I, Aidinis V, et al. Exploring animal models that resemble idiopathic pulmonary fibrosis. *Front Med (Lausanne).* 2017;4:118. doi:10.3389/fmed.2017.00118.

20. Homma S, Azuma A, Taniguchi H, Ogura T, Mochiduki Y, Sugiyama Y, Nakata K, et al. Efficacy of inhaled N-acetylcysteine monotherapy in patients with early stage idiopathic pulmonary fibrosis. *Respirology.* 2012;17(3):467–477. doi:10.1111/j.1440-1843.2012.02132.x.

21. Raghu G, Anstrom KJ, King TE, Jr, Lasky JA, Martinez FJ. Idiopathic pulmonary fibrosis clinical research, network. Prednisone, azathioprine, and N-acetylcysteine for pulmonary fibrosis. *N Engl J Med.* 2012;366(21):1968–1977. doi:10.1056/NEJMoa1113354.

22. Raghu G, Rochwerg B, Zhang Y, Garcia CA, Azuma A, Behr J, Brozek JL, et al. An official ATS/ERS/JRS/ALAT clinical practice guideline: Treatment of idiopathic pulmonary fibrosis. An update of the 2011 clinical practice guideline. *Am J Resp Crit Care.* 2015;192(2):e3–e19. doi:10.1164/rccm.201506-1063ST.

23. Garbuzenko OB, Ivanova V, Kholodovych V, Reimer DC, Reuhl KR, Yurkow E, Adler D, Minko T. Combinatorial treatment of idiopathic pulmonary fibrosis using nanoparticles with prostaglandin E and siRNA(s). *Nanomedicine.* 2017;13(6):1983–1992. doi:10.1016/j.nano.2017.04.005.

24. Diaz KT, Skaria S, Harris K, Solomita M, Lau S, Bauer K, Smaldone GC, Condos R. Delivery and safety of inhaled interferon-gamma in idiopathic pulmonary fibrosis. *J Aerosol Med Pulm Drug Deliv.* 2012;25(2):79–87. doi:10.1089/jamp.2011.0919.

25. Skaria SD, Yang J, Condos R, Smaldone GC. Inhaled interferon and diffusion capacity in idiopathic pulmonary fibrosis (IPF). *Sarcoidosis Vasc Diffuse Lung Dis.* 2015;32(1):37–42.

26. Rasooli R, Rajaian H, Pardakhty A, Mandegary A. Preference of aerosolized pirfenidone to oral intake: An experimental model of pulmonary fibrosis by paraquat. *J Aerosol Med Pulm Drug Deliv.* 2017. doi:10.1089/jamp.2016.1342.

27. Seto Y, Suzuki G, Leung SS, Chan HK, Onoue S. Development of an Improved Inhalable Powder Formulation of Pirfenidone by Spray-Drying: In Vitro Characterization and Pharmacokinetic Profiling. *Pharm Res.* 2016;33(6):1447–1455. doi:10.1007/s11095-016-1887-3.

28. Onoue S, Seto Y, Kato M, Aoki Y, Kojo Y, Yamada S. Inhalable powder formulation of pirfenidone with reduced phototoxic risk for treatment of pulmonary fibrosis. *Pharm Res.* 2013;30(6):1586–1596. doi:10.1007/s11095-013-0997-4.

29. SURBER MW, inventor; Genoa Pharmaceuticals, Inc., assignee. Aerosol pirfenidone and pyridone analog compounds and uses thereof US patent US20120192861 A1. 2012.

30. Vartiainen V, Raula J,Koli K,Kauppinen E, Myllraniemi M. Inhalable Drug Formulations for Idiopathic Pulmonary Fibrosis. *American Thoracic Society 2017 International Conference*; May 23; Washington DC: American Thoracic Society, 2017.

31. Lepparanta O, Tikkanen JM, Bespalov MM, Koli K, Myllarniemi M. Bone morphogenetic protein-inducer tilorone identified by high-throughput screening is antifibrotic in vivo. *Am J Respir Cell Mol Biol.* 2013;48(4):448–455. doi:10.1165/rcmb.2012-0201OC.

32. Brode SK, Ling SC, Chapman KR. Alpha-1 antitrypsin deficiency: A commonly overlooked cause of lung disease. *CMAJ.* 2012;184(12):1365–1371. doi:10.1503/cmaj.111749.

33. White ES, Borok Z, Brown KK, Eickelberg O, Guenther A, Jenkins RG, Kolb M, Martinez FJ, Roman J, Sime P, American Thoracic Society Respiratory C, Molecular Biology Assembly Working Group on Pulmonary F. An American Thoracic Society Official Research Statement: Future Directions in Lung Fibrosis Research. *Am J Respir Crit Care Med.* 2016;193(7):792–800. doi:10.1164/rccm.201602-0254ST.

34. Amara N, Goven D, Prost F, Muloway R, Crestani B, Boczkowski J. NOX4/NADPH oxidase expression is increased in pulmonary fibroblasts from patients with idiopathic pulmonary fibrosis and mediates TGF beta 1-induced fibroblast differentiation into myofibroblasts. *Thorax.* 2010;65(8):733–738. doi:10.1136/thx.2009.113456.

35. du Bois RM. Strategies for treating idiopathic pulmonary fibrosis. *Nat Rev Drug Discov.* 2010;9(2):129–140. doi:10.1038/nrd2958.

36. Hecker L, Logsdon NJ, Kurundkar D, Kurundkar A, Bernard K, Hock T, Meldrum E, et al. Reversal of persistent fibrosis in aging by targeting Nox4-Nrf2 redox imbalance. *Sci Transl Med.* 2014;6(231):231ra47. doi:10.1126/scitranslmed.3008182.

37. Hecker L, Vittal R, Jones T, Jagirdar R, Luckhardt TR, Horowitz JC, Pennathur S, Martinez FJ, Thannickal VJ. NADPH oxidase-4 mediates myofibroblast activation and fibrogenic responses to lung injury. *Nat Med.* 2009;15(9):1077–1081. doi:10.1038/nm.2005.

38. Liu YM, Nepali K, Liou JP. Idiopathic pulmonary fibrosis: Current status, recent progress, and emerging targets. *J Med Chem.* 2017;60(2):527–553. doi:10.1021/acs.jmedchem.6b00935.

39. Banerjee ER, Laflamme MA, Papayannopoulou T, Kahn M, Murry CE, Henderson WR, Jr. Human embryonic stem cells differentiated to lung lineage-specific cells ameliorate pulmonary fibrosis in a xenograft transplant mouse model. *PLoS One.* 2012;7(3):e33165. doi:10.1371/journal.pone.0033165.

40. Lan YW, Choo KB, Chen CM, Hung TH, Chen YB, Hsieh CH, Kuo HP, Chong KY. Hypoxia-preconditioned mesenchymal stem cells attenuate bleomycin-induced pulmonary fibrosis. *Stem Cell Res Ther.* 2015;6:97. doi:10.1186/s13287-015-0081-6.

41. Tzouvelekis A, Paspaliaris V, Koliakos G, Ntolios P, Bouros E, Oikonomou A, Zissimopoulos A, et al. A prospective, non-randomized, no placebo-controlled, phase Ib clinical trial to study the safety of the adipose derived stromal cells-stromal vascular fraction in idiopathic pulmonary fibrosis. *J Transl Med*. 2013;11:171. doi:10.1186/1479-5876-11-171.

42. Yu G, Tzouvelekis A, Wang R, Herazo-Maya JD, Ibarra GH, Srivastava A, de Castro JPW, et al. Thyroid hormone inhibits lung fibrosis in mice by improving epithelial mitochondrial function. *Nat Med*. 2018;24(1):39–49. doi:10.1038/nm.4447.

43. Australia NZCTR. Australia New Zealand Clinical Trials Registry [March 7, 2018]. Available from http://www.anzctr.org.au/.

44. Elsevier. Elsevier; [March 7, 2018]. Available from www.embase.com.

45. European MA. European Medicines Agency; [March 7, 2018]. Available from https://www.clinicaltrialsregister.eu/.

46. Springer I. Springer International; [March 7, 2018]. Available from http://adisinsight.springer.com/.

47. US NLoM. U.S National Library of Medicine; [March 7, 2018]. Available from www.clinicaltrials.gov.

19

Therapeutics in pulmonary hypertension

MARIA F. ACOSTA, DON HAYES, JR., JEFFREY R. FINEMAN, JASON X.-J. YUAN, STEPHEN M. BLACK, AND HEIDI M. MANSOUR

Introduction	313
Prevalence	313
Pathophysiology	313
Cellular factors involved in PH	315
Molecular factors	315
Genetics of PH	316
Biochemical markers	316
Current therapies for pulmonary hypertension	316
Ongoing investigational research therapeutics in pulmonary hypertension	318
Approved inhalation products	318
Supportive therapies	318
Other approaches for the treatment of pulmonary hypertension	319
Conclusion	319
References	319

INTRODUCTION

Pulmonary hypertension (PH) is a pathophysiological condition associated with multiple clinical conditions and obfuscates the majority of cardiovascular and respiratory diseases (1). PH is characterized by the increase in blood pressure in the pulmonary arteries. Mean systemic blood pressure for a healthy adult is 120/80 millimeters of mercury (mmHg). The pulmonary artery blood pressure in a healthy state at rest is 8–20 mmHg. If the mean pulmonary arterial pressure of a patient surpasses 25 mmHg at rest or 30 mmHg during physical activity, he or she can be diagnosed with PH. Many complications may be observed if the PH persists or become even higher. In general, the major damage is to the right ventricle (RV) of the heart, which supplies blood to the pulmonary arteries. When PH exists, the RV of the heart becomes incapable of pumping blood effectively, and the patient experiences symptoms that include shortness of breath, loss of energy, and edema, which is the main sign of right heart failure. The World Health Organization (WHO) divides PH into five groups, which are organized based on the cause of the condition. It is important to note that group 1 is called pulmonary arterial hypertension (PAH) and groups 2 through 5 are called PH (1,2).

Prevalence

The exact prevalence of all types of PH is not well established (3). However, epidemiologic studies have estimated a prevalence of 97 persons per million, with a female/male ratio of 1.8, and the mortality rate ranges from 4.5 to 12.3 per 100,000 population (4). Thus, PH usually affects women more than men. PH that occurs subsequently or in parallel with other diseases is more common. The disease normally develops between the ages of 20 and 60, but it can occur at any age. The average age of diagnosis is 36 years, and 3-year survival after diagnosis is approximately 50% (3). Signs and symptoms of PH may include shortness of breath during routine activity, tiredness, chest pain, a racing heartbeat, pain on the upper right side of the abdomen, and decreased appetite. As PH gets worse, other signs and symptoms appear, such as feeling lightheaded, fainting at times, swelling of legs and ankles, and bluish color on the lips and skin (5).

Pathophysiology

One of the principal characteristics is the response of the pulmonary vascular system to hypoxia (low tissue oxygen levels) (6). The main function of the lungs is to distribute oxygen to the peripheral organs. When oxygen levels are low, the pulmonary arteries constrict while the systemic arteries dilate. This pulmonary vasoconstrictive reaction to hypoxic conditions is inherent only in the lungs and is present in all mammals, maintaining a ventilation-perfusion balance between the air that reaches the alveoli and the blood that reaches the alveoli via the capillaries (6). Oxygen is delivered to the alveolus by alveolar ventilation, and it is removed from the alveolus as it diffuses into the pulmonary capillary blood and is carried away by the pulmonary blood flow. Likewise, carbon dioxide is perfused to the alveolus in the mixed venous blood and diffuses into the alveolus in the pulmonary capillary. The carbon dioxide is removed from the alveolus by alveolar ventilation (7). Pulmonary vasoconstriction due to hypoxia is important because it reduces the perfusion of poorly ventilated areas of the lung and decreases pulmonary shunting, that is, parts of the lung that are unventilated although still perfused (8), preventing the circulation of mixed venous blood to the body (6).

PH is characterized by excessive vasoconstriction, due to the imbalance in the production of vasodilators, such as nitric oxide (NO) and prostacyclin, and vasoconstrictors, such as endothelin-1 (ET-1) and serotonin, produced by the endothelium (9). Other factors involved include inflammation, thrombosis (due to endothelial dysfunction and platelet aggregation (9), and the remodeling of the vasculature due to the proliferation and the inhibition of the apoptosis of endothelial and vascular smooth muscle cells (10). These changes that occur between the normal and hypertensive pulmonary vessels can be visualized in Figure 19.1 (11). Intima and media proliferation and the resulting pulmonary vascular obstruction are considered key elements in the pathogenesis of PH. Vasoconstriction, vascular remodeling, and thrombosis are also factors that increase pulmonary vascular resistance in PH (12). These processes involve a multitude of cellular and molecular elements (12). In addition, oxidative stress, mitochondrial

dysfunction, and an increase in reactive oxygen species (ROS) production have all been observed (13–15).

Overall PH is driven by an initial vascular injury leading to the deregulation of normal cellular processes in the pulmonary vasculature and modifications in proliferation, differentiation, inflammation, and cell death program (16), which in turn cause to excessive vasoconstriction and abnormal remodeling of pulmonary vessels, progressive increase in pulmonary arterial pressure (PAP), and vascular rigidity (16). If maintained, these result in right ventricular hypertrophy (RVH), progressive right heart failure, low cardiac output, and ultimately death (17,18). The process of pulmonary vascular remodeling is accompanied by endothelial dysfunction, activation of fibroblasts and smooth muscle cells, crosstalk between cells within the vascular wall, and recruitment of circulating progenitor cells (19). Moreover, overproduction of ROS contributes to the damage of pulmonary vascular endothelium, pulmonary arterial vasoconstriction, and pulmonary vascular remodeling. ROS can upregulate the expression of several factors that modify vascular remodeling, such as endothelial growth factor, platelet activating factor, and mitogen-activated protein kinase. The mitogenic effect of ET-1 and substance P on pulmonary smooth muscle cells is also mediated by ROS (20). PH is also characterized by a decrease in NO signaling due to the malfunction of the enzyme nitric oxide synthase (NOS) responsible for its generation. Indeed, in PH, the endothelial isoform, eNOS becomes "uncoupled," producing a shift from

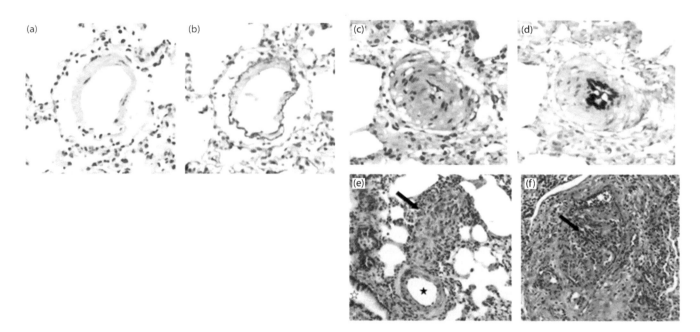

Figure 19.1 Histological changes in the lungs of rats with pulmonary hypertension. Vascular changes were investigated in rats with pulmonary hypertension compared to controls. Small pulmonary arteries of control animals look normal. There is no evident endothelial proliferation and/or hypertrophy (a) and (b). In contrast, pulmonary hypertensive animals developed occlusive vasculopathy with prominent media hypertrophy and endothelial proliferation (c) and (d). Also, plexiform lesions, complex vascular formations that sprouted from small pulmonary arteries, were detected in the pulmonary hypertension group (e) (arrow, plexiform lesion; black star, pulmonary artery; white star, bronchus). These mimicked plexiform lesions found in human patients with severe pulmonary arterial hypertension (f) (arrow, plexiform lesion in human). (Reproduced from Rafikova, O. et al., *Free Radical Biol. Med.*, 56, 28–43, 2013. With permission.)

NO generation to ROS production. In addition, to uncoupled eNOS, the aberrant generation of ROS during the development of PH is complex and involves several systems. These include nicotinamide adenine dinucleotide phosphate (NADPH) oxidase, dysfunctional mitochondria, and xanthine oxidase. In PH, there is also evidence of an interaction between the pulmonary and the cardiovascular system. However, this interaction is not well defined because of the deficiency of arduous investigations and inadequate diagnostic capabilities (21).

Cellular factors involved in PH

In all forms of PH, proliferation of smooth muscle cells (SMCs) in the small pulmonary arteries is evident. In some models of PH, fibroblasts of the adventitia migrate to the media and intima, where proliferation and production of matrix proteins are observed. Neovascularization, mainly of the adventitia, occurs parallel to the thickening of the vascular walls. External factors such as hypoxia, inflammation, shear stress, drugs, viral infections, and genetic susceptibility lead to proliferation of endothelial cells (ECs) (12). Other extrapulmonary cells (fibrocytes and c-kit cells) are also involved in the vascular remodeling of the pulmonary arteries. These cells appear to migrate from the bone marrow and differentiate into vascular cells and/or produce proangiogenic factors that participate in the pathogenesis of PH, leading to the formation of plexiform lesions (endothelial cells, matrix proteins, and fibroblasts that destroy the vascular lumen) (12). Patients with PH have increased levels of inflammatory cytokines such as interleukin 1 (IL-1) and interleukin-6 (IL-6), and chemokines such as fractalkine and Monocyte chemoattractant protein-1 (MCP-1) (22). Inflammatory cells, including B and T cells, macrophages, mastocytes and dendritic cells, have also been found in plexiform lesions associated with severe PH (12).

Molecular factors

Many molecular factors are involved in the physiopathology of PH. Pulmonary vasoconstriction is a very early step in the process of PH. Vasoconstriction has been associated with an abnormal function of the endothelium. This endothelial dysfunction is characterized by a decrease in the production of vasodilators such as NO and prostacyclin and by an increase in the production of vasoconstrictors like ET-1 and serotonin (5-Hydroxytryptamine, 5-HT).

NO inhibits smooth cell proliferation and decreases platelet aggregation through the activation of guanylate cyclase (GC), cyclic adenosine monophosphate (cAMP), and cyclic guanosine monophosphate (cGMP) (12). Prostacycline, on the other hand, inhibits smooth cell proliferation and decreases platelet aggregation only through the activation of cyclic adenosine monophosphate. While prostacyclin through the cyclic adenosine monophosphate (cAMP) pathway. The production of prostacyclin is reduced in patients with PH (12) and as mentioned above, PH is characterized by a decreased in the expression of endothelial NO synthase

(eNOs) and inhibition of its enzymatic activity. Moreover in patients with PH, the activity of guanylate cyclase is reduced and also there is a decrease in the synthesis of cGMP (the second messenger of NO). The principal enzyme in charge of the degradation of cGMP is called phosphodiesterase type five (PDE-5). The lack of NO in patients with PH is due to the upregulation of the production of PDE-5 (23).

ET-1 is an endothelially derived peptide that has two receptor subtypes: endothelin A (ETA) and endothelin B (ETB). ETA is expressed exclusively in the smooth muscle cells of pulmonary arteries, while ETB can be found on both smooth muscle cells and endothelial cells. When ET-1 is ligated to the Endothelin A receptor (ETRA), intracellular calcium levels are increased and the protein kinase C pathway is activated. The consequence is that pulmonary vasoconstriction is augmented, accompanied by the stimulation of mitosis of the arterial smooth muscle cells, leading to pulmonary vasculature remodeling. Serotonin levels are elevated in the plasma of PH patients (24), which is thought to contribute to the remodeling of the pulmonary vasculature and the stimulation of vasoconstriction (12).

GTPases such as Rho-A have also been implicated in the progression of PH. The downstream activation of the Rho kinases disrupts the regulation of a number of essential cellular tasks including contraction, migration, proliferation, and apoptosis (12). The activity of both RhoA and Rho kinase are increased in PH, and the inhibition of Rho kinase has been shown to counteract vasoconstriction associated with PH (6).

Hypoxia inducible factor-1 (HIF-1) is a transcription factor that primarily regulates cellular adaptation to hypoxia but also regulates several genes implicated in angiogenesis, erythropoiesis, cellular metabolism, and survival (25). The immunohistological analysis of human plexiform lesions of patients with severe PH has identified an overexpression of HIF-1 alpha in the proliferating endothelial cells presented (26).

One of the main functions of mitochondria, the oxidation of glucose, is suppressed in endothelial and smooth muscle cells of patients with PH. This suppression has multiple consequences, such as resistance to apoptosis, increased cellular proliferation, and inflammation due to the activation of some transcription factors that is triggered by the increase of mitochondrial (mt)-ROS and the progression to mitochondrial dysfunction (27). The Mitochondria of pulmonary arterial smooth muscle cells (PASMCs) are slightly different than mitochondria of systemic arteries. PASMCs mitochondria are the basis of the pulmonary response. In hypoxia conditions, the mitochondria alter the production mitochondria reactive oxygen species (mROS), which regulate different redox targets. These targets are involved in PASMCs contraction and in the initiation of a response to hypoxia via the activation of HIF-1 alpha genes. PASMCs mitochondria also regulate apoptosis, induce proliferation and inflammatory responses, and respond to many other stress signals. With this knowledge, the mitochondria of the pulmonary arteries could be a novel target for proapoptotic and antiproliferative therapies for the treatment of PH (27).

Genetics of PH

Mutations in genes that encode proteins involved in the Tumor necrosis factor β (TNF-β) signaling pathway are implicated in the development of PH. These mutations include Bone morphogenetic protein receptor type 2 (BMPR2), Activin A receptor like type 1 (ACVRL1), Endoglin (ENG), Smad8, Smad1, Smad5, and *Caveolin-1*. TNF-β signaling pathway controls growth, differentiation, and apoptosis of various cell types including pulmonary vascular (ECs) and SMCs (12). Thus, mutations in genes involved in the TGF-β signaling pathway may be responsible for the abnormal proliferation of pulmonary vascular SMCs and may promote ECs apoptosis (12).

BIOCHEMICAL MARKERS

Biomarkers that could specifically indicate the disease stage and the treatment response would be ideal tools for the optimization of PH management. However, there is still no specific marker for PH or pulmonary vascular remodeling, although a wide variety of biomarkers have been explored in the field (28). The biomarkers can be separated into different categories:

- Vascular dysfunction markers: asymmetric dimethylarginine (ADMA), ET-1, angiopoeitins, and von Willebrand factor (1,29,30)
- Inflammation markers: C-reactive protein, interleukin 6, chemokines, interleukin 1, tumor necrosis factor (1,31–33)
- Myocardial stress markers: atrial natriuretic peptide (ANP), brain natriuretic peptide (BNP)/NT-proBNP, troponins (1,34–36)
- Hypoxia markers: pCO_2, uric acid, growth differentiation factor 15 (GDF15), osteopontin (37,38)
- Secondary organ damage markers: creatinine, bilirubin (36,39)

Current therapies for pulmonary hypertension

Although none of the currently approved therapies can reverse or cure PH, the care and the quality of life of PH patients has improved. Since a substantial number of molecules are implicated in the pathogenesis of PH, several approaches to the treatment of PH are currently available (40). These are discussed below.

Phosphodiesterase type 5 (PDE-5) inhibitors: As described above, the lack of the NO vasodilator is one of the main abnormalities that triggers PH. PDE-5, which is amply expressed in the lungs, is the main cause of the imparity on the amount of NO in patients with PH. Therefore, the inhibition of PDE-5 is one of the select treatments currently used for patients with PH. PDE-5 inhibitors include sildenafil and tadalafil (approved), and a third PDE-5 inhibitor, vardenafil (in investigation). (23). The side effects encountered by using PDE-5 inhibitors, usually minor and temporary, include headache, flushing, nasal congestion, digestive disorders, and myalgia (23).

Prostacyclin and prostacyclin analogs: Prostacyclin is a prostanoid metabolized from endogenous arachidonic acid through the cyclooxygenase (COX) pathway (41). It is a potent vasodilator identified as one of the most effective drugs for the treatment of PH. Prostanoids are potent vasodilators and possess antithrombotic, antiproliferative, and anti-inflammatory properties (42). In the pulmonary circulation, prostacyclin is released by endothelial cells in the pulmonary artery. The binding of prostacyclin to its receptor activates the G-protein and increases intracellular cAMP, which activates protein kinase A. This causes inhibition of platelet aggregation, relaxation of smooth muscle, and vasodilation of the pulmonary arteries (41). Clinical studies for patients with PH are being performed with epoprostenol, iloprost, beraprost, and treprostinil (42). Currently, treprostinil is available in the market, either administered by nebulization (Tyvaso®), intravenously (Remodulin®), and orally (Orenitram®). It is important to note that treprostinil Phase 3 trial of Liquidia Technologies' LIQ861 treprostinil DPI for the treatment of (PH) is underway. LIQ861, a dry powder formulation based on Liquidia's particle replication in nonwetting templates (PRINT) particle engineering technology, is one of two products in the company. At least one other dry powder formulation for inhalation developed by Liquidia and licensed to GSK is in development, and it is expected to be on the market in 2019 (43). Furthermore, MannKind Corporation will start enrollment for a Phase 1 trial to test its treprostinil inhaled therapy for the treatment of PH. The company's Treprostinil Technosphere (TreT) combines the active ingredient treprostinil in a dry powdered formulation that is inhaled via a novel delivery system (technospheres). The dry powder formulation consists of particles with the proper size for delivery into the deep lung. It is designed to be administered through MannKind's breath-powered inhalation devices, which are small, easy-to-use inhalers that require only the patient's breath to deliver the right powder dose (44).

Endothelin receptor antagonists (ERAs): By inhibiting endothelin receptors, vasodilation and antiproliferation of cells can be achieved; therefore a remodeling of the pulmonary arteries can be possible with the administration of these type of drug in patients with PH. As described above, there are two main endothelin receptors: type A (ET-A) and type B (ET-B). ET-As are expressed on SMCs, and they increase intracellular calcium; therefore, vasoconstriction is induced. Conversely, ET-Bs are present principally on endothelial cells, and they allow the release of the vasodilators, NO, and prostacyclin. However, ET-Bs are also present in SMCs and where they also induce vasoconstriction. Hence, the selective or the nonselective inhibition of the receptors is another approach to treat PH (45). Some ET-1 receptor antagonists currently used are sitaxentan, abrisentan, macitentan, and bosentan (46). Chemical structures are shown in Figure 19.2. Currently marketed products are listed in Table 19.1 (40).

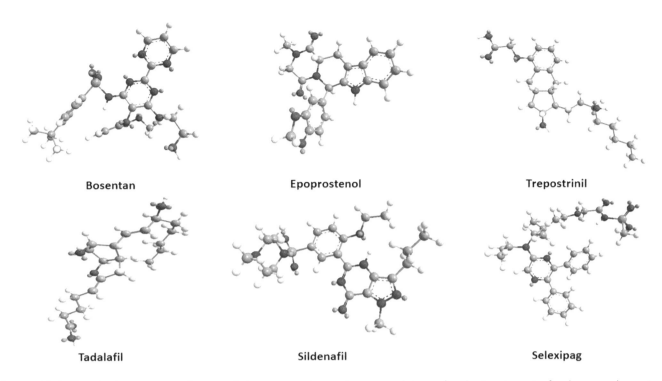

Bosentan	Epoprostenol	Trepostrinil
Tadalafil	Sildenafil	Selexipag

Figure 19.2 Chemical structures of some of the commonly used approved drugs for the treatment of pulmonary hypertension. (Chem3D Ver. 16.0.; CambridgeSoft, Cambridge, MA.)

Table 19.1 Currently marketed medicines for the treatment of pulmonary hypertension

Category	Function	Examples	Route of administration
Endothelin receptor antagonists (ERAs)	Prevention of the blood vessels narrowing	Ambrisentan (Letairis®) Bosentan (Tracleer®) Macitentan (Opsumit®)	Oral
Phosphodiesterase type 5 (PDE-5) inhibitors	Allow the production of the NO vasodilator in the lungs	Sildenafil (Revatio™) Sildenafil (Revatio™) Tadalafil (Adcirca®)	Oral
Prostacyclin analogues	Relaxation of the blood vessels Antithrombotic, antiproliferative, and anti-inflammatory properties	Trepostrinil (Orenitram®)	Oral
Selective IP receptor agonist	Targets and activates the prostacyclin receptor, promoting vasodilation	Selexipag (Uptravi®)	Oral
Soluble guanylate cyclase stimulators	Allow the interaction of soluble guanylate cyclase with nitric oxide, promoting vasodilation	Riociguat (Adempas®)	Oral
Nitric oxide	Vasodilation	Nitric oxide gas	Inhalation
Prostacyclin analogues	Relaxation of the blood vessels Antithrombotic, antiproliferative, and anti-inflammatory properties	Iloprost (Ventavis®) Trepostrinil (Tyvaso®)	Inhalation
Prostacyclin analogues	Relaxation of the blood vessels Antithrombotic, antiproliferative, and anti-inflammatory properties	Trepostrinil (Remodulin®) Epoprostenol (Flolan®) Room temperatura stable Epoprostenol (Veletri®)	Intravenous
Prostacyclin analogues	Relaxation of the blood vessels Antithrombotic, antiproliferative, and anti-inflammatory properties	Trepostrinil (Remodulin®)	Subcutaneous

Source: https://phassociation.org/patients/treatments/.

Ongoing investigational research therapeutics in pulmonary hypertension

Rho-kinase inhibitors: The small GTPases such as RhoA and its target, the Rho-kinase, have significant effects in the prevention of vasoconstriction and in the remodeling of the vascular vessels (47). As explained above, PH is characterized by an imbalance in vasoconstriction-vasodilation. This imbalance is caused by the overproduction and underproduction of vasoconstrictors and vasodilators, respectively. Some vasoconstrictors involved in the development of PH also mediate the Rho/Rho kinase pathway, and hence there is a downregulation of the eNOS and an exacerbation in the pulmonary vascular remodeling. Inhibitors of the Rho-kinase pathway can also contribute as an antioxidant, anti-inflammatory, antithrombotic, and immunomodulatory agents for the treatment of PH (47). Some Rho-kinase inhibitors that are currently in trials include statins (simvastatin, pravastatin, atorvastatin, rosuvastatin) and fasudil.

Selective serotonin reuptake inhibitors (SSRIs): Serotonin promotes the proliferation of PASMCs and fibroblasts and increases vasoconstriction and local thrombosis, all of which are features of PH. The effect of serotonin in the development of PH is mediated through its interaction with the serotonin transporters and receptors, mainly with serotonin transporter (SERT), which plays an important role in the development of the disease (48). SERT overexpression is well ligated with PH. SSRIs act via blockade of SERT, resulting in an extracellular accumulation of serotonin and increased activation of serotonin receptors (49). Fluoxetine, sertraline, paroxetine, and escitalopram are some of the SSRIs proposed for the treatment of PH.

NRF2 activators: The NF-κB pathway can be activated by oxidants and the subsequently produced inflammatory cytokines have been shown to be stimulators of an endothelial-mesenchymal transition (EndMT) (50). NF-E2-related factor 2 (Nrf2), is the main regulatory factor of the antioxidant response through regulating expression of a series of antioxidant enzymes, including heme oxygenase-1 (HO-1). In response to oxidative stress or electrophiles, Nrf2 separates from Kelch-like ECH-associated protein 1 (Keap1), a key Nrf2 inhibitory factor of Nrf2/HO-1 pathway, translocates into the nucleus, and induces the expression of antioxidant proteins (50). Nrf2 activators could be used to bind cysteine residue of Keap1 and promote de-methylation of Nrf2 promoter, giving pharmacological activities in the cardiovascular system, including adjunctive treatment of microcirculation protection, endothelial protection, myocardial preservation, and antioxidation (50).

Metabolic modulators: Since glucose oxidation is suppressed in patients with PH, and glucose levels are augmented in endothelial and smooth muscle cells, there are currently studies showing that drugs such as metformin (commonly used for the treatment of diabetes type II), which decrease the glucose levels, have positive effects for the decrease in PAH (51).

Approved inhalation products

Since PH is a disease that directly affects the lung, treatment targeted manner through inhalation is currently approved. At present, there are three FDA-approved inhalation products for the treatment of PH.

VENTAVIS® (iloprost) inhalation solution is an inhaled prostacyclin analog used to treat PH (Group 1). It simulates some of the effects of natural prostacyclin in the body such as opening up pulmonary arteries (vasodilation), and also affects platelet aggregation, allowing blood to flow more easily and thus putting less stress on the heart. It is administered through nebulization using a breath-activated vibrating mesh nebulizer device that delivers precise individualized dosing only during the personal inspiratory phase with continuous monitoring and adjustment. The aerosolized droplets have an aerodynamic size under 3 microns. This type of nebulizer device is small, hand-held, portable, and battery-operated. After using the device, it should be cleaned with distilled water and liquid detergent (no dishwasher or microwave) (52).

It is available in various dosing options (53): 1 mL of sterile aqueous solution in single-use glass ampule per dose contains 0.01 mg iloprost, 0.81 mg EtOH, 0.121 mg tromethamine, 9.0 mg NaCl, and approximately 0.51 mg HCl (for pH adjustment = 8.1) in WFI (water for injection). All components are inhalable (52).

The dosing frequency is high: 6 to 9 inhalations daily during waking hours (no more than once every 2 hours). This is due to short plasma $t_{1/2}$ within 30 minutes to 1 hour. The standard treatment time is 4 to 10 minutes (52).

TYVASO® (treprostinil) inhalation solution is another inhaled prostacyclin analog used to treat PH (Group 1). TYVASO can improve the ability to exercise in people who also take bosentan or sildenafil (54). The dosage form is a sterile solution for oral inhalation as a 2.9 mL ampule containing 1.74 mg treprostinil (0.6 mg per mL) (54). Dosing frequency is 4 times daily (2–3 minutes each). A single breath of TYVASO delivers about 6 μg of iloprost. Treprostinil is also delivered by nebulization using an Optineb ultrasonic device. The inhaled excipients are sodium chloride, sodium citrate, sodium hydroxide, hydrochloric acid, and water for injection (pH 6.0–7.2). It is important to mention that treprostinil is a photosensitive drug; therefore, it should be protected from light (55).

INOmax® nitric oxide gas for inhalation: Improves ventilation/perfusion matching by reducing pulmonary vascular resistance and decreasing pulmonary artery pressure. When inhaled, nitric oxide selectively dilates the pulmonary vasculature and has minimal effect on the systemic vasculature by targeting only the pulmonary bed (56).

Supportive therapies

Oral anticoagulants: Postmortem examinations in patients with PH have shown a high occurrence of vascular thrombotic lesions as well as abnormalities in coagulation and fibrinolytic pathways. Venous thromboembolism, heart failure, and immobility have also been observed. Given these observations, oral anticoagulation has been used for the treatment of PH (1). The most commonly prescribed anticoagulant is warfarin. More recent alternative options have been approved, including rivaroxaban, apixaban, edoxaban and dabigatran, collectively known as either novel oral anticoagulants (NOACs) or direct oral anticoagulants (DOACs) (57).

Diuretics: Right heart failure leads to fluid retention, increased central venous pressure, hepatic failure, ascites, and peripheral edema. The use of diuretics in patients presenting these symptoms have given notable symptomatic benefits. Common diuretics used for the treatment of PH are furosemide, bumetanide, metolazone, spironolactone, amiloride (58).

Aldosterone antagonists: Since mechanisms of right heart failure are highly associated with PH, the administration of the aldosterone antagonists may be beneficial for the improvement in the treatment of PH.

Calcium channel blockers (CCBs): CCBs relax muscles around blood vessels, thus reducing blood pressure. They are often use to treat systemic high blood pressure. It is also prescribed for patients with PH; however the doses needed are higher than for systemic blood pressure, causing often systemic hypotension and body water retention. The most used CCBs for PH are nifedipine, diltiazem, nicardipine, amlodipine (59).

Supplementary oxygen (O_2) therapy: With this therapy, air with a higher concentration of O_2 is inhaled. O_2 therapy increases the amount of O_2 in the blood (from lower to more normal levels). It is also useful for the relaxation of lung arteries. O_2 therapy can reduce fatigue and breathing difficulty in some people with PH. It can improve the lifestyle of some patients with PH. O_2 is supplied in many different ways such as compressed oxygen in cylinders, liquid oxygen in cylinders, oxygen concentrator machine (extracts oxygen from the air). Oxygen is delivered intranasally from cylinders or concentrator by plastic tubing to a mask or through soft tubes (60).

Other approaches for the treatment of pulmonary hypertension

Stem cell therapies: Stem cell therapies have revealed encouraging results in the repair and regeneration of lung blood vessels for the treatment of PH. Stem-like cells (endothelial progenitor cells) are being genetically manipulated in order to produce molecular factors that play important roles in vascular restore and regeneration (61).

Lung transplantation: Transplantation must be considered when the therapies previously mentioned fail for the improvement of PH. Lung or heart-lung transplant is the best option for patients who are not responding to standard therapies and who are experiencing a poor or declining quality of life. It can elongate survival, improve quality of life, and offer a potential cure for patients with PH. As with all transplant surgeries, however, they carry several risks and significant complications. Hence many factors have to be contemplated before moving forward with the transplantation (1).

Combination therapy: Since many molecular and cellular mechanism are involved in the pathogenesis of PH, the majority of patients do not show an improvement in the therapy using a single class of drug for PH. Hence, physicians are prescribing more than one class of drug to treat this severe disease with the hope of seeing better results and elongating the survival of patients.

CONCLUSION

PH is a very complex and multifactorial disease with multiple molecular and cellular mechanisms involved in its pathogenesis. A substantial number of novel drugs have been approved by the FDA in recent years. Patient compliance with many of the currently approved therapies for long-term chronic PH management is hindered by several factors, including (1) a short biological half-life, (2) a lack of selectivity resulting in serious off-target side effects, and (3) the need to target two or more pathways to effectively stem disease progression. In addition, all of the current therapies target reversal of the disease symptoms and not the underlying pathogenic mechanisms; thus, there is no cure for this fatal disease.

Since this disease directly affects the pulmonary vasculature, the development of inhaled targeted medicines would be the best approach for a better and more efficient treatment. Targeting therapeutic agents directly to the lung allows for the lowering of drug doses, which would exert a successful therapeutic effect while minimizing systemic effects. Also, combining more than one class of drug for PH in the same formulation can potentially cure this disease since many different mechanisms are involved. Currently, only nebulizers are approved and on the market for the targeted treatment of PH. However, many researchers and pharmaceutical companies are investing in the development of successful formulations and novel inhaler devices, such as dry powder inhalers, for the treatment and prevention of the progression of PH by using other therapeutic aerosol delivery systems for the lungs.

REFERENCES

1. Galiè N, Humbert M, Vachiery J-L, Gibbs S, Lang I, Torbicki A, Simonneau G et al. 2015 ESC/ERS guidelines for the diagnosis and treatment of pulmonary hypertension the joint task force for the Diagnosis and Treatment of Pulmonary Hypertension of the European Society of Cardiology (ESC) and the European Respiratory Society (ERS): Endorsed by: Association for European Paediatric and Congenital

Cardiology (AEPC), International Society for Heart and Lung Transplantation (ISHLT). *European Heart Journal.* 2016;37(1):67–119. doi:10.1093/eurheartj/ehv317.

2. Gary H. Gibbons MD. National Heart, Blood, and Lung Institute, https://www.nhlbi.nih.gov/health/health-topics/topics/pah, 2016.

3. Hyduk A, Croft JB, Ayala C, Zheng K, Zheng ZJ, Mensah GA. Pulmonary hypertension surveillance: United States, 1980–2002. *MMWR Surveill Summ.* 2005;54(5):1–28.

4. Zhang M-Z, Qian D-H, Xu J-C, Yao W, Fan Y, Wang C-Z. Statins may be beneficial for patients with pulmonary hypertension secondary to lung diseases. *Journal of Thoracic Disease.* 2017;9(8):2437–2446. doi:10.21037/jtd.2017.07.06.

5. Aerosols ns, metered-dose inhalers, and dry powder inhalers monograph. In. USP 29-NF 24 The United States Pharmacopoeia and The National Formulary: The Official Compendia of Standards. Rockville, MD: The United States Pharmacopeial Convention, Inc., 2006, pp. 2617–2636.

6. Weir EK, Lopez-Barneo J, Buckler KJ, Archer SL. Acute oxygen-sensing mechanisms. *The New England Journal of Medicine.* 2005;353(19):2042–2055. doi:10.1056/NEJMra050002.

7. Levitzky MG. *Pulmonary Physiology.* New York: McGraw-Hill, 2013.

8. Fraser R. *Diagnosis of Diseases of the Chest.* Philadelphia, PA: Saunders, 1988, p. 139.

9. Katsiki N, Wierzbicki AS, Mikhailidis DP. Pulmonary arterial hypertension and statins: An update. *Current Opinion in Cardiology.* 2011;26(4):322–326. doi:10.1097/HCO.0b013e32834659bf.

10. Loirand G, Pacaud P. The role of Rho protein signaling in hypertension. *Nature Reviews Cardiology.* 2010;7(11):637–647. doi:10.1038/nrcardio.2010.136.

11. Rafikova O, Rafikov R, Kumar S, Sharma S, Aggarwal S, Schneider F, Jonigk D, Black SM, Tofovic SP. Bosentan inhibits oxidative and nitrosative stress and rescues occlusive pulmonaryhypertension. *Free Radical Biology and Medicine.* 2013;56:28–43. doi:10.1016/j.freeradbiomed.2012.09.013.

12. Montani D, Günther S, Dorfmüller P, Perros F, Girerd B, Garcia G, Jaïs X et al. Pulmonary arterial hypertension. *Orphanet Journal of Rare Diseases.* 2013;8:97. doi:10.1186/1750-1172-8-97.

13. Iqbal M, Cawthon D, Wideman RF, Jr., Bottje WG. Lung mitochondrial dysfunction in pulmonary hypertension syndrome. I. Site-specific defects in the electron transport chain. *Poultry Science.* 2001;80(4):485–495.

14. Iqbal M, Cawthon D, Wideman RF, Jr, Bottje WG. Lung mitochondrial dysfunction in pulmonary hypertension syndrome. II. Oxidative stress and inability to improve function with repeated additions of adenosine diphosphate. *Poultry Science.* 2001;80(5):656–665.

15. Tan X, Hu SH, Wang XL. The effect of dietary l-carnitine supplementation on pulmonary hypertension syndrome mortality in broilers exposed to low temperatures. *Journal of Animal Physiology Animal Nutrition (Berlin).* 2008;92(2):203–210. doi:10.1111/j.1439-0396.2007.00727.x.

16. Pullamsetti SS, Perros F, Chelladurai P, Yuan J, Stenmark K. Transcription factors, transcriptional coregulators, and epigenetic modulation in the control of pulmonary vascular cell phenotype: Therapeutic implications for pulmonary hypertension (2015 Grover Conference series). *Pulmonary Circulation.* 2016;6(4):448–464. doi:10.1086/688908.

17. Runo JR, Loyd JE. Primary pulmonary hypertension. *Lancet.* 2003;361(9368):1533–1544. doi:10.1016/s0140-6736(03)13167-4.

18. Crosswhite P, Sun Z. Nitric oxide, oxidative stress and inflammation in pulmonary arterial hypertension. *Journal of Hypertension.* 2010;28(2):201–212. doi:10.1097/HJH.0b013e328332bcdb.

19. Morrell NW, Adnot S, Archer SL, Dupuis J, Jones PL, MacLean MR, McMurtry IF et al. Cellular and molecular basis of pulmonary arterial hypertension. *Journal of the American College of Cardiology.* 2009;54(1 Suppl):S20–S31. doi:10.1016/j.jacc.2009.04.018.

20. Tan X, Hu SH, Wang XL. The effect of dietary l-carnitine supplementation on pulmonary hypertension syndrome mortality in broilers exposed to low temperatures. *Journal of Animal Physiology and Animal Nutrition.* 2008;92(2):203–210. doi:10.1111/j.1439-0396.2007.00727.x.

21. Hayes DJ, Tobias JD, Mansour HM, Kirkby S, McCoy KS, Daniels CJ, Whitson BA. Pulmonary hypertension in cystic fibrosis with advanced lung disease. *American Journal of Respiratory and Critical Care Medicine.* 2014;190(8):898–905.

22. Ogata T, Iijima T. Structure and pathogenesis of plexiform lesion in pulmonary hypertension. *Chinese Medical Journal.* 1993;106(1):45–48.

23. Montani D, Chaumais MC, Savale L, Natali D, Price LC, Jais X, Humbert M, Simonneau G, Sitbon O. Phosphodiesterase type 5 inhibitors in pulmonary arterial hypertension. *Advances in Therapy.* 2009;26(9):813–825. doi:10.1007/s12325-009-0064-z.

24. Herve P, Launay JM, Scrobohaci ML, Brenot F, Simonneau G, Petitpretz P, Poubeau P et al. Increased plasma serotonin in primary pulmonary hypertension. *The American Journal of Medicine.* 1995;99(3):249–254.

25. Ziello JE, Jovin IS, Huang Y. Hypoxia-Inducible Factor (HIF)-1 regulatory pathway and its potential for therapeutic intervention in malignancy and ischemia. *The Yale Journal of Biology and Medicine.* 2007;80(2):51–60.

26. Semenza GL. HIF-1 and mechanisms of hypoxia sensing. *Current Opinion in Cell Biology.* 2001;13(2):167–171.

27. Sutendra G, Michelakis ED. Pulmonary arterial hypertension: Challenges in translational research and a vision for change. *Science Translational Medicine*. 2013;5(208):208sr5. doi:10.1126/scitranslmed.3005428.

28. Foris V, Kovacs G, Tscherner M, Olschewski A, Olschewski H. Biomarkers in pulmonary hypertension: What do we know? *Chest*. 2013;144(1):274–283. doi:10.1378/chest.12-1246.

29. Barst RJ, Chung L, Zamanian RT, Turner M, McGoon MD. Functional class improvement and 3-year survival outcomes in patients with pulmonary arterial hypertension in the REVEAL registry. *Chest*. 2013;144(1):160–168. doi:10.1378/chest.12-2417.

30. Pullamsetti S, Kiss L, Ghofrani HA, Voswinckel R, Haredza P, Klepetko W, Aigner C et al. Increased levels and reduced catabolism of asymmetric and symmetric dimethylarginines in pulmonary hypertension. *FASEB Journal: Official Publication of the Federation of American Societies for Experimental Biology*. 2005;19(9):1175–1177. doi:10.1096/fj.04-3223fje.

31. Balabanian K, Foussat A, Dorfmuller P, Durand-Gasselin I, Capel F, Bouchet-Delbos L, Portier A et al. CX(3)C chemokine fractalkine in pulmonary arterial hypertension. *American Journal of Respiratory and Critical Care Medicine*. 2002;165(10):1419–1425. doi:10.1164/rccm.2106007.

32. Quarck R, Nawrot T, Meyns B, Delcroix M. C-reactive protein: A new predictor of adverse outcome in pulmonary arterial hypertension. *Journal of the American College of Cardiology*. 2009;53(14):1211–1218. doi:10.1016/j.jacc.2008.12.038.

33. Humbert M, Monti G, Brenot F, Sitbon O, Portier A, Grangeot-Keros L et al. Increased interleukin-1 and interleukin-6 serum concentrations in severe primary pulmonary hypertension. *American Journal of Respiratory and Critical Care Medicine*. 1995;151(5):1628–1631. doi:10.1164/ajrccm.151.5.7735624.

34. Nagaya N, Nishikimi T, Uematsu M, Satoh T, Kyotani S, Sakamaki F, Kakishita M et al. Plasma brain natriuretic peptide as a prognostic indicator in patients with primary pulmonary hypertension. *Circulation*. 2000;102(8):865–870.

35. Torbicki A, Kurzyna M, Kuca P, Fijałkowska A, Sikora J, Florczyk M, Pruszczyk P, Burakowski J, Wawrzyńska L. Detectable serum cardiac troponin T as a marker of poor prognosis among patients with chronic precapillary pulmonary hypertension. *Circulation*. 2003;108(7):844–848. doi:10.1161/01.cir.0000084544.54513.e2.

36. Nickel N, Golpon H, Greer M, Knudsen L, Olsson K, Westerkamp V, Welte T, Hoeper MM. The prognostic impact of follow-up assessments in patients with idiopathic pulmonary arterial hypertension. *The European Respiratory Journal*. 2012;39(3):589–596. doi:10.1183/09031936.00092311.

37. Nagaya N, Uematsu M, Satoh T, Kyotani S, Sakamaki F, Nakanishi N, Yamagishi M, Kunieda T, Miyatake K. Serum uric acid levels correlate with the severity and the mortality of primary pulmonary hypertension. *American Journal of Respiratory and Critical Care Medicine*. 1999;160(2):487–492. doi:10.1164/ajrccm.160.2.9812078.

38. Nickel N, Kempf T, Tapken H, Tongers J, Laenger F, Lehmann U, Golpon H et al. Growth differentiation factor-15 in idiopathic pulmonary arterial hypertension. *American Journal of Respiratory and Critical Care Medicine*. 2008;178(5):534–541. doi:10.1164/rccm.200802-235OC.

39. Leuchte HH, El Nounou M, Tuerpe JC, Hartmann B, Baumgartner RA, Vogeser M, Muehling O, Behr J. N-terminal pro-brain natriuretic peptide and renal insufficiency as predictors of mortality in pulmonary hypertension. *Chest*. 2007;131(2):402–409. doi:10.1378/chest.06-1758.

40. Pulmonary Hypertension Association (PHA). 2015. Available at: https://phassociation.org/patients/treatments/. (Accessed August 2018).

41. Ruan C-H, Dixon RAF, Willerson JT, Ruan K-H. Prostacyclin therapy for pulmonary arterial hypertension. *Texas Heart Institute Journal*. 2010;37(4):391–399.

42. Gomberg-Maitland M, Olschewski H. Prostacyclin therapies for the treatment of pulmonary arterial hypertension. *The European Respiratory Journal*. 2008;31(4):891–901. doi:10.1183/09031936.00097107.

43. Orally inhaled and nasal drug products (OINDP news). Available at: http://www.oindpnews.com/2018/01/liquidiaannounces-initiation-of-phase-3-trial-of-trepostinildpi-for-pah/].Onc (Accessed August 2018).

44. Pulmonary hypertension news. Available at: https://pulmonaryhypertensionnews.com/2018/03/09/mannkind-starts-enrollment-phase-1-trial-treprostinilpah. (Accessed August 2018).

45. Liu C, Chen J, Gao Y, Deng B, Liu K. Endothelin receptor antagonists for pulmonary arterial hypertension. *The Cochrane Database of Systematic Reviews*. 2013;2:Cd004434. doi:10.1002/14651858.CD004434.pub5.

46. Connolly MJ, Aaronson PI. Key role of the RhoA/Rho kinase system in pulmonary hypertension. *Pulmonary Pharmacology & Therapeutics*. 2011;24(1):1–14. doi:10.1016/j.pupt.2010.09.001.

47. Duong-Quy S, Bei Y, Liu Z, Dinh-Xuan AT. Role of Rho-kinase and its inhibitors in pulmonary hypertension. *Pharmacology & Therapeutics*. 2013;137(3):352–364. doi:10.1016/j.pharmthera.2012.12.003.

48. MacLean MR. The serotonin hypothesis in pulmonary hypertension revisited: Targets for novel

therapies (2017 Grover Conference Series). *Pulmonary Circulation.* 2018;8(2):2045894018759125. doi:10.1177/2045894018759125.

49. Sadoughi A, Roberts KE, Preston IR, Lai GP, McCollister DH, Farber HW, Hill NS. Use of selective serotonin reuptake inhibitors and outcomes in pulmonary arterial hypertension. *Chest.* 2013;144(2):531–541. doi:10.1378/chest.12-2081.

50. Chen Y, Yuan T, Zhang H, Yan Y, Wang D, Fang L, Lu Y, Du G. Activation of Nrf2 attenuates pulmonary vascular remodeling via inhibiting endothelial-to-mesenchymal transition: An insight from a plant polyphenol. *International Journal of Biological Sciences.* 2017;13(8):1067–1081. doi:10.7150/ijbs.20316.

51. Dean A, Nilsen M, Loughlin L, Salt IP, MacLean MR. Metformin reverses development of pulmonary hypertension via aromatase inhibition. *Hypertension (Dallas, Tex: 1979).* 2016;68(2):446–454. doi:10.1161/hypertensionaha.116.07353.

52. Ventavis® iloprost INHALATION SOLUTION [August 21, 2018]. Available from https://www.actelionpathways.com/hcp/ventavis-patient-assistance/ventavis-distribution?gclid=EAIaIQobChMI4aGsv9__3AIVD8NkCh2n3AYeEAAYASAAEgIAlfD_BwE.

53. Inhaled Ventavis® (iloprost) INHALATION SOLUTION. Available at: https://www.4ventavis.com/. (Accessed August 2018).

54. TYVASO® (treprostinil) INHALATION SOLUTION. Available at: https://www.tyvaso.com/hcp/?gclid=EAIaIQobChMItfOQ0uL_3AIVkWV-Ch0JIQYTEAAYASAAEgLDePD_BwE. (Accessed August 2018).

55. TYVASO® (TREPROSTINIL) INHALATION SOLUTION [August 21, 2018]. Available from https://www.tyvaso.com/hcp/?gclid=EAIaIQobChMItfOQ0uL_3AIVkWV-Ch0JIQYTEAAYASAAEgLDePD_BwE.

56. INOmax (nitric oxide) gas for inhalation. Available at: http://inomax.com/about-inomax/treating-hypoxiarespiratory-failure/dosing. (Accessed August 2018).

57. Johnson SR, Mehta S, Granton JT. Anticoagulation in pulmonary arterial hypertension: A qualitative systematic review. *European Respiratory Journal.* 2006;28(5):999–1004. doi:10.1183/09031936.06.00015206.

58. Stamm JA, Risbano MG, Mathier MA. Overview of current therapeutic approaches for pulmonary hypertension. *Pulmonary Circulation.* 2011;1(2):138–159. doi:10.4103/2045-8932.83444.

59. Fan Z, Chen Y, Liu H. Calcium channel blockers for pulmonary arterial hypertension. *The Cochrane Database of Systematic Reviews.* 2015;9:Cd010066. doi:10.1002/14651858.CD010066.pub2.

60. Palmisano JM, Martin JM, Krauzowicz BA, Truman KH, Meliones JN. Effects of supplemental oxygen administration in an infant with pulmonary artery hypertension. *Heart & Lung: The Journal of Critical Care.* 1990;19(6):627–630.

61. Patel NM, Burger CD. Two cases of stem cell therapy for pulmonary hypertension: A clinical report. *Respiratory Medicine CME.* 2011;4(2):70–74. doi:10.1016/j.rmedc.2010.09.002.

20

Overview of lung surfactant and respiratory distress syndrome

HEIDI M. MANSOUR, DEBRA DROOPAD, AND JULIE G. LEDFORD

Pulmonary surfactant	323	References	325
Lung surfactant replacement and drug carriers	324		

PULMONARY SURFACTANT

Pulmonary surfactant (PS) is a phospholipid-protein complex that lines the airways as a monomolecular layer of only a few nanometers. It is a vital component in respiration because it decreases the work of breathing through lowering surface tension, which is the major contributor to the work of breathing. Lung surfactant is also vital in preventing alveolar collapse, which is also known as atelectasis. In addition, PS is vital in lung fluid homeostasis, clearance mechanisms, and immunomodulation in the airways.

PS is an elegant and complex mixture of 90% phospholipids and 10% surface-active protein. There are four known lung surfactant proteins, that is, surfactant-specific proteins: SP-A, SP-B, SP-C, and SP-D. Of the phospholipid content, 55%–60% is dipalmitoylphosphatidylcholine (DPPC), in addition to the anionic phospholipid palmitoyloleoylphosphatidylglycerol (POPG), and palmitoyloleoylphosphatidylcholine (POPC), which are all important in the spreading mechanisms (1,2) and stability. SP-A and SP-D proteins depend on calcium and are large hydrophilic proteins. SP-A and SP-D proteins are critical in pulmonary immunity, alveolar macrophage stimulation, and regulating pulmonary immune response. In contrast to SP-A and SP-D proteins, SP-B and SP-C proteins are hydrophobic proteins and are relatively smaller in size. SP-B and SP-C proteins are needed in lung surfactant spreading mechanisms, lung surfactant stability, and the normal function of lung surfactant.

PS aides in gas exchange and reduces surface tension in the alveoli to prevent airway collapse. Alveolar stability (3,4) depends on lung surfactant surface tension variability (5–7) and its ability to reach low surface tension (8). Lung surfactant is synthesized by the pulmonary Type II cell

(9,10) packaged into multilamellar bodies, which are then secreted into the thin aqueous layer where they become tubular myelin upon hydration and then spread. Spreading occurs at the air-liquid interface to form the lung surfactant monolayer, which is a nanolayer.

SP-A is the most abundant of the four surfactant proteins and is an important mediator of innate and adaptive immunity in the lung. In humans, SP-A is comprised of gene products from *SFTPA1* (SP-A1) and *SFTPA2* (SP-A2) that oligomerize into six trimeric subunits to form an octadecomer (11). As a member of the collectin family of proteins, SP-A contains a collagen-like domain and highly conserved carbohydrate recognition domain (CRD). The CRD enables SP-A to bind to components of bacterial cell walls, thereby enhancing their uptake by resident macrophages.

Although SP-A is perhaps best known as a mediator in host defense, many diverse roles have been ascribed to SP-A that begin in utero. Once the fetal lung is nearing the end of development, SP-A protein is secreted from alveolar type II cells, where it activates macrophages to signal the initiation of labor (12). However, in many preterm newborns prior to 35 weeks gestation, the immature lungs are unable to secrete enough PS to prevent alveoli collapse, which leads to respiratory distress syndrome (RDS). The leading cause of mortality in premature infants, RDS was the first lung disease to be directly attributed to the absence or abnormality in lung surfactant (13).

Despite the discovery that the lack of PS is a driver of preterm newborn RDS a half-century ago, preterm birth and associated RDS remain a major cause of neonatal mortality throughout the world if not treated appropriately. Therefore, it is not surprising that the World Health Organization (WHO) lists pulmonary surfactant replacement on the "model list of essential medicines," which is reserved for the most relevant medications needed in a basic health system. For several decades, pulmonary surfactant replacement therapy has offered animal-derived surfactants as well as synthetic surfactants. However, while containing the essential phospholipids, these medications lack SP-A as a component. As new discoveries reveal new vital roles of SP-A in mediating chronic lung diseases such as idiopathic pulmonary fibrosis (14,15), lung cancer (16), and asthma (17,18), attention has turned to SP-A replacement therapies in addition to the standard phospholipid surfactant replacement. Difficulties may arise from delivery of a full-length oligomeric SP-A into the airspace due to the large size; therefore, much enthusiasm in the field revolves around potential therapeutic replacement of SP-A with specific peptides derived from active regions that can be delivered by conventional inhaler devices.

LUNG SURFACTANT REPLACEMENT AND DRUG CARRIERS

Lung surfactant replacement therapeutics have included synthetic phospholipid colloidal dispersions, animal lung surfactant extracts, and recombinant human surfactant peptides. They are typically administered to intubated premature babies by endotracheal instillation. Table 20.1 lists the lung surfactant replacement pharmaceutical products with dosing information and formulation composition details.

The animal extracts can have relatively high variability in composition but have improved spreading properties, since they contain SP-B and SP-C residual proteins. However, there is the potential for immunogenic responses that can develop with animal extracts due to being an animal source. Dosing is in mL/kg given this special patient population.

Table 20.1 Lung surfactant replacement pharmaceutical products with composition, single dose, maximum dose, and dosing regimen

Product brand name	Single dose (mL/kg)	Maximum dose (mL/kg)	Dosing regimen	Composition	Company
Alveofact®	1.2	4	A single dose within the first hour after birth and up to 3 subsequent doses	Bovine lung surfactant extract/phospholipid, sodium chloride, sodium hydrogen carbonate, and water	Boehringer Ingelheim
Curosurf®	2.5	5	An initial dose divided into 2 aliquots within 15 hours after diagnosis of RDS up to 2 subsequent doses of 1.25 mL/kg	Porcine lung surfactant extract/phospholipid, sodium chloride, sodium hydrogen carbonate, and water	Dey
Exosurf® (discontinued in 2008)	5	10	An initial dose divided into 2 aliquots within the first 30 minutes after birth up to 2 subsequent doses of 2.5 mL/kg	Synthetic phospholipid, acetyl alcohol, colfosceril palmitic acid (PA), and tyloxapol	GlaxoSmithKline
Infasurf®	3	6	An initial dose divided into 2 aliquots within the first 30 minutes after birth up to 2 subsequent doses of 1.5 mL/kg	Bovine lung surfactant extract/phospholipid, sodium chloride, and water	Ony Inc.
Surfaxin® (discontinued in 2015)	5.8	23.2	A single dose within the first hour after birth up to 4 subsequent doses of 5.8 mL/kg	Synthetic (recombinant human 21-amino acid peptide) SP-B peptide/phospholipid, palmitic acid (PA), sinapultide in tromethamine, sodium chloride, and acetic acid	Drug Discovery Labs
Survanta®	4	4	A single dose divided into 4 aliquots within the first hour after birth	Bovine lung surfactant extract/phospholipid, sodium chloride, palmitic acid (PA), dipalmitoylphosphatidylcholine (DPPC), tripalmitin, sodium hydroxide, hydrochloride acid, and water	Abbott Labs

A single dose is given and typically in aliquots. Then multiple doses can be given. These formulations spontaneously spread in the lungs down to the alveolar region due to the inherent surface activity properties.

Lung surfactant replacement therapeutics can also be aerosolized provided the appropriate interactions between the formulation and specific inhaler device are optimized. They can be aerosolized by vibrating mesh nebulizers and dry powder inhalers. There is much research interest in using lung surfactant replacement-mimic formulations as inhaled carriers (19–24) of drugs given the unique spreading and aerosol properties of these advanced formulations. Since many drugs are surface-active and/or hydrophobic, lung surfactant carriers can efficiently encapsulate them as carrier systems. In addition, using recombinant human technology to create lung surfactant peptide mimics (25) of these lung surfactant proteins represents an exciting and innovative therapeutic platform for the treatment of RDS as well as other lung diseases where protein dysfunction and/or abnormal lung surfactant properties exist.

REFERENCES

1. Mansour H, Wang D-S, Chen C-S, Zografi G. Comparison of bilayer and monolayer properties of phoshpholipid systems containing dipalmitoylphosphatidylglycerol and dipalmitoylphosphatidylinositol. *Langmuir.* 2001;17(21):6622–6632.
2. Mansour HM, Zografi G. Relationships between equilibrium spreading pressure and phase equilibria of phospholipid bilayers and monolayers at the air-water interface. *Langmuir.* 2007;23(7):3809–3819.
3. Clements JA, Hustead RF, Johnson RP, Gribetz I. Pulmonary surface tension and alveolar stability. *J. Appl. Physiol.* 1961;16:444–450.
4. Schurch S, Qanbar R, Bachofen H, Possmayer F. The surface-associated surfactant reservoir in the alveolar lining. *Biol. Neonate.* 1995;67(suppl 1):61–76.
5. Schurch S, Goerke J, Clements JA. Determination of surface tension in the lung. *Proc. Natl. Acad. Sci. USA.* 1976;73:4698–4702.
6. Clements JA. Surface tension of lung extracts. *Proc. Soc. Exp. Biol. Med.* 1957;95:170–172.
7. Clements J. Lung surfactant: A personal perspective. *Annu. Rev. Physiol.* 1997;59:1–21.
8. Pattle RE. Properties, function and origin of the alveolar lining layer. *Nature.* 1955;175:1125–1126.
9. Wright JR, Clements JA. Metabolism and turnover of lung surfactant. *Am. Rev. Respir. Dis.* 1987;135:426–444.
10. Wright JR, Dobbs LG. Regulation of pulmonary surfactant secretion and clearance. *Ann. Rev. Physiol.* 1991;53:395–414.
11. Nathan N, Taytard J, Duquesnoy P, Thouvenin G, Corvol H, Amselem S, Clement A. Surfactant protein A: A key player in lung homeostasis. *Int. J. Biochem. Cell Biol.* 2016;81(Pt A):151–155.

12. Mendelson CR, Montalbano AP, Gao L. Fetal-to-maternal signaling in the timing of birth. *J. Steroid Biochem. Mol. Biol.* 2017;170:19–27.
13. Avery ME, Mead J. Surface properties in relation to atelectasis and hyaline membrane disease. *Am. J. Dis. Child.* 1959;97:517–523.
14. Goto H, Ledford JG, Mukherjee S, Noble PW, Williams KL, Wright JR. The role of surfactant protein A in bleomycin-induced acute lung injury. *Am. J. Respir. Crit. Care. Med.* 2010;181(12):1336–1344.
15. Nathan N, Giraud V, Picard C, et al. Germline SFTPA1 mutation in familial idiopathic interstitial pneumonia and lung cancer. *Hum. Mol. Genet.* 2016;25(8):1457–1467.
16. Mitsuhashi A, Goto H, Kuramoto T, et al. Surfactant protein A suppresses lung cancer progression by regulating the polarization of tumor-associated macrophages. *Am. J. Pathol.* 2013;182(5):1843–1853.
17. Lugogo N, Francisco D, Addison KJ, et al. Obese asthmatic patients have decreased surfactant protein A levels: Mechanisms and implications. *J. Allergy Clin. Immunol.* 2018;141(3):918–926 e913.
18. Wang Y, Voelker DR, Lugogo NL, et al. Surfactant protein A is defective in abrogating inflammation in asthma. *Am. J. Physiol. Lung. Cell Mol. Physiol.* 2011;301(4):L598–L606.
19. Wu X, Zhang W, Hayes DJ, Mansour HM. Physicochemical characterization and aerosol dispersion performance of organic solution advanced spray-dried cyclosporine A multifunctional particles for dry powder inhalation aerosol delivery. *Int. J. Nanomed.* 2013;8:1269–1283.
20. Wu X, Hayes DJ, Zwischenberger JB, Kuhn RJ, Mansour HM. Design and physicochemical characterization of advanced spray-dried tacrolimus multifunctional particles for inhalation. *Drug Des. Dev. Ther.* 2013;7:59–72.
21. Meenach SA, Vogt FG, Anderson KW, Hilt JZ, McGarry RC, Mansour HM. Design, physicochemical characterization, and optimization of organic solution advanced spray-dried inhalable dipalmitoylphosphatidylcholine (DPPC) and dipalmitoylphosphatidylethanolamine poly(ethylene glycol) (DPPE-PEG) microparticles and nanoparticles for targeted respiratory nanomedicine delivery as dry powder inhalation aerosols. *Inter. J. Nanomed.* 2013;8:275–293.
22. Meenach SA, Anderson KW, Hilt JZ, McGarry RC, Mansour HM. High-performing dry powder inhalers of paclitaxel DPPC/DPPG lung surfactant-mimic multifunctional particles in lung cancer: Physicochemical characterization, in vitro aerosol dispersion, and cellular studies. *AAPS Pharm. Sci. Tech.* 2014;15(6):1574–1587.
23. Meenach SA, Anderson KW, Zach Hilt J, McGarry RC, Mansour HM. Characterization and aerosol dispersion performance of advanced spray-dried chemotherapeutic PEGylated phospholipid particles for dry powder inhalation delivery in lung cancer. *Eur. J. Pharm. Sci.* 2013;49(4):699–711.

24. Duan J, Vogt FG, Li X, Hayes D, Jr, Mansour HM. Design, characterization, and aerosolization of organic solution advanced spray-dried moxifloxacin and ofloxacin dipalmitoylphosphatidylcholine (DPPC) microparticulate/nanoparticulate powders for pulmonary inhalation aerosol delivery. *Int. J. Nanomed.* 2013;8:3489–3505.

25. Mansour HM, Damodaran S, Zografi G. Characterization of the *in situ* structural and interfacial properties of the cationic hydrophobic heteropolypeptide, KL_4, in lung surfactant bilayer and monolayer models at the air-water interface: Implications for pulmonary surfactant delivery. *Mol. Phar.* 2008;5(5):681–695.

21

Surfactant aerosol therapy for nRDS and ARDS

DONOVAN B. YEATES

Introduction to neonatal respiratory distress syndrome and acute respiratory distress syndrome	327	Delivery of surfactant to neonates	334
		Endotracheal surfactant bolus instillation	334
Prevalence and pathophysiology of neonatal respiratory distress syndrome	328	Minimally invasive surfactant bolus instillation	334
		Aerosol delivery through catheters	335
Prevalence and pathophysiology of ARDS	329	Surfactant aerosol delivery and noninvasive ventilation	335
Surfactant formulations	330		
Effective dose of surfactant aerosol	331	Delivery of surfactant for the treatment of ARDS	336
Aerosol concentration and particle size	331	Technological advances in surfactant aerosol delivery	336
Intra-airway deposition distribution and spreading to the lung periphery	331	Utility of heliox for the generation and delivery of respirable aerosols in nRDS and ARDS	337
Wet or dry surfactant aerosol?	332	Conclusion	337
Effects of electric charge on wet and dry aerosols	333	Conflicts of interest	338
Device-patient interface aerosol losses	333	Acknowledgments	338
Surfactant aerosol generation: general considerations	334	References	338

INTRODUCTION TO NEONATAL RESPIRATORY DISTRESS SYNDROME AND ACUTE RESPIRATORY DISTRESS SYNDROME

Neonatal respiratory distress syndrome (nRDS) and acute respiratory distress syndrome (ARDS) are acute conditions that are associated with insufficient surfactant in the peripheral lungs. When there is insufficient surfactant, more force is required to open and expand the airways and create sufficient surface area for adequate gas exchange to support respiratory homeostasis. In the case of neonatal respiratory distress, the surfactant deficiency is due to the lack of surfactant production in infants born prematurely, and, as expected, the incidence of nRDS increases inversely in proportion to gestational age. In near-term births, meconium aspiration and pneumonia are the most frequent predispositions for infant ARDS. In patients with ARDS, the deficiency in surfactant results from inflammation-induced degradation of the surfactant and the resulting edema. This leads to collapse of the alveoli and small airway bilateral infiltrates, and rapid deterioration of oxygenation. ARDS is still associated with a high mortality rate.

Both nRDS and ARDS patients feature pathogenic mechanisms other than surfactant deficiency. While these mechanisms require further elucidation and investigation into their clinical relevance, the presence of functional surfactant in the distal airways and alveoli is essential to the resolution of this respiratory dysfunction. Surfactant administration decreases the surface tension and consequently the pressure required to open atelectatic airways and collapsed alveoli, which increases respiratory capacity and improves gas exchange. In addition to these beneficial biophysical surface tension–lowering properties, surfactant also has anti-inflammatory and anti-infective properties.

Only in pediatric indications is surfactant instillation approved for administration through an endotracheal tube. In adult ARDS, despite the proven mechanistic functions and associated physiologic benefits of surfactant, neither surfactant instillation nor aerosol administration of surfactant has resulted in sustained, reproducible improvements in clinical outcomes or mortality.

To reduce or eliminate the adverse effects of traumatic intubation procedures in neonates, pediatricians prefer to maintain very preterm neonates on noninvasive ventilator support, such as continuous positive airway pressure (CPAP). Administration of surfactant through an invasive endotracheal tube thwarts this gentle approach. Promising developments, such as less invasive surfactant administration (LISA), have improved pulmonary outcomes but have not reduced the need and drive for neonatologists to be able to administer surfactant noninvasively as an aerosol.

This chapter highlights the technical and physiologic issues relating to the administration of aerosolized surfactant replacement therapy for both nRDS and ARDS. Identifying the substantial limitations related to the delivery of clinically relevant doses of surfactant to the distal lungs and the physiologic role of surfactant in the resolution of these syndromes provides insights on needed improvements in surfactant aerosol delivery to save lives and improve the short- and long-term respiratory disabilities for these patients.

PREVALENCE AND PATHOPHYSIOLOGY OF NEONATAL RESPIRATORY DISTRESS SYNDROME

The World Health Organization (WHO) estimates that, of the 15 million premature babies born around the world each year, 1 million die within the first month of life, and many of the 14 million survivors will be faced with a lifetime of serious health complications. Both morbidity and mortality are much higher in the developing world than in developed countries (1). In the United States, 140,000 babies are born earlier than 34 weeks' gestation every year. In preterm infants, nRDS is the single most important cause of morbidity and mortality. The prevalence of nRDS, the incidence of subsequent bronchopulmonary dysplasia (BPD), the long-term adverse respiratory deficits, and the cost of healthcare increases with decreasing gestational age.

The characteristics of the neonatal patient population that benefit from surfactant replacement therapy are shown in Figure 21.1. As expected, the number of babies born increases with increasing gestational age up to 38 to 42 weeks. However, the survival at discharge from hospital decreases from 98% at 33 weeks to 88% at 27 weeks and to 46% at 24 weeks' gestational age (2). As expected, in a cohort of 6628 infants studied between 2000 and 2013 in Denmark, the percentage of babies with RDS treated with surfactant therapy

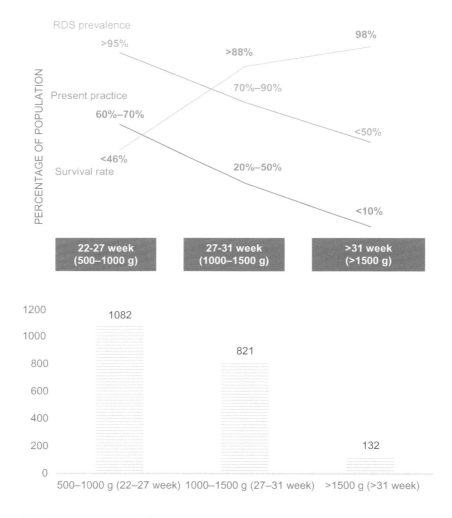

Figure 21.1 Results of multicenter study of all (6628) inborn preterm infants in Denmark from 2000 to 2013. The top panel shows the trends with gestation age of the relative prevalence of nRDS, the percentage treated with surfactant, and the overall survival rate of infants. The bottom panel shows the number of infants treated with surfactant as a function of gestational age. (The data has been extracted from Wiingreen, R., et al., *Neonatology.*, 111, 331–336, 2017.)

decreased with increasing gestational age between 23 and 33 weeks, such that the number of babies treated with surfactant instillation is highest in the 22- to 30-week age group (2). Early surfactant administration to infants with nRDS requiring assisted ventilation, compared to delaying treatment of such infants until they develop worsening nRDS, led to a lower risk of acute pulmonary injury (decreased risk of pneumothorax and pulmonary interstitial emphysema) and lower risk of neonatal mortality and chronic lung disease. Surfactant replacement therapy is also likely to reduce the risk of BPD. In addition, the success rate of surfactant instillation is higher in low birth weight babies compared to those born near term. In infants born near term, this could be due to other confounding factors, such as coexistent pneumonia, infections, or meconium aspiration.

Treatment with mechanical ventilation and high levels of inspired oxygen negatively affect the pathology, inflammation, structural development, and alveolarization of the lungs (3). The introduction of surfactant instillation has reduced the severity of this pathology, but long-term respiratory issues including BPD, chronic obstructive lung disease, and increased prevalence of asthma remain (3).

In premature babies with nRDS, both surfactant instillation into the lungs and CPAP have been shown to improve clinical outcomes; however, the complication rate, comorbidities, and mortality rate due to intubation remain unacceptably high (4). By avoiding the detrimental effects of mechanical ventilation, high inspired oxygen fractions, and direct and collateral damage due to tracheal intubation, clinical care could be improved and healthcare costs reduced. By eliminating intubation, invasive mechanical ventilation, and high inspired oxygen fractions, the need for acute care and progression of nRDS to PBD, obstructive lung disease, and other long-term sequelae could be reduced. Toward these ends, less invasive modalities for surfactant instillation (5,6) are being developed that may allow surfactant administration as an aerosol and could therefore be fully noninvasive and avoid difficult administration procedures reserved for highly practiced neonatologists.

At birth, the lungs must rapidly reverse the transepithelial transport of water from secretion to absorption. The mechanical clearance and absorption of fluid from the airways is essential to establish effective gas exchange. Fluid retention in the airways can contribute to the pathophysiology of nRDS (7). In the newborn, the transepithelial transport of water across the pulmonary epithelium is affected through upregulation of both the apical epithelial sodium channels (ENaCs) and the basolateral Na-K-ATPase channels, together with aquaporin (AQP-5) (8). The ENaC and Na-K-ATPase channels help to actively regulate the transport of water across the respiratory epithelia (9). However, the upregulation of these mechanisms is not fully active in the premature neonate. These transport mechanisms may also be further impaired by respiratory acidosis. Although an increased fluid load resulting from instillation of several milliliters of fluid containing the surfactant represents an additional challenge to the newborn, it appears that the

physiologic responses due to the addition of the surfactant largely override this insult. Administration of surfactant aerosols offers a potentially attractive alternative or in addition to pharmaceutical activation of water absorption in the neonate.

In neonates who have not developed sufficient respiratory drive, intubation and positive pressure ventilation are mandated. At present, these patients are well served with instilled surfactant, given that the traumatic procedure is unavoidable. The most urgent need is to deliver surfactant less invasively or noninvasively to preterm neonates who can be maintained on noninvasive ventilatory support, such as CPAP. Babies less than 29 weeks' gestation lack surfactant. Supplementation of extrinsic surfactant is indicated but needs to be balanced against the harm inflicted by the administration procedure. Provision of a fully noninvasive surfactant aerosol treatment modality, which is efficient enough to provide sufficient doses within a short period of time, would shift the paradigm toward immediate postnatal surfactant administration. The aerosolization and application systems are likely the most difficult to develop for babies weighing as little as 500 grams. These babies have the highest need but require low-caliber tubes and uncompromising safety requirements. Such systems would increase the armamentarium of the neonatologist, save lives, and address the unmet need to improve healthcare for these fragile patients. Past approaches to surfactant nebulization had little success due to inefficient aerosol devices, resulting in low intrapulmonary delivery of surfactant (10).

PREVALENCE AND PATHOPHYSIOLOGY OF ARDS

Worldwide, ARDS is an underdiagnosed entity, with 10.4% of all patients admitted to the intensive care unit (ICU) fulfilling the ARDS criteria (11). According to older studies, ARDS occurs in approximately 200,000 Americans each year (12). The primary risk factors for the development of ARDS include pneumonia, aspiration, major trauma, sepsis, and inhalation injury. According to the Berlin criteria (13), to qualify as suffering from ARDS, a patient must have new or worsening respiratory symptoms within 1 week of such an insult, bilateral opacities on chest imaging, pulmonary edema not fully explained by cardiac failure or fluid overload, and oxygenation failure. Severity is classified according to arterial oxygen saturation (PaO_2)/fraction of inspired oxygen (FiO_2) ratio, with 5 cm H_2O of CPAP or positive end-expiratory pressure (PEEP). The three categories of ARDS are mild (PaO_2/FiO_2: 200 to 300 mmHg), moderate (PaO_2/FiO_2: 100 to 200 mmHg), and severe ($PaO_2/FiO_2 \leq 100$ mmHg), with mortality rates of 34.9%, 40.3%, and 46.1%, respectively (11).

Hypoxia develops due to the reduced volume of aerated lung that is available for gas exchange as a consequence of edema or dense atelectasis that are found predominantly in dependent lung regions (14,15) due to thickening of the alveolar wall with inflammatory processes. Despite sophisticated

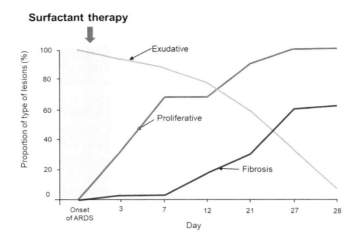

Figure 21.2 Pathological time course in 159 patients who died at the Hospital Universitario de Getafe, Madrid, Spain, between January 1, 1991 and December 31, 2010. Proposed early aerosol surfactant therapy is indicated by the arrow. (Reproduced from Thille, AW, et al., *Lancet Respir. Med.*, 1, 395–401, 2013. With permission.)

intensive care, many patients with mild hypoxemia (PaO_2/FiO_2 between 200 and 300 mmHg) deteriorate to more severe ARDS (16). Although the etiology of ARDS is often multifactorial (17), common to patients with ARDS is impaired surfactant function and continued inflammation-induced degradation of the surfactant's surface tension–lowering activity (18–21). To date, neither surfactant preparations nor any other pharmacologic interventions are approved for the treatment of ARDS. Current treatment is comprised of supportive care and lung protective, low tidal volume ventilation.

The temporal characteristics of the pathologic finding in patients with ARDS are shown in Figure 21.2. The initial inflammatory-induced edematous phase is followed by increased inflammation and subsequent development of fibrosis (22). Early surfactant aerosol therapy, to help arrest the development of these pathogenic processes, represents an attractive possibility. Such promising properties have been demonstrated in animal experiments.

As noted, in ARDS, fluid infiltration into the lungs occurs early in the pathologic sequence. Attempts to resolve this edema in ARDS through modulation of the ENaC and Na-K-ATPase channels have failed to improve edema clearance, although there is reason for hope (23). However, the addition of surfactant to a surfactant-deficient lung reduces the surface tension and increases the diameter of the respiratory airspaces and thus reduces the hydrostatic pressure that contributes to alveolar flooding.

The physiologic rationale for administering surfactant to lungs whose surfactant is impaired (18) remains strong and still holds a great deal of promise. In addition to opening respiratory air spaces, surfactant can facilitate the opening of conducting airways (24). Administration of surfactant as an aerosol could be one key to success. Clear advantages include avoidance of the administration-related side effects that occur with bolus instillation and the likelihood of improved surfactant functionality with less surfactant when delivered as an aerosol. Prerequisites to successfully developing an aerosolized surfactant include thorough

preclinical work, evaluation of the properties and aerosol characteristics exiting the aerosolizer (25,26), and quantitative measurements of surfactant deposition and function in the lung (27) followed by prudent Phase II work establishing a dose-effect relationship together with high-quality Phase III studies. These clinical studies must take into account the vast body of knowledge regarding how to conduct and, more important, how not to conduct large critical care studies. This is especially pertinent to those related to surfactant aerosol therapy. This could lead to the long-awaited, life-saving pharmacologic intervention for patients with ARDS.

SURFACTANT FORMULATIONS

The various surfactant preparations consist of either pure lipids, animal-derived surfactants, or synthetically manufactured surfactants, each of these having different physicochemical properties. Exosurf, a mixture of phospholipids that lacks the apoproteins SP-B and SP-C, is not as effective as preparations containing one or both of these proteins and has been withdrawn from clinical use. The properties of proteins in the surfactant are important for both its surface activity as well as its anti-inflammatory, anti-infective, and lung-protective functions (28). Surfactants with SP-A, SP-B, SP-C, and SP-D proteins exhibit superior properties compared to some early surfactants where these proteins were either absent or markedly reduced (29–33). These proteins also contribute to the resistance of surfactant to metabolic breakdown, which makes them more attractive for use in the treatment of ARDS (34); CLSE (Infasurf) is the most resilient to degradation (35). Of these, SP-B and SP-C are the most important proteins that aid in the lowering of dynamic surface tension and surfactant spreading. In synthesized surfactants, one or both of these has been replaced by mimetics, such as KL4 (36) or by peptide analogs, such as Minipeptide in Minisurf (Molecular Express) (29). Synsurf incorporates two polymers to mimic the hydrophilic and hydrophobic nature of SP-B in a phospholipid mixture (37). The mixture was shown to be partly effective in improving lung function in an adult rabbit lung washout model of lung injury. Inclusion of polymers dextran and hyaluronan has also been demonstrated to improve the effectiveness of a bovine calf-derived surfactant, Infasurf (38). The polymers change both the viscosity of the surfactant suspensions and the morphology of these suspensions in manners that are surfactant-, concentration-, and temperature-dependent (39). It has been proposed that the interaction of surfactant with hyaluronan leads to irreversible structural changes that result in a surfactant with better surface activity and the potential to overcome inactivation (40). The synthetic surfactant, CHF 5633, which includes SP-B and SP-C mimetics, when instilled in multiple doses of 200 mg/kg into a premature lamb model that had been previously treated with the known surfactant inhibitor, albumin, resulted in improved lung compliance, lung morphology, and survival compared to poractant alfa (31).

EFFECTIVE DOSE OF SURFACTANT AEROSOL

Due to the surfactant's biophysical mode of action and the large intrapulmonary surface area, extrinsic surfactant must be delivered in larger masses than treatments that target receptor interactions. Animal models of surfactant depletion by repeated lung lavages or by acid instillation have established 100 to 200 mg/kg of surfactant phospholipids to be a dose range leading to rapid recovery of oxygenation. For instance, in rabbit models, where surfactant was depleted by repeated lavage or by acid instillation, instillation of 35 mg/mL for doses of 100 or 200 mg/kg of surfactant into the tracheobronchial tree initiated a dramatic and early temporal improvement in PaO_2 (41,42). Instillation of 53 mg/kg was shown to be very effective (43). When the surfactant was administered via aerosol, the temporal physiologic responses, when present, were delayed and of lower magnitude. In these cases, the delivery of the surfactant aerosol to the lungs was likely insufficient to elicit a meaningful physiologic response (44,45). Lewis and colleagues (1991) (46) showed that delivery of 2 mg/kg of surfactant aerosol produced some physiologic benefit in neonatal lambs. This was 1/20 of the instilled dose. Gordon and colleagues (2003) (47) claimed that 2.5 to 7.5 mg/kg aerosol delivery was effective in neonatal lambs. Similar doses were shown to be marginally effective in a preterm lamb model (27) in which the amount of rare-earth-spiked surfactant in the lungs was measured postmortem. Most others have failed to document the mass of surfactant leaving the device interface to be inhaled by the animal, let alone measure pulmonary deposition. It has been suggested, on a theoretical basis, that there is a maximum dose that would be clinically effective (48) However, given that 200 mg/kg, aerosolized directly into the tracheobronchial airways in preterm lambs, was shown to be effective suggests that this maximum may be quite high (49,50). The mass of surfactant in healthy lungs has been estimated to be 5 to 10 mg/kg and 20 mg/kg in newborns at term (43), and 20 mg/kg in a 6-hour-old, normally breathing lamb. Thus, a target dose of surfactant aerosol deposited in the periphery

of the neonatal lungs should be 7 to 20 mg/kg. In ARDS, the inactivation of the surfactant by proteins and phospholipases (51) indicates that a higher dose may be desirable. Thus, we can deduce from physiologic amounts in the lung and the few reliable reports that are available that the efficacy related to aerosol delivery of surfactant is an order of magnitude below the amounts needed with instillation of suspensions. These surfactant administration therapies should be repeatable as often as clinically indicated. However, the delivery of these masses of surfactant to the peripheral lung via aerosol in a short treatment time remains a challenge.

AEROSOL CONCENTRATION AND PARTICLE SIZE

As can be inferred from the above discussion, delivery of a sufficient mass of aerosolized surfactant to the peripheral respiratory bronchi and alveoli to treat either the absence of surfactant and/or its continued depletion has been a recalcitrant problem. A substantial mass of surfactant needs to be deposited within the periphery of the lungs to elicit the desired physiologic response. To achieve this therapeutically effective dose in a meaningful treatment time (minutes, not hours), aerosols with a high particle concentration are required. The larger the mass of surfactant per aerosol particle, the lower the number particles at a given total dose and the less likely that agglomeration of the aerosol will occur and cause a reduction in peripheral lung deposition. A solid-phase surfactant aerosol contains over 25 times the mass of an aqueous aerosol of the same diameter containing surfactant from <40 mg/mL surfactant suspensions. This factor is high enough to substantially reduce the treatment time and/or increase the mass deposited. Due to the marked anatomical size differences between adults and neonates, the optimal particle size is likely in the range of 2.5 to 4 μm mass median aerodynamic diameter (MMAD) for maximizing peripheral deposition in adults, and 1.5 to 2.5 μm MMAD for maximizing peripheral deposition in prematurely born infants. In the generation and delivery of very high concentrations of aerosols, the effect of agglomeration due to particle-particle interaction increases with both particle number concentration and decreasing particle size. Thus, for high masses to be delivered, there is a trade-off between the mass delivered by larger particles and the potential for agglomeration when delivering very-fine-particle aerosols. The efficient generation of high masses of pure surfactant aerosols suitable for inhalation, especially in the 1.5 to 2.5 μm diameter range, is a challenge, although the initial data support this possibility (52).

INTRA-AIRWAY DEPOSITION DISTRIBUTION AND SPREADING TO THE LUNG PERIPHERY

As noted, the fundamental prerequisite for surfactant to exhibit its physiologic benefits of opening airways, preventing alveolar collapse on expiration, reducing the work of breathing, and improving gas exchange is the need for sufficient surfactant to line the surfaces of the distal airways and alveoli. The spreading of surfactant deposited on a surface has been shown to be linearly dependent on the mass deposited on the test surface (53). This spreading has two phases: a rapid phase of Marangoni flow lasting about 10 seconds and a slower surfactant flow that lasts several minutes. This slower phase is associated with the combined interaction of surfactant spreading from many high surface concentrations (53). In this way, surfactant may spread into constricted airways. However, in many cases, low surface concentrations of surfactant in distal airways may be insufficient to exhibit the above additive effect (54). In bench experiments with non-nebulized and nebulized surfactant, the surface spreading of the nebulized surfactant took up to 50 seconds, just 20 seconds longer than the non-nebulized surfactant (55). This may be related to the prolonged aerosol delivery time of 20 to 30 seconds. The low surface tension properties of surfactant and its spreading indicate that the physiologic responses to aerosolized surfactant should be observed immediately following the deposition of a clinically relevant surfactant aerosol dose, as observed by Jorch and colleagues (1997) (56) and Ruppert and colleagues (56,57).

Grotberg and colleagues (58) and Filoche and colleagues (48) have proposed that the failure of recent surfactant replacement studies in patients with ARDS to achieve the positive clinical responses observed in earlier studies has been due to insufficient volume of surfactant administration to coat both the conducting airways and alveoli. However, this is not the case in neonates. Through the computational modeling of the spreading of surfactant suspensions instilled into the trachea and its distal transport along the branching airways toward the lung periphery, Grotberg and colleagues have shown that 1 to 4 mL/kg of surfactant administered to neonates provides sufficient surfactant to coat the 40 cm^2 of conducting airways, reach the distal acini, and have its predicted beneficial physiologic effects. However, in adults, when reduced volumes (approximately 35 mL into each lung in the left and right decubitus positions) of 1 mL/kg of more concentrated surfactants (i.e., higher viscosities) were administered (32,59) the expected clinical benefits observed in earlier clinical trials (60–62) were absent. They attribute this to the inability of relatively small volumes of more viscous surfactant to coat the longer and considerably larger surface area of the longer pathways related to the greater number of generations of branching airways in the adult lungs as well as the much larger surface area of the conducting airways (4500 cm^2) compared to 40 cm^2 in neonatal lungs (58). They refer to this as the "coating cost." The flow of surfactant due to gravity when instilled into the conducting airways also limits the broad distribution of this surfactant throughout the alveoli. The failure of delivery of aqueous aerosols containing surfactant (63) was due, at least in part, to insufficient surfactant being delivered to the alveolar regions of the lungs. This can be largely, if not completely, mitigated by inhalation of pure surfactant aerosols and targeting their deposition to the alveolar regions of the lungs.

WET OR DRY SURFACTANT AEROSOL?

The physical and electrical properties of the aerosol in which the surfactant is administered may affect both its regional deposition within the respiratory tract and the resultant physiologic responses.

Ellyett and coworkers (1996) (64) showed that the same surfactant, when delivered as a submicron aerosol of warmed pure surfactant in humidified air to rabbits, improved survival, an effect that was not apparent when the surfactant was delivered as an aqueous aerosol. In pig lungs, both aqueous surfactant aerosol and warmed "dry" surfactant aerosol on which water condensed on cooling were both effective in opening airways, with the advantage given to the "hygroscopic" aerosol (65). Conversely, Hutten and colleagues (66) reported that, when surfactant was administered to preterm lambs over 3 hours using an eFlow nebulizer, an aqueous surfactant aerosol produced positive results. However, when this aerosol was generated with dry air, but still humidified, it was unexpectedly ineffective. In these experiments, the difference in PaO$_2$ was only significant at the 3-hour timepoint and was coincident with a marked decrease in the PaO$_2$ of the saline control (66). In a neonatal porcine acid-induced lung inflammation model, administration of 1.35 grams of aerosolized KL4 surfactant delivered to the ventilator circuit over 60 minutes resulted in improved physiologic and pathogic responses and short-term survival compared to instillation of approximately 315 mg (175 mg/kg) of KL4 surfactant (67). The deposition efficiency of ≥3 grams of surfactant powder, aerosolized, humidified, and delivered to neonatal lambs, was <1% (27). In these preterm lambs, between 1.1 and 7.7 mg/kg body weight of surfactant phospholipids was deposited into the lungs during CPAP-supported spontaneous ventilation. This resulted in a reduction of breathing effort and lower postmortem lung weights (27). High concentrations of dry surfactant aerosols (MMAD = 1.6 µm) produced dramatic and immediate improvements of both PaO$_2$/FiO$_2$ and compliance, observed in lung washout and bleomycin-induced rabbit models of respiratory distress following <1 minute of surfactant aerosol generation (57). In these experiments, neither gas flow rate nor efficiency are known. These studies indicate that surfactant, given either as an aqueous or solid-phase aerosol, can improve respiratory function and gas exchange, but results are inconclusive with regard to the optimum form for delivery of the aerosolized surfactant. Likely there are technical issues regarding the aerosol delivery of each that need to be resolved.

A common theme of aerosol surfactant delivery studies is that when sufficient surfactant was delivered rapidly (<30 minute) to the lung periphery, positive results were obtained no matter whether the surfactant in the aerosol was delivered within an aqueous aerosol or a solid-phase surfactant aerosol.

Inherent in delivering an aerosol generated from a dry surfactant powder is the necessity for spray drying a surfactant to produce very fine surfactant powder and collect it in a dry, and preferably sterile, environment. Surfactant readily absorbs 16% of its weight of water and becomes more difficult to aerosolize. This preprocessing and the storage and reaerosolization of such dry powders can be costly and involve further technical barriers. These factors are important based on the initial size of the surfactant market.

Insights into the effect of aerosol deposition on the physical form of the aerosol being delivered may be gleaned from a discussion of the observations of Pohlmann and colleagues (25). In this system, a surfactant aerosol was generated by dispersion of a dry surfactant powder from a hopper using pulses of compressed air. Pohlmann found that high concentrations of dry surfactant aerosol of 3 μm in diameter suspended in a dry gas and delivered via a thin catheter inserted through an endotracheal tube directly into the trachea formed locally deposited masses in the lower trachea. Adding a humidifier after the surfactant aerosol generation prevented the localized clumps of surfactant powder in the airways but reduced the efficiency by about 50%. This phenomenon was attributed to the hygroscopicity of the surfactant. However, additional electrostatic mechanisms may contribute to these observations, as discussed below.

EFFECTS OF ELECTRIC CHARGE ON WET AND DRY AEROSOLS

In the process of aerosolizing dry powders, the shear forces between particles with disparate physicochemical properties as well as with the container produce electrostatic charges on the particles due, at least in part, to triboelectrification. High shear forces related to the dispersion of dry powders with dry compressed gas, as in the case of the device used by Pohlmann and colleagues, induces charges that will be higher than those found in breath-actuated, dry powder inhalers. Powdered surfactant likely has a very high resistivity. The rates of decay of such charges from the particle surface would be slow, taking several minutes or even hours to complete discharge. These charges may reach thousands of electrons per particle (68), especially with jet-related aerosol generation, as noted in metered-dose inhalers (MDIs) (69). The charge on an aerosol can increase deposition in the airways, especially when charges of over 30 electrons per particle are encountered. The deposition of charged particles is affected by both the image charge force and space charge force. The image charge force depends on the attraction of particles to image charges of opposite polarity on the wall of a vessel or airway. The space-charge force is a repulsive force that is proportional to the square of the distance between the aerosol particles. The space charge is important for aerosol deposition in the upper airways (70), whereas image forces are generally the predominant forces in the smaller airways. Even when ignoring the space-charge effect, deposition of low concentrations of 3 to 6 μm diameter charged particles showed more proximal deposition, with aerosol deposition increasing several times (71). Particle deposition in the nose was shown to increase many times for particles in the 1 to 10 μm range with highly charged particles (72). The space-charge effect is dominant in aerosols of high particle density (>10^5 particles/mL), such as the dry surfactant aerosols generated by Pohlmann and colleagues (25) and by Ruppert (57), and the particle densities are several orders of magnitude larger than this. Turbulence distal to a thin catheter in the trachea causes a local increase in aerosol deposition. Although the charges on these surfactant aerosols were unknown, the observation that an increase in humidity eliminated the proximal airway accumulation of surfactant aerosol (25) is consistent with the effects of electrical charge on aerosol deposition as well as the observation that increasing humidity dissipates charges on aerosol particles.

The process of atomization of an aqueous fluid also induces charges on the surface of the droplets. This is due to charge separation as the liquid surface is disrupted or as the liquid flows along a solid surface. As expected, the charge level increases with the compressed gas flow rate (73). However, using computational modeling, it was concluded that the droplet charges were too low to influence lung deposition. The increase in conductivity due to the addition of an ionic component to the solution to be aerosolized decreases the charges on the particles produced (74). Surfactant suspensions, such as Infasurf, contain 0.9% sodium chloride. Thus, aerosols generated from aqueous suspensions with ions present are less likely to be susceptible to increased and unpredictable deposition due to electrical charges.

DEVICE-PATIENT INTERFACE AEROSOL LOSSES

As noted, the generation of both liquid aerosols and dry powder aerosols can result in an electrostatic charge on the aerosol that can affect the pattern of aerosol deposition within the respiratory tract. These charges can also cause substantial and variable particle losses in the plastic delivery tubing that is most often used for aerosol administration in a clinical setting. It should be noted that the standard delivery tubing and configurations are designed to deliver gases to the patient, not aerosols. This is particularly evident in the case of nasal CPAP in neonates. The electrical charges on aqueous aerosols will be largely dissipated due to the high humidity and electrolyte composition of the aerosolized product. The electrical charges on dry powder aerosols, however, may cause them to be depleted from the aerosol delivery tubing due to electrostatic charges on the tubing. This effect can be highly variable. Factors that have a negative impact on the delivery and efficacy of aqueous suspensions include (1) rain-out in the delivery tubing and patient interface, (2) high nasopharyngeal deposition, (3) a small percentage of the aerosolized surfactant being delivered to the lungs, (4) an insufficient surfactant dose to the lung periphery, and (5) unreliable dose deposited: All of these factors contribute to questionable and variable efficacy. Further improvement in aerosol delivery can be attained through the aerodynamic design of the aerosol generator to patient interface (75–77).

SURFACTANT AEROSOL GENERATION: GENERAL CONSIDERATIONS

Aerosols containing surfactant can be generated as aqueous suspensions of surfactant using a jet atomizer (78), mesh-type nebulizer (79), or ultrasonic nebulizer (57), or by condensation of water vapor on a surfactant nucleus using a capillary aerosol generator (CAG) (67). Dry powder surfactant aerosols have been generated by a rudimentary device (57) and by a pulsed, gas-driven reaerosolization of spray-dried surfactant powder (25,27). Venturi jet type nebulizers that produce ≤3 μm particles have a low output (≤0.3 mL/min) (78). In these devices, the larger particles are collected and recirculated. This reaerosolizing of the fluid increases the surfactant concentration as well as the viscosity, resulting in a continually decreasing output. In addition, foaming can further reduce the output. New technologies have demonstrated that aqueous suspensions of surfactant can been aerosolized and delivered as a concentrated, pure, solid-phase, fine-particle aerosol (52), as discussed below.

Vibrating mesh nebulizers, such as the eFlow and MicroAir, have meshes with 2 to 3 μm diameter holes. Mesh-type nebulizers have very limited fill volumes (1 to 9 mL). Porcine surfactant suspension has been aerosolized up to 40 mg/mL using a Pari eFlow at 0.25 mL/min (55). With an Aeroneb Pro, synthetic 30 mg/mL surfactant preparations were nebulized up to at 0.1 mL/min (41). These nebulizers function well for solutions with a viscosity <2 centipoise (cP) (80). The output of mesh-type nebulizers decreases with increasing viscosity up to approximately 4 centistokes (cSt), at which point aerosolization ceases (Table 21.1) (81). The surfactant output from an eFlow neonatal nebulizer system aerosolizing Curosurf decreased from 0.33 mL/min to 0.18 mL/min over 3 hours (66). Due to this limited ability to aerosolize viscous surfactant suspensions and their tendency to clog, mesh-type nebulizers are more suitable for delivering low-dose rates for short periods (10,41,79).

Aerosol generation of micronized particles from a metered-dose, dry powder inhaler has been reported with a single shot output of 25 mg in 10 seconds with a 25% efficiency (82).

Table 21.1 Output of vibrating mesh nebulizers is limited by viscosity (sorbitol molecular weight = 183 Daltons)

Concentration (mg/mL)	Viscosity (CSt)	Relative respirable output (mg fluid/min)	
		Aeroneb Go	eFlow Rapid
75	1.3	170	520
150	1.6	180	650
300	2.7	150	500
400	3.8	65	

Source: Chan, J. G., et al., J. Aerosol. Med. Respir. Drug Deliv., 25, 297–305, 2012.

DELIVERY OF SURFACTANT TO NEONATES

Given that the spreading time of the deposited surfactant is likely on the order of seconds to minutes (53,54), the physiologic response to surfactant deposition should be observable within minutes following the delivery of a physiologically effective dose of aerosol. Surfactant spreading is enhanced with SP-B or SP-C compared to phospholipids alone.

ENDOTRACHEAL SURFACTANT BOLUS INSTILLATION

In this procedure, the neonate is intubated, and surfactant suspensions with concentrations between 30 mg/mL and 80 mg/mL are instilled distal to the endotracheal tube—first with the neonate in one lateral decubitus position and then in the other. A total dose of 100 to 200 mg/kg of phospholipid is administered. This procedure can take between a few minutes and 1 hour. Retreatment may be indicated at approximately 12-hour intervals. An average of 1.8 treatments are administered. While this therapy has reduced morbidity and mortality in neonates born prematurely, its success rate, as measured by the time to extubation, is only about 40%. The complications of this procedure include vagally induced bradycardia, temporary oxygen desaturation, pneumothorax, cardiac intraventricular hemorrhage, decreased cerebral blood flow, disturbed electroencephalograms, and the development of bronchopulmonary dysplasia (83,84). The delay in response due to surfactant bolus instillation may be both due to the adverse responses to this procedure as well as the need for absorption of the excess fluid instilled. Thus, minimally invasive, less invasive, and noninvasive administration of surfactant to the premature neonate are being actively evaluated.

MINIMALLY INVASIVE SURFACTANT BOLUS INSTILLATION

In the pursuit of reducing the adverse effects of intubation in the neonate, surfactant has been administered during a brief intubation (intubation-surfactant-extubation [INSURE]) (42,85) or approaches summarized as minimally invasive surfactant therapy (MIST) or less invasive surfactant application (LISA). In the latter procedure, surfactant is administered using a fine tube with a tip that is briefly located distal to the vocal cords (5,6,86–88). MIST has been shown to increase lung volume and oxygenation. In neonates born between 23.0 and 26.8 weeks of gestation, the minimally invasive delivery of surfactant results in less intubation, fewer days on mechanical ventilation, a decrease in pneumothorax and intraventricular hemorrhage, and improved survival without major complications. However, it did not result in an increase in survival without BPD (5).

AEROSOL DELIVERY THROUGH CATHETERS

To reduce aerosol deposition losses in the oral cavity or nasopharynx, several catheters have been developed in which the aerosols are generated at the tip of the catheter. The tip of the catheter can be placed either proximal or distal to the larynx or within the lobar bronchi (89–93). When using these catheters, the surfactant suspension is delivered through a central channel while the compressed air is delivered circumferentially or through channels in close juxtaposition to the periphery of this central channel. The fluid aerosolization occurs due to the shearing forces of the gas on the liquid external to the catheter. In this configuration, the particle size and distribution of the aerosol generated is very dependent on the viscosity of the surfactant suspension, with higher viscosities resulting in larger particles with broader size distributions. An aerosol catheter (Aeroprobe, Trudell Medical), with a very high compressed gas driving pressure (approximately 100 psi) has been used to deliver aerosolized surfactant to the lobes of the lungs in premature lambs (49). In this study, aerosolizing 200 mg/kg into the trachea, in the absence of control data, appears to be as effective as the same dose given as a bolus instillation. AeroProbe was stated to deliver 0.4 mL/min, with 80% of the particle being below 5 μm in diameter. However, using Curosurf 80 mg/mL of lipids, Aeroprobe was shown to produce aerosols of 8.3 to 10.6 μm MMAD (91). In the case of the device described by Dellaca (92), fluid flows of 150 to 300 μL/min, with gas flow of less than 1 L/min at approximately 0.75 bar, are targeted. Median particle size of 91 μm was reported with treatment times of ≥45 minutes. In a study involving premature neonatal sheep, 9.6 mL (0.77 gram surfactant) of Curosurf at 0.7 L/min was nebulized at a rate of 400 μL/min during inhalation over 53 minutes. These large droplets deposit locally in the proximal airways by impaction and sedimentation. Such a device, when placed proximal to the larynx, results in high laryngeal deposition, and when placed distal to the larynx, results in high proximal deposition in the tracheobronchial tree. Synchronizing aerosolizing of the surfactant with this device during inspiration reduces the volume of surfactant required as well as surfactant deposition on the vocal cords and upper airways. When 200 mg/kg of surfactant was aerosolized intratracheally in preterm lambs, the physiologic responses were similar to the same dose delivered as in instilled bolus in preterm lambs (50). The delayed physiologic response observed (92) was likely due to both the time required for the proximally deposited surfactant to redistribute in the peripheral lung together with the time required to deposit sufficient surfactant for an observable physiologic response. Another catheter designed for intrapulmonary surfactant aerosolization consists of two concentric tubes, with the center tube comprising a 30-gauge needle. Compressed air at 40 to 120 psi was aerosolized 50 to 250 μL/min surfactant suspensions to produce droplets with mass median diameters of 3.2 to 4.1 μm at velocities

of 5 to 30 m/second (94), velocities that result in deposition by impaction. The surfactant flow rate increases with applied pressure from 30 to 100 μL/minute. The risk of generating high-velocity aerosols from aerosolizing nozzles at 40 to 100 psi in the fragile airways of patients with nRDS or ARDS raises the potential for inducing complications. In addition, the inevitable deposition of surfactant within the large airways raises the question as to how much of this surfactant just coats the airways and how much penetrates to the respiratory acini and alveolar regions.

SURFACTANT AEROSOL DELIVERY AND NONINVASIVE VENTILATION

Noninvasive, transnasal aerosol surfactant replacement therapy has the potential to provide an effective therapeutic treatment for nRDS. In this case, the size of surfactant aerosol needs to be small enough to have minimal deposition in the nasal turbinates and large enough to deposit in the peripheral regions of the neonatal lungs. In this approach, some of the aerosol may be exhaled, and a higher percentage of aerosol is deposited peripherally with improved reproducibility and reliability. Transnasal aerosol delivery has been advocated by a number of investigators (76,95–97). However, the percentage of the aerosol output that is lost within the aerosol generator and within the delivery apparatus and tubing ranges between 40% and 98% (45,98–101). This issue is exacerbated with low flow rates (i.e., 1 to 3 L/min) to the developing lung (95). When a low fraction of the aerosolized surfactant is delivered to the patient, this can result in much greater uncertainty of the dose delivered to the lungs, as small changes in the percent deposited can lead to a large change in dose delivered.

A suspension of Aerosurf 20 mg/mL was aerosolized with an Aeroneb Pro and delivered to neonates at a rate of 0.4 mg phospholipids per minute through nasal prongs over a 3-hour period (79). The nebulizer was cleaned every 30 minutes. The dose of the 1.9 ± 0.3 μm diameter aerosol was associated with approximately 3.5 mL of water. A total of about 35 mL of surfactant was nebulized. The estimated dose delivered at the nose was 72 mg. The mass deposited in the peripheral lung was likely considerably less than this. The dose and procedure were apparently well tolerated.

In clinical studies using a capillary condensation aerosol generator for transnasal surfactant aerosol delivery, the efficiency of delivery appears to be very low. When aerosolizing 60 mL of 30 mg/mL of KL4 (Lucinactant) surfactant at 1.2 mL/min over 50 minutes, 80 mg of the original 1.8 grams of phospholipid was aerosolized. The aerosolized surfactant was delivered to the neonate at 100 mg of phospholipid per hour through nasal prongs at 3 L/min. Based on a minute ventilation of 300 mL/min, just 0.16 mg/min phospholipid in the 2.8 μm MMAD aqueous aerosol would have been inhaled. In monkeys, when this aerosol was delivered through nasal prongs at 3 L/min at 5 cm water nPAP, over 5- to 9-minute period, regionally 80% was deposited in the nose and mouth and 11% was deposited in the lungs

(102,103). Also, during a 50-minute treatment period, it is estimated that 2.8 mL may be presented to the nasal passages. There is a possibility that the accumulated fluid in the nasal passages could cause irritation and/or obstruction. It is possible that the lack of additional benefits observed following 2 hours rather than 1 hour of surfactant administration in a clinical trial was due to adverse effects associated with this lengthy treatment regimen rather than too much phospholipid. In this regard, KL4 surfactant was aerosolized and emitted at a rate of 22.5 mg/min in 6 L/min (1.356 grams) at the ventilator connector over a period of 1 hour and delivered to 1.8 kg newborn pigs using oropharyngeal CPAP (67). The phospholipid concentration of the aerosolized surfactant was 3.7 mg/L. The aerosolized KL4 surfactant was superior to the KL4 given by instillation. In a recent clinical trial by Windtree, the endpoints were not met. However, when Windtree conducted a post-hoc analysis of the neonatal data, they claimed that a subsection of this treated population, in which aerosol treatment was not compromised by technical difficulties, showed an increase in the time to intubation as well as a corresponding decrease in the need for intubation.

DELIVERY OF SURFACTANT FOR THE TREATMENT OF ARDS

Initial studies evaluating surfactant replacement therapy included patients with ARDS resulting from sepsis, with two studies including patients with sepsis of both pulmonary and nonpulmonary origin. They also included patients with a direct lung injury by aspiration and indirect lung injury due to trauma, surgery, transfusion, pancreatitis, burns, and toxic sources (104). As noted, the beneficial effects of surfactant therapy were not evident in these trials. A randomized study in which an aqueous aerosol of artificial surfactant, Exosurf, containing 13% dipalmitoylphosphatidylcholine (DPPC) in 0.45% saline was administered in intubated patients with sepsis-related ARDS showed no clinical benefits to the procedure (105). This failure could be attributed to any of the following: (1) the use of a simplified surfactant in which the only phospholipid was DPPC, (2) the inability to deliver sufficient surfactant to elicit a physiologic response (as none was seen), and (3) the selection and severity of ARDS in the patients studied, or (4) some combination thereof.

Post-hoc analyses of these studies (62) showed that improvement with surfactant administration was confined to patients with direct lung injury on the alveolar side of the alveolar-capillary membrane. These lung injuries were precipitated by either pneumonia, aspiration, or near drowning. Similarly, a post-hoc analysis of several clinical studies with intratracheal instillations of rSP-C surfactant, in mechanically ventilated patients with a direct lung injury due to pneumonia or aspiration, showed a pronounced improvement in oxygenation and a 13% reduction in mortality. This finding was evident in patients with moderate-to-severe lung injury, as indicated by the area under the curve (AUC) of the PaO_2/FiO_2 ratio near 100 mmHg (106) rather than in patients with higher PaO_2/FiO_2 ratios. In these studies, age was identified as a confounder for mortality. Immunocompromise has also been identified as another risk factor (62).

Some of the factors as to why surfactant instillation may have not prevented or at least reduced the mortality in many of the ARDS clinical trials include, but are not limited to, the following:

- Inclusion of patients with indirect, in addition to direct, causes of ARDS
- Severity of ARDS at the time of testing
- Procedural complications
- The lack of use of lung-protective, low-tidal-volume ventilation
- Use of surfactant lacking important associated protein(s)
- Surfactant degradation
- Inadequate surfactant delivery to the lung periphery
- Need for multiple surfactant treatments

Based on the strong rationale regarding the use of extrinsic surfactant in ARDS and the promising preclinical results in lung lavage and lipopolysaccharide-induced respiratory distress, several surfactant preparations were advanced into clinical studies. Unfortunately, despite several promising Phase II studies (35,59,107,108) and in-depth data analyses (106), none of the pivotal Phase III studies escaped the common fate of pharmacologic studies in critical care indications, specifically, failure to establish efficacy (32,105,107,109). It may be tempting to believe that the surfactant preparations just did not have the right composition, that the liquid boli associated with the surfactant suspension may have caused more harm than benefit, or other sophisticated reasons. However, most of these studies failed due to "ICU study killer reasons." Many of these are well established and include inadequate patient selection; statistical "noise" due to concomitant conditions determining the fate of most of the critically ill patients, regardless of the treatment intervention; rushing into Phase III after studying as few as 36 patients in Phase II (110); using immature administration technology (105); and/or introduction of inadequately understood changes in the preparation of a modality as complex as a surfactant suspension (32). None of these studies have conclusively shown, however, that surfactant as a therapeutic principle should not be further pursued.

TECHNOLOGICAL ADVANCES IN SURFACTANT AEROSOL DELIVERY

Synchronization of aerosol delivery has been proposed for surfactant delivery from a vibrating mesh device (111), a dry powder device (25), and an "aerosol catheter (50)."

Breath-synchronized surfactant delivery using aerosolizing catheters (91) has been tested in premature lambs to deliver surfactant aerosol either proximal (89) or distal (50) to the larynx. Its implementation in a neonate could be challenging and result in prolongation of the treatment time.

A new class of aerosolization and delivery system (SUPRAER®) has emerged as a laboratory device (26,52,112,113) that provides the required high concentrations of very-fine-particle aerosols. In this system, the aerosol is generated from a liquid surfactant suspension and delivered as a concentrated solid-phase aerosol. A syringe pump supplies an aqueous surfactant suspension to an aerosolizing nozzle. This nozzle aerosolizes 100% of the suspension to form a liquid aerosol with a narrow size distribution ($\sigma g < 2$). The aerosol plume exits the aerosol exit orifice surrounded by a sheath of particle-free gas, and thus the nozzle neither clogs nor drips. The aerosol plume is arrested with a co-axial counterflow of gas. The fluid is evaporated from the particles using a combination of warm compressed gas and dilution gas, together with infrared radiation with a wavelength that is optimized for the absorption band of water. The resultant aerosol is concentrated using a virtual impactor (concentrator). In this way, the output aerosol is comprised of a high concentration of particles in a smaller volume of gas. The diameter of the initial droplets is selected by choosing the nozzle aerosol exit orifice diameter, compressed gas pressure, suspension concentration, and rate of aerosolization. Surfactant viscosities up to 34 cp have been readily aerosolized with this device. A 3 μm MMAD pure surfactant aerosol was produced by generating a 6 μm diameter aqueous aerosol from a 103 mg/mL surfactant suspension. Such an aerosol contains >20 times the mass of surfactant of a 3 μm MMAD aqueous aerosol generated from a 2% to 3% (w/v) surfactant suspension, thus requiring a less concentrated aerosol than that of liquid systems to deliver the same dose of surfactant. As this device can aerosolize surfactant at up to 3 mL/min, its fluid throughput is approximately 10 times higher than jet atomizers and mesh-type nebulizers and much higher than the device used by Windtree Therapeutics. In the nozzles used in SUPRAER, the atomization processes occur within an aerosolization space and exits through the aerosol exit orifice in a sheaf of essentially particle-free gas. The water is evaporated from the aerosol, and most of the resultant gas is removed from the aerosol using a virtual impactor. During this process, the charges on the particles will likely dissipate. In this way high concentrations of particles at high delivery rates can be achieved.

UTILITY OF HELIOX FOR THE GENERATION AND DELIVERY OF RESPIRABLE AEROSOLS IN nRDS AND ARDS

Heliox is a mixture of helium and oxygen, most often 80% helium and 20% oxygen, with other mixtures containing higher percentages of oxygen being available. When patients with compromised lung function breathe heliox, the work associated with breathing is reduced and gas exchange improves due to the decreased flow resistance resulting from the lower density of helium compared to air and the decrease in turbulence. As the viscosity of heliox and air are similar, the ratio of the inertial forces compared with the viscous forces is markedly lower for heliox than air. The clinical, physiologic benefits of using heliox compared to air are as follows:

- Low Reynolds number leads to less turbulence in the conducting airways (98)
- Decreased work of breathing (114)
- Reduction of airway inflammation (115,116)
- Improvement of oxygenation and CO_2 removal (118)
- Increased peripheral aerosol penetration (118,119)

In addition, noninvasive ventilation with heliox has been found to decrease the incidence of intubation in preterm infants suffering from nRDS (120).

Due to its low density, high kinematic viscosity, high specific heat, and high thermal conductivity compared to air, heliox in SUPRAER (1) produces smaller diameter particles, (2) improves heat and mass transfer, (3) reduces wall losses, (4) enhances the efficiencies of the aerosol concentrators, and (5) enables the delivery of higher payloads. This results in the delivery of aerosols 1.1 to 2.2 μm MMAD at up to 3.4 mg/second for total output doses up to 2.2 grams being delivered in 10 minutes with efficiencies greater than 70% (52,113).

CONCLUSION

New insights into the pathogenic mechanisms involved in both nRDS and ARDS will continue to add new therapeutic modalities for the treatment of these syndromes. Elucidation of the technical issues related to surfactant aerosol generation and delivery, together with the generation of new technologies to address these issues, provide optimism for practical and clinically relevant solutions. The efficient generation of high concentrations of fine-particle, pure surfactant aerosols provides the possibility of new, rapid, and effective treatment modalities for both nRDS and ARDS. Given our understanding of the reasons why surfactant administration in ARDS, especially related to aerosol delivery of aerosolized surfactant, has not resulted in the hoped-for improvement in life expectancy provides the basis for resolving these issues with improved aerosol generation and delivery technology, insightful patient selection, and carefully designed clinical studies with realistic endpoints. Success in demonstrating the efficacy of inhaled surfactant aerosols will lead to the inclusion of co-delivery of other therapeutics or agents targeting the other underlying pathologies of these syndromes.

CONFLICTS OF INTEREST

Donovan Yeates is the CEO and major shareholder of KAER Biotherapeutics, a company developing technologies to deliver surfactant to patients with nRDS and ARDS. KAER Biotherapeutics has a substantial international patent portfolio, of which KAER Biotherpaeutics is the beneficiary.

ACKNOWLEDGMENTS

The author is grateful for constructive comments and discussions with Xin Heng, PhD, and Friedemann Taut, MD, MBA.

This chapter was, in part, supported by the National Heart, Lung and Blood Institute of the National Institutes of Health under Award Number R43HL127834. The content is solely the responsibility of the author and does not necessarily represent the official views of the National Institutes of Health.

REFERENCES

1. Sankar, MJ, Gupta, N, Jain, K, Agarwal, R, Paul, VK. Efficacy and safety of surfactant replacement therapy for preterm neonates with respiratory distress syndrome in low- and middle-income countries: A systematic review. *J Perinatol.* 2016;36(Suppl 1):S36–S48.

2. Wiingreen, R, Greisen, G, Ebbesen, F, et al. Surfactant need by gestation for very preterm babies initiated on early nasal CPAP: A Danish observational multicentre study of 6,628 infants born 2000–2013. *Neonatology.* 2017;111(4):331–336.

3. O'Reilly, M, Sozo, F, Harding, R. Impact of preterm birth and bronchopulmonary dysplasia on the developing lung: Long-term consequences for respiratory health. *Clin Exp Pharmacol Physiol.* 2013;40(11):765–773.

4. Verder, H, Bohlin, K, Kamper, J, Lindwall, R, Jonsson, B. Nasal CPAP and surfactant for treatment of respiratory distress syndrome and prevention of bronchopulmonary dysplasia. *Acta Paediatr.* 2009;98(9):1400–1408.

5. Kribs, A. Minimally invasive surfactant therapy and noninvasive respiratory support. *Clin Perinatol.* 2016;43(4):755–771.

6. Lau, CSM, Chamberlain, RS, Sun, S. Less invasive surfactant administration reduces the need for mechanical ventilation in preterm infants: A meta-analysis. *Glob Pediatr Health.* 2017;4:2333794×17696683.

7. Helve, O, Pitkanen, O, Janer, C, Andersson, S. Pulmonary fluid balance in the human newborn infant. *Neonatology.* 2009;95(4):347–352.

8. Li, Y, Marcoux, MO, Gineste, M, et al. Expression of water and ion transporters in tracheal aspirates from neonates with respiratory distress. *Acta Paediatr.* 2009;98(11):1729–1737.

9. Phillips, JE, Wong, LB, Yeates, DB. Bidirectional transepithelial water transport: Measurement and governing mechanisms. *Biophys J.* 1999;76(2):869–877.

10. Pillow, JJ, Minocchieri, S. Innovation in surfactant therapy II: Surfactant administration by aerosolization. *Neonatology.* 2012;101(4):337–344.

11. Bellani, G, Laffey, JG, Pham, T, et al. Epidemiology, patterns of care, and mortality for patients with acute respiratory distress syndrome in intensive care units in 50 countries. *JAMA.* 2016;315(8):788–800.

12. Rubenfeld, GD, Caldwell, E, Peabody, E, et al. Incidence and outcomes of acute lung injury. *N Engl J Med.* 2005;353(16):1685–1693.

13. Force, ADT, Ranieri, VM, Rubenfeld, GD. Acute respiratory distress syndrome: The Berlin definition. *JAMA.* 2012;307(23):2526–2533.

14. Beitler, JR, Goligher, EC, Schmidt, M, et al. Personalized medicine for ARDS: The 2035 research agenda. *Intensive Care Med.* 2016;42(5):756–767.

15. Pelosi, P, D'Andrea, L, Vitale, G, Pesenti, A, Gattinoni, L. Vertical gradient of regional lung inflation in adult respiratory distress syndrome. *Am J Respir Crit Care Med.* 1994;149(1):8–13.

16. Bakowitz, M, Bruns, B, McCunn, M. Acute lung injury and the acute respiratory distress syndrome in the injured patient. *Scand J Trauma Resusc Emerg Med.* 2012;20:54.

17. Calfee, CS. ARDS in 2015: New clinical directions, new biological insights. *Lancet Respir Med.* 2015;3(12):912–913.

18. Gunther, A, Ruppert, C, Schmidt, R, et al. Surfactant alteration and replacement in acute respiratory distress syndrome. *Respir Res.* 2001;2(6):353-364.

19. Gregory, TJ, Longmore, WJ, Moxley, MA et al. Surfactant chemical composition and biophysical activity in acute respiratory distress syndrome. *J Clin Invest.* 1991;88(6):1976–1981.

20. Pison, U, Seeger, W, Buchhorn, R, et al. Surfactant abnormalities in patients with respiratory failure after multiple trauma. *Am Rev Respir Dis.* 1989;140(4):1033–1039.

21. Hallman, M, Spragg, R, Harrell, JH, Moser, KM, Gluck, L. Evidence of lung surfactant abnormality in respiratory failure. Study of bronchoalveolar lavage phospholipids, surface activity, phospholipase activity, and plasma myoinositol. *J Clin Invest.* 1982;70(3):673–683.

22. Thille, AW, Esteban, A, Fernandez-Segoviano, P, et al. Chronology of histological lesions in acute respiratory distress syndrome with diffuse alveolar damage: A prospective cohort study of clinical autopsies. *Lancet Respir Med.* 2013;1(5):395–401.

23. Huppert, LA, Matthay, MA. Alveolar fluid clearance in pathologically relevant conditions: In vitro and in vivo models of acute respiratory distress syndrome. *Front Immunol.* 2017;8:371.

24. Yamaguchi, E, Giannetti, MJ, Van Houten, MJ, et al. The unusual symmetric reopening effect induced by pulmonary surfactant. *J Appl Physiol (1985)*. 2014;116(6):635–644.

25. Pohlmann, G, Iwatschenko, P, Koch, W, et al. A novel continuous powder aerosolizer (CPA) for inhalative administration of highly concentrated recombinant surfactant protein-C (rSP-C) surfactant to preterm neonates. *J Aerosol Med Pulm Drug Deliv*. 2013;26(6):370–379.

26. Yeates, D, Heng X. Generation of respirable particles from surfactant suspensions and viscous solutions at high dose rates. *Drug Deliv Lungs*. 2016;27:205–208.

27. Rahmel, DK, Pohlmann, G, Iwatschenko, P, et al. The non-intubated, spontaneously breathing, continuous positive airway pressure (CPAP) ventilated preterm lamb: A unique animal model. *Reprod Toxicol*. 2012;34(2):204–215.

28. Han, S, Mallampalli, RK. The role of surfactant in lung disease and host defense against pulmonary infections. *Ann Am Thorac Soc*. 2015;12(5):765–774.

29. Walther, FJ, Hernandez-Juviel, JM, Gordon, LM, Waring, AJ. Synthetic surfactant containing SP-B and SP-C mimics is superior to single-peptide formulations in rabbits with chemical acute lung injury. *PeerJ*. 2014;2:e393.

30. Schurch, D, Ospina, OL, Cruz, A, Perez-Gil, J. Combined and independent action of proteins SP-B and SP-C in the surface behavior and mechanical stability of pulmonary surfactant films. *Biophys J*. 2010;99(10):3290–3299.

31. Seehase, M, Collins, JJ, Kuypers, E, et al. New surfactant with SP-B and C analogs gives survival benefit after inactivation in preterm lambs. *PLoS One*. 2012;7(10):e47631.

32. Spragg, RG, Taut, FJ, Lewis, JF, et al. Recombinant surfactant protein C-based surfactant for patients with severe direct lung injury. *Am J Respir Crit Care Med*. 2011;183(8):1055–1061.

33. Sato, A, Ikegami, M. SP-B, and SP-C containing new synthetic surfactant for treatment of extremely immature lamb lung. *PLoS One*. 2012;7(7):e39392.

34. Taeusch, HW, Keough, KM. Inactivation of pulmonary surfactant and the treatment of acute lung injuries. *Pediatr Pathol Mol Med*. 2001;20(6):519–536.

35. Seeger, W, Grube, C, Gunther, A, Schmidt, R. Surfactant inhibition by plasma proteins: Differential sensitivity of various surfactant preparations. *Eur Respir J*. 1993;6(7):971–977.

36. Cochrane, CG, Revak, SD, Merritt, TA, et al. The efficacy and safety of KL4-surfactant in preterm infants with respiratory distress syndrome. *Am J Respir Crit Care Med*. 1996;153(1):404–410.

37. van Zyl, JM, Smith, J, Hawtrey, A. The effect of a peptide-containing synthetic lung surfactant on gas exchange and lung mechanics in a rabbit model of surfactant depletion. *Drug Des Devel Ther*. 2013;7:139–148.

38. Lu, KW, Taeusch, HW, Clements, JA. Hyaluronan with dextran added to therapeutic lung surfactants improves effectiveness in vitro and in vivo. *Exp Lung Res*. 2013;39(4–5):191–200.

39. Lu, KW, Taeusch, HW. Combined effects of polymers and KL(4) peptide on surface activity of pulmonary surfactant lipids. *Biochim Biophys Acta*. 2010;1798(6):1129–1134.

40. Lopez-Rodriguez, E, Cruz, A, Richter, RP, Taeusch, HW, Perez-Gil, J. Transient exposure of pulmonary surfactant to hyaluronan promotes structural and compositional transformations into a highly active state. *J Biol Chem*. 2013;288(41):29872–29881.

41. Walther, FJ, Hernandez-Juviel, JM, Waring, AJ. Aerosol delivery of synthetic lung surfactant. *Peer J*. 2014;2:e403.

42. Ricci, F, Catozzi, C, Murgia, X, et al. Physiological, biochemical, and biophysical characterization of the lung-lavaged spontaneously-breathing rabbit as a model for respiratory distress syndrome. *PLoS One*. 2017;12(1):e0169190.

43. Ikegami, M, Adams, FH, Towers, B, Osher, AB. The quantity of natural surfactant necessary to prevent the respiratory distress syndrome in premature lambs. *Pediatr Res*. 1980;14(9):1082–1085.

44. Ikegami, M, Hesterberg, T, Nozaki, M, Adams, FH. Restoration of lung pressure-volume characteristics with surfactant: Comparison of nebulization versus instillation and natural versus synthetic surfactant. *Pediatr Res*. 1977;11(3 Pt 1):178–182.

45. Fok, TF, al-Essa, M, Dolovich, M, Rasid, F, Kirpalani, H. Nebulisation of surfactants in an animal model of neonatal respiratory distress. *Arch Dis Child Fetal Neonatal Ed*. 1998;78(1):F3–F9.

46. Lewis, JF, Ikegami, M, Jobe, AH, Tabor, B. Aerosolized surfactant treatment of preterm lambs. *J Appl Physiol (1985)*. 1991;70(2):869–876.

47. Gordon, MS, Tarara, T, Weers, J. Inhalation surfactant therapy. 2003; Patent application 60333729.

48. Filoche, M, Tai, CF, Grotberg, JB. Three-dimensional model of surfactant replacement therapy. *Proc Natl Acad Sci U S A*. 2015;112(30):9287–9292.

49. Rey-Santano, C, Mielgo, VE, Andres, L, et al. Acute and sustained effects of aerosolized vs. bolus surfactant therapy in premature lambs with respiratory distress syndrome. *Pediatr Res*. 2013;73(5):639–646.

50. Milesi, I, Tingay, DG, Zannin, E, et al. Intratracheal atomized surfactant provides similar outcomes as bolus surfactant in preterm lambs with respiratory distress syndrome. *Pediatr Res*. 2016;80(1):92–100.

51. Simonato, M, Baritussio, A, Ori, C, et al. Disaturated-phosphatidylcholine and surfactant protein-B turnover in human acute lung injury and in control patients. *Respir Res.* 2011;12:36.

52. Yeates, D, Heng, X. Augmentation of the generation, processing and delivery of surfactant and macromolecule aerosols with heliox. *J Aerosol Med Pul Drug Deliv.* 2017;30:3.

53. Khanal, A, Sharma, R, Corcoran, TE, et al. Surfactant driven post-deposition spreading of aerosols on complex aqueous subphases. 1: High deposition flux representative of aerosol delivery to large airways. *J Aerosol Med Pulm Drug Deliv.* 2015;28(5):382–393.

54. Sharma, R, Khanal, A, Corcoran, TE, et al. Surfactant driven post-deposition spreading of aerosols on complex aqueous subphases. 2: Low deposition flux representative of aerosol delivery to small airways. *J Aerosol Med Pulm Drug Deliv.* 2015;28(5):394–405.

55. Minocchieri, S, Knoch, S, Schoel, WM, Ochs, M, Nelle, M. Nebulizing poractant alfa versus conventional instillation: Ultrastructural appearance and preservation of surface activity. *Pediatr Pulmonol.* 2014;49(4):348–356.

56. Jorch, G, Hartl, H, Roth, B, et al. Surfactant aerosol treatment of respiratory distress syndrome in spontaneously breathing premature infants. *Pediatr Pulmonol.* 1997;24(3):222–224.

57. Ruppert, C, Kuchenbuch, T, Boensch, M, et al. Dry powder aerosolization of a recombinant surfactant protein-C-based surfactant for inhalative treatment of the acutely inflamed lung. *Crit Care Med.* 2010;38(7):1584–1591.

58. Grotberg JB, Filoche, M, Willson DF, Raghavendran K, Notter RH. Did reduced alveolar delivery of surfactant contribute to negative results in adults with acute respiratory distress syndrome? *Am J Respir Crit Care Med.* 2017;195(4):538–540.

59. Spragg, RG, Lewis, JF, Walmrath, HD, et al. Effect of recombinant surfactant protein C-based surfactant on the acute respiratory distress syndrome. *N Engl J Med.* 2004;351(9):884–892.

60. Willson, DF, Zaritsky, A, Bauman, LA, et al. Instillation of calf lung surfactant extract (calfactant) is beneficial in pediatric acute hypoxemic respiratory failure. Members of the Mid-Atlantic Pediatric Critical Care Network. *Crit Care Med.* 1999;27(1):188–195.

61. Gregory, TJ, Steinberg, KP, Spragg, R, et al. Bovine surfactant therapy for patients with acute respiratory distress syndrome. *Am J Respir Crit Care Med.* 1997;155(4):1309–1315.

62. Willson, DF, Thomas, NJ, Markovitz, BP, et al. Effect of exogenous surfactant (calfactant) in pediatric acute lung injury: A randomized controlled trial. *JAMA.* 2005;293(4):470–476.

63. Anzueto, A, Jubran, A, Ohar, JA, et al. Effects of aerosolized surfactant in patients with stable chronic bronchitis: A prospective randomized controlled trial. *JAMA.* 1997;278(17):1426–1431.

64. Ellyett, KM, Broadbent, RS, Fawcett, ER, Campbell, AJ. Surfactant aerosol treatment of respiratory distress syndrome in the spontaneously breathing premature rabbit. *Pediatr Res.* 1996;39(6):953–957.

65. Ellyett, KM, Cragg, PA, Broadbent, RS. Effect of surfactant deficiency and surfactant replacement on airway patency in the piglet lung. *Respir Physiol Neurobiol.* 2006;150(2–3):173–181.

66. Hutten, MC, Kuypers, E, Ophelders, DR, et al. Nebulization of Poractant alfa via a vibrating membrane nebulizer in spontaneously breathing preterm lambs with binasal continuous positive pressure ventilation. *Pediatr Res.* 2015;78(6):664–669.

67. Lampland, AL, Wolfson, MR, Mazela, J, et al. Aerosolized KL4 surfactant improves short-term survival and gas exchange in spontaneously breathing newborn pigs with hydrochloric acid-induced acute lung injury. *Pediatr Pulmonol.* 2014;49(5):482–489.

68. Telko, MJ, Hickey, AJ. Aerodynamic and electrostatic properties of model dry powder aerosols: A comprehensive study of formulation factors. *AAPS PharmSciTech.* 2014;15(6):1378–1397.

69. Kwok, PC, Glover, W, Chan, HK. Electrostatic charge characteristics of aerosols produced from metered dose inhalers. *J Pharm Sci.* 2005;94(12):2789–2799.

70. Balachandran, W, Machowski, W, Gaura E, Hudson, C. Control of drug aerosol in human airways using electrostatic forces. *J Electrostatics.* 1997;40–41:579–584.

71. Majid, H, Winker-Heil, R, Madl, P, Hofmann, W, Alam, K. Effect of oral pathway on charged particles deposition in human bronchial airways. *J Aerosol Med Pulm Drug Deliv.* 2015.

72. Xi, J, Si, X, Longest, W. Electrostatic charge effects on pharmaceutical aerosol deposition in human nasal-laryngeal airways. *Pharmaceutics.* 2014;6(1):26–35.

73. Hashish, AH, Bailey, A. Administration of drugs using nebulizers: Effect of electrostatic charge on aerosols. *Inst Phys Conf Ser.* 1987;85:81–86.

74. Rosell, J, Gondal, I, Schuster, J, Liu, K. Use of electrolytes (ions in solution) to suppress charging of inhalation aerosols. U.S. Patent Application 09/733,610; 2002.

75. Longest, PW, Walenga, RL, Son, YJ, Hindle, M. High-efficiency generation and delivery of aerosols through nasal cannula during noninvasive ventilation. *J Aerosol Med Pulm Drug Deliv.* 2013;26(5):266–279.

76. Longest, PW, Golshahi, L, Behara, SR, et al. Efficient nose-to-lung (N2L) aerosol delivery with a dry powder inhaler. *J Aerosol Med Pulm Drug Deliv.* 2015;28(3):189–201.

77. Longest, PW, Azimi, M, Golshahi, L, Hindle, M. Improving aerosol drug delivery during invasive mechanical ventilation with redesigned components. *Respir Care.* 2014;59(5):686–698.

78. Sun, Y, Yang, R, Zhong, JG, et al. Aerosolised surfactant generated by a novel noninvasive apparatus reduced acute lung injury in rats. *Crit Care.* 2009;13(2):R31.

79. Finer, NN, Merritt, TA, Bernstein, G, et al. An open label, pilot study of Aerosurf(R) combined with nCPAP to prevent RDS in preterm neonates. *J Aerosol Med Pulm Drug Deliv.* 2010;23(5):303–309.

80. Ghazanfari, T, Elhissi, AM, Ding, Z, Taylor, KM. The influence of fluid physicochemical properties on vibrating-mesh nebulization. *Int J Pharm.* 2007;339(1–2):103–111.

81. Chan, JG, Traini, D, Chan, HK, Young, PM, Kwok, PC. Delivery of high solubility polyols by vibrating mesh nebulizer to enhance mucociliary clearance. *J Aerosol Med Pulm Drug Deliv.* 2012;25(5):297–305.

82. Young, PM, Thompson, J, Woodcock, D, Aydin, M, Price, R. The development of a novel high-dose pressurized aerosol dry-powder device (PADD) for the delivery of pumactant for inhalation therapy. *J Aerosol Med.* 2004;17(2):123–128.

83. Hentschel, R, Jorch, G. Acute side effects of surfactant treatment. *J Perinat Med.* 2002;30(2):143–148.

84. Shangle, CE, Haas, RH, Vaida, F, Rich, WD, Finer, NN. Effects of endotracheal intubation and surfactant on a 3-channel neonatal electroencephalogram. *J Pediatr.* 2012;161(2):252–257.

85. Oncel, MY, Arayici, S, Uras, N, et al. Nasal continuous positive airway pressure versus nasal intermittent positive-pressure ventilation within the minimally invasive surfactant therapy approach in preterm infants: A randomised controlled trial. *Arch Dis Child Fetal Neonatal Ed.* 2016;101(4):F323–F328.

86. Dargaville, PA, Ali, SKM, Jackson, HD, Williams, C, De Paoli, AG. Impact of minimally invasive surfactant therapy in preterm infants at 29–32 weeks gestation. *Neonatology.* 2018;113(1):7–14.

87. Aguar, M, Cernada, M, Brugada, M, et al. Minimally invasive surfactant therapy with a gastric tube is as effective as the intubation, surfactant, and extubation technique in preterm babies. *Acta Paediatr.* 2014;103(6):e229–e233.

88. Aguar, M, Nunez, A, Cubells, E, et al. Administration of surfactant using less invasive techniques as a part of a non-aggressive paradigm towards preterm infants. *Early Hum Dev.* 2014;90(Suppl 2):S57–S59.

89. Milesi, I, Tingay, DG, Lavizzari, A, et al. Supraglottic atomization of surfactant in spontaneously breathing lambs receiving continuous positive airway pressure. *Pediatr Crit Care Med.* 2017;18(9):e428–e434.

90. Murgia, X, Gastiasoro, E, Mielgo, V, et al. Surfactant and perfluorocarbon aerosolization during different mechanical ventilation strategies by means of inhalation catheters: An in vitro study. *J Aerosol Med Pulm Drug Deliv.* 2012;25(1):23–31.

91. Murgia, X, Gastiasoro, E, Mielgo, V, et al. Surfactant and perfluorocarbon aerosolization by means of inhalation catheters for the treatment of respiratory distress syndrome: An in vitro study. *J Aerosol Med Pulm Drug Deliv.* 2011;24(2):81–87.

92. Dellaca, R, Milesi, I, DiCecio, M, Sewell, R, Taylor, D. Improved method and system for the administration of a pulmonary surfactant by atomization. Patent Application US 2016/02633332016.

93. ONY. Comparison of aerosol delivery of Infasurf to usual care in spontaneously breathing RDS patients. Clinical trials.gov Identifier NCT03058666.

94. Syedain, ZH, Naqwi, AA, Dolovich, M, Somani, A. In vitro evaluation of a device for intra-pulmonary aerosol generation and delivery. *Aerosol Sci Technol.* 2015;49(9):747–752.

95. Amirav, I, Newhouse, MT. Deposition of small particles in the developing lung. *Paediatr Respir Rev.* 2012;13(2):73–78.

96. Mazela, J, Polin, RA. Aerosol delivery to ventilated newborn infants: Historical challenges and new directions. *Eur J Pediatr.* 2011;170(4):433–444.

97. Zeman, KL, Balcazar, JR, Fuller, F, et al. A transnasal aerosol delivery device for efficient pulmonary deposition. *J Aerosol Med Pulm Drug Deliv.* 2017;30(4):223–229.

98. Corcoran, TE, Gamard, S. Development of aerosol drug delivery with helium oxygen gas mixtures. *J Aerosol Med.* 2004;17(4):299–309.

99. Ari, A, Fink, JB, Dhand, R. Inhalation therapy in patients receiving mechanical ventilation: An update. *J Aerosol Med Pulm Drug Deliv.* 2012;25(6):319–332.

100. Farney, KD, Kuehne, BT, Gibson, LA, Nelin, LD, Shepherd, EG. In vitro evaluation of radio-labeled aerosol delivery via a variable-flow infant CPAP system. *Respir Care.* 2014;59(3):340–344.

101. Michotte, JB, Jossen, E, Roeseler, J, Liistro, G, Reychler, G. In vitro comparison of five nebulizers during noninvasive ventilation: Analysis of inhaled and lost doses. *J Aerosol Med Pulm Drug Deliv.* 2014;27(6):430–440.

102. Gregory, T, Irshad, H, Chand, R, Kuehl, P. Regional distribution of aerosolized lucinactant in non-human primates. *International Society for Aerosols in Medicine, 21st Congress.* 2017; Santa Fe, NM, June 3–7, 2017.

103. Gregory, T, Irshad, H, Chand, R, Kuehl, P. Non-invasive delivery of aerosolized lucinactant in non-human promotes (NHPS). *International Society for Aerosols in Medicine, 21st Congress.* 2017;Santa Fe, NM, June 3–7, 2017.

104. Davidson, WJ, Dorscheid, D, Spragg, R, et al. Exogenous pulmonary surfactant for the treatment of adult patients with acute respiratory distress syndrome: Results of a meta-analysis. *Crit Care.* 2006;10(2):R41.

105. Anzueto, A, Baughman, RP, Guntupalli, KK, et al. Aerosolized surfactant in adults with sepsis-induced acute respiratory distress syndrome. Exosurf Acute Respiratory Distress Syndrome Sepsis Study Group. *N Engl J Med.* 1996;334(22):1417–1421.

106. Taut, FJ, Rippin, G, Schenk, P, et al. A search for subgroups of patients with ARDS who may benefit from surfactant replacement therapy: A pooled analysis of five studies with recombinant surfactant protein-C surfactant (Venticute). *Chest.* 2008;134(4):724–732.

107. Willson, DF, Truwit, JD, Conaway, MR, Traul, CS, Egan, EE. The adult calfactant in acute respiratory distress syndrome trial. *Chest.* 2015;148(2):356–364.

108. Spragg, RG. The future of surfactant therapy for patients with acute lung injury—new requirements and new surfactants. *Biol Neonate.* 2002;81(Suppl 1):20–24.

109. Kesecioglu, J, Beale, R, Stewart, TE, et al. Exogenous natural surfactant for treatment of acute lung injury and the acute respiratory distress syndrome. *Am J Respir Crit Care Med.* 2009;180(10):989–994.

110. Kesecioglu, J, Schultz, MJ, Haitsma, JJ, den Heeten, GJ, Lachmann, B. Lodixanol inhibits exogenous surfactant therapy in rats with acute respiratory distress syndrome. *Eur Respir J.* 2002;19(5):820–826.

111. Fink, J, Ivri, Y. Method and composition for the treatment of lung surfactant deficiency or dysfunction. US Grant US7201167B2. 2004.

112. Yeates, DB. High dose rate generation of fine particle aerosols of antibodies with SUPRAER(R) compared to two mesh nebulizers. *Respiratory Drug Deliv.* 2013:313–316.

113. Yeates, DB, Heng, X. Targeting the optimal particle size and output for aerosol drug delivery using SUPRAER(R). *Respiratory Drug Deliv.* 2016:395–400.

114. Beurskens, CJ, Wosten-van Asperen, RM, Preckel, B, Juffermans, NP. The potential of heliox as a therapy for acute respiratory distress syndrome in adults and children: A descriptive review. *Respiration.* 2015;89(2):166–174.

115. Yilmaz, S, Daglioglu, K, Yildizdas, D, et al. The effectiveness of heliox in acute respiratory distress syndrome. *Ann Thorac Med.* 2013;8(1):46–52.

116. Nawab, US, Touch, SM, Irwin-Sherman, T, et al. Heliox attenuates lung inflammation and structural alterations in acute lung injury. *Pediatr Pulmonol.* 2005;40(6):524–532.

117. Jaber, S, Fodil, R, Carlucci, A, et al. Noninvasive ventilation with helium-oxygen in acute exacerbations of chronic obstructive pulmonary disease. *Am J Respir Crit Care Med.* 2000;161(4 Pt 1):1191–1200.

118. Peterson, JB, Prisk, GK, Darquenne, C. Aerosol deposition in the human lung periphery is increased by reduced-density gas breathing. *J Aerosol Med Pulm Drug Deliv.* 2008;21(2):159–168.

119. Svartengren, M, Anderson, M, Philipson, K, Camner, P. Human lung deposition of particles suspended in air or in helium/oxygen mixture. *Exp Lung Res.* 1989;15(4):575–585.

120. Long, C, Li, W, Wanwei, L, Jie, L, Yuan, S. Noninvasive ventilation with Heliox for respiratory distress syndrome in preterm infant: A systematic review and meta-analysis. *Can Respir J.* 2016;2016:9092871.

22

Fundamentals in nasal drug delivery

ZACHARY WARNKEN, YU JIN KIM, HEIDI M. MANSOUR, ROBERT O. WILLIAMS, III, AND HUGH D.C. SMYTH

Introduction	343	Current therapies using intranasal administration	347
Nasal anatomy and physical barriers to delivery	343	Intranasal delivery of peptides and proteins	348
Variability between individuals, genders, ethnicities, and ages	343	Intranasal drug delivery to the CNS	348
		Strategies used for enhancing nasal drug absorption	350
Nasal clearance	344	Drug delivery technologies for nasal administration	353
Effect of disease on nasal drug delivery	345	Conclusion	353
Enzyme metabolism in nasal drug delivery	345	References	354
In vitro models used to evaluate nasal drug delivery	346		

INTRODUCTION

The nasal route of delivery is favorable for the treatment of local symptoms of diseases such as allergy rhinitis and nasal congestion. In addition, nasal drug administration has several demonstrated and potential advantages for the treatment of local, systemic, and central nervous system (CNS) diseases as well. Systemic drug delivery of small molecules, peptides, and proteins has been achieved by noninvasive measures using nasal drug delivery. In addition, the innervation of the nasal cavity provides pathways that can promote drug delivery to the brain, potentially circumventing the blood-brain barrier (BBB) in specific cases. As with any route of delivery, the advantages of the administration method meet with particular challenges associated with the route of delivery. This chapter overviews the fundamentals to delivering drugs by the nasal route of administration, and includes discussion of the barriers to nasal drug delivery as well as the formulation and device technologies that have been invented in order to overcome these barriers.

NASAL ANATOMY AND PHYSICAL BARRIERS TO DELIVERY

Various aspects of the nasal cavity anatomy lend themselves to either enhancing or inhibiting the absorption of drugs. The structure of the nasal cavity, comprised of two halves split at a midline known as the septum, functions to entrap particulates on the surface of the nasal epithelium to filter them before they enter the lower respiratory tract. This function of the nasal cavity promotes selective deposition of drugs onto the nasal epithelium, limiting lung exposure. Once deposited in the nasal mucosa, other barriers such as mucociliary clearance, permeability limitations, and enzymatic activity of the mucosa effect the drug absorption. The influence and importance of the structure and physiology of the nasal mucosa as they relate to drug delivery are discussed in the following sections. Detailed anatomic descriptions of the nasal cavity have been reviewed previously by Illum (1) and Gizurason (2), and only aspects relevant to drug delivery are discussed.

VARIABILITY BETWEEN INDIVIDUALS, GENDERS, ETHNICITIES, AND AGES

Much of our understanding of the deposition of particles in the nasal cavity is based on research taken from a toxicology perspective. Because of the focus of these studies, most research has been performed on the regions of deposition and deposition efficiencies of smaller particles that are influenced by the inspiratory airflow of individuals (typically 10 microns and smaller). These research findings directly relate to drug deposition from specific dosage forms that have or produce particles in similar size ranges and that are influenced by the same forces as the particles being studied. An important aspect of nasal deposition studies, as it relates to drug delivery, is the influence of the nasal airway geometry on the regional deposition of particles in the nasal cavity. The nasal cavity can be segmented into three main parts: the olfactory region, responsible for our sense of smell and comprised of the olfactory neuroepithelium; the respiratory region, which makes up the greatest amount of surface area of the nasal cavity; and the vestibule/nasal valve area (3). The nasal valve is responsible for the highest resistance of airflow within the nasal cavity and is a narrow opening that delineates the anterior and posterior portions of the nasal cavity. The posterior portion, largely comprised of the respiratory region, is generally the target for therapeutics that work locally and for those intended to be absorbed systemically. The respiratory region possesses at least three turbinates, the inferior, middle, and superior turbinates, that function to alter the airflow assisting air conditioning and increase surface area for filtration of inhaled particulates (2). The region in which drugs deposit on the nasal mucosa can have an influence on their bioavailability, their efficacy, and their brain tissue distribution (4,5).

Deposition efficiencies in the nasal cavity can be affected by the size of the particles within a spray or aerosol; generally, particles larger than 10 microns are completely retained in the nasal cavity during inspiration and do not enter the lung (6). Garcia et al. report, under certain conditions, the highest deposition of inhaled nanoparticles to the olfactory region to be in the 1–2 nm range; however, this deposited amount was only about 1%, potentially limiting the usefulness for targeting drug delivery to this region by particle size alone with simple inhalation due to dose considerations (7). Similarly, studies accessing the deposition of inhaled micron-size particles found a maximum of 3% deposition to the olfactory region and about 20% to the respiratory region of the nasal cavity (8). The studies by Garcia and Schroeter were based, however, on the results from a single individual. More recently, Calmet et al. tested the deposition of inhaled micron-size particles in three individuals, and only one of the three showed any deposition in the olfactory region, and the total deposition efficacies were highly variable between individuals (9).

The variability in total deposition efficiencies and regional deposition presents a significant challenge in nasal drug delivery. Differences in nasal deposition efficiencies have been reported in several studies, showing differences between individuals of similar ages (10–12), different ages (13,14), and ethnicities (15). The variability in deposition between individuals reflects the variation in the nasal cavity anatomy between individuals. The geometric complexity of the nasal cavity with various measurable anatomical parameters explains the variability on the total deposition efficiencies of ultrafine particles in a small subset of individuals (16,17). In trying to understand the relationship between the anatomical parameters of the nasal cavity and particle deposition, it becomes evident that the growth of the nasal cavity from adolescence to adulthood affects particle deposition in the nasal cavity. The general dimensions and airflow in the nasal cavity differ between genders as one grows, being larger in women than men in adolescence and reciprocally true in adulthood (18–20). Differences in age affect nasal drug delivery in more than just deposition patterns based on nasal geometry sizes. Doughty et al. characterized the actuation parameters of children and adults for meter pump nasal spray devices and found significant differences in both the actuation parameters between the groups and the resulting spray characteristics generated when reproducing the different actuation parameters mechanically (21,22). In addition to variability in nasal drug delivery resulting from differences in ages, the variability and deposition patterns differ between ethnic groups (23). While differences in airflow between individuals of different ethnic groups influences particles deposition between individuals (19,20,24), nasal drug delivery may also be influenced by other differences in physiology of the nasal cavity, such as differences in pH. Ireson et al. report significantly higher pH values in Caucasians compared to people of African origin which may affect the release or absorption of drugs in the nasal cavity depending on their respective physicochemical properties (25).

NASAL CLEARANCE

Particles that have been entrapped on the nasal mucosa surface are cleared from the nasal cavity and eventually swallowed. In the olfactory region, the cilia are extensions of the olfactory neurons and are nonmotile. Clearance from this region is governed by the flow of the mucous layer. Reports of the mean residence time of drugs deposited within the olfactory region vary depending on the formulation; however, they are often in the range of 8–14 minutes (26,27). However, the respiratory region has active ciliated cells that contain about 100–250 cilia per cell and beat at nearly 1000 times per minute (28). The controlled and rhythmic beating of the cilia results in mucus transport/clearance rates that may vary from 1 to 20 mm/min and appear to be age dependent, decreasing with age (29,30). Mucociliary clearance is a barrier to nasal drug delivery for two opposing reasons. First, the relatively rapid clearance from the nasal cavity surfaces decreases the time for dissolution and absorption of drugs across the nasal mucosa and time for active ingredients to work locally on the tissue, depending on the intent of delivery. On the other hand, the mucociliary clearance plays a vital role in maintain the respiratory tract. Individuals born without functional cilia have an increased risk of bronchial infection and chronic rhinitis. Some drugs and excipients in formulations can inhibit ciliary function, which is likely to result in similar diseases in those individuals born with dysfunctional cilia (31,32). The clearance rate can be influenced without irreversible harm to the cilia and is a relevant formulation strategy for nasal drug delivery and is discussed later. Various substances can either inhibit or promote nasal clearance by altering the rheology of the mucus or changing the ciliary beat frequency. Examples of these substances and their effect on the mucociliary

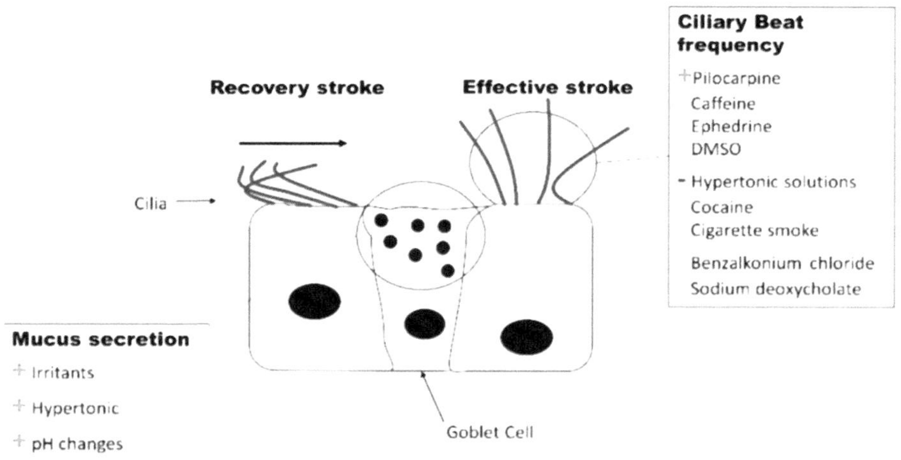

Figure 22.1 Mucociliary clearance of the respiratory epithelium and examples of chemicals and excipients which stimulate or inhibit the clearance rate. (From Gizurarson, S., *Biol. Pharm. Bull.*, 38, 497–506, 2015.)

clearance are presented in Figure 22.1 (33,34). The mean residence time for a formulation can depend on its formulation and its location of deposition. Considering the entire nasal passage, spray dosage forms can have residence time half-lives of around an hour and half. Particles deposited in the anterior section of the nose, which is not ciliated, can be retained longer than those deposed in the posterior section if the formulation remains in the cavity and does not flow out of the front (35,36).

EFFECT OF DISEASE ON NASAL DRUG DELIVERY

Anatomical and physiological factors of the nasal cavity can be influenced by the presence of various disease states. Successful drug delivery by the nasal route requires a complete understanding of the nasal cavity environment in both disease and healthy individuals. Diseases can influence the anatomical structure of the nasal cavity for local diseases such as nasal allergies. A deviated nasal septum, for example, can hinder the ability of intranasal sprays to deposit drugs to their intended target tissues (37,38). The physiology of the nasal cavity can also be influenced by diseases, leading to differences in mucociliary clearance rates and therefore the efficacy and absorption of nasally administered drugs. The effect of diseases on nasal drug delivery can be a function of the symptoms of the patient. In addition to deposition differences, patients with nasal congestion have reduced clearance of drugs from the nasal cavity. For patients experiencing increased mucus production resulting in a runny nose, clearance can be rapidly increased compared to baseline (39,40). However, there is conflicting evidence on the effect of rhinitis on the mucociliary clearance time. Another study suggests the clearance is longer due to influences in both mucus rheological properties and cilia activity (41). Treatment with guaifenesin, a drug intended to alter the rheological properties of

mucus by thinning it and promoting its clearance from the respiratory tract, had no effect in the mucociliary clearance time (42). Nasal drug clearance may also be influenced by nonlocal diseases. For instance, Delehaye et al. report a correlation between the nasal mucociliary clearance time and gastroesophageal reflux disease. HIV-positive individuals have been shown to have significantly prolonged mucociliary clearance times compared to HIV-negative individuals. The mucociliary clearance can also be affected by the widespread chronic diseases, diabetes, and hypertension (43). While these diseases influenced the mucociliary clearance time, blood pressure and glucose level were not associated with prolonged clearance times. The influence that these relatively common diseases have on nasal clearance times may contribute to the variability associated with nasal drug delivery.

ENZYME METABOLISM IN NASAL DRUG DELIVERY

The nasal mucosa has a relatively high enzymatic activity in local tissues and serves as a metabolic defensive barrier against xenobiotics. It has even been reported that cytochrome P450 enzyme activity exceeds that of the liver when normalized for tissue protein content (29). The high metabolic capacity of the nasal mucosa creates a pseudo-first-pass metabolism for drugs intended to be systemically delivered or delivered to the central nervous system. In addition to cytochrome P450 enzymes, several phase 1 and phase 2 metabolism enzymes are present in the nasal mucosa, including carbonic anhydrases, carboxylesterases, epoxide hydrolases, flavin-containing monooxygenases, glucuronyl and sulfate transferases, glutathione transferase, and proteases (44). The enzymatic activity in the nasal mucosa can influence both small and large molecule delivery. Dhamanar et al. studied expression of cytochrome P450s and the metabolism of melatonin in bovine respiratory and olfactory epithelium (45,46). Melatonin is a substrate for CYP1A2 and is based on the rate of 6-hydroxy–melatonin, its primary metabolite, Dhamanar et al. showed both olfactory and respiratory epithelium were metabolically active toward melatonin, with high activity being present in the respiratory epithelium. Enzyme degradation of peptides contributes to the relatively low bioavailability of salmon calcitonin when delivered intranasally (47). In other cases, the rate of enzymatic degradation compared to the short residence time in the nasal cavity results in negligible loss by degradation, such as insulin degradation by nasal mucosa aminopeptidases, and may be an aspect of nasal drug delivery that will have growing relevance as new technologies increase the residence time for drugs in the nasal cavity (48).

In addition to enzymes, the olfactory epithelium also contains binding proteins, which bind hydrophobic odorants and mediate internalization of the substances into lysosomes within the supporting cells of the epithelium, the sustentacular cells (29,49). This also leads to rapid clearance of hydrophobic odorants and may play a role in the clearance of hydrophobic drugs from the tissue. The enzymes in the olfactory epithelium are largely located in the sustentacular cells, the olfactory receptor neurons having very little xenobiotic-metabolizing capacity. Enzyme differences between species may play an important role in studying drug delivery in animal models. cytochrome P450 family 2 subfamily G (CYP2G), for example, has two copies in humans; however, neither function in the majority of individuals. However, Cynomolgus moneys have a functional copy expressed that is active toward coumarin, a common fluorescent molecule used for testing intranasal drug delivery systems. While the enzyme locations in specific cell types are similar across various species, the distribution and concentrations of enzymes can vary greatly (29,44).

IN VITRO MODELS USED TO EVALUATE NASAL DRUG DELIVERY

As with other routes of delivery, the process of formulation and device design for nasal drug delivery relies on accurate and predictive *in vitro* models. Various *in vitro* models have been used over time to study and determine the deposition pattern, absorption mechanisms, and metabolism of drugs in the nasal cavity (50). As technology progresses, the use of new, more rapid, and more accurate *in vitro* tests have been implemented in nasal drug delivery. Possibly the most straightforward for assessing drug deposition in the nasal cavity is found in the FDA guidance for bioequivalence of nasal products. In this test, a 2 L round bottom flask with an opening for a nasal spray is placed onto a cascade impactor to measure the amount of product that could reach the lungs of patients (51). The safety profile for excipients and drugs in the nasal cavity may differ from that of the lungs; thus, it is important to formulation or design devices that maintain

nasal products in the nasal cavity. During development of a formulation or device, it is often useful to gain more detailed information about the deposition pattern of the drug due the effects it will have on the absorption, residence time, and tissue distribution of the drug. Over the years, nasal models have been developed that more and more closely resemble the nasal cavity. This allows testing and assessment of deposition in the nasal cavity, with the need for testing in humans with every iteration of development. An early example was published by Hallworth et al., who studied regional deposition using a glass model nose that was based on anatomic measurements made from autopsies (52). This allowed simplified production and easy visualization of nasal deposition compared to some of the earlier plastic models made from cadavers beforehand. While the simplified glass-model nose was useful in determining the region of deposition with nasal sprays at the time, it lacked turbinates and the complexity of structures found in the nasal cavity for assessing deposition of other dosage forms. Casts developed from cadavers possessed accurate shape and configurations of the nasal airways, but they failed to capture the airway in its normal physiological state and were limited by the results obtained after fixation of the tissue (53). This led to the development of realistic anatomical nasal casts developed from medical imaging such as magnetic resonance imaging (MRI) and computed tomography (CT) scans. Models from medical images remain a popular choice for anatomically realistic nasal models However, the manufacturing implementation of the models has changed over time to reduce artifacts created in the manufacturing process. Early implementation involved cutting sheets of plastic for every cross-sectional image and aligning them to create the nasal cast (14,54,55). More recently, physical models of the casts have been manufactured using 3D-printing technologies with increasing accuracy (13,56–58). The use of this relatively rapid production process has expanded the testing of nasal products from single individuals in studies to multiple individuals with both healthy and disease-modified nasal anatomies (12). Nasal geometries based on the averages of more than 30 individuals have been created and may be useful in the development of devices for nasal drug delivery (59,60). Recent studies into the subject-variability effects of micron-size particle deposition have shown the importance of understanding the variability between individuals (9). For example, some patients may exhibit deposition in the olfactory region, while others do not; this could result in the average amount deposited to the olfactory region appearing acceptable. However, in individual patients, the deposition and delivery to the brain can be markedly different. In addition to physical models made from medical imaging, modeling software has used this data to study the airflow and deposition of particles in nasal cavities with varying conditions such as deviated septum and surgical effects (7,37,61–64).

Research on the mechanisms of absorption and screening between formulations is performed using *in vitro* and *ex vivo* techniques using grown or excised nasal tissue to evaluate the permeation of drug across the membrane (65,66). The use of excised tissue from mammals such as goats, sheep, cattle, and pigs have been used to study the permeation of drugs before *in vivo* testing using diffusion cells (66–71). Research using excised tissues has improved our understanding of the transport mechanisms and transporters present in both the olfactory and respiratory tissues. Using excised bovine olfactory mucosa, Kandimalla and Donovan described the role of passive diffusion in the transport of particular small molecules that are not affected by P-glycoprotein efflux pumps on the olfactory epithelium (66). Similar studies have been performed with atrazine, chlorpheniramine, and chlorcyclizine, drugs that are affected by efflux pumps in olfactory and respiratory epithelium, and the significance of efflux transporters on drug delivery has been explored using these models (72,73). Excised porcine tissue has been used to explore the mechanism of nanoparticle transport for drug delivery across the olfactory epithelium to determine if drug release from nanoparticles or direct transport of nanoparticles is possible. Mistry et al. report seeing increased nanoparticle uptake into the olfactory mucosa with specific particles but no detectable nanoparticles in the receiving reservoir of their diffusion cell system (69). The use of studies with freshly excised tissues will continue to be useful as research is dedicated to understanding the transport of other nanoparticle types as well as drug transport for new

chemical entities intended for both systemic and brain drug delivery. An additional benefit of using excised tissue and cell-cultured olfactory or respiratory tissue is for evaluation of potential irritation and toxicities associated with either the formulation or drug on the nasal mucosa (74–76).

CURRENT THERAPIES USING INTRANASAL ADMINISTRATION

Nasal drug delivery has specific advantages for the treatment of local, systemic, and CNS-related diseases. Over the last three decades, a number of intranasal products have been approved by the FDA for both the treatment of local diseases such as allergic rhinitis or for systemic absorption and action elsewhere in the body. While more nasal products intended for the treatment of local diseases have been approved, around 60% of approved products since 1977, both local- and systemic-acting nasal products have been approved across this period (Figure 22.2). The relatively small number of diseases currently treated with intranasal products is summarized in Table 22.1. While the use of nasal drug delivery to treat local disease is intuitive, this dosage form is also favorable for drugs intended to treat CNS disorders that do not readily cross the BBB or have systemic side effects, for diseases requiring rapid onset of action, for drugs that undergo high first-pass metabolism, or for drugs that would be unstable via other routes of administration as well as for proteins and peptides.

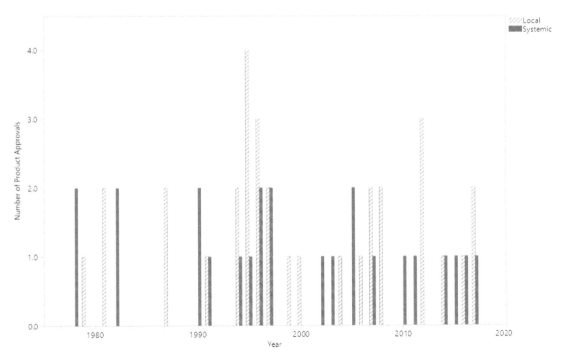

Figure 22.2 Number of approved nasal products since 1977 with indications for local treatment or systemic/central nervous system drug delivery. (From Drugs@FDA [Internet], U.S. Food and Drug Administration, 2018.)

Table 22.1 FDA-approved indications for nasal drug products of current and past nasal products

Treatment location	Indication	Number of product approvals
Local	Allergic rhinitis	26
	Rhinorrhea	3
	Nasal polyps	6
	Nasal congestion	2
	Nasal MRSA colonization	1
	Anesthesia	2
Systemic	Hypogonadism	1
	Central cranial diabetes insipidus	1
	Vitamin B_{12} deficiency	3
	Central precocious puberty	1
	Endometriosis	1
	Hemophilia A	1
	Von Willebrand's disease (Type I)	1
	Nocturia	1
	Paget's disease of the bone	1
	Hypercalcemia	1
	Postmenopausal osteoporosis	1
Central Nervous System	Opioid overdose	1
	Pain management	3
	Smoke cessation	1
	Migraine	4

Source: From Drugs@FDA [Internet], U.S. Food and Drug Administration, 2018.

INTRANASAL DELIVERY OF PEPTIDES AND PROTEINS

Oral administration is the most convenient and standard route for many drugs. However, it is not an effective delivery route for proteins and peptides due to their large molecular size, poor absorption/permeation, and rapid metabolism in the gastrointestinal (GI) tract (77,78). Currently, a parenteral route such as subcutaneous, intramuscular, and intravenous injection is considered as a major route for delivering most protein and peptide drugs in the market. However, other noninvasive (needle-free) routes such as pulmonary, nasal, ocular, transdermal, buccal, and vaginal delivery routes have also been extensively investigated as alternatives. The nasal route has emerged as a promising delivery route for proteins and peptides.

The nasal cavity provides a large surface area for drug absorption and rapid onset of action. Hepatic first-pass metabolism and drug degradation in the GI environment can be prevented via this route (78,79). Currently, several peptide-based drugs have been approved by the Food and Drug Administration (FDA) for nasal delivery (Table 22.2). Fortical® is a metered nasal spray pump for the delivery of calcitonin salmon prepared in liquid solution and used for the treatment of postmenopausal osteoporosis. Synarel® is a nasal spray solution of nafarelin acetate and indicated for the treatment of endometriosis. There are four marketed products, Minirin®, DDAVP®, Noctiva™, and Stimate®,

for the nasal delivery of desmopressin acetate. Minirin®, DDAVP, and Noctiva are indicated for the treatment of polyuria and polydipsia, and are delivered in nasal spray solutions (Minirin and DDAVP) or spray emulsion (Noctiva). Stimate is a nasal spray pump containing liquid solution of desmopressin acetate, which is indicated for the treatment of bleeding in patients with hemophilia A or von Willebrand disease. Chemical structures of these marketed products are presented in Figure 22.3. With the success of these products, a wide range of proteins and peptides is currently in development. Examples of therapeutics currently in clinical trials are listed in Table 22.3.

INTRANASAL DRUG DELIVERY TO THE CNS

The nasal route is advantageous for the delivery of small molecules, proteins, and peptides to the CNS, and can be used for the treatment of acute pain, migraines, smoking (nicotine addiction), or various neurodegenerative diseases such as Alzheimer's disease and Parkinson's disease. Once drugs are delivered into the nasal cavity and reach the cribriform plate, the substances can be delivered to the brain through the olfactory bulbs or trigeminal nerve (direct pathways) or through the lymphatic system (indirect pathway) (80). Although the direct pathway circumvents the BBB, drugs transported via the lymphatic system and drained into the circulation may enter the brain if the substances pass through the BBB (80). Multiple factors influence the transport of drug substances

Table 22.2 Marketed nasal peptide and protein delivery products approved by the U.S. FDA

Product	Drug	Dosage form	Indications	Company
Calcitonin salmon	Calcitonin salmon	Nasal spray solution	Postmenopausal osteoporosis	Apotex Inc., Par Pharmaceutical Inc.
Fortical	Calcitonin salmon	Nasal spray solution	Postmenopausal osteoporosis	Upsher Smith Laboratories
Synarel	Nafarelin acetate	Nasal spray solution	Endometriosis	Pfizer Inc.
Minirin	Desmopressin acetate	Nasal spray solution	Primary nocturnal enuresis, central cranial diabetes insipidus, polyuria and polydipsia	Ferring Pharmaceuticals Inc.
DDAVP	Desmopressin acetate	Nasal spray solution	The management of central cranial diabetes insipidus, and temporary polyuria and polydipsia following head trauma or surgery in the pituitary region	Ferring Pharmaceuticals Inc.
Noctiva™	Desmopressin acetate	Nasal spray oil-in-water emulsion	Nocturnal polyuria	Avadel Pharmaceuticals, Serenity Pharmaceuticals
Stimate	Desmopressin acetate	Nasal spray pump solution	Bleeding in patients with hemophilia A or von Willebrand disease	Ferring Pharmaceuticals Inc., BDI Pharma Inc.

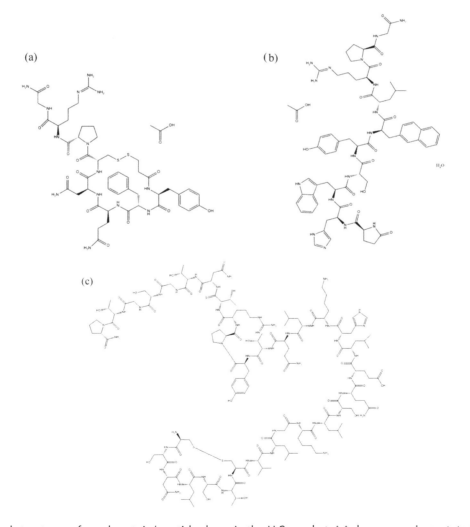

Figure 22.3 Chemical structures of nasal protein/peptide drugs in the U.S. market: (a) desmopressin acetate (mol. wt.: 1129.28 g/mol) (140), (b) nafarelin acetate (mol. wt.: 1400.56 g/mol) (140), and (c) calcitonin salmon (mol. wt.: 3431.90 g/mol). (From ChemicalBook—Chemical Search Engine 2018, http://www.chemicalbook.com/ProductIndex_EN.aspx.)

Table 22.3 Intranasal delivery of proteins and peptides currently in clinical trials in the United States (www.clinicaltrial.gov)

Proteins/ peptides	Molecular weight (mol. wt.), g/mol	Treatment	Current status
Oxytocin	1007.19	Obstructive sleep apnea	Phase 2, recruiting
		Schizophrenia	Phase 2, active
		Unit cohesion	Phase 1, recruiting
Insulin	5733.55	Alzheimer's disease, mild cognitive impairment	Phase 1, recruiting
Insulin (Humulin)	5807.63	Amnestic mild cognitive impairment, Alzheimer's disease	Phase 2 & 3, active
Insulin detemir	5916.89	Alzheimer's disease, mild cognitive impairment	Phase 2, active
Davunetide	824.93	Predicted tauopathies, progressive supranuclear palsy, frontotemporal dementia with Parkinsonism linked to chromosome 17, corticobasal degeneration syndrome, progressive nonfluent aphasia	Phase 2, active
Neuropeptide Y	4254.70	Mood disorder, anxiety disorders	Phase 2, completed

across the BBB. In general, lipophilic compounds with molecular weight less than 500 Da and low numbers of hydrogen bond donors and acceptors are favorable for passive diffusion (81). Absorption enhancers are commonly employed to improve the transport of hydrophilic macromolecules like proteins and peptides to target areas in the brain (79,82). The applications of PEGylated nanoparticles and colloidal nanocarrier systems such as liposomes, micelles, and emulsions to the nasal delivery of peptide therapeutics are other possible options (79,81,83). These strategies to improve the intranasal delivery of protein and peptide drugs are reviewed in the next section.

The intranasal delivery of insulin to the CNS is one of the promising research areas for the treatment of Alzheimer's disease. Preclinical and clinical evaluations have shown that the intranasal administration of insulin improved memory and cognitive processes (84–86). Investigations of intranasal insulin are ongoing to elucidate its delivery mechanisms to the brain such as delivery via the olfactory pathway (87). Several clinical trials have been completed or are ongoing to demonstrate the mechanisms or effects of intranasal insulin on memory or cognitive function in Alzheimer's disease. Nasal delivery of other proteins and peptides such as oxytocin (88), nerve growth factor (89), leptin (90), angiotensin II (91), and interferonsβ-1b (IFNβ-1b) (92) have also been extensively studied.

There have been efforts to deliver small molecules to the brain and/or vasculature via a nasal route (Table 22.4). Imitrex® (GlaxoSmithKline) is a nasal spray solution of sumatriptan approved by the FDA in 1997; it is indicated for the treatment of migraine. There are reports showing that an oral dose of sumatriptan may induce GI disturbances, nausea, and/or vomiting during the migraine attack (93–95). Furthermore, sumatriptan is subjected to first-pass metabolism, resulting in low bioavailability in animal models (93). Hence, nasal administration may be advantageous for patients suffering from adverse effects after an oral dose of sumatriptan. Nasal formulations of Zomig® (AstraZeneca) and Migranal® (Valeant Pharmaceuticals) are also beneficial to overcome potential

side effects of the oral medications for migraine. Zomig is a single-use metered spray device for the nasal delivery of zolmitriptan solution, which was approved by the FDA in 2013. Its good tolerability and efficacy in long-term use have been demonstrated in the clinical stage (96). Migranal, approved in 1997, is a single-use metered spray pump device containing a solution form of dihydroergotamine mesylate. Nasal administration is beneficial to overcome poor oral bioavailability of dihydroergotamine mesylate, since it has been known that oral dihydroergotamine mesylate has low bioavailability due to incomplete drug absorption across the GI mucosa and first-pass metabolism (97). Narcan® (Adapt Pharma, Inc.) is an FDA-approved (in 2015) nasal spray solution that contains naloxone for the treatment of opioid overdose. The MAD Nasal™ Mucosal Atomizer (Teleflex Inc.) with a pre-filled cartridge of naloxone solution is an alternative device for the nasal delivery of naloxone, but it is not approved by the FDA. Nicotrol® (Pfizer Inc.), a metered nasal spray solution containing nicotine, was approved by the FDA in 1996. It is indicated for the treatment of smoking cessation. The primary advantage of the nasal form of nicotine over other forms, such as transdermal, gum, sublingual, and oral inhaler, is its rapid action (98). Goprelto® (Genus Lifesciences Inc.) was approved by the FDA in late 2017. It is a nasal solution of cocaine hydrochloride, and it is used for the induction of local anesthesia of the mucous membranes. Chemical structures of these products are presented in Figure 22.4.

STRATEGIES USED FOR ENHANCING NASAL DRUG ABSORPTION

The cells of the nasal epithelium are connected by tight junctions, creating a limiting barrier for drug absorption across the membrane. Drug absorption across the nasal epithelium favors small lipophilic molecules that can passively diffuse across the membrane for uptake into the blood and lymphatic system. Larger, more hydrophilic molecules such as proteins and peptides are limited in their absorption by their poor permeability across the nasal epithelium. The use of absorption

Table 22.4 FDA-approved nasal small molecule drug (nonprotein/nonpeptide) products delivered to the brain

Product	Drug	Dosage form/devices	Indications	Company
Imitrex	Sumatriptan	Nonpressurized metered nasal spray solution, single use	Migraine	GlaxoSmithKline
Sumatriptan	Sumatriptan	Nasal spray solution, single use	Migraine	Lannett Company, Inc.
ONZETRA Xsail	Sumatriptan succinate	Nasal dry powder delivery device, single use	Migraine	Avanir Pharmaceuticals, Inc.
Zomig	Zolmitriptan	Nonpressurized metered nasal spray solution, single use	Migraine	AstraZeneca
Migranal	Dihydroergotamine mesylate	Metered nasal spray pump solution, single use	Migraine	Valeant Pharmaceuticals
Narcan	Naloxone hydrochloride	Nasal spray solution delivered by Narcan spray device (Adapt Pharma, Inc., approved by the FDA) or a mucosal nasal atomizer with a prefilled cartridge of naloxone (not approved by the FDA), single use	Opioid overdose	ADAPT Pharma, Inc.
Butorphanol tartrate	Butorphanol tartrate	Nasal spray solution, multiple use	Pain management	Apotex Corp., Mylan Pharmaceutical Inc.
Nicotrol	Nicotine	Metered nasal spray solution, multiple use	Smoke cessation	Pfizer Inc.
Goprelto	Cocaine hydrochloride	Nasal solution	Induction of local anesthesia of the mucous membranes	Genus Lifesciences Inc.

enhancers is a frequent option to improve the nasal absorption of polar small molecules and macromolecules (99). Several compounds have been evaluated as absorption enhancers for the nasal route, including surfactants such as laureth-9, bile salts and derivatives such as sodium glycocholate and sodium tauro-24,25-dihydrofusidate, phospholipids such as didecanoyl-L-α-phosphatidylcholine, cyclodextrins, and cationic polymers such as chitosan (82). Absorption enhancers have been commercially developed by companies for nasal drug delivery (100,101). For example, CriticalSorb™ (Critical Pharmaceuticals Ltd.) is hydroxy fatty acid ester of polyethylene glycol that promotes the nasal absorption of hydrophilic small molecules, proteins, and peptides across mucosal epithelial cells (101). Preclinical studies have demonstrated the effectiveness of CriticalSorb in the nasal absorption of insulin and human growth hormone (101). It is used in marketed oral and intravenous products, and it is available in liquid and powder drug formulations. ChiSys® (Archimedes Pharma Ltd.) is a chitosan-based absorption enhancer that was developed for the nasal delivery of various drugs. Chitosan is bioadhesive due to its positive charge that extends drug residence time in the nasal cavity (101). There are studies demonstrating that chitosan transiently opens tight junctions in a mucosal membrane with its bioadhesive property, which enhances the nasal absorption of drugs (100–102). Intravail® (Aegis Therapeutics Inc.), a class of alkylsaccharides, is a nontoxic and nonirritating agent that

can be employed as a nasal delivery system for small polar molecules, proteins, and peptides (100,101). Tetradecyl maltoside (TDM) is a class of alkylsaccharides and its effectiveness has been evaluated in a preclinical model. Previous studies have shown that TDM improved the nasal absorption of insulin and leptin, and increased their bioavailability (101,103). However, it should be noted that absorption enhancers may cause irritation and possibly irreversible damage of nasal tissues (1,101). Hence, it may need to be cautiously applied, and it especially may not be suitable for multiple dosing and/or long-term treatments. Formulation development is another critical approach to improve the nasal delivery of proteins and peptides. Different formulations, including microparticles, nanoparticles, and liposomes, have been developed and evaluated in a preclinical stage for their utilization in a nasal drug delivery system (104–113).

One of the barriers to nasal drug delivery discussed previously is mucociliary clearance. Rapid clearance from the nasal cavity decreases the time for drug dissolution and absorption to occur. Several formulation strategies have been utilized to increase drug residence time and thus improve nasal absorption. One such strategy is to incorporate polymers into the formulation, which increases the formulation's viscosity and can act as a mucoadhesive. A balance between viscosity and mucoadhesion is necessary as high viscosity solutions are difficult to administer to the

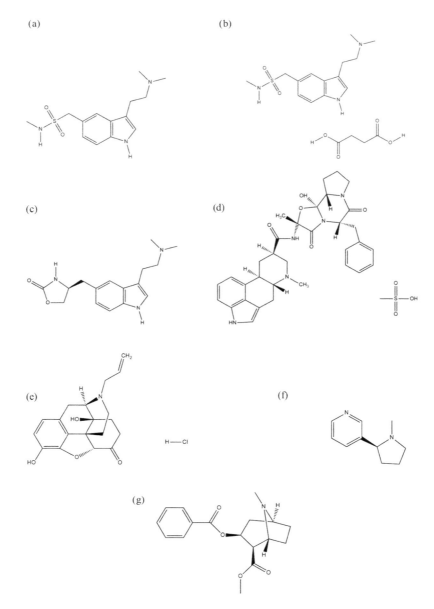

Figure 22.4 Chemical structures of nasal nonprotein/nonpeptide drugs targeting the brain in the U.S. market: **(a)** sumatriptan (mol. wt.: 295.40), **(b)** sumatriptan succinate (mol. wt.: 413.49 g/mol), **(c)** zolmitriptan (mol. wt.: 287.36 g/mol), **(d)** dihydroergotamine mesylate (mol. wt.: 679.79 g/mol), **(e)** naloxone hydrochloride (mol. wt.: 363.84 g/mol), **(f)** nicotine (mol. wt.: 162.24 g/mol), and **(g)** cocaine hydrochloride (mol. wt.: 339.82 g/mol). (From National Center for Biotechnology Information, PubChem Compound Database [Internet], National Institutes of Health [NIH], 2018.)

nasal cavity and limit drug diffusion, which has a negative impact on drug absorption (114). Similar viscosities between polymers do not always reflect similar mucoadhesion to the nasal mucosa as the function groups on the polymer and polymer structure play an important role in the formulation's interaction with nasal mucus and mucosa (115). Another strategy for increasing formulation residence time while maintaining ease of administration is the use of *in situ* gelling formulations. Incorporation of poloxamer in formulations has been utilized to create thermo-reversible *in situ* gels, which remain liquid at room temperature and gel at the temperatures found in the nasal cavity (116,117). *In situ* gels can also be formed by taking advantage of other

changes in the nasal cavity environment. The incorporation of deacetylated gellan gum and low methoxyl pectin in the formulation have gelling properties when in the presence of divalent cations in the nasal mucus (118–120).

Many of the formulation techniques for improving nasal drug bioavailability improve absorption for drugs across both the olfactory and respiratory epithelium. A few specific formulation strategies that are unique to improving drug delivery across the olfactory membrane for brain targeting have been reported (121). Co-administering drug with a vasoconstrictor has been shown to increase brain targeting after intranasal administration by decreasing the amount of drug available for transport into the blood. This method may be of particular importance for drugs that possess high systemic toxicity (122). The production rate of the cerebrospinal fluid can be reduced in the presence of acetazolamide, resulting in decreased clearance rate of cerebrospinal fluid. Preadministration with acetazolamide has been shown to increase cerebrospinal fluid levels of some small molecules after intranasal delivery (123,124). Nose-to-brain drug delivery can also be improved with the use of matrix metalloprotease-9 (MMP-9) as an absorption enhancer. MMP-9 breaks down the extracellular matrix of cells, improving the delivery of macromolecules across the olfactory epithelium (125,126).

DRUG DELIVERY TECHNOLOGIES FOR NASAL ADMINISTRATION

There are primarily two targeted regions for nasal drug delivery: the respiratory region and the olfactory region. The respiratory region is targeted due to its high surface area, vascularization, and its being the site of action for local therapeutics. The olfactory region is the targeted site for enhanced brain targeting to take advantage of the direct pathway between the neuroepithelium and the cerebrospinal fluid and brain parenchyma. Both of these target sites are hindered by the narrow geometric size of the nasal valve region, separating the anterior and posterior sections of the nasal cavity (127). Currently, the most common delivery device for nasal drug delivery is the meter-dosed pump spray. This device can produce straightforward, accurate, and reproducible dosing by patients with a variety of volumes between 25 and 200 μL. The characteristics of the spray emitted from the device can be influenced by the device design, formulation, and patient actuation parameters (22,128). Nasal formulations with higher viscosity produce sprays with larger droplets and more narrow plume geometry angles that, when administered to the nasal cavity at particular administration angles, result in greater deposition to the posterior portions of the nasal cavity (55,58). Several studies have reported that a majority of the droplets from nasal spray devices are deposited in the anterior section of the nasal cavity; however, this depends on the device, formulation, and administration angles greater than 70% of deposition to the respiratory region and can be achieved with a particular combination of parameters (54,55,129,130). While nasal sprays have shown their efficacy for both local and systemic delivery by delivering effective amounts of drug to their intended site, they are ineffective at depositing drug in the olfactory region. While nasal drops are capable of reaching the olfactory region and effectively coating large regions of the respiratory epithelium, their delivery is hindered by difficulties in accurate dosage delivery and higher clearance from the nasal cavity, and they require patients to use complex maneuvers for proper administration (131).

The development of various types of nasal drug delivery devices raises interest in intranasal delivery of proteins and peptides. These substances are commonly prepared in the form of solutions, suspensions, emulsions, or dry powders. Aqueous solutions with preservatives are the most frequently used for systemic delivery of peptide-based therapeutics. Dry powder nasal formulations and devices have several advantages over liquid formulations: (1) Dry powder provides chemical stability since drugs are delivered in a powder form without being solubilized in a liquid phase, and (2) nasal irritation may be reduced because preservatives may not be required for dry powder formulations (132). Liquid-based delivery systems include nasal drops, aerosols, gels, squeezed bottle, instillation and rhinyle catheter, vapor inhaler, metered-dose spray pumps, syringe spray, pressurized metered-dose inhaler, and nebulizers. Powder-based delivery systems include dry powder inhalers, insufflators, pressurized metered-dose inhalers, and dry powder sprays (132,133). Optinose, Inc. provides two FDA-approved exhalation delivery systems: ONZETRA® Xsail® (licensed to Avanir Pharmaceuticals, Inc. affiliated with Otsuka Pharmaceutical Co., Ltd.) and XHANCE™ metered nasal spray (www.optinose.com). ONZETRA Xsail is the first nasal dry powder product approved by the FDA in 2016 for the treatment of migraine headache, and it contains sumatriptan succinate. It is supplied as a disposable (single-use) nosepiece with a hypromellose capsule filled with sumatriptan succinate in a dry powder form and a reusable delivery device body. XHANCE was approved by the FDA in late 2017 for the treatment of nasal polyps; it contains fluticasone propionate in a solution form. OPN-300, which combines their exhalation delivery system with oxytocin, is currently in phase 1 clinical trials (www.optinose.com). Another example of a nasal device is the nasal delivery of insulin via the ViaNase™ Electronic Atomizer (Kurve Technology, Inc.), which is also in clinical trials (www.kurvetech.com/devices.asp).

Targeting of the olfactory region utilizes many of the same novel devices discussed above for protein and peptide drug delivery. Optinose, Inc. has developed a dry powder and liquid nasal drug delivery device for targeting the olfactory region. As the force for actuation of the device is provided by exhalation, this results in closure of the soft palate, thus disconnecting the nasal cavity from the lungs during administration. This allows for use of smaller particle sizes, which can benefit deposition and dissolution within the nasal cavity without concern for additional toxicity to the lung tissue (134). The precision olfactory delivery (POD) device by Impel Neuropharma utilizes actuation force from pressurized gases such as those used with pressurized metered-dose inhalers to propel drug past the nasal valve and reach the olfactory region. The device can also be used with liquid or powder dosage forms and has been used in both human and animal studies (135–137).

CONCLUSION

Nasal drug delivery provides many advantages for administration of therapeutically active drugs for both small and large molecules. The high vascularity and immediate contact of drugs with the membrane for absorption promotes rapid response drugs for treating diseases such as migraines and as a route for emergency rescue therapies. Absorption bypassing the GI tract and liver make it a viable route for drugs that undergo high first-pass metabolism and proteins and peptides. In addition, the olfactory neuroepithelium provides pathways for direct nose-to-brain drug delivery, overcoming the barriers associated with the BBB. Although there are many advantages to nasal drug delivery, there are also many challenges. The variability in nasal cavity anatomy, relatively rapid clearance, volume limitation, and enzymatic activity of the nasal mucosa can limit the success of nasal drug delivery and provide opportunities for formulation and device technologies. Several formulation strategies for overcoming the barriers associated with nasal drug delivery have been used successfully for local, systemic, and CNS delivery of small molecules and proteins/peptides. These strategies continue to be investigated, with exploration of new avenues to safely improve drug efficacy after intranasal administration. As knowledge about particle deposition, anatomic structure, and absorption mechanisms in the nasal cavity expands, novel devices continue to be developed to deliver drug formulations to their intended target and maximize their intended purpose.

REFERENCES

1. Illum L. Nasal drug delivery—possibilities, problems and solutions. *Journal of Controlled Release*. 2003;87:187–198. doi:10.1016/S0168–3659(02)00363–2.
2. Gizurarson S. Anatomical and histological factors affecting intranasal drug and vaccine delivery. *Current Drug Delivery*. 2012;9(6):566–582. doi:10.2174/156720112803529828.
3. Clerico D, To W, Lanza D. Anatomy of the human nasal passages. In Doty RL, ed., *Handbook of Olfaction and Gustation*. New York: CRC Press, 2003, pp. 1–16.
4. Dhuria SV, Hanson LR, Frey WH. Intranasal delivery to the central nervous system: Mechanisms and experimental considerations. *Journal of Pharmaceutical Sciences*. 2010;99:1654–1673. doi:10.1002/jps.21924.
5. Ruigrok MJR, de Lange ECM. Emerging insights for translational pharmacokinetic and pharmacokinetic-pharmacodynamic studies: Towards prediction of nose-to-brain transport in humans. *The AAPS Journal*. 2015. doi:10.1208/s12248–015-9724-x.
6. Brown JS. Chapter 27: Deposition of particles A2. In Parent RA, ed., *Comparative Biology of the Normal Lung*, 2nd ed. San Diego, CA: Academic Press, 2015, pp. 513–536.
7. Garcia GJM, Schroeter JD, Kimbell JS. Olfactory deposition of inhaled nanoparticles in humans. *Inhalation Toxicology*. 2015;27(8):394–403. doi:10.3109/08958378.2015.1066904.
8. Schroeter JD, Kimbell JS, Asgharian B. Analysis of particle deposition in the turbinate and olfactory regions using a human nasal computational fluid dynamics model. *Journal of Aerosol Medicine*. 2006;19(3):301–313. doi:10.1089/jam.2006.19.301.
9. Calmet H, Kleinstreuer C, Houzeaux G, Kolanjiyil AV, Lehmkuhl O, Olivares E, Vázquez M. Subject-variability effects on micron particle deposition in human nasal cavities. *Journal of Aerosol Science*. 2018;115:12–28. doi:10.1016/j.jaerosci.2017.10.008.
10. Kesavanathan J, Bascom R, Swift DL. The effect of nasal passage characteristics on particle deposition. *Journal of Aerosol Medicine*. 1998;11(1):27–39.
11. Kesavanathan J, Swift DL. Human nasal passage particle deposition: The effect of particle size, flow rate, and anatomical factors. *Aerosol Science and Technology*. 1998;28(5):457–463. doi:10.1080/02786829808965537.
12. Garcia GJ, Tewksbury EW, Wong BA, Kimbell JS. Interindividual variability in nasal filtration as a function of nasal cavity geometry. *Journal of Aerosol Medicine and Pulmonary Drug Delivery*. 2009;22(2):139–156.
13. Zhou Y, Guo M, Xi J, Irshad H, Cheng Y-S. Nasal deposition in infants and children. *Journal of Aerosol Medicine and Pulmonary Drug Delivery*. 2014;27(2):110–116.
14. Swift D. Inspiratory inertial deposition of aerosols in human nasal airway replicate casts: Implication for the proposed NCRP lung model. *Radiation Protection Dosimetry*. 1991;38(1–3):29–34.
15. Hsu D-J, Chuang M-H. In-vivo measurements of micrometer-sized particle deposition in the nasal cavities of Taiwanese adults. *Aerosol Science and Technology*. 2012;46(6):631–638. doi:10.1080/02786826.2011.652749.
16. Cheng K-H, Cheng Y-S, Yeh H-C, Guilmette RA, Simpson SQ, Yang Y-H, Swift DL. In vivo measurements of nasal airway dimensions and ultrafine aerosol deposition in the human nasal and oral airways. *Journal of Aerosol Science*. 1996;27(5):785–801.
17. Cheng Y, Yeh H, Guilmette R, Simpson S, Cheng K, Swift D. Nasal deposition of ultrafine particles in human volunteers and its relationship to airway geometry. *Aerosol Science and Technology*. 1996;25(3):274–291.
18. Samoliński BK, Grzanka A, Gotlib T. Changes in nasal cavity dimensions in children and adults by gender and age. *The Laryngoscope*. 2007;117(8):1429–1433. doi:10.1097/MLG.0b013e318064e837.
19. Bennett WD, Zeman KL, Jarabek AM. Nasal contribution to breathing and fine particle deposition in children versus adults. *Journal of Toxicology and Environmental Health Part A*. 2008;71(3):227–237. doi:10.1080/15287390701598200.

20. Bennett WD, Zeman KL, Jarabek AM. Nasal contribution to breathing with exercise: Effect of race and gender. *Journal of Applied Physiology (Bethesda, Md: 1985)*. 2003;95(2):497–503. doi:10.1152/japplphysiol.00718.2002.

21. Doughty DV, Vibbert C, Kewalramani A, Bollinger ME, Dalby RN. Automated actuation of nasal spray products: Determination and comparison of adult and pediatric settings. *Drug Development and Industrial Pharmacy*. 2011;37(3):359–366. doi:10.3109/03639045.2010.520321.

22. Doughty DV, Hsu W, Dalby RN. Automated actuation of nasal spray products: Effect of hand-related variability on the in vitro performance of Flonase nasal spray. *Drug Development and Industrial Pharmacy*. 2014;40(6):711–718. doi:10.3109/03639045.2013.777735.

23. Keeler JA, Patki A, Woodard CR, Frank-Ito DO. A computational study of nasal spray deposition pattern in four ethnic groups. *Journal of Aerosol Medicine and Pulmonary Drug Delivery*. 2015;29(2):153–166. doi:10.1089/jamp.2014.1205.

24. Bennett WD, Zeman KL. Effect of race on fine particle deposition for oral and nasal breathing. *Inhalation Toxicology*. 2005;17(12):641–648. doi:10.1080/08958370500188984.

25. Ireson NJ, Tait JS, MacGregor GA, Baker EH. Comparison of nasal pH values in black and white individuals with normal and high blood pressure. *Clinical Science (London, England: 1979)*. 2001;100(3):327–333.

26. Djupesland PG, Skretting A. Nasal deposition and clearance in man: Comparison of a bidirectional powder device and a traditional liquid spray pump. *Journal of Aerosol Medicine and Pulmonary Drug Delivery*. 2012;25(5):280–289. doi:10.1089/jamp.2011.0924.

27. Charlton S, Jones NS, Davis SS, Illum L. Distribution and clearance of bioadhesive formulations from the olfactory region in man: Effect of polymer type and nasal delivery device. *European Journal of Pharmaceutical Sciences*. 2007;30:295–302. doi:10.1016/j.ejps.2006.11.018.

28. Gizurarson S. The effect of cilia and the mucociliary clearance on successful drug delivery. *Biological & Pharmaceutical Bulletin*. 2015;38:497–506.

29. Ding X, Xie F. Olfactory mucosa: Composition, enzymatic localization, and metabolism. In: Doty RL, editor. *Handbook of Olfaction and Gustation*. Hoboken, NJ: John Wiley & Sons, Inc., 2015, pp. 63–92.

30. Paul P, Johnson P, Ramaswamy P, Ramadoss S, Geetha B, Subhashini AS. The effect of ageing on nasal mucociliary clearance in women: A pilot study. *ISRN Pulmonology*. 2013;2013:5. doi:10.1155/2013/598589.

31. Donovan MD, Zhou M. Drug effects on in vivo nasal clearance in rats. *International Journal of Pharmaceutics*. 1995;116(1):77–86. doi:10.1016/0378–5173(94)00274–9.

32. Marttin E, Schipper NGM, Verhoef JC, Merkus FWHM. Nasal mucociliary clearance as a factor in nasal drug delivery. *Advanced Drug Delivery Reviews*. 1998;29(1–2):13–38. doi:10.1016/S0169–409X(97)00059–8.

33. Workman AD, Cohen NA. The effect of drugs and other compounds on the ciliary beat frequency of human respiratory epithelium. *American Journal of Rhinology & Allergy*. 2014;28(6):454–464. doi:10.2500/ajra.2014.28.4092.

34. Homer JJ, Dowley AC, Condon L, El-Jassar P, Sood S. The effect of hypertonicity on nasal mucociliary clearance. *Clinical Otolaryngology & Allied Sciences*. 2000;25(6):558–560. doi:10.1046/j.1365–2273.2000.00420.x.

35. Fry FA, Black A. Regional deposition and clearance of particles in the human nose. *Journal of Aerosol Science*. 1973;4(2):113–124. doi:10.1016/0021–8502(73)90063–3.

36. Schipper NGM, Verhoef JC, Merkus FWHM. The nasal mucociliary clearance: Relevance to nasal drug delivery. *Pharmaceutical research*. 1991;8(7):807–814. doi:10.1023/a:1015830907632.

37. Frank DO, Kimbell JS, Cannon D, Pawar SS, Rhee JS. Deviated nasal septum hinders intranasal sprays: A computer simulation study. *Rhinology*. 2012;50(3):311–318. doi:10.4193/Rhin.

38. Merkus P, Ebbens FA, Muller B, Fokkens WJ. Influence of anatomy and head position on intranasal drug deposition. *European Archives of Oto-Rhino-Laryngology and Head & Neck*. 2006;263(9):827–832.

39. Bond SW, Hardy JG, Wilson CG. Deposition and clearance of nasal sprays. *Presented at the 2nd International Congress of Biopharmaceutics and Pharmacokinetics*, Salamanca, Spain, 1984.

40. Illum L. Nasal clearance in health and disease. *Journal of Aerosol Medicine*. 2006;19(1):92–99. doi:10.1089/jam.2006.19.92.

41. Rusznak C, Devalia JL, Lozewicz S, Davies RJ. The assessment of nasal mucociliary clearance and the effect of drugs. *Respiratory Medicine*. 1994;88(2):89–101. doi:10.1016/0954–6111(94)90020–5.

42. Sisson JH, Yonkers AJ, Waldman RH. Effects of guaifenesin on nasal mucociliary clearance and ciliary beat frequency in healthy volunteers. *Chest*. 1995;107(3):747–751.

43. de Oliveira-Maul JP, de Carvalho HB, Goto DM, Maia RM, Fló C, Barnabé V, Franco DR, Benabou S, Perracini MR, Jacob-Filho W. Aging, diabetes,

and hypertension are associated with decreased nasal mucociliary clearance. *CHEST Journal.* 2013;143(4):1091–1097.

44. Sarkar MA. Drug metabolism in the nasal mucosa. *Pharmaceutical Research.* 1992;9(1):1–9. doi:10.1023/a:1018911206646.

45. Dhamankar V, Assem M, Donovan MD. Gene expression and immunochemical localization of major cytochrome P450 drug-metabolizing enzymes in bovine nasal olfactory and respiratory mucosa. *Inhalation Toxicology.* 2015;27(14):767–777.

46. Dhamankar V, Donovan MD. Modulating nasal mucosal permeation using metabolic saturation and enzyme inhibition techniques. *Journal of Pharmacy and Pharmacology.* 2017;69(9):1075–1083. doi:10.1111/jphp.12749.

47. Na DH, Youn YS, Park EJ, Lee JM, Cho OR, Lee KR, Lee SD, Yoo SD, DeLuca PP, Lee KC. Stability of PEGylated salmon calcitonin in nasal mucosa. *Journal of Pharmaceutical Sciences.* 2004;93(2):256–261. doi:10.1002/jps.10537.

48. Gizurarson S, Bechgaard E. Study of nasal enzyme activity towards insulin. In vitro. *Chemical & Pharmaceutical Bulletin.* 1991;39(8):2155–2157. doi:10.1248/cpb.39.2155.

49. Débat H, Eloit C, Blon F, Sarazin B, Henry C, Huet J-C, Trotier D, Pernollet J-C. Identification of human olfactory cleft mucus proteins using proteomic analysis. *Journal of Proteome Research.* 2007;6(5):1985–1996. doi:10.1021/pr0606575.

50. Schmidt MC, Peter H, Lang SR, Ditzinger G, Merkle HP. In vitro cell models to study nasal mucosal permeability and metabolism. *Advanced Drug Delivery Reviews.* 1998;29:51–79. doi:10.1016/S0169–409X(97)00061–6.

51. FDA U. *Draft Guidance for Industry: Bioavailability and Bioequivalence Studies for Nasal Aerosols and Nasal Sprays for Local Action.* Food and Drug Administration, Center for Drug Evaluation and Research (CDER), 2003.

52. Hallworth GW, Padfield JM. A comparison of the regional deposition in a model nose of a drug discharged from metered serosel and metered-pump nasal delivery systems. *Journal of Allergy and Clinical Immunology.* 1986;77(2):348–353. doi:10.1016/S0091–6749(86)80116–6.

53. Guilmette RA, Wicks JD, Wolff RK. Morphometry of human nasal airways in vivo using magnetic resonance imaging. *Journal of Aerosol Medicine.* 1989;2(4):365–377. doi:10.1089/jam.1989.2.365.

54. Cheng Y, Holmes T, Gao J, Guilmette R, Li S, Surakitbanharn Y, Rowlings C. Characterization of nasal spray pumps and deposition pattern in a replica of the human nasal airway. *Journal of Aerosol Medicine.* 2001;14(2):267–280.

55. Foo MY, Cheng YS, Su WC, Donovan MD. The influence of spray properties on intranasal deposition. *Journal of Aerosol Medicine: The Official Journal of the International Society for Aerosols in Medicine.* 2007;20(4):495–508. doi:10.1089/jam.2007.0638.

56. Kelly JT, Asgharian B, Kimbell JS, Wong BA. Particle deposition in human nasal airway replicas manufactured by different methods. Part I: Inertial regime particles. *Aerosol Science and Technology.* 2004;38:1063–1071. doi:10.1080/027868290883360.

57. Xi J, Yuan JE, Zhang Y, Nevorski D, Wang Z, Zhou Y. Visualization and quantification of nasal and olfactory deposition in a sectional adult nasal airway cast. *Pharmaceutical Research.* 2016;33(6):1527–1541. doi:10.1007/s11095–016-1896–2.

58. Pu Y, Goodey AP, Fang X, Jacob K. A comparison of the deposition patterns of different nasal spray formulations using a nasal cast. *Aerosol Science and Technology.* 2014;48(9):930–938. doi:10.1080/02786826.2014.931566.

59. Liu Y, Johnson MR, Matida EA, Kherani S, Marsan J. Creation of a standardized geometry of the human nasal cavity. *Journal of Applied Physiology.* 2009;106(3):784–795.

60. Liu Y, Matida EA, Johnson MR. Experimental measurements and computational modeling of aerosol deposition in the Carleton-Civic standardized human nasal cavity. *Journal of Aerosol Science.* 2010;41:569–586. doi:10.1016/j.jaerosci.2010.02.014.

61. Schroeter JD, Garcia GJ, Kimbell JS. Effects of surface smoothness on inertial particle deposition in human nasal models. *Journal of Aerosol Science.* 2011;42(1):52–63.

62. Kimbell JS, Segal RA, Asgharian B, Wong BA, Schroeter JD, Southall JP, Dickens CJ, Brace G, Miller FJ. Characterization of deposition from nasal spray devices using a computational fluid dynamics model of the human nasal passages. *Journal of Aerosol Medicine.* 2007;20(1):59–74. doi:10.1089/jam.2006.0531.

63. Patel RG, Garcia GJ, Frank-Ito DO, Kimbell JS, Rhee JS. Simulating the nasal cycle with computational fluid dynamics. *Otolaryngology–Head and Neck Surgery: Official Journal of American Academy of Otolaryngology-Head and Neck Surgery.* 2015;152(2):353–360. doi:10.1177/0194599814559385.

64. Rhee JS, Pawar SS, Garcia GJM, Kimbell JS. Towards personalized nasal surgery using computational fluid dynamics. *Archives of Facial Plastic Surgery.* 2011;13(5):305–310. doi:10.1001/archfacial.2011.18.

65. Zhang L, Du S-Y, Lu Y, Liu C, Tian Z-H, Yang C, Wu H-C, Wang Z. Puerarin transport across a Calu-3 cell monolayer – an in vitro model of nasal mucosa permeability and the influence of paeoniflorin and menthol. *Drug Design, Development and Therapy.* 2016;10:2227–2237. doi:10.2147/DDDT.S110247.

66. Kandimalla KK, Donovan MD. Transport of hydroxyzine and triprolidine across bovine olfactory mucosa: Role of passive diffusion in the direct nose-to-brain uptake of small molecules. *International Journal of Pharmaceutics.* 2005;302:133–144. doi:10.1016/j.ijpharm.2005.06.012.

67. Abdelbary GA, Tadros MI. Brain targeting of olanzapine via intranasal delivery of core–shell difunctional block copolymer mixed nanomicellar carriers: In vitro characterization, ex vivo estimation of nasal toxicity and in vivo biodistribution studies. *International Journal of Pharmaceutics.* 2013;452:300–310. doi:10.1016/j.ijpharm.2013.04.084.

68. Abdelrahman FE, Elsayed I, Gad MK, Elshafeey AH, Mohamed MI. Response surface optimization, Ex vivo and In vivo investigation of nasal spanlastics for bioavailability enhancement and brain targeting of risperidone. *International Journal of Pharmaceutics.* 2017;530(1–2):1–11. doi:10.1016/j.ijpharm.2017.07.050.

69. Mistry A, Stolnik S, Illum L. Nose-to-brain delivery: Investigation of the transport of nanoparticles with different surface characteristics and sizes in excised porcine olfactory epithelium. *Molecular Pharmaceutics.* 2015;12(8):2755–2766. doi:10.1021/acs.molpharmaceut.5b00088.

70. Shah BM, Misra M, Shishoo CJ, Padh H. Nose to brain microemulsion-based drug delivery system of rivastigmine: Formulation and ex-vivo characterization. *Drug Delivery.* 2014:1–13. doi:10.3109/10717544.2013.878857.

71. Tas C, Ozkan CK, Savaser A, Ozkan Y, Tasdemir U, Altunay H. Nasal absorption of metoclopramide from different Carbopol® 981 based formulations: In vitro, ex vivo and in vivo evaluation. *European Journal of Pharmaceutics and Biopharmaceutics.* 2006;64(2):246–254.

72. Al Bakri W. The role of the efflux transporters in the direct nose-to-brain transport of atrazine and 2,4-D following nasal inhalation. *Presented at AAPS Annual Meeting,* San Diego, CA, 2017.

73. Kandimalla KK, Donovan MD. Carrier mediated transport of chlorpheniramine and chlorcyclizine across bovine olfactory mucosa: Implications on nose-to-brain transport. *Journal of Pharmaceutical Sciences.* 2005;94(3):613–624. doi:10.1002/jps.20284.

74. Nour SA, Abdelmalak NS, Naguib MJ, Rashed HM, Ibrahim AB. Intranasal brain-targeted clonazepam polymeric micelles for immediate control of status epilepticus: In vitro optimization, ex vivo determination of cytotoxicity, in vivo biodistribution and pharmacodynamics studies. *Drug Delivery.* 2016:1–15. doi:10.1080/10717544.2016.1223216.

75. Dhamankar V. Cytochrome P450-mediated drug metabolizing activity in the nasal mucosa [Dissertation]. University of Iowa, 2013.

76. Harikarnpakdee S, Lipipun V, Sutanthavibul N, Ritthidej GC. Spray-dried mucoadhesive microspheres: Preparation and transport through nasal cell monolayer. *AAPS PharmSciTech.* 2006;7(1):E79–E88. doi:10.1208/pt070112.

77. Patel A, Cholkar K, Mitra AK. Recent developments in protein and peptide parenteral delivery approaches. *Therapeutic Delivery.* 2014;5(3):337–365.

78. Bruno BJ, Miller GD, Lim CS. Basics and recent advances in peptide and protein drug delivery. *Therapeutic Delivery.* 2013;4(11):1443–1467.

79. Ghori MU, Mahdi MH, Smith AM, Conway BR. Nasal drug delivery systems: An overview. *American Journal of Pharmacological Sciences.* 2015;3(5):110–119.

80. Meredith ME, Salameh TS, Banks WA. Intranasal delivery of proteins and peptides in the treatment of neurodegenerative diseases. *The AAPS Journal.* 2015;17(4):780–787.

81. Lalatsa A, Schatzlein AG, Uchegbu IF. Strategies to deliver peptide drugs to the brain. *Molecular Pharmaceutics.* 2014;11(4):1081–1093.

82. Davis SS, Illum L. Absorption enhancers for nasal drug delivery. *Clinical Pharmacokinetics.* 2003;42(13):1107–1128.

83. Lu C-T, Zhao Y-Z, Wong HL, Cai J, Peng L, Tian X-Q. Current approaches to enhance CNS delivery of drugs across the brain barriers. *International Journal of Nanomedicine.* 2014;9:2241.

84. Guo Z, Chen Y, Mao Y-F, Zheng T, Jiang Y, Yan Y, Yin X, Zhang B. Long-term treatment with intranasal insulin ameliorates cognitive impairment, tau hyperphosphorylation, and microglial activation in a streptozotocin-induced Alzheimer's rat model. *Scientific Reports.* 2017;7:45971.

85. Benedict C, Hallschmid M, Hatke A, Schultes B, Fehm HL, Born J, Kern W. Intranasal insulin improves memory in humans. *Psychoneuroendocrinology.* 2004;29(10):1326–1334.

86. Reger M, Watson G, Frey Wn, Baker L, Cholerton B, Keeling M, Belongia D, Fishel M, Plymate S, Schellenberg G. Effects of intranasal insulin on cognition in memory-impaired older adults: modulation by APOE genotype. *Neurobiology of Aging.* 2006;27(3):451–458.

87. Renner DB, Svitak AL, Gallus NJ, Ericson ME, Frey WH, Hanson LR. Intranasal delivery of insulin via the olfactory nerve pathway. *Journal of Pharmacy and Pharmacology.* 2012;64(12):1709–1714.

88. Neumann ID, Maloumby R, Beiderbeck DI, Lukas M, Landgraf R. Increased brain and plasma oxytocin after nasal and peripheral administration in rats and mice. *Psychoneuroendocrinology.* 2013;38(10):1985–1993.

89. Tian L, Guo R, Yue X, Lv Q, Ye X, Wang Z, Chen Z, Wu B, Xu G, Liu X. Intranasal administration of nerve growth factor ameliorate β-amyloid deposition after traumatic brain injury in rats. *Brain Research.* 2012;1440:47–55.

90. Fliedner S, Schulz C, Lehnert H. Brain uptake of intranasally applied radioiodinated leptin in Wistar rats. *Endocrinology.* 2006;147(5):2088–2094.

91. Derad I, Willeke K, Pietrowsky R, Born J, Fehm HL. Intranasal angiotensin II directly influences central nervous regulation of blood pressure. *American Journal of Hypertension.* 1998;11(8):971–977.

92. Ross T, Martinez P, Renner J, Thorne R, Hanson L, Frey WN. Intranasal administration of interferon beta bypasses the blood–brain barrier to target the central nervous system and cervical lymph nodes: A non-invasive treatment strategy for multiple sclerosis. *Journal of Neuroimmunology.* 2004;151(1):66–77.

93. Fuseau E, Petricoul O, Moore KH, Barrow A, Ibbotson T. Clinical pharmacokinetics of intranasal sumatriptan. *Clinical Pharmacokinetics.* 2002;41(11):801–811.

94. Dahlöf C. How does sumatriptan perform in clinical practice? *Cephalalgia.* 1995;15(S15):21–28.

95. Dahlöf C, Boes-Hansen S, Cederberg C, Hardebo J, Henriksson A. How does sumatriptan nasal spray perform in clinical practice? *Cephalalgia.* 1998;18(5):278–282.

96. Dowson AJ, Charlesworth BR, Purdy A, Becker WJ, Boes-Hansen S, Färkkilä M. Tolerability and consistency of effect of zolmitriptan nasal spray in a long-term migraine treatment trial. *CNS Drugs.* 2003;17(11):839–851.

97. Rapoport AM, Bigal ME, Tepper SJ, Sheftell FD. Intranasal medications for the treatment of migraine and cluster headache. *CNS Drugs.* 2004;18(10):671–685.

98. Wadgave U, Nagesh L. Nicotine replacement therapy: An overview. *International Journal of Health Sciences.* 2016;10(3):425.

99. Mansour HM, Xu Z, Meenach S, Park C-W, Rhee Y-S, DeLuca PP. Book chapter 5: Novel drug delivery systems. In Mitra AK, ed., *Drug Delivery.* Burlington, MA: Jones & Bartlett, 2015.

100. Casettari L, Illum L. Chitosan in nasal delivery systems for therapeutic drugs. *Journal of Controlled Release.* 2014;190:189–200.

101. Illum L. Nasal drug delivery—recent developments and future prospects. *Journal of Controlled Release.* 2012;161(2):254–263.

102. Amidi M, Mastrobattista E, Jiskoot W, Hennink WE. Chitosan-based delivery systems for protein therapeutics and antigens. *Advanced Drug Delivery Reviews.* 2010;62(1):59–82.

103. Arnold JJ, Ahsan F, Meezan E, Pillion DJ. Correlation of tetradecylmaltoside induced increases in nasal peptide drug delivery with morphological changes in nasal epithelial cells. *Journal of Pharmaceutical Sciences.* 2004;93(9):2205–2213.

104. Sintov AC, Levy HV, Botner S. Systemic delivery of insulin via the nasal route using a new microemulsion system: In vitro and in vivo studies. *Journal of Controlled Release.* 2010;148(2):168–176.

105. Law S, Shih C. Characterization of calcitonin-containing liposome formulations for intranasal delivery. *Journal of Microencapsulation.* 2001;18(2):211–221.

106. Law S, Huang K, Chou V, Cherng J. Enhancement of nasal absorption of calcitonin loaded in liposomes. *Journal of Liposome Research.* 2001;11(2–3):165–174.

107. Law S, Huang K, Chou H. Preparation of desmopressin-containing liposomes for intranasal delivery. *Journal of Controlled Release.* 2001;70(3):375–382.

108. Mitra R, Pezron I, Chu WA, Mitra AK. Lipid emulsions as vehicles for enhanced nasal delivery of insulin. *International Journal of Pharmaceutics.* 2000;205(1):127–134.

109. Morimoto K, Katsumata H, Yabuta T, Iwanaga K, Kakemi M, Tabata Y, Ikada Y. Evaluation of gelatin microspheres for nasal and intramuscular administrations of salmon calcitonin. *European Journal of Pharmaceutical Sciences.* 2001;13(2):179–185.

110. Fernández-Urrusuno R, Calvo P, Remuñán-López C, Vila-Jato JL, Alonso MJ. Enhancement of nasal absorption of insulin using chitosan nanoparticles. *Pharmaceutical Research.* 1999;16(10):1576–1581.

111. Li J, Feng L, Fan L, Zha Y, Guo L, Zhang Q, Chen J, Pang Z, Wang Y, Jiang X. Targeting the brain with PEG–PLGA nanoparticles modified with phage-displayed peptides. *Biomaterials.* 2011;32(21):4943–4950.

112. Marazuela E, Prado N, Moro E, Fernández-García H, Villalba M, Rodriguez R, Batanero E. Intranasal vaccination with poly (lactide-co-glycolide) microparticles containing a peptide T of Ole e 1 prevents mice against sensitization. *Clinical & Experimental Allergy.* 2008;38(3):520–528.

113. Simon M, Wittmar M, Kissel T, Linn T. Insulin containing nanocomplexes formed by self-assembly from biodegradable amine-modified poly (vinyl alcohol)-graft-poly (L-lactide): Bioavailability and nasal tolerability in rats. *Pharmaceutical Research.* 2005;22(11):1879–1886.

114. Furubayashi T, Inoue D, Kamaguchi A, Higashi Y, Sakane T. Influence of formulation viscosity on drug absorption following nasal application in rats. *Drug Metabolism and Pharmacokinetics.* 2007;22(3):206–211.

115. Chaturvedi M, Kumar M, Pathak K. A review on mucoadhesive polymer used in nasal drug delivery system. *Journal of Advanced Pharmaceutical Technology & Research*. 2011;2:215–222. doi:10.4103/2231-4040.90876.

116. Shelke S, Shahi S, Jalalpure S, Dhamecha D. Poloxamer 407-based intranasal thermoreversible gel of zolmitriptan-loaded nanoethosomes: Formulation, optimization, evaluation and permeation studies. *Journal of Liposome Research*. 2016;26(4):313–323. doi:10.3109/08982104.2015.1132232.

117. Xu X, Shen Y, Wang W, Sun C, Li C, Xiong Y, Tu J. Preparation and in vitro characterization of thermosensitive and mucoadhesive hydrogels for nasal delivery of phenylephrine hydrochloride. *European Journal of Pharmaceutics and Biopharmaceutics*. 2014;88(3):998–1004. doi:10.1016/j.ejpb.2014.08.015.

118. Cai Z, Song X, Sun F, Yang Z, Hou S, Liu Z. Formulation and evaluation of in situ gelling systems for intranasal administration of gastrodin. *AAPS PharmSciTech*. 2011;12:1102–1109. doi:10.1208/s12249-011-9678-y.

119. Wang S, Chen P, Zhang L, Yang C, Zhai G. Formulation and evaluation of microemulsion-based in situ ion-sensitive gelling systems for intranasal administration of curcumin. *Journal of Drug Targeting*. 2012;20:831–840. doi:10.3109/10611 86X.2012.719230.

120. Li X, Du L, Chen X, Ge P, Wang Y, Fu Y, Sun H, Jiang Q, Jin Y. Nasal delivery of analgesic ketorolac tromethamine thermo-and ion-sensitive in situ hydrogels. *International Journal of Pharmaceutics*. 2015;489(1–2):252–260.

121. Warnken ZN, Smyth HDC, Watts AB, Weitman S, Kuhn JG, Williams III RO. Formulation and device design to increase nose to brain drug delivery. *Journal of Drug Delivery Science and Technology*. 2016;35:213–222. doi:10.1016/j.jddst.2016.05.003.

122. Dhuria SV, Hanson LR, Frey WH. Novel vasoconstrictor formulation to enhance intranasal targeting of neuropeptide therapeutics to the central nervous system. *Journal of Pharmacology and Experimental Therapeutics*. 2009;328:312–320. doi:10.1124/jpet.108.145565.

123. Shingaki T, Hidalgo IJ, Furubayashi T, Katsumi H, Sakane T, Yamamoto A, Yamashita S. The transnasal delivery of 5-fluorouracil to the rat brain is enhanced by acetazolamide (the inhibitor of the secretion of cerebrospinal fluid). *International Journal of Pharmaceutics*. 2009;377:85–91. doi:10.1016/j.ijpharm.2009.05.009.

124. Shingaki T, Inoue D, Furubayashi T, Sakane T, Katsumi H, Yamamoto A, Yamashita S. Transnasal delivery of methotrexate to brain tumors in rats: A new strategy for brain tumor chemotherapy. *Molecular Pharmaceutics*. 2010;7:1561–1568. doi:10.1021/mp900275s.

125. Lochhead JJ, Wolak DJ, Pizzo ME, Thorne RG. Rapid transport within cerebral perivascular spaces underlies widespread tracer distribution in the brain after intranasal administration. *Journal of Cerebral Blood Flow and Metabolism*. 2015;35:371–381. doi:10.1038/jcbfm.2014.215.

126. Appu AP, Arun P, Krishnan JKS, Moffett JR, Namboodiri AMA. Rapid intranasal delivery of chloramphenicol acetyltransferase in the active form to different brain regions as a model for enzyme therapy in the CNS. *Journal of Neuroscience Methods*. 2016;259:129–134. doi:10.1016/j.jneumeth.2015.11.027.

127. Warnken Z, Smyth HD, Williams III RO. Route-specific challenges in the delivery of poorly water-soluble drugs. In Williams III RO, Watts AB, Miller D, eds., *Formulating Poorly Water Soluble Drugs*. New York: Springer, 2016, pp. 1–39.

128. Dayal P, Shaik MS, Singh M. Evaluation of different parameters that affect droplet-size distribution from nasal sprays using the Malvern Spraytec®. *Journal of Pharmaceutical Sciences*. 2004;93(7):1725–1742. doi:10.1002/jps.20090.

129. Djupesland PG, Skretting A, Winderen M, Holand T. Breath actuated device improves delivery to target sites beyond the nasal valve. *The Laryngoscope*. 2006;116(3):466–472.

130. Suman JD, Laube BL, Dalby R. Comparison of nasal deposition and clearance of aerosol generated by a nebulizer and an aqueous spray pump. *Pharmaceutical Research*. 1999;16(10):1648–1652.

131. Hardy JG, Lee SW, Wilson CG. Intranasal drug delivery by spray and drops. *The Journal of Pharmacy and Pharmacology*. 1985;37(5):294–297.

132. Djupesland PG. Nasal drug delivery devices: Characteristics and performance in a clinical perspective: A review. *Drug Delivery and Translational Research*. 2013;3(1):42–62.

133. Kublik H, Vidgren M. Nasal delivery systems and their effect on deposition and absorption. *Advanced Drug Delivery Reviews*. 1998;29(1):157–177.

134. Djupesland PG. Nasal drug delivery devices: Characteristics and performance in a clinical perspective: A review. *Drug Delivery and Translational Research*. 2013;3:42–62. doi:10.1007/s13346-012-0108-9.

135. Hoekman JD, Ho RJY. Effects of localized hydrophilic mannitol and hydrophobic nelfinavir administration targeted to olfactory epithelium on brain distribution. *AAPS PharmSciTech*. 2011;12(2):534–543. doi:10.1208/s12249-011-9614-1.

136. Hoekman JD, Ho RJY. Enhanced analgesic responses after preferential delivery of morphine and fentanyl to the olfactory epithelium in rats. *Anesthesia & Analgesia*. 2011:1. doi:10.1213/ANE.0b013e3182239b8c.

137. SPECT Imaging of Direct Nose-to-Brain Transfer of MAG-3 in Man [Poster]. AAPS2013.

138. Drugs@FDA [Internet]. U.S. Food and Drug Administration; 2018 [cited January 22, 2018].

139. National Center for Biotechnology Information. PubChem Compound Database [Internet]. National Institutes of Health (NIH); 2018 [cited June 2, 2018].

140. ChemicalBook—Chemical Search Engine 2018. Available from http://www.chemicalbook.com/ProductIndex_EN.aspx.

23

Inhaled therapeutics against TB: The promise of pulmonary treatment and prevention strategies in the clinic

DOMINIQUE N. PRICE, NITESH K. KUNDA, ELLIOTT K. MILLER, AND PAVAN MUTTIL

A recent resurgence of an old epidemic	361	Vaccines	365
Clinical pathology of infection	362	TuBerculosis Vaccine Initiative (TBVI),	
Stalled progress—Current antibiotic regimens and		GlaxoSmithKline (GSK)	365
vaccination strategies	362	Antibiotics	367
Current antibiotic regimens	362	Immunotherapy	367
The rise of antibiotic-resistant MTB	362	Future of pulmonary therapeutics in TB	368
Vaccine: Bacille Calmette-Guérin	363	Challenges of inhaled therapy to the clinic	368
Advantages of the pulmonary route of delivery		Devices for pulmonary drug delivery	368
compared to parenteral route	364	Regulatory approval	369
Rationale for pulmonary delivery	364	Aerosol drugs	369
Devices available	365	Aerosol vaccines	369
Targeting alveolar macrophages	365	Speculation on aerosol treatments	370
Pulmonary drugs and vaccines in clinical development	365	References	370

A RECENT RESURGENCE OF AN OLD EPIDEMIC

Tuberculosis (TB) has been known by many names. Ancient Hindu texts termed the disease *Rogaraj*, meaning "king of all diseases," and *Rajayakshma*, meaning "disease of kings" (1). The Greek physician Hippocrates (460–370 BC) called tuberculosis *Phthisis*, derived from phthinein, meaning "to waste away" into death, and described it as the most prominent disease of his time (2). Shortly thereafter, the disease was known as *consumption* because of its ability to "consume" its victims. During the nineteenth century, names became even more poetically grim as the illness continued to spread worldwide: the white plague or the white death, captain of all these men of death, graveyard cough, and the king's evil (3).

Mention in historical texts, representation in art and artifacts, and pathology on ancient human remains have prompted many scientists to propose that TB is the oldest and the most formidable pathogen humanity has ever faced. Tubercular DNA has been recovered from the mummies of ancient Egypt, and signs of tubercular decay have been observed on 500,000-year-old *Homo erectus* skeletal remains found in Turkey (4,5). While the precise time of TB's origin remains unknown, history tells us that TB has always plagued humanity, and it has done so without prejudice both geographically and economically.

It wasn't until 1882, when German microbiologist Robert Koch discovered the tubercle bacillus, that an infectious bacterium was declared the causative agent of these diseases of old (6). After Koch's discovery, a vaccine and different antibiotic treatments against the bacteria followed. TB, like smallpox, was presumed to be on the path of eradication (7). However, the onset of the human immunodeficiency virus (HIV) epidemic in the 1980s, along with the rise of drug resistance to first-line TB drugs, shattered any hopes of worldwide TB elimination. In 1993, the World Health Organization (WHO) declared TB a global emergency, calling the disease humanity's greatest killer (8).

Over two decades later, TB is still a global epidemic. WHO estimates that over a third of the world has the disease (9). Yearly disease incidence is up to 10.4 million people with active TB, leading to a mortality rate of 1.7 million people every year (9). These dismal statistics rank TB as the second leading cause of death due to a single infectious agent, just behind HIV (10).

To address this epidemic, research efforts in the TB field have shifted from commonly used therapeutic interventions (such as antibiotics, chemotherapy, and radiation) to immunotherapies, drug repurposing, and vaccines (11–13). Specifically, in this work, we will discuss various pulmonary treatments and preventions being used and developed by the medical community.

CLINICAL PATHOLOGY OF INFECTION

The majority of TB infections result from the inhalation of droplet nuclei carrying small amounts of infective mycobacteria (14–18). However, humans can also be infected through the gastrointestinal tract from ingestion or cutaneously through a cut or wound (16). While many species are susceptible to infection by *Mycobacterium tuberculosis* (MTB), the primary reservoir for MTB is humans (16). A single cough or sneeze can generate up to 3000 aerosolized infectious droplets, and it takes less than 10 bacteria to cause infection (14,16,18). After aerosolization, droplets less than 5–10 μm can stay suspended in the air for several hours (16,17). Thus, the risk of infection is associated with closeness of contact and ventilation (16).

Once the bacterium has been inhaled and deposited in the lung, it is phagocytosed by alveolar macrophages (15–21). However, MTB escapes destruction by preventing fusion of the phagosome with the lysosome, and multiplies within the nonactivated macrophages (15–18,22–26). Infection migrates out of the lungs, first to the mediastinal lymph nodes, then throughout the body, including the liver, spleen, kidney, bone, and brain (16–18,20,27). After 2–4 weeks of infection MTB-specific cell-mediated immunity initiates (15–18,20,21). Cytotoxic T cells kill infected macrophages and release mycobacterial proteins, which trigger a delayed-type hypersensitivity (DTH) response via phagocytes, fluid, and digestive enzymes (16–18,20,28). The DTH response is destructive to the lung and other tissues due to chronic inflammation, and it is the primary source of injury in TB (16). The magnitude of the DTH is closely associated with the magnitude of infection and is also the basis for the tuberculin skin test (16).

Clusters of macrophages, lymphocytes, fibroblasts, and giant cells encase MTB, forming granulomas in the lung and other tissues (15–18,22–26). In most cases, the bacteria cease to multiply in the anaerobic environment of the granuloma, bacterial numbers slowly decrease, and the lesions heal via fibrosis (16–18,20,22,24). However, it is suspected that a small amount of MTB becomes dormant, called latent TB, and survives in the healed lesions (16–18,21,29). Reactivation of latent TB can occur years later especially in immunocompromised individuals.

The immunological responses from patient to patient seem to be highly variable, and the balance between an appropriate inflammatory response to infection and an overabundance of tissue-damaging inflammatory mediators seems to be critical (15–17). Th1 responses are required to clear the infection, and yet it is the DTH response that is responsible for morbidity to the patient (16,18,20,21,27,30,31). Some researchers have suggested that establishing lung immunity is critical to clearing TB infections (18,32–36). These researchers argue that the best way to limit TB dissemination is to generate strong lung immunity with pulmonary vaccination.

STALLED PROGRESS—CURRENT ANTIBIOTIC REGIMENS AND VACCINATION STRATEGIES

Current antibiotic regimens

For many, TB is a treatable infection. Beginning with the discovery of streptomycin in 1944, a steady stream of antibiotics were approved for TB treatment, ending with the discovery of ofloxacin in 1980. Since then, antibiotic discovery has been largely unproductive, with bedaquiline and delamanid being the only new approved TB antibiotics in the last 40 years.

Currently, 14 drugs are approved by the U.S. Food and Drug Administration (FDA) and/or European Medicines Agency (EMA) for the treatment of TB (Table 23.1). These antibiotics are always used in combination to mitigate drug resistance. Standard treatment usually takes place over a 6-month period and is antithetically referred to as "short-course" anti-TB therapy (37,38). For the first 2 months (initial phase), patients take 3 to 4 of the first-line drugs. During the final 4 months (continuation phase), they receive only rifampicin and isoniazid. Adding together, the daily doses for a typical adult patient equals more than one-third of a kilogram of the multidrug mixture (oral administration) in a series of 182 total daily dosages (38). Comparatively, uncomplicated community-acquired bacterial pneumonia or similar infections take 2–5 grams in a series of 5–7 total dosages (38).

The rise of antibiotic-resistant MTB

As previously stated, the same TB antibiotics have been used for decades, with only two new TB antibiotics approved by the US FDA in the last 40 years (39). In 2015, 480,000 people developed multidrug-resistant TB (MDR-TB), and it is estimated that 9.5% of these cases were actually extensively-drug-resistant TB (XDR-TB) (40). Even more terrifying were recent reports of the emergence of totally-drug-resistant strains of TB (TDR-TB) in India, which are potentially untreatable with existing drugs (41).

MDR-TB is defined as a strain of MTB that is resistant to the two most powerful first-line drugs: isoniazid and rifampin (42). MDR-TB is treatable, but second-line drugs must be incorporated in the treatment regimen. These antibiotics generally have severe side effects, require longer

Table 23.1 Antibiotics used for the treatment of TB

Drug	Year of discovery	Molecular target	Effect	Reported resistance	Ref
First-line drugs					
Isoniazid (INH)	1952	Enoyl-acyl carrier protein reductase	Inhibition of mycolic acid synthesis	Yes	(13,45,46)
Pyrazinamide (PZA)	1954	S1 component of the 30S ribosomal subunit	Inhibition of translation; acidification of the cytoplasm	Yes	(13,47,48)
Ethambutol (EMB)	1961	Arabinosyl transferases	Inhibition of arabinogalactan biosynthesis	Yes	(13,45,49)
Rifampicin (RIF)	1963	Beta subunit of RNA polymerase	Inhibition of transcription	Yes	(13,45,50)
Second-line drugs					
Streptomycin	1944	S12 and 16S rRNA components of the 30S ribosomal subunit	Inhibition of protein synthesis	Yes	(13,45,51)
Para-amino salicylic acid	1948	Dihydropteroate synthase	Inhibition of folate biosynthesis	Yes	(13,52,53)
Cycloserine	1955	d-alanine racemase and ligase	Inhibition of peptidoglycan synthesis	Yes	(13,54–56)
Kanamycin	1957	30S ribosomal subunit	Inhibition of protein synthesis	Yes	(13,57,58)
Ethionamide	1961	Enoyl-acer carrier protein reductase	Inhibition of mycolic acid biosynthesis	Yes	(13,45,59)
Capreomycin	1963	Interbridge B2a between the 30S and 50S ribosomal subunits	Inhibition of protein synthesis	Yes	(13,58,60)
Amikacin	1972	30S ribosomal subunit	Inhibition of protein synthesis	Yes	(13,58,60)
Ofloxacin	1980	DNA gyrase and DNA topoisomerase	Inhibition of DNA supercoiling	Yes	(13,45,61,62)
Bedaquiline	1997	C-subunit of the F0 complex of ATP synthase	Inhibition of ATP synthase	Yes	(63–67)
Delamanid	2006	Methoxy mycolic and ketomycolic acid	Inhibition of mycolic acid synthesis	Yes	(67,68–70)

treatment times, and can cost up to nine times more than first-line antibiotic therapies (average of $150,000 for MDR patient treatment versus $17,000 for drug-susceptible TB patient treatment in the United States) (43,44). If the MTB strain develops further resistance to second-line drugs, specifically any fluoroquinolone and at least one of the three injectable drugs (kanamycin, capreomycin, amikacin), then it is termed XDR-TB (42). Patients with XDR-TB not only have limited treatment options but endure complicated anti-TB regimens that are 28 times more expensive than standard short-course therapy ($480,000 for XDR patient treatment in the United States) (43,44). If the strain of TB develops resistance to all first- and second-line therapies, the patient is diagnosed with TDR-TB; antibiotic options are minimal, and the clinical outlook is grim.

Vaccine: Bacille Calmette-Guérin

In 1921, the first vaccine against TB was administered to infants. The vaccine was developed through the continuous passage of *Mycobacterium bovis*, resulting in diminished bacterial virulence and some retained antigenicity. The vaccine was named after the scientists credited with its development: Albert Calmette and Camille Guérin (71).

Today, 100 million doses of Bacille Calmette-Guérin (BCG) are given each year (72). WHO recommends that BCG be given at or shortly after birth, and 157 countries include the vaccine as part of their childhood vaccination program (72). However, studies assessing the efficacy of the vaccine suggest that the protection afforded against TB is highly variable, ranging from 0% to 80% (73–76).

This variability in protection has been associated with many factors, including the route of BCG immunization, environmental exposures to helminths and nontubercular mycobacteria (NTM), and use of different vaccine strains.

One of the most compelling arguments concerning the failure of BCG is that the vaccine should be given by the pulmonary route instead of the current intradermal delivery route. The BCG vaccine was initially administered orally and was given to children in milk (77). However, after accidental contamination of vaccine stocks with MTB led to the death of 67 infants in Lübeck, Germany, the oral route was deemed unsafe (71,77). Today, the BCG vaccine is given by the intradermal route as a single dose (77). Ongoing study and discussion continue to explore the best administration route for BCG, including intranasal, pulmonary, and oral routes. Aerosolized BCG has been shown to increase protection and enhance lung-specific immunity, and it has the potential to be more effective in humans (36,78–80). Further, some argue that pulmonary immunization resembles a natural MTB infection to the lung, and therefore using the pulmonary route of immunization can be considered a form of biomimicry (18,33,81).

Another widely studied hypothesis of BCG failure is environmental exposure. BCG protection varies with geography, which prompted research looking for environmental exposures that may be modulating vaccine efficacy in TB-burdened areas of the world (73,82). Since then, both helminths and NTMs have been shown to modulate immunity to BCG. Helminths alter the immune environment of their host, changing the inflammatory responses required to generate protective immunity (83,84). In contrast, NTMs modulate protective immunity by generating immunosuppression within the hosts to BCG (36,85–89). Animal studies have suggested that immunity against NTMs is an oral tolerance mechanism that is cross-reactive to the vaccine itself, thus preventing the host from developing protective immunity to BCG (36).

In addition to the hypotheses involving administration routes and environmental exposures, some researchers have hypothesized that the vaccine itself may have variable antigenicity. The BCG vaccine is not standardized in terms of strain or preparation (77). After its discovery and later utilization in the early 1900s, *M. bovis BCG* was passaged over 1173 times for maintenance because there was no cold-chain storage or lyophilization at the time (77). Today over 13 documented strains of BCG exist, and each has its own molecular and genetic fingerprints (77,90). Different regions of the world use different strains of the vaccine to vaccinate their population, leading some researchers to suggest that the protective variability of BCG may be due to differences in strains.

ADVANTAGES OF THE PULMONARY ROUTE OF DELIVERY COMPARED TO PARENTERAL ROUTE

Rationale for pulmonary delivery

The most commonly used treatment strategies for TB containment utilize either oral or parenteral routes of administration. However, systemic routes of delivery usually lead to sub-therapeutic drug levels in the lungs (Figure 23.1a). This effect is exaggerated in regions of the lungs that are poorly vascularized, with oral and parenteral routes of drug delivery clearing the infection less effectively in these areas (91). On the other hand, direct delivery of anti-TB drugs (ATDs) to the lungs allows for high local concentration of drug at the primary site of MTB infection (92) (Figure 23.1b). Further, aerosolized particulate drug delivery systems allow for effective targeting of alveolar macrophages (AMs), thereby enhancing intracellular bactericidal activity (93). Moreover, the lungs have a large surface area with extensive vasculature from which the ATDs can enter the systemic circulation and reach therapeutic

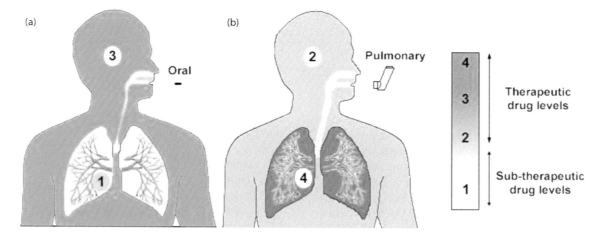

Figure 23.1 Schematic representation of drug levels in the lungs and systemic circulation when administered by (a) oral route, more drug in the systemic circulation (therapeutic drug levels) compared to lungs (sub-therapeutic drug levels) and (b) pulmonary route, more drug in the lungs compared to systemic circulation with both compartments having therapeutic drug levels. *Color intensity represents drug levels.* (Adapted from Muttil, P., et al., *Pharm. Res.*, 2401–2416, 2009.)

levels in the blood to target extrapulmonary mycobacteria. Systemic side effects are also reduced when ATDs are delivered by the pulmonary route, compared to direct systemic administration, since only a portion of the drug reaches the systemic circulation. In addition, ATDs avoid the hepatic first-pass metabolism when delivered by the pulmonary route (94).

The pulmonary route is the appropriate delivery route for TB vaccines. Having immunity in the lungs, that is, at the MTB entry site, offers better immune protection and enhanced clearance rates of MTB from the lungs compared to immunization by the systemic route.

Devices available

Drug delivery to the lungs is usually achieved by either using nebulizers, metered-dose inhalers (MDIs), or dry powder inhalers (DPIs). Nebulizers emit micron-sized droplets of drug-containing solution or suspension for inhalation, and these devices are usually prescribed to children and the elderly. However, challenges with formulating multiple drugs, the stability of the active ingredient in a liquid form, and the bulkiness of the product limit the applicability of these devices for an effective TB therapy (95). MDIs are the most widely used device for inhaled therapy for many local and systemic disorders; however, the amount of drug needed to achieve effective TB treatment is not realized with these devices, thereby limiting their applicability in developing novel TB inhalation treatments (96). DPIs administer ATDs in a dry form and thus offer more stability to ATDs than the liquid formulations in nebulizers and MDIs. In addition, DPIs aerosolize particles suitable for inhalation (1–3 μm size range) and deposition in the airways (94). DPIs can have multiple drug combinations as dry powders, and they demonstrate increased portability compared to nebulizers and MDIs.

Targeting alveolar macrophages

Targeting ATDs to the lung delivers huge drug payloads to infected AMs and has the potential to further enhance the phagocytic capability of AMs and result in activation of infected macrophages. For successful delivery and targeting to AMs, the drug delivery vehicle should possess appropriate physicochemical and surface characteristics (97). Particulate systems with a size range of 1–3 μm are suitable for deposition in the respirable airways and are optimum for phagocytosis by AMs (98). It has also been shown that particles made of hydrophobic materials such as polystyrene are less efficiently phagocytosed by AMs compared to less hydrophobic materials such as poly(lactic-co-glycolic) acid (99). See the reviews by Muttil et al. (93), Das et al. (96), Hickey et al. (100), and Giovagnoli et al. (101), which discuss the formulation trials and preclinical and clinical studies that evaluate inhaled ATDs as a potential therapy for TB.

PULMONARY DRUGS AND VACCINES IN CLINICAL DEVELOPMENT

Vaccines

Design and development of novel vaccines that are more efficacious than the current *M. bovis* BCG are of utmost importance. These vaccines should aim to reduce TB infections by protecting from the initial infection, limit transmission of disease from one individual to another, generate specific immune responses against MTB independent of environmental mycobacteria exposure, and minimize chances of progression of TB from a dormant state to an active disease state (102). However, the complex interplay between the human immune system and MTB makes it challenging to develop an effective vaccine. Unlike vaccines against most infectious diseases, where neutralizing antibodies are sufficient to contain the disease, a successful vaccine against TB requires a robust cellular immune response for protection (18,102,103). The majority of the clinical vaccine candidates employ vector-antigen combinations with adjuvants that result in the induction of pro-inflammatory cytokines such as Interferon-gamma (IFNγ) or Tumor necrosis factor-alpha (TNFα).

Clinical trials of new vaccines against TB are designed to evaluate two primary outcomes: prevention of infection (POI) and prevention of recurrence (POR). POI evaluates the ability of vaccines to prevent infection, whereas POR evaluates the ability of vaccines to prevent re-infection (104). The Treatment Action Group (TAG) 2017 pipeline contains 14 vaccine candidates under clinical development, with four subunit vaccines combined with adjuvants, five viral-vectored vaccines, and five whole-cell or extract vaccines (Figure 23.2) (104). These vaccines are further classified into three categories: (1) prophylactic pre-exposure vaccines, which target newborns, and are aimed at administering prior to any exposure to MTB; (2) prophylactic post-exposure vaccines, for individuals who have potentially been exposed to MTB or had prior BCG vaccination (these vaccines mostly target latently infected patients to reduce disease progression to active TB); and (3) therapeutic vaccines, to treat active TB patients and to be administered as an adjunct to ATDs (105,106). Figure 23.2 lists different vaccine candidates currently in clinical trials with a brief description of each candidate.

TuBerculosis Vaccine Initiative (TBVI), GlaxoSmithKline (GSK)

Despite the many advantages of pulmonary administration of vaccines, the majority of the current vaccine candidates in development vary in antigen and carrier and are almost exclusively administered systemically. MVA85A was the first study to show safety and immunogenicity in BCG-vaccinated healthy adults when delivered as aerosols (107). This phase I, double-blinded trial was performed (NCT01497769) to compare the safety

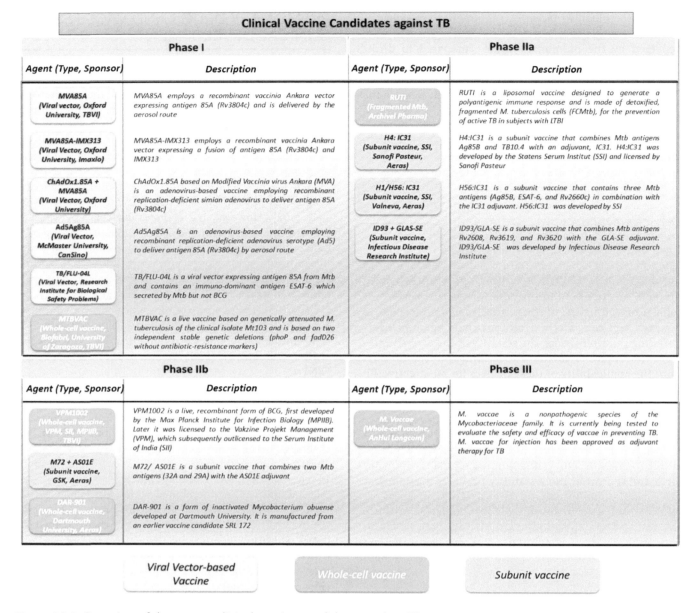

Figure 23.2 Overview of the current clinical vaccine candidates against TB.

and immunogenicity of MVA85A when administered as an aerosol (107). The primary outcome of this study was safety evaluated by assessing vaccine-related local and systemic adverse events. The secondary outcome of the study was immunogenicity evaluated by assessing cell-mediated immunity markers in the blood and bronchoalveolar lavage fluid (BALF). Intradermal administration had mild local injection-site reactions, whereas the aerosol adverse events were mild. Systemic adverse events did not differ between the immunization groups, with mild fatigue and mild to moderate headache as the most common symptoms. Both routes of vaccination induced MVA CD4$^+$ and CD8$^+$ T cell responses, with the aerosol group reporting higher CD4$^+$ T cell responses than the intradermal group. The aerosol group induced a higher number of Ag85A-specific CD4$^+$ T cell cytokines. The study concluded with

the observation that aerosol administration induced equally strong systemic immune responses and significantly stronger BALF immune responses compared to intradermal vaccination (107). Based on the promising results from this study, another aerosol trial is underway to fully characterize the mucosal and systemic immune responses to the MVA85A vaccine and to evaluate safety in latent TB patients (NCT02532036).

Similarly, in a murine model of pulmonary TB, mucosal administration of the vaccine Ad5Ag85A elicited higher T cell responses in the lung and correlated with enhanced protection over cutaneous BCG vaccination (108). In another study by Santosuosso et al., mucosal, but not intramuscular, immunization with Ad5Ag85A elicited significant CD8$^+$ T cells in the airway lumen of mice (109). Following these encouraging results from preclinical studies, wherein it was evident that aerosol administration offered the optimum immune response for protection against TB, the current ongoing clinical trial (NCT02337270) is evaluating the safety and immunogenicity of Ad5Ag85A administered as an aerosol. In this Phase I study, with a completion date of late 2019 to early 2020, healthy volunteers with prior BCG immunization have been recruited. The results from these aerosol immunization studies in humans will have a significant impact on the progress of pulmonary vaccination for TB.

Antibiotics

The concept of inhaled antibiotics to treat TB is not recent. In 1950, Miller JB et al. published a study that followed 12 children with advanced pulmonary TB and treated them with inhaled streptomycin. The patients were administered 2 g of streptomycin per day for 3 to 6 months and reported achieving high concentrations of streptomycin in the lungs. The results of the study showed 9 children cleared the infection, while 3 children developed atelectatic lesions. However, no significant toxicity was observed in any of the patients (110).

In another study in the 1990s, inhaled kanamycin was administered along with conventional ATDs to treat five patients who were admitted for MDR-TB. The findings reported that the inhalation therapy was well tolerated and that sputum conversions were observed for all patients within 60 days of initiating the treatment (111). In the early 2000s, Sacks et al. published a study wherein they treated patients with drug-resistant (12 individuals) and drug-susceptible (7 individuals) TB, who were smear and culture positive for MTB even after months of conventional ATDs, with inhaled aminoglycosides as an adjunct therapy. The results showed that 13 of 19 patients (6 of 7 with drug-susceptible TB and 7 of 12 with drug-resistant TB) converted to smear negative in less than a month of treatment (112). More recently, in 2013, Dharmadhikari et al. published data from a Phase I, single-dose, dose-escalating study of inhaled dry powder capreomycin as a therapy against MDR-TB. Five healthy adults per group were recruited to self-administer either 25, 75, 150, or 300 mg of dry powder capreomycin using a simple handheld inhaler device. All subjects showed no changes in lung function, audiometry, or other laboratory parameters evaluated, and dry powder inhalations were well tolerated. Peak and mean drug plasma concentrations were dose proportional and only exceeded the systemic Minimum Inhibitory Concentration (MIC) (2 μg/mL) for MTB when administered at the highest dose (113).

These studies suggest a great potential for inhaled therapy as a novel approach for treating pulmonary TB. Despite these successes and growing interest in the inhalational delivery of antibiotics, there is a lack of consensus on the clinical significance of inhaled ATD therapy in controlling TB. In addition, lack of approved pharmaceutical excipients for pulmonary delivery limits the translation of the large number of preclinical studies to clinical

trials (101). Considerations of factors such as patient's age, health condition, breathing pattern, lung physiology, physicochemical properties of the formulation, device performance, and cost-effectiveness of the final product add to the complexity in the development of a successful inhalation product for treating pulmonary TB.

Immunotherapy

In 2015, MDR and XDR-TB contributed to 10% of TB-related deaths (9). Evolution of drug-resistance has long been attributed to poor patient compliance resulting from long-term treatment regimens. Recent studies have also shown poor drug penetration into TB lesions as a reason for the emergence of resistance. Variable drug penetration in lesions usually leads to monotherapy or suboptimal drug levels near bacterial populations in spite of multidrug therapy. The rise in drug-resistant TB has led to renewed interest in host-directed immunotherapy (HDT). HDT works by mounting a protective host immune response against MTB. This mechanism is different from direct MTB targeting with ATDs in that inducing the host immunity may not increase the probability of bacterial resistance. The immune response generated by HDT is capable of reversing the balance between bacterial persistence and host defense from favoring the pathogen during infection to favoring the host (114). Therefore, HDT may be beneficial against active TB, which is known to emerge from either a primary infection or from immune suppression where MTB may have long persisted in the host. HDTs use host cellular mechanisms such as autophagy, apoptosis, and pyroptosis to kill intracellular MTB and have been used in clinical trials when delivered by the subcutaneous, intramuscular, and pulmonary routes (115).

The cytokine IFNγ was one of the first HDTs to be evaluated by the pulmonary route (116). IFNγ is a soluble factor critical for host defense against MTB and is known to stimulate autophagy by activating macrophages (117). Inhaled IFNγ has been shown to be safe in MDR-pulmonary TB patients and led to sputum smear conversion in various clinical trials (116,118,119). However, the sputum reverted back to positive after cessation of HDT, leading the authors to suggest that the timing and dosing of aerosolized IFNγ needs to be further optimized (118). Nebulized IFNγ as an adjunct to conventional treatment decreased symptoms such as night sweats and fever, and further increased MTB clearance from sputum (120). The proposed mechanism of targeted IFNγ to the lung is the release of IP-10, which increases lymphocyte recruitment and decreases neutrophil-mediated inflammation (121); this leads to better MTB clearance and less tissue damage, respectively. Ultimately, HDT approaches against TB will be best served as adjuncts to anti-TB drugs to shorten the treatment duration, possibly minimize the risk of reinfection in immunosuppressed individuals, and in cases where conventional therapy has failed (122).

FUTURE OF PULMONARY THERAPEUTICS IN TB

In earlier sections, we outlined the advantages of inhaled TB therapy compared to other conventional routes of treatment modalities. We discuss below some of the challenges that pulmonary delivery against TB could potentially face when evaluated in clinical and field trials.

Challenges of inhaled therapy to the clinic

One of the challenges with the pulmonary route relates to the cost of the combined device-formulation product and the ability of patients to use inhalers consistently and properly to achieve treatment compliance. Since TB primarily affects low- and middle-income countries, it is important to develop treatment and preventive strategies that are cost-effective. Current inhalers in the market (for diseases such as asthma) are expensive and complicated to use without proper medical supervision; this makes it challenging to use a similar strategy against TB, especially if it requires long-term inhaler use. Adherence to treatment also entails patient's satisfaction with the inhaler device, which is influenced by convenience of daily use, patient age, adverse effects observed during treatment, and overall treatment cost. For inhaled therapy to be successful against TB, affordable inhalers should be made available on a large scale in TB-affected nations. In the section below, we discuss the inhaler devices for drugs and vaccines separately since it requires different development and use strategies.

Devices for pulmonary drug delivery

Lung deposition of ATDs to the affected areas is determined by the aerodynamic particle size distribution, particle mass, and patients' inspiratory flow (123). Aerodynamic particle size distribution is optimized when the aerodynamic diameter is between 1 and 3 μm, a limitation that is easily overcome in the formulation aspect of inhalable products. Similarly, particle mass is affected by the added excipients, which can be optimized for deep lung delivery, for uptake by alveolar macrophages, and to minimize mucociliary clearance. One major limitation to the pulmonary route of administration, however, is the individual variation observed among patients, such as inspiratory flow rate, tidal volume, ability to hold breath after performing the inhalation maneuver, and so on (124,125). Such differences in patient-specific factors can be affected by many variables, such as age and disease states (i.e., chronic obstructive pulmonary disease [COPD]), and these variations can potentially lead to differences in clinical outcomes between patients despite using the same inhaler device–ATDs combination.

Historically, the aerosol devices used for pulmonary delivery have been nebulizers, MDIs, and DPIs (see the section called "Devices available"). One major limitation to using nebulizers is that these systems require lengthy treatment time and waste much of the drug. Here, drug loss to the environment is observed as the patient passively breathes, or the drug is retained within the device; only an average of 10% of the drug is deposited into the lung (126). In comparison, MDIs promise to provide more drug deposition; however, the effectiveness of this system is highly variable among patients. Drug deposition is largely affected by the inspiratory flow rate, in which faster inhalations may cause a significant amount of the drug to be deposited via inertial impaction in conducting airways and oropharyngeal regions (127). Issues regarding a patient's ability to coordinate actuation of the device and inspiration remains a frequent complication while using MDIs (128). Introduction of spacer and valve holding chambers have helped minimize complications regarding hand-eye coordination; this is achieved by slowing the aerosol velocity, which reduces drug deposited at the oropharynx (129). However, the use of auxiliary attachments to MDIs has previously led to compliance concerns with chronic use, especially in pediatric patients. In contrast, DPIs are designed to decrease the coordination difficulties associated with MDIs. This system also relies on the patient's inspiratory flow rate, however, and can be negatively affected by humidity and changes in temperature (130,131). Lung deposition from DPIs is further affected by the ability of the drug to deaggregate from the carrier particles (i.e., lactose), or by the patient's inability to hold her or his breath after the inhalation maneuver, which may be compromised in TB patients. Aerosol ATD formulations are further limited by the excipients that are currently approved for pulmonary delivery. Pulmonary TB therapeutics using novel but non-approved excipients, such as biodegradable polymers that are used to formulate nano- and microparticles, require additional safety and toxicological data. In addition, many excipients that are generally recognized as safe (GRAS) by other routes of administration are not approved for pulmonary delivery because of the potential safety, toxicity, and pathological inflammation concerns (132).

Interest in DPIs has arisen more recently due to the delivery platform's ability to generate high local drug concentration in the lungs, as well as the improved stability of the powders compared to drug solutions. Dry powder formulations encompass a few promising strategies for optimal inhalational TB therapy, with liposomal, microparticle, and nanoparticle dry powders at the forefront of this research (91). Liposomes encapsulating anti-TB drugs can be utilized for pulmonary delivery as they are not immunogenic (133). Micro-and nanoparticles formulated with polymeric excipients such as poly(l-lactic) acid and poly(lactic-co-glycolic) acid may potentially have a positive impact on the pharmacokinetic and pharmacodynamic parameters of ATDs. Such polymer-based formulations would allow for a less frequent dosing regimen by prolonging the drug release profiles and leading to better patient compliance. Poly(l-lactic) acid microparticles, for example, have displayed a slow *in vitro* release, where only 70% the encapsulated ATDs was released in 10 days (134). Conversely, particles delivered in the nano-size range are not suitable for inhalation purposes and must be formulated into a larger, micron-size particles (135).

Regulatory approval

For aerosol drugs and vaccines against TB, appropriate regulatory and manufacturing guidelines need to be established. Developers should consider the target population and the region where the product will ultimately be used, regardless where the product will be manufactured or approved by the regulatory authorities. At present, the highly controlled regulatory environment, especially in western countries, is a hindrance to the clinical testing of inhaled therapies against TB.

In a recent workshop convened by National Institute of Allergy and Infectious Diseases (NIAID) and the nonprofit organization Aeras, entitled "Developing Aerosol Vaccines for *Mycobacterium tuberculosis*," no major regulatory barriers were identified for aerosol TB vaccines (136). However, the research community needs to consider a few challenges associated with aerosol vaccines before evaluating them in large human trials. It is critical to demonstrate that the vaccine remains potent and safe following aerosolization. There is a possibility that the vaccine will degrade during aerosolization, especially when a nebulizer-type device is used. The biological product along with the delivery device (inhaler-formulation combination) should therefore demonstrate safety and effectiveness in clinical trials. Further, we need to address wasting the vaccine to the environment and the subsequent consequences of such contamination. Monitoring environmental contamination from the aerosolized vaccine product becomes essential in a mass immunization setting where significant vaccine exposure to the healthcare provider and the environment is possible. Another regulatory concern is the potential for adverse events from an aerosol vaccine, especially when administered in infants and young children. This issue could be addressed by first titrating the vaccine doses in human adults in order to demonstrate safety (7).

Aerosol drugs

As previously stated, it is critical that inhaled delivery achieves sufficient ATD concentration not only in the non-vascularized lung lesions where MTB resides during infection, but the drug should also permeate the lipid-rich cell membrane of the mycobacteria in sufficient concentration and for the required duration (137). A recent Phase I study in healthy individuals evaluated capreomycin dry powder as an inhaled therapy; the powder formulation was well tolerated, with only mild to moderate transient cough observed at the highest dose (113). The highest dose (300 mg) was able to achieve plasma drug concentration similar to that achieved by the control group (intramuscular delivery). However, the correlation between drug concentrations in plasma versus lung was not considered during this trial. This is further complicated by the TB pathology that consists of a broad range of lesions with heterogeneous architecture; in spite of multidrug therapy, this could potentially lead to local and temporal monotherapies in specific MTB lesions that could

in turn cause the emergence of drug resistance (137). Drug concentration in the human lung can be evaluated from the BALF fluid; however, this process is challenging since it involves an invasive procedure.

Approximately 20% of all TB cases involve extrapulmonary pathologies (138). Extrapulmonary manifestations of TB can result in lymphadenitis, central nervous system (CNS) penetration; peritonitis; pericarditis; and skeletal, genitourinary, and disseminated TB infections (91). Therefore, there is a risk for inducing resistance with subtherapeutic drug concentrations in the circulation; regulatory approval for inhalational TB therapies will require some proof of therapeutic systemic concentrations of the inhaled drug. This prerequisite often requires delivery of a massive amount of ATDs into the lungs or divided doses of the ATDs. However, divided doses are generally avoided in clinical practice for TB treatment because direct supervision of each dosage administration is considered a necessary standard of care (113). Ultimately, implementing the use of drug combinations, using aerosols as an adjunct to the conventional delivery route, and optimization of the pharmacokinetic and pharmacodynamic parameters of the ATDs will potentially lead to superior clinical outcomes for the pulmonary route of administration (100).

Aerosol vaccines

The development of an aerosol TB vaccine has similar goals to that of aerosol drugs: that is, to prevent TB transmission by immunizing adults and adolescents who are at high risk of transmitting TB to healthy individuals. However, pulmonary immunization using BCG, or other live vaccines, has the potential to be associated with adverse reactions such as ulcerative lesions due to the persistence of the live-cell vaccines within the body and lung. Aerosolized live vaccines may therefore be inappropriate in immunocompromised patients for fear of conversion of an avirulent bacteria to a virulent state (139). Recently, the vaccine candidate, MVA85A (see the section called "Pulmonary drugs and vaccines in clinical development"), completed a Phase I trial with delivery by the pulmonary route, with promising results. Rare adverse events included cough, which occurred at the same frequency as the placebo group (107). Further safety studies of inhalable vaccines need to be completed before the regulatory agencies could approve aerosol vaccines against TB (18). Other theoretical limitations to pulmonary delivery of live vaccines include irreversible inflammation, infection of other bodily systems (i.e., CNS), and risk of pathogen escape during aerosolization into the environment and potentially vaccinating unintended bystanders (140). Specific to TB, there are strong concerns with the ease of accessibility and use of pulmonary vaccines in countries with high TB disease burden and suboptimal healthcare access. Immunization occurs most often in the early years of childhood, which further necessitates easy-to-use devices with minimal actuation-inhalation coordination. Vaccine efficacy, formulation stability, ease of device use, and cost of therapy must be major considerations when formulating such aerosolized vaccines. Methods to overcome these challenges, including spray drying and lyophilization of vaccine formulations for stability and creation of cheap and easy-to-use, single-use inhaler devices, are already being actively pursued (141–143).

Speculation on aerosol treatments

The aerosol route of drug and vaccine delivery against TB offers many advantages over oral and parenteral delivery routes as discussed earlier (see the section called "Rationale for pulmonary delivery"). The inhaled administration of drugs should initially be adapted on a small scale, possibly in patients that have already failed conventional treatment, especially patients who harbor drug-resistant strains of MTB. In 2015, MDR and XDR-TB patients contributed 10% of TB-related deaths (9). Drug-resistant TB usually happens due to poor patient compliance for lengthy treatment regimens. The potential to incorporate inhaled therapy along with conventional treatment could shorten treatment duration and possibly improve patient compliance. Supplementing inhaled therapy along with conventional treatment modalities will also ensure that therapeutic concentrations of the drug are achieved to treat both pulmonary and extrapulmonary TB. For aerosol vaccines, the best evaluation should consist of human safety and immunogenicity with parallel nonhuman primate challenge, since it is not ethical to challenge humans with any form of mycobacteria. The recent aerosol immunization study in humans using MVA85A vaccine has demonstrated safety and immunogenicity, and aerosol AdAg85A vaccine will complete human trials soon; the successful completion of these studies will open new possibilities for aerosol TB immunization in the near future.

REFERENCES

1. Collins C, Grange JM, Yates M. *Tuberculosis Bacteriology: Organization and Practice*, 2nd ed. Oxford, UK: Taylor & Francis Group, 1997.
2. Daniel TM, Iversen PA. Hippocrates and tuberculosis. *Int J Tuberc Lung Dis*. 2015;19:373–374. doi:10.5588/ijtld.14.0736.
3. Frith J. History of tuberculosis. Part 1: Phthisis, consumption and the White Plague. *J Mil Veterans' Health*. 2014;22(2):29–35.
4. Donoghue HD, Lee OY-C, Minnikin DE, Besra GS, Taylor JH, Spigelman M. Tuberculosis in Dr Granville's mummy: A molecular re-examination of the earliest known Egyptian mummy to be scientifically examined and given a medical diagnosis. *Proc R Soc B Biol Sci*. 2009;277:51–56. doi:10.1098/rspb.2009.1484.
5. Kappelman J, Alçiçek MC, Kazanci N, Schultz M, Ozkul M, Sen S. First Homo erectus from Turkey and implications for migrations into temperate Eurasia. *Am J Phys Anthropol*. 2008;135:110–116. doi:10.1002/ajpa.20739.
6. Sakula A, Robert Koch. Centenary of the discovery of the tubercle bacillus, 1882. *Can Vet J*. 1983;24:127–131.
7. Persson S. *Smallpox, Syphilis and Salvation: Medical Breakthroughs that Changed the World*. Wollombi, Australia: Exisle Publishing, 2010.
8. WHO calls tuberculosis a global emergency. *LA Times*, April 24, 1993.
9. World Health Organization. *Global Tuberculosis Report 2017*. Geneva, Switzerland: Author, 2017.
10. World Health Organization. *Global Tuberculosis Report 2014*. Geneva, Switzerland: Author, 2014.
11. Dannenberg AM. Perspectives on clinical and preclinical testing of new tuberculosis vaccines. *Clin Microbiol Rev*. 2010;23:781–794. doi:10.1128/CMR.00005-10.
12. Beresford B, Sadoff JC. Update on research and development pipeline: Tuberculosis vaccines. *Clin Infect Dis*. 2010;50 Suppl 3:S178–S183. doi:10.1086/651489.
13. Zumla A, Nahid P, Cole ST. Advances in the development of new tuberculosis drugs and treatment regimens. *Nat Rev Drug Discov*. 2013;12:388–404. doi:10.1038/nrd4001.
14. Nicas M, Nazaroff WW, Hubbard A. Toward understanding the risk of secondary airborne infection: Emission of respirable pathogens. *J Occup Environ Hyg*. 2005;2:143–154. doi:10.1080/15459620590918466.
15. Orme IM, Robinson RT, Cooper AM. The balance between protective and pathogenic immune responses in the TB-infected lung. *Nat Immunol*. 2014;16:57–63. doi:10.1038/ni.3048.
16. Ryan KJ. Mycobacteria. In *Sherris Medical Microbiology*, 7th ed. New York: McGraw-Hill Education, 2017.
17. Kasper DL, Fauci AS, Hauser SL, Longo DL, Jameson JL, Loscalzo J. Tuberculosis and other mycobacterial infections. In *Harrison's Manual of Medicine*, 19th ed. New York: McGraw-Hill Education, 2016.
18. Price DN, Muttil P. Directed intervention and immunomodulation against pulmonary tuberculosis. In Torchilin V, editor. *Drug Delivery Systems for Tuberculosis Prevention and Treatment*. Chichester, UK: John Wiley & Sons, 2016, pp. 346–377.
19. Philips JA, Ernst JD. Tuberculosis pathogenesis and immunity. *Annu Rev Pathol*. 2012;7:353–384. doi:10.1146/annurev-pathol-011811-132458.
20. O'Garra A, Redford PS, McNab FW, Bloom CI, Wilkinson RJ, Berry MPR. The immune response in tuberculosis. *Annu Rev Immunol*. 2013;31:475–527.

21. Ernst JD. The immunological life cycle of tuberculosis. *Nat Rev Immunol*. 2012;12:581–591. doi:10.1038/nri3259.

22. Leemans JC, Thepen T, Weijer S, Florquin S, van Rooijen N, van de Winkel JG et al. Macrophages play a dual role during pulmonary tuberculosis in mice. *J Infect Dis* 2005;191:65–74. doi:10.1086/426395.

23. Ehrt S, Schnappinger D. Mycobacterial survival strategies in the phagosome: Defence against host stresses. *Cell Microbiol*. 2009;11:1170–1178. doi:10.1111/j.1462-5822.2009.01335.x.

24. Behar SM, Divangahi M, Remold HG. Evasion of innate immunity by Mycobacterium tuberculosis: Is death an exit strategy? *Nat Rev Microbiol*. 2010;8:668–674. doi:10.1038/nrmicro2387.

25. Divangahi M, Behar SM, Remold H. Dying to live: How the death modality of the infected macrophage affects immunity to tuberculosis. In Divangahi M, editor. *The New Paradigm of Immunity to Tuberculosis*, vol. 783. New York: Springer Science+Business Media, 2013, pp. 103–120.

26. Marino S, Cilfone NA, Mattila JT, Linderman JJ, Flynn JL, Kirschner DE. Macrophage polarization drives granuloma outcome during mycobacterium tuberculosis infection. *Infect Immun*. 2014;83:324–338. doi:10.1128/IAI.02494-14.

27. Cooper AM. Cell-mediated immune responses in tuberculosis. *Annu Rev Immunol*. 2009;27:393–422. doi:10.1146/annurev.immunol.021908.132703.

28. Sud D, Bigbee C, Flynn JL, Kirschner DE. Contribution of CD8+ T cells to control of mycobacterium tuberculosis infection. *J Immunol*. 2006;176:4296–4314. doi:10.4049/jimmunol.176.7.4296.

29. Gill WP, Harik NS, Whiddon MR, Liao RP, Mittler JE, Sherman DR. A replication clock for mycobacterium tuberculosis. *Nat Med*. 2009;15:211–214. doi:10.1038/nm.1915.

30. Orme IM, Andersen P, Boom WH. T cell response to mycobacterium tuberculosis. *J Infect Dis*. 1993;167:1481–1497.

31. North RJ, Jung Y-J. Immunity to tuberculosis. *Annu Rev Immunol*. 2004;22:599–623. doi:10.1146/annurev.immunol.22.012703.104635.

32. Chen L, Wang J, Zganiacz A, Xing Z. Single intranasal mucosal mycobacterium bovis BCG vaccination confers improved protection compared to subcutaneous vaccination against pulmonary tuberculosis. *Infect Immun*. 2004;72:238–246. doi:10.1128/IAI.72.1.238-246.2004.

33. Jeyanathan M, Heriazon A, Xing Z. Airway luminal T cells: A newcomer on the stage of TB vaccination strategies. *Trends Immunol*. 2010;31:247–252. doi:10.1016/j.it.2010.05.002.

34. Xing Z, McFarland CT, Sallenave J-M, Izzo A, Wang J, McMurray DN. Intranasal mucosal boosting with an adenovirus-vectored vaccine markedly enhances the protection of BCG-primed guinea pigs against pulmonary tuberculosis. *PLoS One*. 2009;4:e5856. doi:10.1371/journal.pone.0005856.

35. Horvath CN, Shaler CR, Jeyanathan M, Zganiacz A, Xing Z. Mechanisms of delayed anti-tuberculosis protection in the lung of parenteral BCG-vaccinated hosts: A critical role of airway luminal T cells. *Mucosal Immunol*. 2012;5:420–431. doi:10.1038/mi.2012.19.

36. Price DN, Kusewitt DF, Lino CA, McBride AA, Muttil P. Oral tolerance to environmental mycobacteria interferes with intradermal, but not pulmonary, immunization against tuberculosis. *PLOS Pathog*. 2016;12:e1005614. doi:10.1371/journal.ppat.1005614.

37. American Thoracic Society/Centers for Disease Control/Infectious Diseases Society of America. Treatment of tuberculosis. *MMWR Recomm Reports Morb Mortal Wkly Report Recomm Reports*. 2003;52:1–77. doi:10.1164/ajrccm.161.supplement_3.ats600.

38. Jain S, Lamichhane G. Antibiotic treatment of tuberculosis: Old problems, new solutions. *Microbe*. 2008;3:285–292.

39. Mase S. *New Drug Available to Treat Multidrug-Resistant TB*. Medscape Multispecialty; 2014. http://www.medscape.com/viewarticle/822098. Accessed November 12, 2015.

40. World Health Organization. *TUBERCULOSIS Global Tuberculosis Report 2016*. Geneva, Switzerland: Author, 2016.

41. Udwadia ZF, Amale RA, Ajbani KK, Rodrigues C. Totally drug-resistant tuberculosis in India. *Clin Infect Dis*. 2012;54:579–581. doi:10.1093/cid/cir889.

42. Koch A, Mizrahi V, Warner DF. The impact of drug resistance on Mycobacterium tuberculosis physiology: What can we learn from rifampicin? *Emerg Microbes Infect*. 2014;3:e17. doi:10.1038/emi.2014.17.

43. Marks SM, Flood J, Seaworth B, Hirsch-Moverman Y, Armstrong L, Mase S et al. Treatment practices, outcomes, and costs of multidrug-resistant and extensively drug-resistant tuberculosis, United States, 2005-2007. *Emerg Infect Dis*. 2014;20:812–821. doi:10.3201/eid2005.131037.

44. The White House. *National Action Plan for Combating Antibiotic-Resistant Bacteria*. Washington, DC: Author, 2015, p. 62.

45. Pym AS, Cole ST. Mechanism of drug resistance in mycobacterium tuberculosis. In Wax RG, Lewis K, Salyers A, Taber H, ed., *Bacterial Resistance to Antimicrobials*, 2nd ed. Boca Raton, FL: CRC Press, 2008, p. 448.

46. Miesel L, Rozwarski DA, Sacchettini JC, Jacobs WR. Mechanisms for isoniazid action and resistance. *Novartis Found Symp*. 1998;217:209–220; discussion 220–221.

47. Shi W, Zhang X, Jiang X, Yuan H, Lee JS, Barry CE, et al. Pyrazinamide inhibits trans-translation in mycobacterium tuberculosis. *Science*. 2011;333:1630–1632. doi:10.1126/science.1208813.

48. Budzik JM, Jarlsberg LG, Higashi J, Grinsdale J, Hopewell PC, Kato-Maeda M, et al. Pyrazinamide resistance, mycobacterium tuberculosis lineage and treatment outcomes in San Francisco, California. *PLoS One*. 2014;9:e95645. doi:10.1371/journal.pone.0095645.

49. Sreevatsan S, Stockbauer KE, Pan X, Kreiswirth BN, Moghazeh SL, Jacobs WR, et al. Ethambutol resistance in mycobacterium tuberculosis: Critical role of embB mutations. *Antimicrob Agents Chemother*. 1997;41:1677–1681.

50. Kurbatova E V, Cavanaugh JS, Shah NS, Wright A, Kim H, Metchock B, et al. Rifampicin-resistant mycobacterium tuberculosis: Susceptibility to isoniazid and other anti-tuberculosis drugs. *Int J Tuberc Lung Dis*. 2012;16:355–357. doi:10.5588/ijtld.11.0542.

51. Tudó G, Rey E, Borrell S, Alcaide F, Codina G, Coll P, et al. Characterization of mutations in streptomycin-resistant mycobacterium tuberculosis clinical isolates in the area of Barcelona. *J Antimicrob Chemother* 2010;65:2341–2346. doi:10.1093/jac/dkq322.

52. Chakraborty S, Gruber T, Barry CE, Boshoff HI, Rhee KY. Para-aminosalicylic acid acts as an alternative substrate of folate metabolism in mycobacterium tuberculosis. *Science*. 2013;339:88–91. doi:10.1126/science.1228980.

53. Mathys V, Wintjens R, Lefevre P, Bertout J, Singhal A, Kiass M, et al. Molecular genetics of para-aminosalicylic acid resistance in clinical isolates and spontaneous mutants of mycobacterium tuberculosis. *Antimicrob Agents Chemother*. 2009;53:2100–2109. doi:10.1128/AAC.01197-08.

54. Bruning JB, Murillo AC, Chacon O, Barletta RG, Sacchettini JC. Structure of the mycobacterium tuberculosis D-alanine:D-alanine ligase, a target of the antituberculosis drug D-cycloserine. *Antimicrob Agents Chemother*. 2011;55:291–301. doi:10.1128/AAC.00558-10.

55. David HL. Resistance to D-cycloserine in the tubercle bacilli: Mutation rate and transport of alanine in parental cells and drug-resistant mutants. *Appl Microbiol*. 1971;21:888–892.

56. Hong W, Chen L, Xie J. Molecular basis underlying mycobacterium tuberculosis D-cycloserine resistance: Is there a role for ubiquinone and menaquinone metabolic pathways? *Expert Opin Ther Targets*. 2014;18:691–701. doi:10.1517/14728222.2014.902937.

57. Salian S, Matt T, Akbergenov R, Harish S, Meyer M, Duscha S, et al. Structure-activity relationships among the kanamycin aminoglycosides: Role of ring I hydroxyl and amino groups. *Antimicrob Agents Chemother*. 2012;56:6104–6108. doi:10.1128/AAC.01326-12.

58. Jugheli L, Bzekalava N, de Rijk P, Fissette K, Portaels F, Rigouts L. High level of cross-resistance between kanamycin, amikacin, and capreomycin among mycobacterium tuberculosis isolates from Georgia and a close relation with mutations in the rrs gene. *Antimicrob Agents Chemother*. 2009;53:5064–5068. doi:10.1128/AAC.00851-09.

59. Brossier F, Veziris N, Truffot-Pernot C, Jarlier V, Sougakoff W. Molecular investigation of resistance to the antituberculous drug ethionamide in multidrug-resistant clinical isolates of mycobacterium tuberculosis. *Antimicrob Agents Chemother*. 2011;55:355–360. doi:10.1128/AAC.01030-10.

60. Sirgel FA, Tait M, Warren RM, Streicher EM, Böttger EC, van Helden PD, et al. Mutations in the rrs A1401G gene and phenotypic resistance to amikacin and capreomycin in mycobacterium tuberculosis. *Microb Drug Resist*. 2012;18:193–197. doi:10.1089/mdr.2011.0063.

61. Sirgel FA, Warren RM, Streicher EM, Victor TC, van Helden PD, Böttger EC. gyrA mutations and phenotypic susceptibility levels to ofloxacin and moxifloxacin in clinical isolates of mycobacterium tuberculosis. *J Antimicrob Chemother*. 2012;67:1088–1093. doi:10.1093/jac/dks033.

62. Mokrousov I, Otten T, Manicheva O, Potapova Y, Vishnevsky B, Narvskaya O, et al. Molecular characterization of ofloxacin-resistant Mycobacterium tuberculosis strains from Russia. *Antimicrob Agents Chemother*. 2008;52:2937–2939. doi:10.1128/AAC.00036-08.

63. Mahajan R. Bedaquiline: First FDA-approved tuberculosis drug in 40 years. *Int J Appl Basic Med Res*. 2013;**3**:1–2. doi:10.4103/2229-516X.112228.

64. Goel D. Bedaquiline: A novel drug to combat multiple drug-resistant tuberculosis. *J Pharmacol Pharmacother*. 2014;5:76–78. doi:10.4103/0976-500X.124435.

65. Andries K, Villellas C, Coeck N, Thys K, Gevers T, Vranckx L, et al. Acquired resistance of mycobacterium tuberculosis to bedaquiline. *PLoS One*. 2014;9:e102135. doi:10.1371/journal.pone.0102135.

66. Leibert E, Danckers M, Rom WN. New drugs to treat multidrug-resistant tuberculosis: The case for bedaquiline. *Ther Clin Risk Manag*. 2014;10:597–602. doi:10.2147/TCRM.S37743.

67. Lewis K. Platforms for antibiotic discovery. *Nat Rev Drug Discov*. 2013;12:371–387. doi:10.1038/nrd3975.

68. Skripconoka V, Danilovits M, Pehme L, Tomson T, Skenders G, Kummik T, et al. Delamanid improves outcomes and reduces mortality in multidrug-resistant tuberculosis. *Eur Respir J*. 2013;41:1393–1400. doi:10.1183/09031936.00125812.

69. Bloemberg GV, Keller PM, Stucki D, Stuckia D, Trauner A, Borrell S, et al. Acquired resistance to bedaquiline and delamanid in therapy for tuberculosis. *N Engl J Med.* 2015;373:1986–1988. doi:10.1056/NEJMc1505196.

70. Xavier AS, Lakshmanan M. Delamanid: A new armor in combating drug-resistant tuberculosis. *J Pharmacol Pharmacother.* 2014;5:222–224. doi:10.4103/0976-500X.136121.

71. Sakula A. BCG: Who were Calmette and Guérin? *Thorax.* 1983;38:806–812.

72. Trunz BB, Fine P, Dye C. Effect of BCG vaccination on childhood tuberculous meningitis and miliary tuberculosis worldwide: A meta-analysis and assessment of cost-effectiveness. *Lancet.* 2006;367:1173–1180. doi:10.1016/S0140-6736(06)68507-3.

73. World Health Organization. Trial of BCG vaccines in south India for tuberculosis prevention: First report. *Bull World Health Organ.* 1979;57:819–827.

74. Hart PD, Sutherland I. BCG and vole bacillus vaccines in the prevention of tuberculosis in adolescence and early adult life. *BMJ.* 1977;2:293–295. doi:10.1136/bmj.2.6082.293.

75. ten Dam HG, Hitze KL. Does BCG vaccination protect the newborn and young infants? *Bull World Health Organ.* 1980;58:37–41.

76. Colditz GA, Brewer TF, Berkey CS, Wilson ME, Burdick E, Fineberg HV, et al. Efficacy of BCG vaccine in the prevention of tuberculosis. Meta-analysis of the published literature. *JAMA.* 1994;271:698. doi:10.1001/jama.1994.03510330076038.

77. Price DN, Kunda NK, McBride AA, Muttil P. Vaccine preparation: Past, present, and future. *Drug Delivery Systems for Tuberculosis Prevention and Treatment.* Chichester, UK: John Wiley & Sons, 2016, pp. 67–90.

78. BCG vaccine highly protective against pulmonary TB: Study. n.d. http://www.news-medical.net/news/20131220/BCG-vaccine-highly-protective-against-pulmonary-TB-Study.aspx. Accessed February 23, 2015.

79. Price DN. *Pulmonary BCG Vaccination for Uniform Protection Against Tuberculosis in Environmental Mycobacteria Endemic Regions.* University of New Mexico, 2016.

80. Garcia-Contreras L, Wong Y-L, Muttil P, Padilla D, Sadoff J, Derousse J, et al. Immunization by a bacterial aerosol. *Proc Natl Acad Sci U S A.* 2008;105:4656–4660. doi:10.1073/pnas.0800043105.

81. Benyus JM. *Biomimicry: Innovation Inspired by Nature.* New York: William Morrow, 1997.

82. Kamala T, Paramasivan CN, Herbert D, Venkatesan P, Prabhakar R. Isolation and identification of environmental mycobacteria in the Mycobacterium bovis BCG trial area of South India. *Appl Environ Microbiol.* 1994;60:2180–2183.

83. Méndez-Samperio P. Modulation of tuberculosis-related immune responses by helminths. *J Egypt Soc Parasitol.* 2014;44:141–144.

84. Rafi W, Ribeiro-Rodrigues R, Ellner JJ, Salgame P. Coinfection-helminthes and tuberculosis. *Curr Opin HIV AIDS.* 2012;7:239–244. doi:10.1097/COH.0b013e3283524dc5.

85. Brandt L, Feino Cunha J, Weinreich Olsen A, Chilima B, Hirsch P, Appelberg R, et al. Failure of the mycobacterium bovis BCG vaccine: Some species of environmental mycobacteria block multiplication of BCG and induction of protective immunity to tuberculosis. *Infect Immun.* 2002;70:672–678.

86. Demangel C, Garnier T, Rosenkrands I, Cole ST. Differential effects of prior exposure to environmental mycobacteria on vaccination with mycobacterium bovis BCG or a recombinant BCG strain expressing RD1. *Infect Immun.* 2005;73:2190–2196. doi:10.1128/IAI.73.4.2190.

87. Flaherty DK, Vesosky B, Beamer GL, Stromberg P, Turner J. Exposure to mycobacterium avium can modulate established immunity against mycobacterium tuberculosis infection generated by mycobacterium bovis BCG vaccination 2006. doi:10.1189/jlb.0606407.0741-5400/06/0080-1262.

88. Young SL, Slobbe L, Wilson R, Buddle BM, de Lisle GW, Buchan GS. Environmental strains of mycobacterium avium interfere with immune responses associated with Mycobacterium bovis BCG vaccination. *Infect Immun.* 2007;75:2833–2840. doi:10.1128/IAI.01826-06.

89. Poyntz HC, Stylianou E, Griffiths KL, Marsay L, Checkley AM, McShane H. Non-tuberculous mycobacteria have diverse effects on BCG efficacy against mycobacterium tuberculosis. *Tuberculosis (Edinb).* 2014;94:226–237. doi:10.1016/j.tube.2013.12.006.

90. Behr MA, Wilson MA, Gill WP, Salamon H, Schoolnik GK, Rane S, et al. Comparative genomics of BCG vaccines by whole-genome DNA microarray. *Science.* 1999;284:1520–1523.

91. Pham D-D, Fattal E, Tsapis N. Pulmonary drug delivery systems for tuberculosis treatment. *Int J Pharm.* 2015;478:517–529. doi:10.1016/j.ijpharm.2014.12.009.

92. Hickey AJ, Misra A, Fourie PB. Dry powder antibiotic aerosol product development: Inhaled therapy for tuberculosis. *J Pharm Sci.* 2013:3900–3907. doi:10.1002/jps.23705.

93. Muttil P, Wang C, Hickey AJ. Inhaled drug delivery for tuberculosis therapy. *Pharm Res.* 2009:2401–2416. doi:10.1007/s11095-009-9957-4.

94. Kunda NK, Somavarapu S, Gordon SB, Hutcheon GA, Saleem IY. Nanocarriers targeting dendritic cells for pulmonary vaccine delivery. *Pharm Res.* 2013;30:325–341. doi:10.1007/s11095-012-0891-5.

95. Hanif SNM, Garcia-Contreras L. Pharmaceutical aerosols for the treatment and prevention of tuberculosis. *Front Cell Infect Microbiol*. 2012;2:118. doi:10.3389/fcimb.2012.00118.

96. Das S, Tucker I, Stewart P. Inhaled dry powder formulations for treating tuberculosis. *Curr Drug Deliv*. 2015;12:26–39. doi:10.2174/1567201811666140716123050.

97. Misra A, Hickey AJ, Rossi C, Borchard G, Terada H, Makino K, et al. Inhaled drug therapy for treatment of tuberculosis. *Tuberculosis*. 2011;91:71–81. doi:10.1016/j.tube.2010.08.009.

98. Hirota K, Hasegawa T, Hinata H, Ito F, Inagawa H, Kochi C, et al. Optimum conditions for efficient phagocytosis of rifampicin-loaded PLGA microspheres by alveolar macrophages. *J Control Release*. 2007;119:69–76. doi:10.1016/j.jconrel.2007.01.013.

99. Hasegawa T, Hirota K, Tomoda K, Ito F, Inagawa H, Kochi C, et al. Phagocytic activity of alveolar macrophages toward polystyrene latex microspheres and PLGA microspheres loaded with anti-tuberculosis agent. *Colloids Surf B Biointerfaces*. 2007;60:221–228. doi:10.1016/j.colsurfb.2007.06.017.

100. Hickey AJ, Durham PG, Dharmadhikari A, Nardell EA. Inhaled drug treatment for tuberculosis: Past progress and future prospects. *J Control Release*. 2016;240:127–134. doi:10.1016/j.jconrel.2015.11.018.

101. Giovagnoli S, Schoubben A, Ricci M. The long and winding road to inhaled TB therapy: Not only the bug's fault. *Drug Dev Ind Pharm*. 2017;43:347–363. doi:10.1080/03639045.2016.1272119.

102. Evans TG, Schrager L, Thole J. Status of vaccine research and development of vaccines for tuberculosis. *Vaccine*. 2016;34:2911–2914. doi:10.1016/j.vaccine.2016.02.079.

103. Kaufmann SHE, Hussey GD, Lambert P-H. New vaccines for tuberculosis. *Lancet*. 2010;375:2110–2119. doi:10.1016/S0140-6736(10)60393-5.

104. Frick M. *The TB Prevention Pipeline*. New York: Treatment Action Group, 2017.

105. Marinova D, Gonzalo-Asensio J, Aguilo N, Martin C. MTBVAC from discovery to clinical trials in tuberculosis-endemic countries. *Expert Rev Vaccines*. 2017;16:565–576. doi:10.1080/14760584.2017.1324303.

106. Kaufmann SHE, Weiner J, von Reyn F. Novel approaches to tuberculosis vaccine development. *Int J Infect Dis*. 2017;56:263–267. doi:10.1016/J.IJID.2016.10.018.

107. Satti I, Meyer J, Harris SA, Manjaly Thomas Z-R, Griffiths K, Antrobus RD, et al. Safety and immunogenicity of a candidate tuberculosis vaccine MVA85A delivered by aerosol in BCG-vaccinated healthy adults: A phase 1, double-blind, randomised controlled trial. *Lancet Infect Dis*. 2014;14:939–946. doi:10.1016/S1473-3099(14)70845-X.

108. Wang J, Thorson L, Stokes RW, Santosuosso M, Huygen K, Zganiacz A, et al. Single mucosal, but not parenteral, immunization with recombinant adenoviral-based vaccine provides potent protection from pulmonary tuberculosis. *J Immunol*. 2004;173:6357–6365. doi:10.4049/jimmunol.173.10.6357.

109. Santosuosso M, Zhang X, McCormick S, Wang J, Hitt M, Xing Z. Mechanisms of mucosal and parenteral tuberculosis vaccinations: Adenoviral-based mucosal immunization preferentially elicits sustained accumulation of immune protective CD4 and CD8 T cells within the airway lumen. *J Immunol*. 2005;174:7986–7994. doi:10.4049/jimmunol.174.12.7986.

110. Miller JB, Abramson HA, Ratner B. Aerosol streptomycin treatment of advanced pulmonary tuberculosis in children. *Am J Dis Child*. 1950;80:207–237.

111. Turner MT, Haskal R, McGowan K, Nardell E, Sabbag R. Inhaled kanamycin in the treatment of multidrug-resistant tuberculosis: A study of five patients. *Infect Dis Clin Pract*. 1998;7:49–53.

112. Sacks L V., Pendle S, Orlovic D, Andre M, Popara M, Moore G, et al. Adjunctive salvage therapy with inhaled aminoglycosides for patients with persistent smear-positive pulmonary tuberculosis. *Clin Infect Dis*. 2001;32:44–49. doi:10.1086/317524.

113. Dharmadhikari AS, Kabadi M, Gerety B, Hickey AJ, Fourie PB, Nardell E. Phase I, single-dose, dose-escalating study of inhaled dry powder capreomycin: A new approach to therapy of drug-resistant tuberculosis. *Antimicrob Agents Chemother*. 2013;57:2613–2619. doi:10.1128/AAC.02346-12.

114. Kaufmann SHE, Dorhoi A, Hotchkiss RS, Bartenschlager R. Host-directed therapies for bacterial and viral infections. *Nat Rev Drug Discov*. 2017;17:35–56. doi:10.1038/nrd.2017.162.

115. Zumla A, Rao M, Parida SK, Keshavjee S, Cassell G, Wallis R, et al. Inflammation and tuberculosis: Host-directed therapies. *J Intern Med*. 2015;277:373–387. doi:10.1111/joim.12256.

116. Condos R, Rom WN, Schluger NW. Treatment of multidrug-resistant pulmonary tuberculosis with interferon-gamma via aerosol. *Lancet (London, England)*. 1997;349:1513–1515. doi:10.1016/S0140-6736(96)12273-X.

117. Gutierrez MG, Master SS, Singh SB, Taylor GA, Colombo MI, Deretic V. Autophagy is a defense mechanism inhibiting BCG and mycobacterium tuberculosis survival in infected macrophages. *Cell*. 2004;119:753–766. doi:10.1016/j.cell.2004.11.038.

118. Grahmann PR, Braun RK. A new protocol for multiple inhalation of IFN-gamma successfully treats MDR-TB: A case study. *Int J Tuberc Lung Dis*. 2008;12:636–644.

119. Koh W-J, Kwon OJ, Suh GY, Chung MP, Kim H, Lee NY, et al. Six-month therapy with aerosolized interferon-gamma for refractory multidrug-resistant pulmonary tuberculosis. *J Korean Med Sci.* 2004;19:167–171.

120. Dawson R, Condos R, Tse D, Huie ML, Ress S, Tseng C-H, et al. Immunomodulation with recombinant interferon-gamma1b in pulmonary tuberculosis. *PLoS One.* 2009;4:e6984. doi:10.1371/journal. pone.0006984.

121. Condos R, Raju B, Canova A, Zhao B-Y, Weiden M, Rom WN, et al. Recombinant gamma interferon stimulates signal transduction and gene expression in alveolar macrophages in vitro and in tuberculosis patients. *Infect Immun.* 2003;71:2058–2064. doi:10.1128/IAI.71.4.2058-2064.2003.

122. Kaufmann SHE, Lange C, Rao M, Balaji KN, Lotze M, Schito M, et al. Progress in tuberculosis vaccine development and host-directed therapies: A state of the art review. *Lancet Respir Med.* 2014;2:301–320. doi:10.1016/S2213-2600(14)70033-5.

123. Hickey AJ. *Pharmaceutical Inhalation Aerosol Technology.* New York: CRC Press, 2004.

124. Dunber CA, Hickey AJ, Holzner P. Dispersion and characterization of pharmaceutical dry powder aerosols. *KONA Powder Part J.* 1998;16:7–45. doi:10.14356/kona.1998007.

125. Telko MJ, Hickey AJ. Dry powder inhaler formulation. *Respir Care.* 2005;50:1209–1227.

126. O'Callaghan C, Barry PW. The science of nebulised drug delivery. *Thorax.* 1997;52 Suppl 2:S31–S44.

127. Newman SP, Pavia D, Garland N, Clarke SW. Effects of various inhalation modes on the deposition of radioactive pressurized aerosols. *Eur J Respir Dis Suppl.* 1982;119:57–65.

128. Labiris NR, Dolovich MB. Pulmonary drug delivery. Part II: The role of inhalant delivery devices and drug formulations in therapeutic effectiveness of aerosolized medications. *Br J Clin Pharmacol* 2003;56:600–612. doi:10.1046/J.1365-2125.2003.01893.X.

129. Kunda NK, Hautmann J, Godoy SE, Marshik P, Chand R, Krishna S, et al. A novel approach to study the pMDI plume using an infrared camera and to evaluate the aerodynamic properties after varying the time between actuations 2017. doi:10.1016/j.ijpharm.2017.04.051.

130. Newhouse MT, Kennedy A. Condensation due to rapid, large temperature (t) changes impairs aerosol dispersion from Turbuhaler (T). *Am J Respir Cell Mol Biol.* 2000;161:A35.

131. Newhouse MT, Kennedy A. Inspiryl Turbuhaler (ITH) DPI vs. Ventolin MDI + Aerochamber (AC): Aerosol dispersion at high and low flow and relative humidity/temperature (RH/T) in vitro. *Am J Respir Crit Care Med.* 2000;161:A35.

132. Tolman J, Huslig M. Aerosol dosage forms. In Dash A, Singh S, Tolman S, eds., *Pharmaceutics: Basic Principles and Application to Pharmacy Practice.* San Diego, CA: Academic Press, 2014, pp. 225–238.

133. Cosgrove BD, Cheng C, Pritchard JR, Stolz DB, Lauffenburger DA, Griffith LG. An inducible autocrine cascade regulates rat hepatocyte proliferation and apoptosis responses to tumor necrosis factor-alpha. *Hepatology.* 2008;48:276–288. doi:10.1002/hep.22335.

134. Muttil P, Kaur J, Kumar K, Yadav AB, Sharma R, Misra A. Inhalable microparticles containing large payload of anti-tuberculosis drugs. *Eur J Pharm Sci* 2007;32:140–150. doi:10.1016/j.ejps.2007.06.006.

135. Finlay WH, Gehmlich MG. Inertial sizing of aerosol inhaled from two dry powder inhalers with realistic breath patterns versus constant flow rates. *Int J Pharm.* 2000;210:83–95. doi:10.1016/S0378-5173(00)00569-X.

136. Developing aerosol vaccines for mycobacterium tuberculosis. Workshop proceedings. National Institute of Allergy and Infectious Diseases, Bethesda, MD, USA, April 9, 2014. *Vaccine.* 2015;33:3038–3046. doi:10.1016/j.vaccine.2015.03.060.

137. Dartois V. The path of anti-tuberculosis drugs: From blood to lesions to mycobacterial cells. *Nat Rev Microbiol.* 2014;12:159–167. doi:10.1038/nrmicro3200.

138. Lee JY. Diagnosis and treatment of extrapulmonary tuberculosis. *Tuberc Respir Dis (Seoul).* 2015;78:47–55. doi:10.4046/trd.2015.78.2.47.

139. Muttil P, Price D, McBride A. Pulmonary immunization for TB with live cell-based vaccines: The importance of the delivery route. *Ther Deliv.* 2011;2:1519–1522.

140. Agarkhedkar S, Kulkarni PS, Winston S, Sievers R, Dhere RM, Gunale B, et al. Safety and immunogenicity of dry powder measles vaccine administered by inhalation: A randomized controlled Phase I clinical trial. *Vaccine.* 2014;32:6791–6797. doi:10.1016/j.vaccine.2014.09.071.

141. Wong Y-L, Sampson S, Germishuizen WA, Goonesekera S, Caponetti G, Sadoff J, et al. Drying a tuberculosis vaccine without freezing. *Proc Natl Acad Sci U S A.* 2007;104:2591–2595. doi:10.1073/pnas.0611430104.

142. Price DN, Kunda NK, Ellis R, Muttil P. Design and optimization of a temperature-stable dry powder BCG vaccine. Manuscript in Preparation n.d.

143. Lu D, Hickey AJ. Pulmonary vaccine delivery. *Expert Rev Vaccines.* 2007;6:213–226. doi:10.1586/14760584.6.2.213.

Integrated Strategies (Reflecting Combined Elements from Chapters 8 through 23)

24 Inhaled medication: Factors that affect lung deposition   379
    Joy H. Conway
25 A critical perspective on future developments based on the knowledge we have now   389
    Tania F. Bahamondez-Canas, Jasmim Leal, and Hugh D.C. Smyth
26 Ensuring effectiveness and reproducibility of inhaled drug treatment   397
    Anthony J. Hickey
27 Conclusion   405
    Anthony J. Hickey and Heidi M. Mansour

Inhaled medication: Factors that affect lung deposition

JOY H. CONWAY

pMDI	380	CT	382
DPIs	380	MRI	383
Nebulizers and SMIs	381	The influence of disease on deposition/targeting	383
Imaging	381	Using inhalers in real life	385
Scintigraphy, single photon emission computed tomography, and positron emission tomography	381	Conclusion	385
		References	386

There are three general categories of aerosol delivery technology: (a) pressurized metered-dose inhalers (pMDIs), (b) dry powder inhalers (DPIs), and (c) nebulizers. In addition, there are emerging technologies such as soft mist inhalers (SMIs) and mesh-based nebulizers. Each of these systems has unique characteristics in terms of formulation, metering system, and aerosol generation mechanism, resulting in aerosol properties of dose and aerodynamic particle size distribution that may be suitable for specific diseases. Inhalers give the therapeutic advantage of topical drug administration. The prescribed dose can often be given with just one or two breaths from a pMDI or DPI, offering considerable time benefits to patients who are often overloaded with medications and therapies. Other formulations require a liquid base, and nebulizers offer a functional device for those formulations. Nebulizers take longer to deliver a prescribed dose than a pMDI or PDI, but the more recent emergence of vibrating mesh nebulizers has meant that dose delivery times have been significantly reduced. All of the devices have gone through recent design changes aimed at improving lung dose and improving handling errors. There are now multiple choices of inhaler device on the market, often combined with improved formulation design. However, one of the greatest obstacles to effective treatment via inhaler devices is critical handling errors, that is, the patient interface. There are multiple challenges ahead for design: partnerships between inhalers and new drug formulations; targeting inhaled therapeutics to the disease; using new metrics to define therapeutic success; and the potential inclusion of interactive, intelligent feedback to the user.

The majority of commercially available aerosol products are intended for the treatment of the major obstructive lung diseases, asthma, or chronic obstructive pulmonary disease (COPD). Some diseases, such as cystic fibrosis (CF), have historically been uniquely dependent, for a variety of reasons, on a specific delivery system and nebulized antibiotic administration. Once a device is selected and the correct breathing technique taught, the expected deposition of an inhaled drug in the lung then depends on several factors, including airway patency/caliber. A reduction in patency or the deformation of an airway can affect the deposition of an inhaled drug and, as a consequence, can affect the clinical performance of the drug. The pattern of deposition of inhaled drugs within the lungs has been shown by multiple authors to be affected by the presence of airway obstruction. With increasing airway obstruction, inhaled aerosols have been shown to deposit in the more central airways (1–3). For the obstructive lung diseases such as asthma and COPD, bronchospasm, inflammation of the airway wall, and excess airway secretions can reduce airway caliber, even in early disease. Airways can deform with disease progression, becoming bronchiectatic in COPD and CF. The presence of bronchiectatic airways in COPD can be underdiagnosed, and this can have important consequences for therapeutic strategy in terms of controlling chronic bacterial infection and the impact on the natural history of COPD (4). Complete airway obstruction can be present in severe disease. Ventilation and perfusion defects increase with disease severity and are heterogeneous in pattern (5). Breathing patterns become disordered with lung disease progression. Hyperinflation is often described with severe disease (6). All of these factors can affect the site of deposition of an inhaled drug within the lung, and the subsequent absorption and clearance of the inhaled drug and the clinical effect.

pMDI

The pressurized metered-dose inhaler (pMDI) is the most commonly prescribed inhaler device. The traditional pMDI, when used with an optimal inhalation pattern, can achieve a lung dose of approximately 5%–15% of the emitted dose. The speed with which an aerosol is emitted form a pMDI results in a large percentage of the emitted dose deposited in the mouth and pharynx. The pMDI requires good coordination of inspiration and actuation, and this can lead to handling errors, any of which reduces the therapeutic lung dose (7,8). The response to handling errors has led to the development of breath-actuated devices and also the development of spacer devices. Spacer devices reduce oropharyngeal dose by acting as a holding chamber for the aerosol cloud, reducing the speed of the aerosol cloud, and thus allowing the patient to inhale the medication in a controlled manner (9). Spacer devices also allow children and infants to use a pMDI for the delivery of inhaled medication (10). The spacers for the pediatric population are specifically designed with anatomically shaped facemasks to match the contours of the face of different age groups. The subsequent recommendation for spacer devices to be prescribed for patients who have difficulty synchronizing aerosol actuation with inspiration of breath is now in clinical guidelines for the major obstructive lung diseases. The design of spacer devices has improved recently, with additions such as an inhalation indicator, providing confirmation of number of breaths taken, and sounds and visual indicators that show there is a good seal between the device and the patient.

A further development of pMDIs is the improvement in formulations as a result of the switch to hydrofluoroalkanes (HFAs) as the propellant. The resulting extra-fine formulations have a reduced mass median aerodynamic diameter (MMAD) from traditional pMDIs. Inhaled drug deposition, and specifically deposition of the aerosol to the lung periphery, is improved. Lung deposition is shown to increase to 30%–40% from the 5%–15% achieved with traditional pMDIs (11). The development of inhalers containing extra-fine particles has been used to target the small airways.

DPIs

Dry powder devices (DPIs) have been used to treat respiratory conditions since the late 1940s (12). DPIs have multiple designs: Some use a unit dose, some a multi-unit dose (blister pack), and others use a reservoir design. DPIs have varying resistance to an inspiratory effort and can be classified as low-, medium-, or high-resistance devices. The method of aerosolizing the dry powder is usually via the inspiratory

effort of the user, and so efficiency of the device is reliant on a correct inhalation technique. DPIs have found a niche in the inhaler device market. Portability, stability, lack of propellant, and decreased need for hand-inhalation coordination compared to pMDIs are some of the reasons for prescribing DPIs (12). Design improvements for DPIs have included auditory and visual feedback mechanisms to indicate a correct inhalation and/or the number of inhalations taken.

The need for the DPI user to aerosolize the formulation via a forced inhalation has led to the design of so-called active DPI devices, including the Exubra® insulin inhaler (Pfizer). More recently Teva Pharmaceutical Industries Ltd. has released a breath-activated, multidose DPI, the Respiclick™, to deliver albuterol sulphate (salbutamol), fluticasone proprionate, and a combined fluticasone propionate plus salmeterol formulation (13,14). Breath-actuated devices decrease the likelihood of errors between the coordination of the actuation and the inhalation and have previously been applied to the pMDI market (15). This application to the DPI market could simplify DPI use, particularly where there are specific handling errors involving hand coordination.

The need to deliver large unit doses via a DPI has led to the development of novel formulation designs. An example of this approach is PulmoSphere™, which is comprised of phospholipid-based, hollow, light, porous particles (16). This development of low-density particles allows improved flow and dispersion of dry powders. The TOBI® Podhaler® is an example of the use of PulmoSphere particle technology. The TOBI Podhaler delivers tobramycin sulphate as a dry powder for the management of CF, delivering a total dose of 112 mg via 4 capsules, twice a day. These newly developed DPIs can deliver high payloads with a high-percentage fine particle fraction (FPF), and this is particularly relevant to the delivery of dry powder formulations of antibiotics for CF. The Dreamboat™ (MannKind) and the Cyclops inhalers are also good examples of DPIs capable of delivering high unit doses. The Dreamboat inhaler has been used to deliver inhaled insulin (Afrezza®) by combining the inhaler with Technosphere® particle technology (12).

Another approach is the use of rapid vaporization of a dry powder film coated on a metallic substrate (the Staccato® system, Alexza Pharmaceuticals). The Staccato inhaler has been developed for loxapine to treat the agitation associated with psychiatric disorders, such as schizophrenia and bipolar disorder, with other inhaled drugs in the pipeline (12).

The DPI sector has also developed device/formulation combinations to target the small airways. The NEXThaler® (Chiesi) is a breath-actuated reservoir inhaler designed to have a significant percentage of particles in the extra-fine range (<1.5 µm MMAD) range, targeting both greater total lung dose and greater deposition in the peripheral lung region (12,17). The NEXThaler has been developed to deliver an inhaled steroid and long-acting bronchodilator for asthma and COPD.

NEBULIZERS AND SMIs

Jet and ultrasonic nebulizers have a long history of use for the delivery of drugs to the lungs of those with respiratory disease, with jet nebulizers dominating the market. Jet nebulizers have traditionally been used to deliver liquid formulations for those with complex healthcare needs and in an acute setting. The design of nebulizers has improved with the development of novel vibrating mesh devices such as the I-neb AAD system (Philips) and eFlow® (PARI). The vibrating mesh devices can deliver a high percentage of fine particles within a low-velocity aerosol cloud, can achieve high output rates, and can potentially impose less stress on the formulation compared to jet and ultrasonic nebulizers. These vibrating mesh devices can deliver high lung deposition and significant peripheral deposition (18,19). The vibrating mesh devices are used to deliver a variety of inhaled drugs, including antibiotics, hypertonic saline, and DNase for CF, and iloprost for pulmonary arterial hypertension (PAH) (19). The introduction of patient guidance systems, for example, AKITA, can promote long, deep, and slow (e.g., <15 L/min) inhalation and thus can allow peripheral targeting of inhaled formulations (20). The emergence of telehealth related to nebulizer devices may help align these devices to clinical trial needs (21).

SMIs and nebulizers use liquid formulations to deliver inhaled drugs. The Respimat® (Boehringher Ingelheim) device is an SMI and has been developed to deliver inhaled bronchodilators. The aerosol cloud is produced by two converging jets of solution set to collide, generating an aerosol that is slow in velocity, with a significant percentage of fine droplets, and generated over a long duration (22,23). Other examples of this class are the AERx device (Aradigm) and the ADI inhaler (Pharmaero). This technology allows delivery of an effective dose in one or two inhalations. The AERx device has respiratory inhalation products in development for the treatment of CF, biodefense, and tobacco cessation.

IMAGING

Scintigraphy, single photon emission computed tomography, and positron emission tomography

It is important to reflect on the deposition of the drugs in the lungs in order to understand their availability for pharmacological action and ultimately for efficacy in treating disease. Lung imaging is conducted primarily by 2D-planar gamma scintigraphy, but single photon emission computed tomography (SPECT) and positron emission tomography (PET) are employed more and more often for particular applications that require high resolution and 3D-imaging of the lungs. There are also promising new developments for lung imaging using computed tomography (CT) and magnetic resonance imaging (MRI).

Scintigraphy is described in detail in Chapter 2. This imaging technique has allowed the fundamentals of aerosol deposition in the lungs to be assessed. The use of radioisotopes to act as markers for the site of deposition of an inhaled formulation has been utilized for over 40 years and resulted in a mass of literature on deposition patterns. This technique has shown the importance of aerosol particle size and inhalation technique to the final deposition pattern, and the influence of disease on deposition pattern. There has been wide variety in scintigraphic methodology, which has not aided cross-center comparison. Standardized methods are now published for both radiolabeling of the formulation and the imaging/analysis methodology (24,25).

SPECT is based on the same principle as scintigraphy, but the images are acquired by a rotational gamma camera acquisition protocol allowing a three-dimensional (3D) reconstruction of the deposition pattern. SPECT acquisitions are often combined with CT images of the thorax to allow for co-registration of deposition pattern and anatomy. This has then allowed further interrogation of regional deposition within the lung (26). Standardized methods are now published for the use of SPECT in the assessment of aerosol deposition (27). SPECT has been used to give increased information on regional deposition for multiple inhaled formulations. An example is the use of SPECT/CT to assess the respiratory tract deposition of HFA-Beclomethasone and HFA-Fluticasone in asthmatic patients (28). In this study, Leach and colleagues described a significant increase in lung dose of 53% with the HFA steroid formulation (QVAR) compared to 22% for the HFA fluticasone formulation (Flovent). The difference was attributed to the difference in fine particle fraction between the two formulations.

Other centers have used SPECT/CT to describe the deposition of a radiolabeled, inhaled aerosol under varying conditions such as varying particle size, inhalation flow rate, inhaled gas mix (2,3). SPECT can also be used to reconstruct a 3D ventilation/perfusion image. Ventilation images can be gained by inhaling a radioactive gas such as krypton or an ultrafine dispersion (approximately 35 nm) of technetium-labeled carbon (Technegas). Perfusion images can be gained by the injection of technetium-labeled macroaggregated albumin (Tc99m MAA). A gamma camera acquires images through a 360° orbit for both the ventilation and the perfusion phases of the study (5). Using SPECT, ventilation-perfusion images were carried out in a COPD cohort. The investigators found perfusion defects in 32% of the patient cohort (Figure 24.1).

PET is another useful imaging tool for investigating inhaled drug deposition. The positron emitters used most commonly are fluorine-18, carbon-11, and nitrogen-13. Images are acquired using a PET scanner, which provides 3D reconstructed images with higher spatial detail than SPECT. PET radiotracers can be incorporated directly into drug molecules. The development and validation of PET radiolabels is expensive and requires an in-house cyclotron facility, but the advantage of this radiolabeling method is

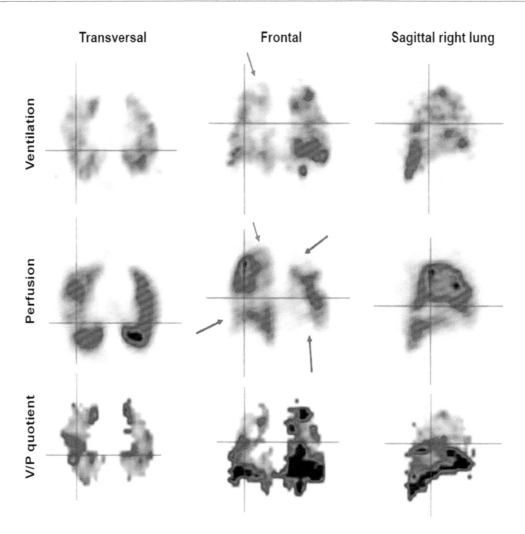

Transversal   **Frontal**   **Sagittal right lung**

Ventilation

Perfusion

V/P quotient

Figure 24.1 Heterogeneity of ventilation in COPD. Note the uneven distribution of ventilation with hot spots (indicating obstructive small airways disease), area with absent ventilation and perfusion in the upper lobe (blue arrows indicating emphysema), as well as an area with absent perfusion and preserved ventilation (mismatch—red arrows indicating pulmonary embolism). (Reproduced from Bajc, M., et al., *Int. J. Chron. Obstr. Pulm. Dis.*, 12, 1579–1587, 2017. With permission.)

that the label is incorporated into the drug, thus allowing an estimation of drug transport/metabolism (29,30). PET images are usually combined with CT in a similar way to SPECT/CT. There are less studies using PET to investigate inhaled aerosol deposition in the lungs than for SPECT due in part to the expense and complexity of the radiolabeling methods.

PET has been used to investigate patterns of lung ventilation and perfusion. Musch et al. (31) was one of several authors to describe a method using PET and intravenously injected $^{13}N_2$ to assess the topographical distribution of pulmonary perfusion and ventilation. Greenblatt et al. (32) investigated a cohort of subjects with mild to moderate asthma who were broncho-constricted with methacholine and imaged with PET/CT while inhaling aerosol carried with He-O_2. Data on deposition and ventilation were acquired using PET, with no difference found for deposition patterns between inhaled air and a helium-oxygen mix.

CT

CT images of the lungs are a mainstay of clinical investigation for lung disease. CT images are acquired and combined with SPECT and PET data to allow for anatomical mapping of aerosol deposition and to provide information on details such as lung outline, and so on. However, direct measurement of the small airways is beyond current CT imaging resolution. One method of indirectly assessing the effects of small airway dysfunction typical of obstructive lung diseases such as COPD is to quantify gas trapping on expiratory CT scans. A technique to quantify gas trapping has been to measure the percentage of voxels on a CT scan of the lungs less than −856 Hounsfield units. The problem with this methodology to assess gas trapping is its inability to distinguish gas trapping due to small airway disease when significant emphysema is present. A recent development is a technique called parametric response mapping (PRM), which matches inspiratory and expiratory lung scans to examine local changes in density. The use of this technique, when image registration of inspiratory and expiratory CT images is combined with CT density thresholds, allows the distinction between functional small airway disease (PRM^fSAD, a measure of nonemphysematous air trapping) and emphysema (PRM^emph) (33). These methods may help future clinical trials establish improvement, or not, of small airway dysfunction as a result of an inhaled therapeutic intervention but require standardization and correlation with clinical outcome measures and lung function indices (33).

CT images can also be used to establish modeling data of inhaled deposition by assessing central airway dimensions and using the lung outline in inspiration and expiration as boundary conditions. One example of this approach is functional respiratory imaging (FRI), which uses data from high-resolution CT (HRCT) combined with computational fluid dynamics (CFD) to create simulations of functional changes within the airways and predict deposition pattern of inhaled drugs. This method allows simulations of deposition studies previously only available via scintigraphy, SPECT, or PET. FRI has been used to investigate variations in inhaler technique, effects of a therapeutic intervention, and other clinical scenarios (11).

MRI

MRI has not traditionally been a tool used for the investigation of lung disease or the assessment of the effects of an inhaled therapy. MRI applied to lung studies has not previously allowed the acquisition of images of sufficient quality or resolution (34). The development of a combination of inhaled hyperpolarized gases and MRI has allowed the description of ventilation patterns in the lung. Hyperpolarized helium (^{3}He) has become an established technique, allowing high-resolution images of ventilation distribution to be obtained. This technique has been used to investigate the obstructive lung diseases, COPD, asthma, and CF (35–37), and to investigate the effect of therapeutic intervention such as the use of ivacaftor for CF (38).

The major advantage of MRI is the avoidance of a radiation dose as opposed to scintigraphy, SPECT, PET, and CT. The disadvantage of hyperpolarized MRI is the complexity of producing hyperpolarized gases and the potential shortage of worldwide supplies of helium. Other hyperpolarized gases such as xenon are used, but these gases are associated with a reduced signal (34,39).

Novel MRI methods have potential for future use as outcome measures for trials involving lung disease and inhaled therapeutics. Fourier decomposition (FD-MRI) methods, as well as oxygen-enhanced MRI (OE-MRI), have shown some initial promise (40,41). These techniques do not use hyperpolarized gases, which makes their application more widely accessible.

The MRI methods outlined here all allow detail on structure and function of the lungs without the need for a radiation dose. This allows repeat imaging, which may be of particular importance in pediatric lung disease

cohorts. Improvement of lung function should follow a successful inhaled therapeutic intervention and so MRI may become a useful, repeated measure of clinical trial success.

THE INFLUENCE OF DISEASE ON DEPOSITION/TARGETING

Each inhaled drug has a proposed optimal site of action in the lungs. Using the device and formulation improvements described, it is possible to alter the amount of drug that gets to the lung, and the preferential site of deposition within the lung. Sometimes the issue is lack of clarity on optimal site for deposition and sometimes the issue is a lack of sufficiently sensitive tools to detect change in the deep lung.

COPD is characterized by small airway disease (SAD); that is, there is increased obstruction with disease in the small airways, i.e., less than 2 mm in diameter (42). McDonough and colleagues (43) used microcomputed tomography (micro-CT) to show that the progression of COPD was characterized by a decrease in the number of terminal bronchioles and wall thickening in the remaining bronchioles. It is considered that small airway disease occurs early in the life course of COPD (44). To target the small airways, both theory and clinical trial data suggest that reducing the average particle size of an inhaled medication will increase the peripheral deposition of that medication. The emergence of inhaled formulations that produce a greater percentage of fine particles has therefore been directed at delivering therapy to the small airways (45).

Currently, the main treatment options for COPD patients are bronchodilators (short-acting beta$_2$ agonists [SABAs], long-acting beta$_2$agonists [LABAs], short-acting muscarinic antagonists [SAMAs], and long-acting muscarinic antagonists [LAMAs]), inhaled corticosteroids (ICSs), and inhibitors of the enzyme phosphodiesterase-4. Recent clinical trials have shown the efficacy of extra-fine inhaled therapy that targets the small airways in patients with COPD. The FORWARD (46), FUTURE (47), TRILOGY (48,49), and TRINITY (50) studies provide information on clinically relevant outcomes with extra-fine aerosol treatment such as symptoms and exacerbations.

The FORWARD study was a randomized, double-blind trial that compared the efficacy and safety of 48 weeks of treatment with extra-fine beclomethasone dipropionate/formoterol fumarate (BDP/FF), 100/6 μg pMDI, 2 inhalations BID, versus FF 12 μg pMDI, 1 inhalation BID, in severe COPD patients with a history of exacerbations. The study concluded that extra-fine BDP/FF significantly reduced the exacerbation rate and improved lung function of patients with severe COPD and history of exacerbations as compared to FF alone.

The FUTURE study was a 12-week multicenter, randomized, double-blind, double dummy study in which 419 patients with moderate/severe COPD were randomized to BDP/FF 200/12 μg or Fluticasine (FP)/salmeterol (S) 500/50 μg twice daily. BDP/FF extra-fine combination provided COPD patients with an equivalent improvement of dyspnea and a faster bronchodilation in comparison to FP/S.

The TRILOGY study evaluated the safety and efficacy of extra-fine BDP/FF/glycopyrronium (GB) versus an ICS/LABA combination for COPD (FEV$_1$ < 50% of predicted). TRILOGY was a 52-week, double-blind, randomized, multicenter, two-arm, active-controlled clinical trial to test the superiority of extra-fine BDP/FF/GB versus a fixed combination of extra-fine BDP plus FF administered via pMD. Extra-fine BDP/FF/GB was found to be superior to BDP/FF for both pre-dose FEV$_1$ and 2-h post-dose FEV$_1$ at week 26, with a positive effect on exacerbation rates.

TRINITY was a 52-week, randomized, parallel group, double-blind, controlled study conducted in 2691 patients with COPD (FEV$_1$ < 50% of predicted). The objective of the TRILOGY study was to compare the efficacy of triple therapy with two long-acting bronchodilators and an inhaled corticosteroid in COPD. This study compared treatment with extra-fine beclometasone dipropionate, formoterol fumarate, and glycopyrronium bromide (BDP/FF/GB; fixed triple) with tiotropium, and BDP/FF plus tiotropium (open triple). The TRINITY study found that treatment with extra-fine fixed triple therapy had clinical benefits, including exacerbation rates, compared with tiotropium in patients with symptomatic COPD, FEV$_1$ of less than 50%, and a history of exacerbations.

The specific effects of extra-fine BDP/FF on small airway geometry in COPD patients were investigated in another study using CT scanning and CFD modeling (51). In this study, there was a reduction in hyperinflation after 6-month treatment of the extra-fine particles to the small airways in COPD.

The small airways are of significant importance in COPD, and extra-fine aerosols have been shown to be able to target peripheral airways in the lungs. A recent analysis from the SPIROMICS study (1843 patients with COPD) identified several novel biomarkers associated with consistent exacerbations, including CT-defined small airway abnormality (52). Small airway function and dysfunction are increasingly recognized as important to disease control in COPD; therefore, treatment targeted to the small airways could have an important role to play in disease stability/progression.

In asthma, airway inflammation is predominantly present within the small airways, and this region is the main contributor to airflow limitation (53). The evidence for small airway dysfunction and the clinical emergence of a small airway phenotype suggest that consideration should be given to treating the small airways when reviewing patients with asthma or COPD clinically. A recent review (54) of the available literature suggests that, in randomized controlled trials, small-particle aerosol therapy is at least as good as large-particle aerosol therapy.

Alongside the development of extra-fine formulations and novel inhalers, there is an ongoing need to develop more sensitive physiological and imaging assessment techniques

directed at the small airways. Imaging technique improvements and novel pulmonary function tests are likely to aid our decisions in the short-term (33).

For those with CF, the majority of inhaled medication is directed at treating infection throughout the bronchial tree. A recent Cochrane review (55) reviewed the evidence of the benefit of inhaled antibiotics against persistent *Pseudomonas aeruginosa* from 18 trials with people with CF aged 5–56 years. The conclusions were that inhaled anti-pseudomonal antibiotic treatment probably improves lung function and reduces exacerbation rate, but the level of benefit were very limited. The best evidence was for inhaled tobramycin. More evidence is needed to determine a better measure of benefit. Longer-term trials are needed to look at the effect of inhaled antibiotics on quality of life, survival, and nutritional outcomes. For those with a complex disease like CF, a device that can offer a single-breath dose offers great time savings over devices that require minutes to complete treatment. For this reason, formulations of antibiotics have moved as quickly as possible to devices like DPIs.

For some inhaled medications, the target site within the lung is the alveolar zone. This can be to treat the alveoli or to maximize absorption through the lung for systemic uptake of an inhaled drug. Inhaled Iloprost, a prostacyclin analog, is used to treat pulmonary arterial hypertension, a life-limiting condition that can lead to right hear failure. Inhaler devices for this context use nebulizer technology with an aerosol bolus of typically 50%–80% of the inhalation followed by "clean" air for the remainder of the inhalation. This pattern of inhalation has been used to promote deposition in the periphery of the lung (56). This example illustrates that the combination of a liquid formulation and a targeted breathing pattern can achieve preferential peripheral lung deposition.

Using the inhaled route to treat restrictive lung diseases is less developed. Idiopathic pulmonary fibrosis (IPF) is a chronic lung disease of unknown cause associated with a median survival of 3–5 years. Treatment for this disease is limited, and the inhaled route is not usually associated with IPF. However a recent clinical trial has demonstrated that, in a small group of patients with varying degrees of severity of IPF, a 1.5 μm diameter monodisperse aerosol particle size is capable of depositing in the peripheral areas of the lung, as opposed to 6 μm particles, which deposited in the throat and central airways (57). These findings are similar to those reported for healthy volunteers and those with obstructive lung disease. This study does demonstrate that inhaled therapies are possible in IPF and that an extra-fine aerosol approach is appropriate in the context of a disease that alters the structure of the lung architecture with peripheral destruction dominant. Inhaled pirfenidone is currently in the development pipeline for the treatment of IPF, so it is possible that the inhaled route may be used in the future for IPF (57).

One aspect of aerosol deposition that can be overlooked is the effect of ventilation heterogeneity that accompanies the airway diseases and also often the disease of the parenchyma.

Aerosol particles have mass and are subject to the laws of physics regarding flow, aerodynamics, and gravity. An aerosol cloud is entrained into the lungs with an inhaled breath, and the speed and volume of that breath has an effect on the site of deposition. Patterns of ventilation within the lung also have an effect on the pattern of deposition. Ventilation patterns in the human lung are affected by gravity, with ventilation tending to prefer dependent lung in spontaneous breathing, older children and adults. There are elegant studies that describe this effect using gravity–free environments (58). For fine particles (approximately 1 μm), both aerosol bolus inhalations and studies in small animals suggest that particles deposit more peripherally in reduced gravity.

It is possible to affect the deposition pattern of an aerosol by simply altering the position of a patient when he or she inhales the aerosol. The positional change affects preferential ventilation by altering the effects of gravity on the lung structure. Sa et al. (59) used scintigraphy to investigate deposition patterns in supine and seated positions. Inhalation of 5 μm particles in the supine posture shifts relative deposition from the alveolar to the bronchial airways, when compared to the seated posture, and is likely driven by changes in functional residual capacity, and airway size, as well as changes in the regional distribution of ventilation between postures. In a later study, Sa et al. (60) used scintigraphy plus OE-MRI to quantify and co-register deposition pattern and ventilation pattern. These results support the hypothesis that alveolar deposition is directly proportional to ventilation for 5 μm particles that are inhaled in the supine posture. This is consistent with previous simulation predictions that show that convective flow is the main determinant of aerosol transport to the lung periphery. Thus, ventilation patterns are a potentially important aspect of aerosol targeting. In the presence of diseases such as COPD, ventilation inhomogeneity is a characteristic of the disease progression, making optimization of aerosol targeting and uptake a future challenge (5).

USING INHALERS IN REAL LIFE

The design improvements for inhalers and formulations and the clinical trials carried out with care about every detail to ensure accurate targeting of deposition within the lung are all completely wasted if the patient fails to take her or his medication or has poor inhaler technique. A study by Melzer et al. (61) reported that, in a cohort of 688 individuals with COPD, 65% had poor technique for at least one device. Inhaler errors were found to be associated with educational achievements and race. Another study of 2935 patients with COPD found over 50% of the cohort had critical handling errors for their inhaler devices (62).

When a treatment is given by the inhaled route, the importance of education and training in inhaler device technique cannot be overemphasized (Table 24.1). Observational studies have identified a significant relationship between poor inhaler use and symptom control in patients with COPD (62,63). Determinants of poor inhaler

Table 24.1 The inhaled route[a]: The importance of education and training to the success of inhaled treatment

- When a treatment is given by the inhaled route, the importance of education and training in inhaler device technique cannot be overemphasized.
- The choice of inhaler device has to be individually tailored and will depend on access, cost, prescriber, and most importantly, patient's ability and preference.
- It is essential to provide instructions and to demonstrate the proper inhalation technique when prescribing a device, to ensure that inhaler technique is adequate and recheck at each visit that patients continue to use their inhaler correctly.
- Inhaler technique (and adherence to therapy) should be assessed before concluding that the current therapy is insufficient.

[a] Taken from the Global Initiative for Chronic Obstructive Lung Disease and Global Initiative for Asthma COPD Guidelines 2018, table 3.6. With permission from www.goldcopd.org.

technique in asthma and COPD patients include socioeconomic status, older age, use of multiple devices, and lack of previous education on inhaler technique (64,65). It is essential to check and recheck that patients continue to use their device correctly.

The main errors in the use of a delivery device relate to problems with inspiratory flow, inhalation duration, coordination, dose preparation, exhalation maneuver prior to inhalation, and breath-holding following dose inhalation (66). Evidence supports a relevant role for e-health in monitoring and improving inhaler use and treatment adherence in asthma. E-health represents a potentially valuable tool for achieving optimal management of lung disease (67).

Studies exploring issues surrounding health literacy and optimizing the benefit of various educational strategies such as use of videos are urgently needed. Without effective educational interventions and strategies to improve compliance, we will fail our patients (68).

CONCLUSION

Both inhaler devices and formulations have had multiple design improvements in recent years. Targeting of inhaled drug to discrete zones in the lung is possible. Imaging has helped to identify the efficiency of inhaled drugs to reach the lung and to describe the regional deposition within the lung. Small airway disease is an important component of several lung diseases but at present we are unable to directly visualize the small airways *in vivo*. There are promising, future developments in imaging that may enhance our understanding of drug targeting within the lung and specifically to the periphery of the lung. One of the immediate issues to overcome, however, is the large numbers of patients who have critical handling errors for inhaler devices. The need for effective educational and motivational interventions must also be a research priority.

REFERENCES

1. Svartengren M, Anderson M, Philipson K, Camner P. Individual differences in regional deposition of 6-micron particles in humans with induced broncho-constriction. *Exp Lung Res.* 1989;15:139–149.

2. Fleming J, Conway J, Majoral C, Katz I, Caillibotte G, Pichelin M, Montesantos S, Bennett M. Controlled, parametric, individualized, 2D and 3D imaging measurements of aerosol deposition in the respiratory tract of asthmatic human subjects for model validation. *J Aerosol Med Pulm Drug Deliv.* 2015;28(6):432–451.

3. Katz I, Pichelin M, Montesantos S, Majoral C, Martin A, Conway J, Fleming J, Venegas J, Greenblatt E, Caillibotte G. Using helium-oxygen to improve regional deposition of inhaled particles: Mechanical principles. *J Aerosol Med Pulm Drug Deliv.* 2014;27(2):71–80.

4. Martinex-Garcia MA, Miravitlles M. Bronchiectasis in COPD patients: More than a comorbidity? *Int J Chron Obstruct Pulmon Dis.* 2017;12:1401–1411.

5. Bajc M, Chen Y, Wang J, Shen WM, Wang CZ, Huang H, Lindqvist A, He XY. Identifying the heterogeneity of COPD by V/P SPECT: A new tool for improving the diagnosis of parenchymal defects and grading the severity of small airways disease. *Int J Chron Obstruct Pulmon Dis.* 2017;12:1579–1587.

6. Gagnon P, Guenette JA, Langer D, Laviolette L, Mainguy V, Maltias F, Ribeiro F, Saey D. Pathogenesis of hyperinflation in chronic obstructive pulmonary disease. *Int J Chron Obstruct Pulmon Dis.* 2014;9:187–201.

7. Chrystyn H, Van der Palen J, Sharma R, Barnes N, Delafont N, Mahajan A, Thomas M. Device errors in asthma and COPD: Systematic literature review and meta-analysis. *NPJ Prim Care Respir Med.* 2017;27:22.

8. Mahon J, Fitzgerald A, Glanville J, Dekhuijzen R, Glatte J, Glanemann S, Torvinen S. Misuse and/or treatment delivery failure of inhalers among patients with asthma or COPD: A review and recommendations for the conduct of future research. *Respir Med.* 2017;129:98–116.

9. Burudpakdee C, Kushnarev V, Coppolo Dm Suggett JA. A retrospective study of the effectiveness of the AeroChamber Plus® Flow-Vu® antistatic valved holding chamber for asthma control. *Pulm Ther.* 2017;3:283–296.

10. Gillette C, Rockich-Winston N, Kuhs JA, Flesher S, Shepherd M. Inhaler technique in children with asthma: A systematic review. *Acad Pediatr.* 2016;16(7):605–615.

11. Van Holsbeke C, De Backer J, Vos W, Marshall J. Use of functional respiratory imaging to characterize the effect of inhalation profile and particle size on lung deposition of inhaled corticosteroid/long-acting β2-agonists delivered via a pressurized metered-dose inhaler. *Ther Adv Respir Dis* 2018;12:1–15.

12. De Boer AH, Hagedoorn P, Hoppentocht M, Buttini F, Grasmeijer F, Frijlink HW. Dry powder inhalation: Past, present and future. *Expert Opin Drug Deliv.* 2017;14(4):499–512.

13. Welch MJ. Pharmacokinetics, pharmacodynamics, and clinical efficacy of albuterol RespiClick(™) dry-powder inhaler in the treatment of asthma. *Expert Opin Drug Metab Toxicol.* 2016;12(9):1109–1119.

14. Paik J, Scott LJ, Pleasants RA. Fluticasone propionate/salmeterol MDPI (AirDuo RespiClick®): A review in asthma. *Clin Drug Investig.* 2018;38(5):463–473.

15. Small CJ, Gillespie M. Pharmacokinetics of beclomethasone dipropionate delivered by breath-actuated inhaler and metered-dose inhaler in healthy subjects. *J Aerosol Med Pulm Drug Deliv.* 2017. doi:10.1089/jamp.2017.1397.

16. Geller DE, Weers J, Heuerding S. Development of an inhaled dry powder formulation of tobramycin using pulmosphere technology. *J Aerosol Pulm Drug Deliv.* 2011;24(4):175–182.

17. Corradi M, Chrystyn H, Cosio BG, Pirozynski M, Loukides S, Loius R, Spinola M, Usmnai O. NEXThaler, an innovative dry powder inhaler delivering and extrafine combination of beclametasone and formoterol to treat large and small airways in asthma. *Expert Opin Drug Deliv.* 2014;11(9):1497–1506.

18. Nikander K. Challenges and opportunities in respiratory drug delivery devices. *Expert Opin Drug Deliv.* 2010;7:1235–1238.

19. Beck-Broichsitter M, Prufer N, Oesterheld N, Seeger W, Schmehl T. Nebulisation of active pharmacveutical ingredients with the eFlow rapid: Impact of formulation variables on aerodynamic characteristics. *J Pharm Sci.* 2014;103(8):2585–2589.

20. Reychler G, Aubriot AS, Depoortere V, Jamar F, Liistro G. Effect of targeting nebulisation on lung deposition: A randomised crossover scintigraphic comparison between central and peripheral delivery. *Respir Care.* 2014;59(10):1501–1507.

21. Elphick M, Von Hollen D, Pritchard JN, Nikander K, Hardaker LE, Hatley RH. Factors to consider when selecting a nebuliser for a new inhaled drug product development program. *Expert Opin Drug Deliv.* 2015;12(8):1375–1387.

22. Dalby R, Spallek M, Voshaar T. A review of the development of Respimat Soft Mist Inhaler. *Int J Pharm.* 2004;283:1–9.

23. Meltzer EO, Berger WE. A review of efficacy and safety of once-daily tiotropium Respimat 2.5 micrograms in adults and adolescents with asthma. *Allergy Asthma Proc.* 2018;39(1):14–26.

24. Devadason SG, Chan HK, Haeussermann S, Kietzig C, Kuehl PJ, Newman S, Sommerer K, Taylor G. Validation of radiolabelling of drug formulations for aerosol deposition assessment of orally inhaled products. *J Aerosol Med Pulm Drug Deliv.* 2012;suppl 1:S6–S9.

25. Newman S, Bennett WD, Biddiscombe M, et al. Standardisation of techniques for using planar (2D) imaging for aerosol deposition assessment of orally onhaled products. *J Aerosol Med Pulm Drug Deliv.* 2012;suppl 1:S10–S28.

26. Fleming J, Conway J, Majotal C, Tossici-Bolt L, Caillibotte G, Perchet D, Muellinger B, Martonen T, Kronenberg P, Apiou-Sbirlea G. The use of combined single photon emission computed tomography and x-ray computed tomography to assess the fate of inhaled aerosol. *J Aerosol Med Pulm Drug Deliv.* 2011;24(1):49–60.

27. Fleming J, Bailey D, Chan HK, Conway J, Kuehl PJ, Laube BL, Newman S. Standardisation of techniques for using single photon emission computed tomography (SPECT) for aerosol deposition assessment of orally inhaled products. *J Aerosol Med Pulm Drug Deliv.* 2012;suppl 1:s29–s51.

28. Leach CL, Kuehl PJ, Chand R, McDonald JD. Respiratory tract deposition of HFA-beclomethasone and HFA fluticasone in asthmatic patients. *J Aerosol Med Pulm Drug Deliv.* 2016;29(2):127–133.

29. Dolovich MB, Bailey DL. Positron emission tomography (PET) for assessing aerosol deposition of orally inhaled drug products. *J Aerosol Med Pulm Drug Deliv.* 2012;suppl 1:s52–s71.

30. Darquenne C, Fleming JS, Katz I, Martin AR, Schoreter J, Usmani O, Venegas J, Schmid O. Bridging the gap between science and clinical efficacy: Physiology, imaging and modelling of aerosol in the lung. *J Aerosol med Pulm Drug Deliv.* 2016;29(2):107–126.

31. Musch G, Layfield DH, Harris RS, Vidal Melo MF, Winkler T, Callahan RJ, Fischman AJ, Venegas JG. Topological distraibution of pulmonary perfusion and ventilation assessed by PET in supine and prone humans. *J Appl Physiol.* 2002;93:1841–1851.

32. Greenblatt EE, Winkler T, Harris RS, Kelly VJ, Krone M, Katz I, Martin A, Caillibotte G, Hess DR, Venegas JG. Regional ventilation and aerosol deposition with helium-oxygen in broncho-constricted asthmatic lungs. *J Aerosol Med Pulm Drug Deliv.* 2016;29:260–272.

33. Gove K, Wilkinson T, Jack S, Ostridge K, Thompson B, Conway J. Systematic review of evidence for relationships between physiological and CT indices of small airways and clinical outcomes in COPD. *Respir Med.* 2018;139:117–125.

34. Biddiscombe MF, Usmani O. The importance of imaging and physiology measurements in assessing the delivery of peripherally targeted aerosolized drugs. *Ther Deliv.* 2012;3(11):1329–1345.

35. Ouriadov A, Lessard E, Sheikh K, Parraga G. Pulmonary MRI morphometry modelling of airspace enlargement in chronic obstructive pulmonary disease and alpha-1 antitrypsin deficiency. *Magn Reson Med.* 2018;79(1):439–448.

36. Leary D, Svenningsen S, Guo F, Bhatawadekar S, Parraga G, Maksym GN. Hyperpolarised 3He magnetic resonance imaging ventilation defects in asthma: Relationship to airway mechanics. *Physiol Rep.* 2016;4(7):e12761. doi:10.14814/phy2.12761.

37. Kolodziej M, De Veer MJ, Cholewa M, Egan GF, Thompson BR. Lung function imaging methods in cystic fibrosis pulmonary disease. *Respir Res.* 2017;18(1):96.

38. Altes TA, Johnson M, Fidler M, Botfield M, Tustison NJ, Leiva-Salinas C De Lange EE, Froh D, Mugler JP. Use of hyperpolarised helium-3 MRI to assess response to ivacaftor treatment in patients with cystic fibrosis. *J Cyst Fibros.* 2017;16(2):267–274.

39. Chan HF, Stewart NJ, Norquay G, Collier GJ, Wild JM. 3D diffusion-weighted 129Xe MRI for whole lung morphometry. *Magn Reson Med.* 2018;79(6):2986–2995.

40. Bauman G, Pusteria O, Bieri O. Ultra-fast steady-state precession pulse sequence for fourier decomposition pulmonary MRI. *Magn Reson Med.* 2016;75(4):1647–1653.

41. Pusteria O, Bauman G, Bieri O. Three-dimensional oxygen-enhanced MRI of the human lung at 1.5T with ultra-fast steady-state free precession. *Magn Reson Med.* 2018;79(1):246–255.

42. Hogg JC, Pare PD, Hackett TL. The contribution of small airway obstruction to the pathogenesis of chronic obstructive pulmonary disease. *Physiol Rev.* 2017;97(2):529–552.

43. McDonough JE, Yuan R, Suzuki M, et al. Small-airway obstruction and emphysema in chronic obstructive pulmonary disease. *N Engl J Med.* 2011;365:1567–1575.

44. Bhatt SP, Soler X, Wang X, et al.; COPDGene Investigators. Association between functional small airway disease and FEV$_1$ decline in chronic obstructive pulmonary disease. *Am J Respir Crit Care Med.* 2016;194:178–184.

45. Singh D. Small airway disease in patients with chronic obstructive pulmonary disease. *Tuberc Respir Dis (Seoul).* 2017;80:317–324.

46. Wedzicha JA, Singh D, Vestbo J, et al. Extrafine beclamethsaone/formoterol in severe COPD patients with history of exacerbations. *Respir Med.* 2014;108(8):1153–1162.

47. Singh D, Nicolini G, Bindi E, et al. Extrafine beclomethasone/formoterol compared to fluticasone/salmeterol combination therapy in COPD. *BMC Pulm Med.* 2014;14:43.

48. Singh D, Corradi M, Spinola M, Petruzzelli S, Papi A. Extrafine beclometasone dipropionate/formoterol fumarate: A review of its effects in COPD. *NPJ Prim Care Respir Med.* 2016;26:16030.

49. Singh D, Papi A, Corradi M, et al. Single inhaler triple therapy versus inhaled cortico- steroid plus long-acting beta2-agonist therapy for chronic obstructive pulmonary disease (TRILOGY): A double-blind, parallel group, randomised controlled trial. *Lancet.* 2016;388:963–973.

50. Vestbo J, Papi A, Corradi M, et al. Single inhaler extrafine triple therapy versus long- acting muscarinic antagonist therapy for chronic obstructive pulmonary disease (TRINITY): A double-blind, parallel group, randomised controlled trial. *Lancet.* 2017;389:1919–1929.

51. De Backer J, Vos W, Vinchurkar S, et al. The effects of extrafine beclometasone/formoterol (BDP/F) on lung function, dyspnea, hyperinflation, and airway geometry in COPD patients: Novel insight using functional respiratory imaging. *J Aerosol Med Pulm Drug Deliv.* 2015;28:88–99.

52. Han MK, Quibrera PM, Carretta EE, et al. Frequency of exacerbation in patients with chronic pulmonary disease: An analysis of the SPIROMICS cohort. *Lancet.* 2017;5(8):619–626.

53. Cottini M, Lombardi C, Micheletto C. Small airway dysfunction and bronchial asthma control: The state of the art. *Asthma Res Pract.* 2015;1:13.

54. Usmani O. Small airway dysfunction in asthma: Evaluation and management to improve asthma control. *Allergy Asthma Immunol Res.* 2014;6(5):376–388.

55. Smith S, Rowbotham NJ, Regan KH. Inhaled antipseudomonal antibiotics for long-term therapy in cystic fibrosis. *Cochrane Database Syst Rev.* 2018;3:CD001021. doi:10.1002/14651858.CD001021.pub3.

56. Hill NS, Preston IR, Roberts KE. Inhaled therapies for pulmonary hypertension. *Respir Care.* 2015;60(6):794–802.

57. Usmani O, Biddiscombe M, Yang S, Meah S, Oballa E, Simpson JK, Fahy WA, Marshall RP, Lukey PT, Maher T. The topical study of inhaled drug (salbutamol) delivery in idiopathic pulmonary fibrosis. *Respir Res.* 2018;19:25.

58. Darquenne C. Aerosol deposition in the human lung in reduced gravity. *J Aerosol Med Pulm Drug Deliv* 2014;27(3):170–177.

59. Sa RC, Zeman KL, Bennett WD, Prisk GK, Darquenne C. Effect of posture on regional deposition of coarse particles in the healthy human lung. *J Aerosol Med Pulm Drug Deliv.* 2015;28(6):423–431.

60. Sa RC, Zeman KL, Bennett WD, Prisk GK, Darquenne C. Regional ventilation is the main determinant of alveolar deposition of coarse particles in the supine healthy human lung during tidal breathing. *J Aerosol Med Pulm Drug Deliv.* 2017;30(5):322–331.

61. Melzer AC, Ghassemieh BJ, Gillespie SE, Lindenauer PK, McBurnie MA, Mularski RA, Naureckas ET, Vollmer WM, Au DH. Patient characteristics associated with poor inhaler technique among a cohort of patients with COPD. *Respir Med.* 2017;123:124–130.

62. Molimard M, Raherison C, Lignot S, Balestra A, Lamarque S, Chartier A, Droz-Perroteau C, Lasalle R, Moore N, Grodet PO. Chronic obstructive pulmonary disease exacerbation and inhaler device handling: Real-life assessment of 2935 patients. *Eur Respir J.* 2017;49:1601794.

63. Melani AS, Bonavia M, Cilenti V, et al. Inhaler mishandling remains common in real life and is associated with reduced disease control. *Respir Med.* 2011;105(6):930–938.

64. Rootmensen GN, van Keimpema AR, Jansen HM, de Haan RJ. Predictors of incorrect inhalation technique in patients with asthma or COPD: A study using a validated videotaped scoring method. *J Aerosol Med Pulm Drug Deliv.* 2010;23(5):323–328.

65. Usmani O, Lavorni F, Marshal J, Dunlop WCN, Heron L, Farington E, Dekhuijzen R. Critical errors in asthma and COPD: A systematic review of impact on health outcomes. *Respir Res.* 2018; 19: 10.

66. Sulaiman I, Cushen B, Greene G, et al. Objective assessment of adherence to inhalers by COPD patients. *Am J Respir Crit Care Med.* 2017;195(10):1333–1343.

67. Bonini M, Usmani OS. Novel methods for device and adherence monitoring in asthma. *Curr Opin Pulm Med.* 2018;24(1):63–69.

68. Sanchis J. Has patient technique improved over time? *Chest.* 2016;150:394.

A critical perspective on future developments based on the knowledge we have now

TANIA F. BAHAMONDEZ-CANAS, JASMIM LEAL, AND HUGH D.C. SMYTH

Introduction   389
Why things happen in the field   390
Challenges in the clinical use of inhaler devices   392
Challenges in devices and formulation stability   392
    Systemic delivery   393

Proteins and peptides   393
Electronic devices   393
Future developments and major advances   394
References   394

INTRODUCTION

Although inhalation therapies date back more than 4000 years (1), the first modern systems are much more recent. For example, the first metered-dose devices were the Medihaler Iso™ and Medihaler Epi™ developed by Riker Laboratories beginning in the mid 1950s. With the first inhaler, pressurized metered-dose inhaler (pMDI), a new era of portable, multidose, metered-dose inhalers began and represented a milestone in the field (2,3). A few decades later, propellant gases used in pMDIs underwent a replacement and reformulation due to chlorofluorocarbon (CFC) ozone depletion issues. The CFC phase-out process was completed in the United States in 2013 (4). Early dry powder inhalers (DPIs) were developed before the first pMDIs (Aerohalor®, Abbott in 1944), but their widespread use was only realized later in response to the phase-out of CFC-propelled pMDIs. Today, DPIs are a widely accepted dosage form, and their use increasing steadily (5). Respimat® is the first of a new generation of active metered-dose devices known as Soft Mist™ Inhalers that have been commercialized and that do not require propellants and/or patient inspiratory effect for actuation (6–8).

In order to speculate on the future developments in the field of inhalation aerosols, it is pertinent to reflect on these developments and others to observe how advances and newer technologies succeed or fail in this specialized field. Figure 25.1 shows a timeline of selected major events in the field of orally inhaled delivery and therapeutics. As we can learn from this perspective, the adoption of novel technologies does not mean necessarily the end of an older technology. Also, the commercialization of newer technologies can often take decades. The pathway is likely strongly correlated to the significance of the unmet need that the technology is addressing and the complexity of the disease/device and associated regulatory hurdles.

By current standards, the development and regulatory approval of the first pMDI was extremely fast. It was approved only few months after the new drug application was filed and about a year after the idea was born. Today, the development and approval time frames can be on the order of about 7 years, and some take up to 19 years. Some examples are the first soft mist inhalers (SMIs), for which a patent was filed in 1995 (9) and approved by the U.S. Food and Drug Administration (FDA) in 2014 (10). The DPI technologies, Diskus® (11,12) and Flexhaler® (13,14), took 7 and 8 years, respectively, to reach the pharmaceutical market in the United States. Indeed, these and other antecedents may have guided the definition of deadlines for the phase-out of CFC-propelled pMDIs. Regulatory agencies respond to advances in the field to ensure the safety and efficacy of the new products. For example, the FDA recognized the importance of dose-counters in inhalers to improve disease management (15,16), by making them mandatory for pMDI products since 2003 (17).

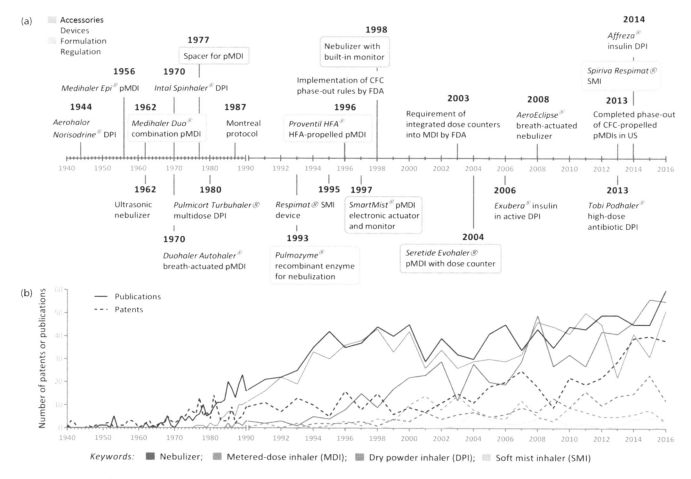

Figure 25.1 Timeline of major events in the field of orally inhaled delivery. (a) Milestones of the field, (b) results of keywords found in the title of patents and publications searched in Google Scholar, by year, from 1940 to 2016.

WHY THINGS HAPPEN IN THE FIELD

Originally, inhalation therapy was designed to treat local lung problems, and the first devices were designed to atomize therapeutics into a breathable mist. Today we have a better, though incomplete understanding of the mechanisms behind aerosolization processes and are uncovering the critical aspects that need to be addressed for a successful treatment from a pharmaceutical perspective. The relationship between particle size and lung deposition is widely understood; however, it is recognized that smaller particles, with much higher surface area, can be more difficult to generate. Also, the velocity of the emitted pMDI plume can make it difficult for some patients to synchronize with the inhalation; therefore, a significant fraction of the emitted dose can have an impact on the back of the throat (18). This issue directly drove the development of breath-actuated devices as well as spacer-type devices as an accessory for pMDIs to markedly reduce the deposition in the back of the throat (19).

Many patents and primary literature reports in the field state the problem of inhalation systems as the low efficiency of the delivery of the drug to the lung. Thus, this issue continues to attract great attention. A major

hindrance in inhalation aerosol development has also been recognized as the limited number of excipients found in approved products administered via the pulmonary route. Both limitations have directed the efforts primarily toward device design, whereas formulation innovation has been secondary, and particularly so in the DPI area. Certainly, mechanisms of dispersion and particle engineering have been widely investigated, but the greatest diversity of commercialized technologies has remained in the device space. This is reflected by the broad variety of DPI devices currently available on the market. Currently, without a significant improvement in the efficacy within recent and future devices, a plateau in device efficiency optimization may be reached, and different efforts are gaining prominence, such as technologies focused on the improvement of patient compliance or patient interface. In this line, more accessories that recognize patients' needs can be envisaged in the future to update current devices and customize the inhalation therapy. Figure 25.2 depicts the main elements that influence the development of the field: patient, formulation, and device.

Other reasons for technological innovations in the field include therapeutic need, intellectual property protection

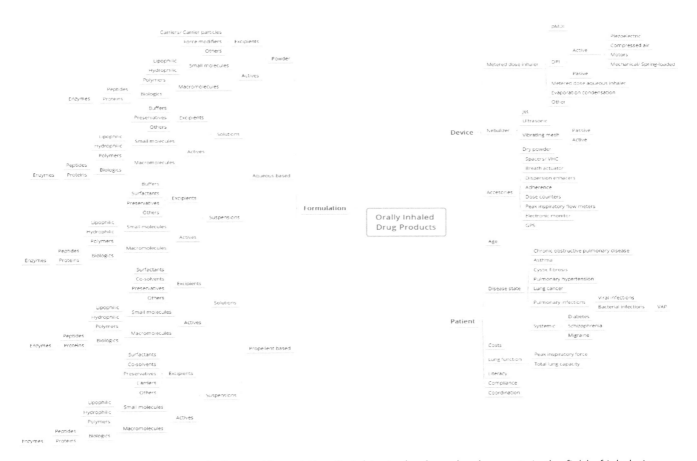

Figure 25.2 Triumvirate of patient, device, and formulation that drive technology developments in the field of inhalation aerosols.

and barriers to genericization, adoption of technologies from other fields, and regulatory pressure, among others. Some of these examples are outlined below.

Between 1850 and 1950, progressive advancements were made with nebulizer technology, with emerging devices able to deliver respirable aerosols for treatment of lung diseases (20), particularly for diseases requiring high pulmonary doses, and for patients with respiratory insufficiency (21). As mentioned previously, the development of the pMDI was instrumental in advancing the field (22–24). Those portable devices were able to deliver a range of different therapeutics to the lungs in a relatively consistent manner (25). Though these new devices had dramatic benefits over existing therapies, limitations of delivery to the lung were recognized (23,26). Thus, recent advances in pMDI technologies have been made in order to circumvent these limitation with the introduction of dose counters, breath-actuated devices, and electronic monitors (21,26,27). The new regulations around CFCs (28–30) also motivated the development and introduction of new and more efficient DPIs (20,23,31). DPI device technology has witnessed several milestones over the past few decades, with the introduction of multiple-unit dose and multi-dose devices and fixed dose combination products (32). Significant effort has been made to

understand the governing mechanisms of powder dispersion and particle interactions in DPIs, such as particle size, surface, density, and morphology, as well as lung deposition patterns (Figure 25.3), although this understanding still relies on significant empirical knowledge. However, this knowledge no doubt has contributed to improved products and the development of particle engineering technologies for improved DPI efficiency. Indeed, it was previously demonstrated that larger particles with low mass density not only are able to deposit in the lungs but also produced two times higher respirable fractions compared to small nonporous particles due to lower particle aggregation, thus efficiently delivering dry powder aerosols to the lungs and increasing the systemic bioavailability of inhaled drugs (33). Surprisingly, highly porous particles with low bulk density have still been a viable approach for higher dose delivery to the lung. One example is the TOBI Podhaler (Novartis), approved in 2013 by the FDA (34) for the treatment of lung infections in cystic fibrosis (CF) patients; it delivers high doses of tobramycin using DPIs (20). In terms of chronic therapies, decreasing the frequency of dosing (either by utilizing fixed-dose combinations or long-acting actives) has provided motivation for new products with potentially improved patient compliance (32).

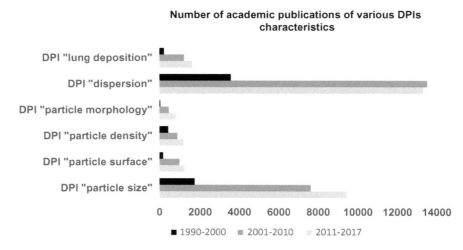

Figure 25.3 Number of academic publications of DPI particles and dispersion characteristics searched by keywords in Google Scholar, including patents and citations.

CHALLENGES IN THE CLINICAL USE OF INHALER DEVICES

Factors that may negatively affect the effectiveness of pulmonary inhalation aerosols include patient factors (coordination sub-optimal inhalation and breathing maneuvers, disease state) inhalation aerosol quality, and drug properties (35). It could be argued that technologies should be developed that obviate patient-related factors so that the success of the product is not dependent on these aspects. Indeed, there is some debate regarding optimal inhalation instructions for patients. For example, in pMDIs and nebulizers, rapid inhalation is not recommended to avoid turbulent and high-speed airflow, which is proposed to increase the deposition in the upper airways by inertial impaction (36). However, this is countered by newer products that are less sensitive to flow rates, such as Qvar®. In particular, Leach et al. showed that inhalation flow rates up to 137 L/min did not influence drug deposition in the airways (37). Similarly, "rules of thumb" for inhalation rates for DPIs may not apply across all devices and even different formulations within similar devices. Currently, inhalation therapy success relies heavily on proper training of correct inhalation technique to the patient by the healthcare professional. Technologies that can eliminate the need for training, ensure intuitive device operation, and enhance compliance are ideal but have yet to be realized.

CHALLENGES IN DEVICES AND FORMULATION STABILITY

Nebulizer formulation parameters such as droplet aerosol properties, viscosity, and surface tension are critical for a successful inhaled nebulizer therapy (21). Advances in the field have paralleled advances in microfabrication technologies, control systems, and patient interface understandings. These advancements are likely to continue for aqueous-based inhalation aerosols as droplet formation mechanisms,

for example, the behavior of non-Newtonian fluids and their influence in the droplet aerosol formation from nebulizers, become better understood (38). In addition, developments in device and formulation design addressing stability of the delivered cargo will be particularly important. Next-generation carriers (e.g., liposomes) as well as biopharmaceuticals such as proteins and peptides are particularly sensitive to shear applied during nebulization and interfacial forces that may cause aggregation, disruption, and stability issues (39,40). A significant challenge in pMDI drug formulations has been to maintain stability of the entire inhaler system over time. Dose and particle size can be affected due to instabilities in the formulation, resulting in inefficient or inconsistent inhalation therapy. For example, some formulations have been shown to react in the presence of aluminum containers, resulting in degradation (41). Also, drug deposition on the canister and metered valves can lead to aggregation and reduced shelf life (21). To reduce issues related with suspension stability, co-solvents such as ethanol have been used to solubilize surfactants and some drugs in pMDIs to yield solution formulations with hydrofluoroalkane (HFA) propellants (42,43). Yet the increase of ethanol concentration in a formulation may affect aerosol quality, particle deposition, and formulation performance. Indeed, it was demonstrated previously that increasing ethanol concentrations in budesonide solution-based pMDIs decreased the fine particle fraction (FPF) by approximately 50% over the ethanol co-solvent range in the study (43). Moreover, a direct correlation between an increase in ethanol concentration and mass median aerodynamic diameter (MMAD) as well as oropharynx deposition was found in the formulations. Advances in suspension-based systems using low-density drug carriers to enhance the physical stability of the suspension have already reached the market. Indeed, the realization that these technologies could then enable fixed-dose combination suspension products has led to the development of triple-drug combinations, which may be therapeutically preferred.

Formulations in DPIs contain internal forces resisting dispersion of the respirable particles into an aerosol of primary particles. During inhalation, the powder undergoes external forces such as airflow shear and drug–drug or drug-device impaction to decrease aggregation and aerosolize the drug powder. Inadequate powder mixtures might remain significantly aggregated due to cohesive and adhesive forces among particles compromising aerosol redispersion. The addition of excipients may help decrease strong cohesive forces, thus improving dispersion and enabling more uniform doses (32,44). Despite the relatively large amount of research into DPI formulations, the field remains in its infancy with regard to being able to develop mechanistic models or a well-defined design space. Significant improvements in our understanding of particle-particle adhesion forces will likely enable advances to be made in the area of detachment forces. In this area, DPI device design plays a major role in the product performance. Inhaler resistance, flow path design, detachment mechanism, and flow parameters remain a significant challenge to attain sufficient and efficient dispersion energy input into the powder (31,45,46).

Systemic delivery

Systemic delivery through the lungs has been in development since 1925 (20). Research in the delivery of insulin and other proteins and peptides increased significantly in the late 1980s. Among some technologies developed to deliver inhaled insulin systemically, Exubera® (Nektar Therapeutics and Pfizer) is of particular significance. Nektar and Pfizer conducted multiple clinical studies of Exubera, including the assessment of potential impacts of inhaled insulin on lung function, the comparative effectiveness study between smokers and nonsmokers, as well as safety and efficacy in asthma and chronic obstructive pulmonary disease (COPD) patients (47). In 2006, the FDA approved Exubera (48), with the condition that clinical trials were extended to monitor the effects of inhaled insulin on the lungs (20). One year later, Pfizer removed Exubera from the market due to a number of factors that have been reported differently (47,49). Despite some negative sentiment, there appears to be a significant increase in interest for the development of novel inhaled therapies for systemic diseases. Several products are in late-stage development, and many others can be found in publicly disclosed early pipelines.

PROTEINS AND PEPTIDES

Delivery of proteins and peptides has also been of interest recently, several being already commercialized or under clinical investigation for a number of diseases. These biologics include monoclonal antibodies, cytokines, hormones, immunoglobulins, interferons, and growth factors, among others (50). The first inhaled biological, Pulmozyme® (Dornase alfa, DNAse), was approved in 1993 for the treatment of CF (39,51). Yet proteins and peptides pose challenges

in the development of inhaled formulations. Stability is a major concern with those macromolecules, along with short half-lives, immunogenicity, and lack of precise dosing (52–54).

While some proteins can remain stable during aerosolization (e.g., DNase), proteins and peptides may be highly susceptible to the shear and stress conditions encountered in inhaler systems. The choice of an optimal inhaler device not only relies on sufficient pulmonary deposition and efficacy but also on the stability of the macromolecule in the aerosolization conditions. Individual molecule properties along with device limitations have to be considered in order to develop successful pulmonary delivery of proteins and peptides. Protein degradation and inactivation depend on the underlying mechanism of aerosol generation (39). In addition, increasing temperatures in ultrasound and vibrating mesh devices might contribute to the loss of protein and peptide activity (39). Proteins and peptides have been shown to lose biological activities after aerosolization (52). Thus, alternative approaches for increasing the stability after formulation and increasing the half-life of proteins and peptides have been used, such as polymers microspheres for sustained release or PEGylation of proteins (54,55). Depending on several factors, it has been estimated that half of the dose of a peptide molecule that reaches the lungs will be absorbed, resulting in low bioavailability (53,54). However, advances on novel pMDIs and DPIs allow the delivery of higher doses to the lungs (21,54).

Development of simple-to-administer, long-lasting, and stable inhaler immunization platforms eliminates the need for cold-chain complex transportation logistics and the potential for transmission of other diseases with the use of needles in remote areas without proper biohazard waste management and qualified trained personnel. Inhaled vaccines have been developed recently with promising results. A respiratory (nasal) recombinant adenovirus-based vaccine for protection against Ebola virus infection was tested in nonhuman primates and protected partially for 62 days after immunization (56). A live-attenuated measles dry powder vaccine delivered without reconstitution using two DPIs resulted in complete protection of rhesus macaques for more than one year (57). Similarly, inhaled vaccines have been developed for tuberculosis (58), and measles, mumps, and rubella (59).

ELECTRONIC DEVICES

In the era of digital technology, electronic smart inhaler devices are improving patient adherence to inhaled therapies (21). Recent improvements in software development and mobile apps allow clinicians to monitor patient treatment and compliance remotely, adding key information to problem-solving strategies related to patient adherence issues. In addition, the use of electronic technologies provides resources for patient self-monitoring, decision making, as well as disease management education, thus creating a shift toward patient-centered, personalized medical treatment (60).

FUTURE DEVELOPMENTS AND MAJOR ADVANCES

A recent informal survey of 25 experts in the field of inhalation aerosols on new technologies and major advances was conducted and sheds some light on potential future developments (61). Responses to this survey were varied but recognized inhalation aerosol technologies that are patient friendly. As mentioned previously, there is significant motivation to obviate patient-related factors so that the success of the product does not depend on controllable but patient-dependent aspects of therapy. The highlights of this survey included technologies related to patient adherence, the rebirth of breath-actuated devices, simple device operation, development of flow rate independent delivery systems, and technologies allowing a reduction in administration time for large doses. In terms of other technologies thought to become important in the future was the increased ability to target small airways and emerging developments of systems for aerosol delivery in the intensive care unit for intubated patients. Clearly, preclinical formulation discoveries made in the past decade are also progressing into late-stage and commercialized products (e.g., particle engineered formulations), but a significant driver of future developments will likely derive from the target product profiles of new chemical entities being developed for inhalation aerosols. The specific design requirements for each product will drive specific technologies toward commercialization. An example of this is the two major inhaled insulin programs that achieved regulatory approval, where engineering of the device and formulation enabled precise dosing of a macromolecule. New disease targets, different new chemical entities (NCEs) with varying physicochemical properties, and changing dose requirements (therapeutic window or higher payload) will drive future technology developments. Of course, these developments will be determined by the perceived regulatory hurdles and the risks of investment.

REFERENCES

1. Nerbrink O. A history of the development of therapy by jet nebulisation. In Gradoń L, Marijnissen J, eds., *Optimization of Aerosol Drug Delivery*. Dordrecht, the Netherlands: Springer, 2003, pp. 1–22.
2. Freedman T. Medihaler® therapy for bronchial asthma: A new type of aerosol therapy. *Postgraduate Medicine*. 1956;20(6):667–673.
3. Sanders M. Pulmonary drug delivery: An historical overview. In Smyth HDC, Hickey AJ, eds., *Controlled Pulmonary Drug Delivery*. New York: Springer, 2011, pp. 51–73.
4. FDA. Seven inhalers that use CFCs being phased out. 2010.
5. Atkins PJ. Dry powder inhalers: An overview. *Respiratory Care*. 2005;50(10):1304–1312.
6. Schürmann W, Schmidtmann S, Moroni P, Massey D, Qidan M. Respimat® Soft Mist™ inhaler versus hydrofluoroalkane metered dose inhaler. *Treatments in Respiratory Medicine*. 2005;4(1):53–61.
7. Ram FS, Carvallho CR, White J. Clinical effectiveness of the Respimat® inhaler device in managing chronic obstructive pulmonary disease: Evidence when compared with other handheld inhaler devices. *International Journal of Chronic Obstructive Pulmonary Disease*. 2011;6:129.
8. Dalby R, Spallek M, Voshaar T. A review of the development of Respimat® Soft Mist™ Inhaler. *International Journal of Pharmaceutics*. 2004;283(1):1–9.
9. Jaeger J, Cirillo P, Eicher J, Geser J.; Boehringer Ingelheim Gmbh., assignee. Device for producing high pressure in a fluid in miniature. United States patent US 5,964,416A. October 4, 1995.
10. US Food and Drug Administration (FDA) Approval Letter Spiriva Respimat NDA 21936. Available at https://www.accessdata.fda.gov/drugsatfda_docs/appletter/2014/021936Orig1s000ltr.pdf (accessed December 4, 2017).
11. Davies MB, Hearne DJ, Rand PK, Walker RI.; Glaxo Group Ltd., assignee. Inhalation device. United States patent US 5,873,360A. March 2, 1990.
12. US Food and Drug Administraion (FDA) Approval Letter Serevent Diskus NDA 20692. Available at https://www.accessdata.fda.gov/drugsatfda_docs/nda/97/020692s000_Serevent_AdminCorres.pdf (accessed December 4, 2017).
13. Dagsland A, Virtanen R.; Astrazeneca Ab., assignee. Inhalation device. United States patent US 7,143,764B1. March 13, 1998.
14. US Food and Drug Administraion (FDA) Approval Letter Pulmicort Flexhaler NDA 21949. Available at https://www.accessdata.fda.gov/drugsatfda_docs/appletter/2006/021949s000ltr.pdf (accessed December 4, 2017).
15. Given J, Taveras H, Iverson H, Lepore M. Prospective, open-label assessment of albuterol sulfate hydrofluoroalkane metered-dose inhaler with new integrated dose counter. *Allergy and Asthma Proceedings*. 2013;34(1):42–51.
16. Sander N, Fusco-Walker SJ, Harder JM, Chipps BE. Dose counting and the use of pressurized metered-dose inhalers: Running on empty. *Annals of Allergy, Asthma & Immunology*. 2006;97(1):34–38.
17. FDA. *Guidance for Industry: Integration of Dose-Counting Mechanisms into MDI Drug Products*. Washington, DC: U.S. Department of Health and Human Services Food and Drug Administration Center for Drug Evaluation and Research (CDER), 2003.
18. Crompton G. The adult patient's difficulties with inhalers. *Lung*. 1990;168:658–662.
19. Dolovich M, Ruffin R, Corr D, Newhouse M. Clinical evaluation of a simple demand inhalation MDI aerosol delivery device. *Chest*. 1983;84(1):36–41.
20. Stein SW, Thiel CG. The history of therapeutic aerosols: A chronological review. *Journal of Aerosol Medicine and Pulmonary Drug Delivery*. 2017;30(1):20–41.

21. Chan JG, Wong J, Zhou QT, Leung SS, Chan HK. Advances in device and formulation technologies for pulmonary drug delivery. *AAPS PharmSciTech.* 2014;15(4):882–897.

22. Grossman J. The evolution of inhaler technology. *Journal of Asthma.* 1994;31(1):55–64.

23. Sanders M. Inhalation therapy: An historical review. *Primary Care Respiratory Journal.* 2007;16(2):71–81.

24. Thiel C. From Susie's question to CFC free: An inventor's perspective on forty years of MDI development and regulation. In *Respiratory Drug Delivery.* Phoenix, AZ: Interpharm Press, Inc., 1996, pp. 115–123.

25. Hickey A. Summary of common approaches to pharmaceutical aerosol administration. In *Pharmaceutical Inhalation Aerosol Technology*, 2nd ed. New York: CRC Press, 2003.

26. Stein SW, Sheth P, Hodson PD, Myrdal PB. Advances in metered dose inhaler technology: Hardware development. *AAPS PharmSciTech.* 2014;15(2):326–338.

27. Bell J, Newman S. The rejuvenated pressurised metered dose inhaler. *Expert Opinion on Drug Delivery.* 2007;4(3):215–234.

28. Vervaet C, Byron PR. Drug–surfactant–propellant interactions in HFA-formulations. *International Journal of Pharmaceutics.* 1999;186(1):13–30.

29. Smyth HD. The influence of formulation variables on the performance of alternative propellant-driven metered dose inhalers. *Advanced Drug Delivery Reviews.* 2003;55(7):807–828.

30. McDonald KJ, Martin GP. Transition to CFC-free metered dose inhalers--into the new millennium. *International Journal of Pharmaceutics.* 2000;201(1):89–107.

31. de Boer AH, Hagedoorn P, Hoppentocht M, Buttini F, Grasmeijer F, Frijlink HW. Dry powder inhalation: Past, present and future. *Expert Opinion on Drug Delivery.* 2017;14(4):499–512.

32. Hoppentocht M, Hagedoorn P, Frijlink HW, de Boer AH. Technological and practical challenges of dry powder inhalers and formulations. *Advanced Drug Delivery Reviews.* 2014;75:18–31.

33. Edwards DA, Hanes J, Caponetti G, Hrkach J, Ben-Jebria A, Eskew ML, Mintzes J, Deaver D, Lotan N, Langer R. Large porous particles for pulmonary drug delivery. *Science.* 1997;276:1868–1871.

34. US Food and Drug Administraion (FDA) Approval Letter Tobi Podhaler NDA 201688. Available at https://www.accessdata.fda.gov/drugsatfda_docs/appletter/2013/201688Orig1s000ltr.pdf (accessed December 4, 2017).

35. Newman SP. Aerosol deposition considerations in inhalation therapy. *Chest.* 1985;88(2 Suppl):152s–160s.

36. Darquenne C. Aerosol deposition in health and disease. *Journal of Aerosol Medicine and Pulmonary Drug Delivery.* 2012;25(3):140–147.

37. Leach C. Effect of formulation parameters on hydrofluoroalkane-beclomethasone dipropionate drug deposition in humans. *Journal of Allergy and Clinical Immunology.* 1999;104(6):s250–s252.

38. Carvalho TC, McCook JP, Narain NR, McConville JT. Development and characterization of phospholipid-stabilized submicron aqueous dispersions of coenzyme Q10 presenting continuous vibrating-mesh nebulization performance. *Journal of Liposome Research.* 2013;23(4):276–290.

39. Hertel SP, Winter G, Friess W. Protein stability in pulmonary drug delivery via nebulization. *Advanced Drug Delivery Reviews.* 2015;93:79–94.

40. Elhissi A. Liposomes for pulmonary drug delivery: The role of formulation and inhalation device design. *Current Pharmaceutical Design.* 2017;23(3):362–372.

41. Wu Z-z, Thatcher ML, Lundberg JK, Ogawa MK, Jacoby CB, Battiste JL, Ledoux KA. Forced degradation studies of corticosteroids with an alumina-steroid-ethanol model for predicting chemical stability and degradation products of pressurized metered-dose inhaler formulations. *Journal of Pharmaceutical Sciences.* 2012;101(6):2109–2122.

42. Saleem IY, Smyth HDC. Tuning aerosol particle size distribution of metered dose inhalers using cosolvents and surfactants. *BioMed Research International.* 2013;2013:7.

43. Zhu B, Traini D, Chan H-K, Young PM. The effect of ethanol on the formation and physico-chemical properties of particles generated from budesonide solution-based pressurized metered-dose inhalers. *Drug Development and Industrial Pharmacy.* 2013;39(11):1625–1637.

44. Wong W, Fletcher DF, Traini D, Chan HK, Crapper J, Young PM. Particle aerosolisation and break-up in dry powder inhalers: Evaluation and modelling of impaction effects for agglomerated systems. *Journal of Pharmaceutical Sciences.* 2011;100(7):2744–2754.

45. Ibrahim M, Verma R, Garcia-Contreras L. Inhalation drug delivery devices: Technology update. *Medical Devices (Auckland, NZ).* 2015;8:131–139.

46. Frijlink HW, De Boer AH. Dry powder inhalers for pulmonary drug delivery. *Expert Opinion on Drug Delivery.* 2004;1(1):67–86.

47. Santos Cavaiola T, Edelman S. Inhaled insulin: A breath of fresh air? A review of inhaled insulin. *Clinical Therapeutics.* 2014;36(8):1275–1289.

48. US Food and Drug Administraion (FDA) Approval Letter Exubera NDA 21868. Available at https://www.accessdata.fda.gov/drugsatfda_docs/appletter/2006/021868s000ltr.pdf (accessed December 4, 2017).

49. Heinemann L. The failure of Exubera: Are we beating a dead horse? *Journal of Diabetes Science and Technology.* 2008;2(3):518–529.

50. Uchenna Agu R, Ikechukwu Ugwoke M, Armand M, Kinget R, Verbeke N. The lung as a route for systemic delivery of therapeutic proteins and peptides. *Respiratory Research*. 2001;2(4):198.

51. US Food and Drug Administration (FDA) Approved Drug Products Pulmozyme BLA 103532. Available at https://www.accessdata.fda.gov/scripts/cder/daf/index.cfm?event=overview.process&applno=103532 (accessed December 4, 2017).

52. Byron PR. Determinants of drug and polypeptide bioavailability from aerosols delivered to the lung. *Advanced Drug Delivery Reviews*. 1990;5(1):107–132.

53. Davis SS. Delivery of peptide and non-peptide drugs through the respiratory tract. *Pharmaceutical Science & Technology Today*. 1999;2(11):450–456.

54. Shoyele SA, Slowey A. Prospects of formulating proteins/peptides as aerosols for pulmonary drug delivery. *International Journal of Pharmaceutics*. 2006;314(1):1–8.

55. Thanoo BC, Sunny MC, Jayakrishnan A. Cross-linked chitosan microspheres: Preparation and evaluation as a matrix for the controlled release of pharmaceuticals. *The Journal of Pharmacy and Pharmacology*. 1992;44(4):283–286.

56. Choi JH, Jonsson-Schmunk K, Qiu X, Shedlock DJ, Strong J, Xu JX, Michie KL, et al. A single dose respiratory recombinant adenovirus-based vaccine provides long-term protection for non-human primates from lethal ebola infection. *Molecular Pharmaceutics*. 2015;12(8):2712–2731.

57. Lin W-H, Griffin DE, Rota PA, Papania M, Cape SP, Bennett D, Quinn B, et al. Successful respiratory immunization with dry powder live-attenuated measles virus vaccine in rhesus macaques. *Proceedings of the National Academy of Sciences*. 2011;108(7):2987–2992.

58. Tyne AS, Chan JG, Shanahan ER, Atmosukarto I, Chan HK, Britton WJ, West NP. TLR2-targeted secreted proteins from Mycobacterium tuberculosis are protective as powdered pulmonary vaccines. *Vaccine*. 2013;31(40):4322–4329.

59. Castro JFd, Bennett JV, Rincon HG, Munoz MTAy, Sanchez LAEP, Santos JI. Evaluation of immunogenicity and side effects of triple viral vaccine (MMR) in adults, given by two routes: Subcutaneous and respiratory (aerosol). *Vaccine*. 2005;23(8):1079–1084.

60. Himes BE, Weitzman ER. Innovations in health information technologies for chronic pulmonary diseases. *Respiratory Research*. 2016;17(1):38.

61. Smyth HD, Colthorpe P, George M, Jansen P, Fuglsang A, Armstrong KE, Lyapustina S. Highlights from the 2017 IPAC-RS/ISAM joint workshop "new frontiers in inhalation technology." *Journal of Aerosol Medicine and Pulmonary Drug Delivery*. 2018;31(4):199–203.

Ensuring effectiveness and reproducibility of inhaled drug treatment

ANTHONY J. HICKEY

Introduction	397	Statistical experimental design	399
General product quality	397	Statistical process control	399
Inhaled pharmaceutical products	398	Risk management	400
Product development considerations	399	Biopharmaceutical considerations	400
Target product profile	399	Conclusion	402
Quality by design	399	References	402
Process analytical technology	399		

INTRODUCTION

The major topics covered in this chapter relate to the product and the patient. The effort expended in controlling product performance establishes the foundation of ruggedness and overall quality that ensures accurate and reproducible dose delivery. General principles of quality by design (QbD) include statistical experimental design, process analytical technology, statistical process control, and risk management. Each of these activities is conducted in a controlled and regulated physical, data, and information environment. The interface of the dosage form with the patient introduces the variability associated with anatomy, physiology, drug disposition, metabolism, and pharmacology. The following discussion initially considers product quality strategies and concludes with patient variables.

GENERAL PRODUCT QUALITY

QbD as a foundation for product development and as a regulatory requirement has increased in prominence in the last decade (1–3). This is of particular importance for the development of inhaled products since the number of variables contributing to the quality and performance of these complex systems are numerous.

The major focus of QbD is to identify important variables influencing the product performance and ultimately affecting quality, efficacy, and safety. In order to explore which variables are important, it is necessary to identify all that impinge on specifications that drive performance. These variables can be assigned to specific product components or procedures.

The approach to product/process optimization was elaborated by Buckminster Fuller in a book describing critical path analysis where the need to capture all variable contributing to the desired product or outcome was emphasized (4). W. Edwards Deming had already identified the need for statistical approaches to the control of quality in product development (5).

A variety of tools are at the disposal of the pharmaceutical scientist in setting specification and performance expectations, including Ishikawa diagrams and GANTT charts (6,7). Ishikawa diagrams are excellent depictions of the relationship between variables and allow for structuring of the outcome of brainstorming sessions and input from a variety of sources before acting to explore the major variables. The impact of certain variables can frequently be assumed based on experience and attention, and these variables can be brought to bear on major variables of unknown impact. However, capturing all variables at the outset is the foundation for further investigation if unusual observations are made during the development process.

GANTT charts allow each process on a development sequence to be divided into its component parts and for clear decision points to be identified along the critical path. The sequence is not necessarily chronological, especially for activities that are not critical, but in broad terms, especially where time is a crucial defining element of the process, such as stability, the sequence does correspond with a time line.

Statistical experimental design can be employed for both product and process optimization. The original concept of multivariate statistical design was first published in the 1930s (8). It was popularized by George Box and colleagues and adopted widely at the end of the last century (9). The ability to explore process space and with sufficient data to define the surface response map with respect to key variables allows the product to be optimized to regions of insensitivity to input variables that make the performance robust, thus reducing the potential for manufacturing deviations from specifications.

Figure 26.1 illustrates the parallel functions of management and technical tools to ensure the quality of the product. Integration of these techniques through human and automated structural monitoring; decision making; and control of management, statistical, scientific, and technical components based on data and expertise ensures the product quality.

Several publications can be cited as examples of inhaled product performance optimization through statistical experimental design (10–12). International pharmaceutical aerosol consortium on regulation and science (IPAC-RS) has also discussed the application of QbD principles to orally inhaled drug product development (13,14).

Once specifications have been set on the product and processes, analytical controls can be used as a risk mitigation strategy. The key to the success of process analytical technology is this: the closer the method is to a real-time measurement, especially if it can be used to modulate input variables, the more likely it is to prevent deviations that can be both costly and time consuming if the need for formal investigation is required. The most common approach is to adopt online or inline methods that measure critical quality attributes defining the possibility/probability of a product meeting specified performance metrics, as shown in Figure 26.1.

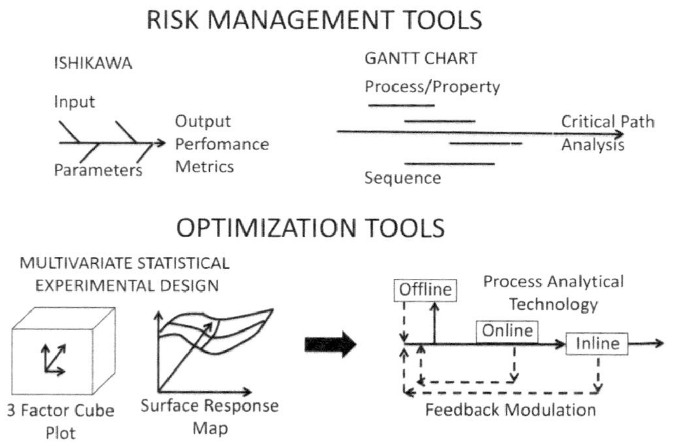

INHALED PHARMACEUTICAL PRODUCTS

Development of inhaled products is inherently a complex process because it represents the conjunction of chemistry, physics, and biology. Figure 26.2 depicts the major barriers to drug delivery. Each drug product consists of essentially three elements: the drug formulation, the metering system, and the aerosol-generating mechanism. The latter is usually an internal feature of the hardware components of the device. This combination of chemical and physical components is employed to create an aerosol of airborne particulates or droplets instantly in a nonequilibrium manner. The physics describing these aerosols dictates the efficiency of delivery (14,15). The aerosol is either directly, or though an auxiliary system directed to the inspiratory flow of the patient. Deposition of the aerosol in the lungs depends on patient effort, age, gender, and disease state. Dissolution and transport of drug depend on the site of deposition and the local conditions of the airways in terms of mucus, airway epithelial lining fluid, architecture, infection, and inflammation. In comparison to oral or parenteral drug delivery, the practical, regulatory, and financial challenge is substantial. However, the benefits for certain diseases outweigh the challenges. The ability to deliver potent therapeutic agents topically to the lung mucosa for direct local therapy, thus minimizing systemic exposure and off-target toxicity, has been shown to be valuable. For asthma and chronic

RISK MANAGEMENT TOOLS

ISHIKAWA

Input

Output
Perfomance
Metrics

Parameters

GANTT CHART

Process/Property

Critical Path
Analysis

Sequence

OPTIMIZATION TOOLS

MULTIVARIATE STATISTICAL
EXPERIMENTAL DESIGN

Offline

Process Analytical
Technology

Online

Inline

3 Factor Cube
Plot

Surface Response
Map

Feedback Modulation

Figure 26.1 Management and process tools applied to process and product development to ensure quality and performance of the dosage form.

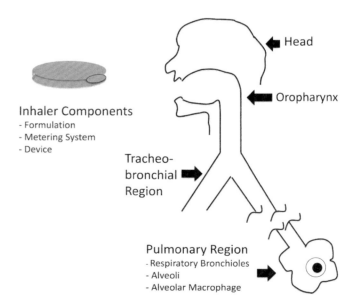

Inhaler Components
- Formulation
- Metering System
- Device

Head

Oropharynx

Tracheo-
bronchial
Region

Pulmonary Region
- Respiratory Bronchioles
- Alveoli
- Alveolar Macrophage

Figure 26.2 The physical elements of drug therapy include the inhaler and its components and the patient anatomy consisting broadly of the oropharynx, tracheobronchial, and pulmonary regions.

obstructive lung disease, enormous benefits have accrued in terms of life expectancy and quality of life for those afflicted with these diseases. A wider range of both local and systemic disease are being shown to be targets for inhaled therapy, and new technologies are being explored as described in earlier chapters of this book.

The task of relieving the symptoms or underlying cause of disease while minimizing undesired side effects is the major thrust of product development, and the need for quality control arises from the understanding of the therapeutic window (16). Ideally the margin of safety, the ratio of the maximum tolerated dose to the minimum effective dose, is large (16). Or more simply stated, therapy can be achieved at a dose that carries little to no risk of toxicity. The development process is guided by the intent to manufacture a product that accurately and reproducibly meets specification for an effective dose and thereby does not exhibit variations that could risk insufficiency for efficacy or exceeding the limit to cause toxicity.

The historical approach to combining these elements was to iterate on specifications and evaluate the performance of batches to establish quality metrics suitable to ensure the delivery of safe and effective doses. Since the beginning of the millennium, regulatory agencies have promoted a QbD approach in which sufficient control over manufacture and assembly is exercised to ensure the quality of the product. The focus on criticality is a major factor in the success of this approach, whether from the perspective of attributes or the development path.

PRODUCT DEVELOPMENT CONSIDERATIONS

Target product profile

The target product profile (TPP) is dictated by the needs of the disease therapy, the limitations and benefits of the desired technology, and potentially by manufacturing and regulatory considerations (3). Safe and effective inhaled therapy requires that an efficacious dose is delivered in a manner that can target the desired site for local (receptor or pathogen) or systemic (pathway for absorption) bioavailability. The performance characteristics over which control can be exercised are delivered dose and aerodynamic particle size distribution.

Quality by design

QbD has been a central tenet of engineering practices for decades, the best example being the implementation of six sigma practices (17). Pharmaceutical engineering has been a relatively late adopter of this general approach, despite the best efforts of process engineers consistent with the rest of their profession. The approach was embraced at the turn of the millennium by the publication of a guidance document by the U.S. Food and Drug Administration (FDA) promoting its use in pharmaceutical development (1,2,18,19). In addition, International

Conference on Harmonization of Technical requirements for Registration of Pharmaceuticals for Human Use (ICH) guidelines also now indicate the need for application of QbD principles (20). General principles have been applied to inhaled products (14,21).

The most effective approach to quality is to invest time and resources in identifying all parameters that might influence the process and the product. These parameters include both those that can be controlled and those that may be subject to limited or no control. The greater the knowledge of the process and the environment, the more likely is the prospect of ensuring the quality of the product.

PROCESS ANALYTICAL TECHNOLOGY

It is perhaps not surprising that the pharmaceutical industry was a latecomer to QbD. Most drug product manufacturing operations have involved batch processes whose input variables may be adjusted (22,23). Analytical instrumentation to monitor these processes has allowed control and modulation of operating conditions (24,25). The use of continuous processes allows for far greater control over the product at various stages of manufacture and allows for integration of risk assessment by monitoring critical attributes of the product (1,3).

STATISTICAL EXPERIMENTAL DESIGN

Statistical experimental design is the foundation of process and product development (26,27). Its basis is the use of multivariate analysis to allow for complete exploration of process or analytical space to identify the attributes that are critical to the final performance of the product (1,3). Once these attributes have been identified, they can be closely monitored and controlled to ensure that the product performance remains within the desired outcome specification for which regulatory approval was given.

STATISTICAL PROCESS CONTROL

Statistical process control is applied across the broad range of factors that contribute to a variety of outcomes that are important for the process and for the success of the product (28). Figure 26.3 illustrates the factors that might be considered in a typical process. In addition to the complex interplay of equipment, materials, and operational conditions (including the environment), other elements must be controlled. Staff expertise and training must be documented. Training logs establish that staff members are familiar with certain standard operating procedures (SOPs), and oversight processes must be in place. Documents and information must be controlled through validated electronic or paper repositories. These documents, whether they are SOPs, protocols, or drug manufacturing files (DMFs), become part of the output record to accompany output data and information.

Statistical process control assumes an understanding of some basic principles. First, all work to develop the product and maintain the environment involves process. Consequently, all engaged in these activities share the responsibility for quality management. Second, stability and variation in the process are necessary elements to engage in optimization.

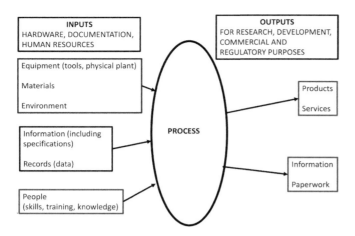

Figure 26.3 Materials, equipment, and human and environment factors influencing the product or service and information outcome of a process.

It is desirable that sufficient understanding of a process is gained before manufacturing to prevent unacceptable deviations and to minimize or eliminate the importance of their detection. Product failure should be treated with the same systematic investigation to address remedial action. Finally, blame has no role to play in decision making and is counterproductive to maintaining management control. Minimal educational requirements and common training of operators is a route to common understanding.

Risk management

The intent of each of the underpinning elements of QbD, including statistical experimental design and process control, is to mitigate the risk of making erroneous interventions or decisions. A systematic approach to implementation of monitoring and control strategies gives clear points of traction for managing the process and minimizing the risk of process or product failure. This has clear implications for consistency and conformity, leading to efficiency, increased productivity, and reduced expense. These outcomes are tied directly through the TPP and specification adherence to quality, safety, and efficacy through metrics defined according to critical quality attributes. As indicated in Figure 26.1, management tools are available to help identify critical steps in the process or product development activity and to adopt a human or automated decision-making strategy to respond in terms of relevant available resources (materials, equipment, staff, environment) to mitigate the risk.

BIOPHARMACEUTICAL CONSIDERATIONS

The interface between the product and the patient requires attention to translate controlled quality as established by performance measures into safe and efficacious therapeutic outcomes. This area has been the topic of significant research and debate over the last decade. An ideal to which many aspire is the development of an *in vitro* method that will predict disposition of drugs to and from the lungs sufficiently to manage the desired clinical outcome. Some progress has been made on this topic, but a standard approach has not emerged.

Figure 26.2 shows the fixed elements of therapy: the inhaler and the patient. The inhaler and its components have been thoroughly defined in terms of qualitative (Q1) and quantitative (Q2) regulatory considerations to ensure quality (29). The composition will have emerged from a thorough evaluation with respect to desired performance characteristics. However, the mechanism of aerosol dispersion and its interaction with the physiology of patient effort are dynamic. The latter is subject to a number of intrinsic variables, such as disease state, age, gender, training, coordination and adherence. Figure 26.4 illustrates these dependent variables. Mechanism of aerosol delivery depends on the product composition, and patient effort depends on the factors identified above and also the overall health of the patient that might influence the strength of the muscles employed in the required effort to breathe and inhale the drug. Patient effort is a work function that can be defined in terms of the combination of pressure drop (ΔP) that has to be overcome in the device to achieve a specific flow rate (Q). The term for this function is *power* ($Q.\Delta P$) or *work done per unit time* (30).

The key performance properties, recognized by regulatory and compendial guidance documents, as influencing the quality and, by inference, the safety and efficacy of orally inhaled drug products (OIDPs) are delivered dose and aerodynamic particle size distribution. The aerosol delivery rate and particle dissolution properties may also play a role in the performance of some OIDPs. Delivered dose dictates the absolute amount of drug that is delivered to the patient. The aerodynamic particle size distribution (APSD) (31–33) and aerosol delivery rate (ADR) (34–36) dictate the site of deposition in the lungs. Dissolution dictates the initial step in bioavailability of the drug once it has deposited (37). Regional deposition and dissolution

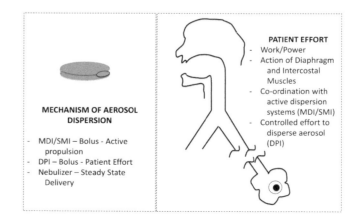

Figure 26.4 Dynamic variables of mechanism of aerosol generation and physiology of patient effort overlaid on the drug product and anatomy to achieve drug delivery.

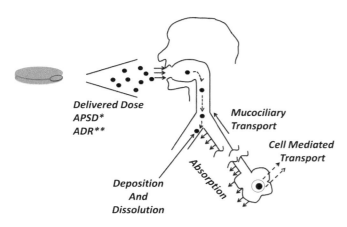

*Aerodynamic Particle Size Distribution
**Aerosol Delivery Rate

Figure 26.5 Performance properties of an aerosolized drug and its influence on deposition and initial disposition (dissolution) in the lungs and mechanisms of clearance that contribute to the overall pharmacokinetics.

rate are important because they dictate the influence that specific clearance mechanisms have on transport of drug. Figure 26.5 shows the impact of the inhaler components and aerosol delivery in combination with the anatomy and physiology of the patient in terms of aerosol properties and lung deposition.

The basis for establishing uniformity of product performance can be generalized up to the point that the specific target, tissue, cell, or receptor needs consideration. As a consequence, it is likely that generalized models of the product quality can extend only to the deposition in the lungs and release of drug in the dissolution process. The performance requirements that are unique to the disease and the patient may result in some adjustment of specifications to accommodate local efficiency of delivery. Figure 26.5 also depicts the dynamic product performance characteristics and the interface with the physiological mechanisms of disposition, absorption, and mucociliary and cell-mediated transport that influence the efficiency and reproducibility of delivery of drug to the site of action (38).

APSD characteristics are major endpoints in establishing the quality of the product since they reflect the accuracy and precision with which an aerosol can be produced and, by inference, ensure reproducible delivery to the lungs (32,33). Indeed, inertial impaction, the method by which APSD is measured, has received QbD consideration (13,39). However, there are significant limitations to the use of inertial impactors as predictors of whole or regional lung deposited dose. Most significantly, inertial impactors are calibrated at fixed flow rates, which do not mimic inspiratory flow cycles. Two methods have been devised to compensate for this deficiency. The first is to use an inspiratory flow cycle to sample through the impactor, which inherently loses the calibration of the instrument and its utility for particle sizing. The second approach is to use a mixing inlet and to generate the aerosol with an inspiratory flow cycle

but allow the impactor to continue to operate at a fixed flow rate, thereby retaining the calibration and allowing particle sizing to occur (40). The latter more accurately reflects the performance of the inhaler as it might be used by the patient but still does nothing to predict the likely deposition in the patient. There is a fortuitous convergence of lung deposition and cascade impaction operated under these conditions at a cut-off size of 3 μm that appears to be predictive (41). The proportion of the aerosol below 3 μm appears to correlate directly with lung deposition. Knowledge of the proportion of the distribution in particle sizes above and below 3 μm seems to be irrelevant to lung deposition.

Others have focused on the way in which the aerosol is sampled and, rather than attempt to superimpose inertial impaction data on lung deposition, have explored the relationship between deposition in oropharyngeal casts representing different sizes (ages) of individual (42). From sampling a number of inhaled products, both dry powder inhaler (DPI) and pressurized metered-dose inhaler (pMDI), for which lung deposition data was available, a correlation was established between cast deposition and *in vivo* lung deposition.

Theoretical and experimental approaches to modeling human lung deposition of pharmaceutical aerosols have a high probability of accurately and reproducibly predicting the lung dose. However, more work is required to refine experimental models sufficiently to predict regional deposition, but theoretical models generate good approximations. Of course, each person exhibits unique deposition based on anatomy and physiology, and all models are, at some level, averaging their results to make population predictions. This source of variation will be overcome only if a personalized medicine approach appears in the coming years.

As depicted in Figure 26.5, clearance plays an important role in the effectiveness of drug delivery to the target site in the lungs. The major clearance mechanisms are absorption and mucociliary and cell-mediated transport. The site of deposition dictates the combination of clearance mechanisms that prevail and other local phenomena that may influence disposition (35,38). Absorption occurs throughout the respiratory tract. In the tracheobronchial region, transport to the bronchial circulation occurs (43). Transport to the pulmonary blood supply, which is in intimate association with the alveoli to support gaseous exchange, happens in the periphery (43). The large surface area and short distance from airways to vasculature resulting from local cell structure in the periphery makes this the target for rapid uptake to treat systemic rather than local disease.

For materials that exhibit delayed dissolution for whatever reason (low solubility, impeded dissolution due to the presence of additives) that deposit in the tracheobronchial airways, mucociliary transport will influence disposition. The magnitude of its effect depends on the dissolution rate of the particle. The region from which transport or translocation to the local site of action occurs requires presentation of the drug in the molecular state. To illustrate the importance of this mechanism, two situations can be considered while recognizing that a range of intermediate phenomena may occur. Highly soluble materials are available for absorption/action at the site of deposition, and they are only influenced by local permeability; poorly soluble materials present at each site where they are cleared by a combination of dissolution and mucociliary transport rates and local permeability.

Materials that exhibit delayed dissolution in the periphery, and depending on their geometric particle size characteristics, are taken up by alveolar macrophages that may act as a depot for release or degrade the drug depending on its composition. As indicated earlier, the extent of the influence of this mechanism depends on the local solubility of the drug and the rate at which it dissolves.

So far, the biological disposition of the drug has been considered at large spatial scales of scrutiny: the whole and regional disposition in the lungs and systemic disposition, through the vascular circulation. It should also be acknowledged that, at a molecular scale, there are further barriers to be overcome at each of the sites of deposition. The thickness and composition of airway lining fluid varies throughout the respiratory tract. Consequently, each site of deposition presents a different dissolution medium. Mucus is a complex material composed of a glyco- and lipo-protein matrix that presents a diffusion barrier with respect to the molecular weight, charge, and other properties of the drug (44–46). In the periphery, a layer of surfactant is the only barrier to penetration to the epithelium (47). Once inside epithelial or surrounding tissue cells, drugs may be subject to the action of efflux transporters or metabolic enzymes that further influence the potential to reach the site of action (48–50). The extent and nature of transport and metabolism depends on the chemical structure of the drug and is usually influenced by its similarity to endogenous substances.

The overall complexity of the challenge facing those in inhaled pharmaceutical product development can be conveyed by combining Figures 26.2, 26.4, and 26.5 to indicate all of the macroscale factors influencing effective and reproducible therapy, as shown in Figure 26.6. Of course, the molecular scale variables add an additional level of complexity. A great deal of progress has been made in understanding and controlling the drug product and aerosol performance characteristics. An effort is underway to translate that into a prediction of the biological disposition and development of appropriate tools to evaluate disposition both in terms of pharmacokinetics and pharmacodynamics, and perhaps to develop an inhaled biopharmaceutical classification system (29,51,52). However, more scientific research into the biology of drug disposition from the lungs is required to define the limits to predictive modeling.

The recent focus on feedback control systems to enable the patient to monitor her or his effort or the use of systems that control patient breathing is likely to improve physiological reproducibility (53–55). In turn, improved uniformity in subsequent biological disposition might emerge. Whether improvement in variability in effort arising from

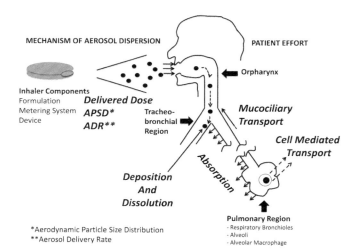

Figure 26.6 Physical and anatomical systems (inhaler and lungs) on which dependent performance and physiological dynamics (aerosol generation and patient effort) are overlaid, thus defining key properties (APSD, delivered dose [DD], ADR) that dictate lung deposition and disposition (dissolution).

the fluctuations in pulmonary function of a single patient can translate to overall improvement in the population being treated will be evident only when sufficient outcome data have been collected.

CONCLUSION

Control of the performance of inhaled pharmaceutical products as measured by uniformity of quality is linked to reproducibility of efficacy and safety. Control may be exercised through practices of QbD in product development and through training and adherence to therapy of the patient. The anatomical, pathophysiological, and pharmacological variability within and between patients mediate between the uniformity of the product and anticipated therapeutic outcomes. The recent focus on patient feedback and breath control systems are steps toward greater physiological reproducibility. The challenge is to extend knowledge sufficiently to define the absolute limit to the ability to predict drug disposition and to effect maximum control over pharmacological performance.

REFERENCES

1. Yu L. Pharmaceutical quality by design. Product and process development, understanding and control. *Pharmaceutical Research.* 2008;25:781–791.
2. Yu L, Amidon G, Khan M, Hong S, Polli J, Raju G, Woolcock J. Understanding pharmaceutical quality by design. *AAPS Journal.* 2014;16:771–783.
3. Pramod K, Tahir A, Charoo N, Ansari S, Ali J. Pharmaceutical product development: A quality by design approach. *International Journal of Pharmaceutical Investigation.* 2016;6:129–138.

4. Fuller RB. *Critical Path*. New York: St. Martin's Press, 1981.

5. Deming W. *Quality, Productivity and Competitive Position*. Cambridge, MA: MIT Press, 1982.

6. Liliana L. A new model of Ishikawa diagram for quality assessment. *IOP Conference Series: Materials Science and Engineering*. 2016;161:012099.

7. Geraldi J, Lechter T. Gantt charts revisited: A critical analysis of its roots and implications to the management of projects today. *International Journal of Managing Projects in Business*. 2012;5:578–594.

8. Cramer E, Rock R. Multivariate analysis. *Review of Educational Research*. 1966;36:604–617.

9. Box G, Hunter W, Hunter J. *Statistics for Experimenters. An Introduction to Design, Data Analysis and Model Building*. New York: John Wiley & Sons, 1978.

10. O'Hara P, Hickey A. Respirable PLGA microspheres containing rifampicin for the treatment of tuberculosis: Manufacture and characterization. *Pharmaceutical Research*. 2000;17:955–961.

11. Taylor M, Hickey A, VanOort M. Manufacture, characterization, and pharmacodynamic evaluation of engineered ipratropium bromide particles. *Pharmaceutical Development and Technology*. 2006;11:321–336.

12. Telko M, Hickey A. Aerodynamic and electrostatic properties of model dry powder aerosols: A comprehensive study of formulation factors. *AAPS PharmSciTech*. 2014;15:1378–1397.

13. Tougas T, Christopher D, Mitchell J, Lyapustina S, Oort MV, Bauer R, VanOort M, Glaab V. Product lifecycle approach to cascade impaction measurements. *AAPS PharmSciTech*. 2011;12:312–322.

14. Bowles N, Cahill E, Haberlin B, Jones C, Mett I, Mitchell J, Muller-Walz R, et al. Application of quality by design to inhalation products. *RDD Europe*. 2007;1:61–70.

15. Xu Z, Hickey A. The physics of aerosol droplet and particle generation from inhalers. In Smyth H, Hickey A, eds., *Controlled Pulmonary Drug Delivery*. New York: Springer, 2011, pp. 75–100.

16. Klaassen C, III JW. *Casarett and Doull's Toxicology The Basic Science of Poisons Companion Handbook*, 5th ed. New York: McGraw-Hill, 1999, pp. 21–23.

17. Schroeder R, Linderman K, Liedtke C, Choo A. Six sigma: Definition and underlying theory. *Journal of Operations Management*. 2008;26:536–554.

18. US Food and Drug Administration. *Guidance for Industry: Q8(R2) Pharmaceutical Development*. Washington DC: US Department of Health and Human Services; 2009.

19. Lionberger R, Lee S, Lee L, Raw A, Yu L. Quality by design concepts for ANDAs. *AAPS Journal*. 2008;10:268–276.

20. http://www.ich.org [Internet].

21. Sallam A, Nazzal S, AlKahatib H, Darwazeh N. Quality by design: Concept for product development of dry powder inhalers. In Nokhodchi A, Martin G, eds., *Pulmonary Drug Delivery Advances and Challenges*. New York: Springer, 2015, pp. 321–338.

22. Lee S, O'Connor T, Yang X, Cruz C, Chatterjee S, Madurawe R, Moore C, Yu L, Woodcock J. Modernizing pharmaceutical manufacturing: From batch to continuous processing. *Journal of Pharmaceutical Innovation*. 2015;10:191.

23. O'Connor T, Yu L, Lee S. Emerging technology: A key enabler for modernizing pharmaceutical manufacturing and advancing product quality. *International Journal of Pharmaceutics*. 2016;25:492–498.

24. Barrett P, Smith B, Worlitschek J, Bracken V, O'Sullivan B, O'Grady D. A review of the use of process analytical technology for the understanding and optimization of production batch crystallization processes. *Organic Process Research and Development*. 2005;9:348–355.

25. Rantanen J, Khinast J. The future of pharmaceutical manufacturing sciences. *Journal of Pharmaceutical Sciences*. 2015;104:3612–3638.

26. Anderson T. *An Introduction to Multivariate Statistical Analysis*. New York: John Wiley & Sons, 1958.

27. Cochran W, Cox G. *Experimental Designs*. New York: John Wiley & Sons, 1957.

28. Oakland J, Followell R. *Statistical Process Control*. 2nd ed. Oxford, UK: Heinnemann Newnes, 1990.

29. Forbes B, Backman P, Christopher D, Dolovich M, Li B, Morgan B. In vitro testing for orally inhaled products: Developments in science-based regulatory approaches. *AAPS Journal*. 2015;17:837–852.

30. Dunbar C, Morgan B, Oort MV, Hickey A. A comparison of dry powder inhaler dose delivery characteristics using a power criterion. *PDA Journal of Pharmaceutical Science and Technology*. 2000;54:478–484.

31. US Food and Drug Administration. Draft Guidance for the industry, metered dose inhaler (MDI) and dry powder inhaler (DPI) chemistry manufacturing and controls documentation. 1998.

32. ICRP Task Group on Lung Dynamics. Deposition and retention models for internal dosimetry of the human respiratory tract. *Health Physics*. 1966;12:173–207.

33. Heyder J, Gebhart J, Rudolf G, Schiller C, Stahlhofen W. Deposition of particles in the human respiratory tract in the size range 0.005–15um. *Journal of Aerosol Science*. 1986;17:811–825.

34. Ziffels S, Durham P, Bemelmans N, Hickey A. In vitro dry powder inhaler formulation performance considerations. *Journal of Controlled Release*. 2015;199:45–52.

35. Hickey A. Controlled delivery of inhaled therapeutic agents. *Journal of Controlled Release*. 2014;190:182–188.

36. Hickey A. Complexity in pharmaceutical powders for inhalation: A perspective. *KONA Powder and Particle Journal*. 2017(35):Advanced pub J-stage.

37. Gray V, Hickey A, Balmer P, Davies N, Dunbar C, Foster T, Olsson B, et al. The inhalation ad hoc advisory panel for the USP performance tests of inhalation dosage forms. *Pharm Forum*. 2008;34:1068–1074.

38. Mortensen N, Hickey A. Targeting inhaled therapy beyond the lungs. *Respiration*. 2014;88:353–364.

39. Mitchell J, Nagel M, Doyle C, Ali R, Avvakoumova V, Christopher J, Quiroz J, Strickland H, Tougas T, Lyapustina S. Relative precision of inhaler aerodynamic particle size distribution (APSD) metrics by full resolution and abbreviated Andersen cascade impactors (ACIs): Part 1. *AAPS PharmSciTech*. 2010;11:845–851.

40. Nadarassan D, Assi K, Chrystyn H. Aerodynamic characterstics of a dry powder inhaler at low flows using a mixing inlet with an Andersen Cascade Impactor. *European Journal of Pharmaceutical Sciences*. 2010;39:348–354.

41. Newman S, Chan H-K. In vitro/In vivo comparisons in pulmonary drug delivery. *Journal of Aerosol Medicine and Pulmonary Drug Delivery*. 2008;21:77–84. doi:10.1089/jamp.2007.0643.

42. Olsson B, Borgstom L, Lundback H, Svensson M. Validation of a general in vitro approach for prediction of total lung deposition in healthy adults for pharmaceutical inhalation products. *Journal of Aerosols in Medicine and Pulmonary Drug Delivery*. 2013;26:355–369.

43. Hickey A, Thompson D. Physiology of the airways. In Hickey A, ed., *Pharmaceutical Inhalation Aerosol Technology*. 2nd ed. New York: Marcel Dekker, 2004, pp. 1–29.

44. Button B, Button B. Structure and function of the mucu clearance system of the lung. *Cold Spring Harbor Perspectives in Medicine*. 2013;3:a009720.

45. Lillehoj E, Kim K. Airway mucus: Its components and function. *Archives of Pharmaceutical Research*. 2002;25:770–780.

46. Rubin B. Physiology of airway mucus clearance. *Respiratory Care*. 2002;47:761–768.

47. Hamm H, Kroegel C, Hohlfeld A. Surfactant: A review of its functions and relevance in adult respiratory distress disorders. *Respiratory Medicine*. 1996;90:251–270.

48. Ehrhardt C, Backman P, Couet W, Edwards C, Forbes B, Friden M, Gumbleton M, et al. Current progress toward a better understanding of drug disposition within the lungs: Summary proceedings of the first workshop on drug transporters in the lungs. *Journal of Pharmaceutical Sciences*. 2017;106:2234–2244.

49. Sporty J, Horalkova L, Ehrhardt C. In vitro cell culture models for the assessment of pulmonary drug disposition. *Expert Opinion on Drug Metabolism & Toxicology*. 2008;4:333–345.

50. Olsson B, Bondesson E, Borgstrom L, Edsbacker S, Eirefelt S, Ekelund K, Gustavsson L, Hegelund-Myrback T. Pulmonary drug metabolism, clearance and absorption. In Smyth H, Hickey A, eds., *Controlled Pulmonary Drug Delivery*. New York: Springer, 2011, pp. 21–50.

51. Hastedt J, Backman P, Clark A, Doub W, Hickey A, Hochhaus G, Kuehl P, et al. Scope and relevance of a pulmonary biopharmaceutical classification system AAPS/FDA/USP Workshop March 16–17th, 2015 in Baltimore, MD. *AAPS Open*. 2016;2:1.

52. Sbirlea-Apiou G, Newman S, Fleming J, Seikmeier R, Ehrmann S, Scheuch G, Hochhaus G, Hickey A. Bioequivalence of inhaled drugs: Fundamentals, challenges and perspectives. *Therapeutic Delivery*. 2013;4:343–367.

53. Geller D, Kesser K. The I-neb adaptive aerosol delivery system enhances delivery of alpha1-antitrypsin with controlled inhalation. *Journal of Aerosol Medicine and Pulmonary Drug Delivery*. 2010;23(Suppl 1):S55–S59.

54. Fischer A, Stegemann J, Scheuch G, Siekmeier R. Novel devices for individualized controlled inhalation can optimize aerosol therapy in efficacy, patient care and power of clincial trials. *European Journal of Medical Research*. 2009;14(Suppl 4):71.

55. Carpenter D, Roberts C, Sage A, George J, Home R. A review of electronic devices to assess inhaler technique. *Current Allergy and Asthma Reports*. 2017;17:17.

27

Conclusion

ANTHONY J. HICKEY AND HEIDI M. MANSOUR

Dose	405	Dissolution	407
Aerodynamic particle size distribution	406	Disease	407
Other	407	References	407
Aerosol delivery rate	407		

An increasing interest in the potential for inhaled therapy for the treatment of a wide range of diseases demands an understanding of the opportunities and challenges that will occur. The foundation of scientific and technical principles on which inhaled therapy is based was established over a period of approximately 50 years and continues to be elaborated as new approaches emerge. There are a large number of introductory and specialized texts on the topics of inhaled medicines, pharmaceutical aerosols, and pulmonary drug delivery. The intent in this text has been to adopt a structure that relates directly to clinical translation.

An overview of the physical chemistry, aerosol physics, biology of drug disposition, and device and product considerations was considered a necessary introduction and reference for the remainder of the text. Subsequent chapters focused on specific diseases and their aerosol treatment, highlighting the specific barriers that need to be overcome and the solutions adopted from the range of options available. Some of these options were developed uniquely for a particular disease therapy. The necessarily diverse discussion arising from each of these diseases has been placed in two integrated contexts. Dosage form and disease general observations may be useful to consider during product development. In addition, their influence on quality, safety, and efficacy should be elements of the overarching development framework.

The development of a target product profile draws on many of the points that have been emphasized throughout this text. Items that should be considered are dose, aerodynamic particle size distribution, and other measures such as aerosol delivery and dissolution rates.

DOSE

The nominal dose of drug required to treat the disease depends on the inherent pharmacology (potency), the nature of the disease, age of the patient, and possibly the gender of the patient. Genotypic and phenotypic differences may also play a role, and the best current examples are cystic fibrosis and drug-resistant microorganisms. There are a number of ways to consider dose, each of which reflects the efficiency of transitioning through delivery of the drug aerosol. Figure 27.1 illustrates terms employed for dose.

Unlike oral drug delivery, where the dose is clear in the sense that the nominal dose in the tablet or capsule is ingested by the patient and there is no equivocation about the amount of drug that is delivered. Inhaled therapy involved multiple steps in which the dose delivered is a function of intervening events. It was noted over two decades ago that the contribution of each of these elements of delivery contributes, through compound functions, to the therapeutic dose (1). The following expression captures the dose in terms of functions of different elements of drug delivery

Dose α f(components) • f(formulation) • f(metering system) • f(device) • f(anatomy) • f(respiratory effort) • f(age) • f(gender) • f(disease state)

As depicted in Figure 27.1, the first step in the reduction in the amount of drug delivered is the role of the combined composition, formulation, metering system, and device in limiting the dose emitted from the device and delivered

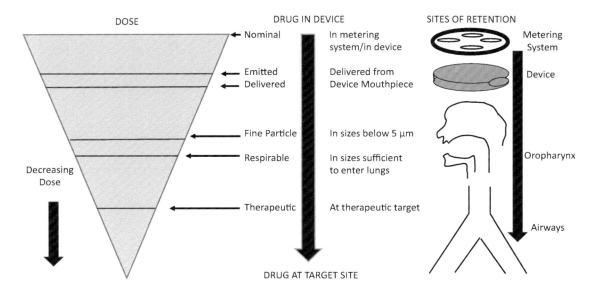

Figure 27.1 Dose segmentation as a result of efficiency of delivery and retention in various locations, including the metering system device and the upper and lower airways.

to the patient. For dry powder inhalers (DPIs), the emitted dose and delivered dose are identical, whereas for pressurized metered-dose inhalers (pMDIs) and nebulizers, there may be minor differences between them, or there may be major differences if, in the case of pMDIs, spacers are employed or, in the case of nebulizers, the aerosol is exhausted between inspiratory cycles. The next major limitation on dose is the proportion of the aerosol that is respirable, that is, the fraction that can pass the oropharynx and enter the lungs. Two terms are often used interchangeably that have completely different definitions and absolute values. The term *fine particle dose* (or *fine particle fraction* if expressed as a percentage of nominal or emitted dose) is a quality measure of particles in a size range that statistically have a high probability of entering the lungs. This can specifically be assigned to the proportion of the aerodynamic particle size distribution (APSD) below 5 μm, or it can be somewhat arbitrarily assigned to particles below a certain cut-off diameter in an inertial sampler such as the Andersen cascade impactor of 5.8 μm at 28.3 L/min 1 American cubic foot per minute (1ACFM) or the two-stage liquid impinger of 6.4 μm at 60 L/min (2). In contrast, the *respirable dose* (or *respirable fraction*) is based on known lung deposition and is a composite term made up of probabilities of all particles below 10 μm depositing in the lungs where smaller particles have a higher probability than larger ones. This approach has significance for determining risk and was first developed by organizations such as the American Conference on Government and Industrial Hygienists (3).

The reduction in dose to the target site up to the point described in the previous paragraph is defined clearly, and all steps are subject to measurement from which quality of performance can be translated into lung delivery. Unfortunately,

the last step, defining the therapeutic dose, is not currently subjected to the same level of scrutiny. The location of certain receptors in the lungs or the likely site of infection can be defined, but the drug availability at the specific site of action is limited by the dissolution of particles and the residence time (as dictated by clearance mechanisms). The instantaneous amount of drug present to act depends on competing kinetic phenomena that are subject only to measurement in *in vitro* models or by inference from the pharmacokinetics of systemic appearance. Consequently, the last step does not allow a formal definition of the therapeutic dose. As a result, bioequivalence testing is currently constrained to a combination of tests that give approximations that have yet to be fully accepted as predictors of performance (4,5).

AERODYNAMIC PARTICLE SIZE DISTRIBUTION

There is a modest opportunity to manipulate APSD to accommodate the perceived barriers to delivery of aerosols in a specific disease. While considerable research has been conducted on the influence of aerodynamic diameter on lung delivery using both monodisperse and polydisperse aerosols, there is no consensus on the ideal particular size distribution. Generally speaking, it is acknowledged that there is sufficient control of aerosol particle delivery to achieve predominantly central or peripheral deposition by adjusting the median diameter between 1 and 5 μm. However, it is not clear that deposition at a specific level of branching within the lungs is either feasible or desirable. Moreover, the desired target for therapeutic agents for specific diseases has not been localized to specific airway generations.

OTHER

Aerosol delivery rate

Two other measures of inhaled product performance might be valuable in narrowing down dose delivery estimations sufficiently to give an adequate approximation of likely bioavailability: aerosol delivery rate and dissolution. First, the aerosol delivery rate relating to the point at which the aerosol is introduced on the inspiratory flow has an impact on the site of deposition (6,7). This is particularly important for DPIs and pMDIs. Capsule or blister emptying may affect the rate of delivery and thereby likely the site of drug deposition from DPIs. pMDIs often require coordination, and if the patient does not coordinate correctly with delivery, the point on the inspiratory flow that the aerosol is placed dictates how far into the lungs the drug can penetrate. Nebulizers are not affected by this phenomenon because the aerosol is inhaled from a near steady-state dispersion.

Dissolution

When solid particles deposit in the airways, dissolution is required for the drug to be available in the molecular state at the site of action (8–10). For highly soluble, rapidly dissolving drugs, this step is presumably not a barrier to bioavailability. However, given the limited airway lining fluid for dissolution if a substance with low solubility and slow dissolution dissolves, this may well become a significant barrier to bioavailability and therapeutic effect. There is no evidence for existing products that this phenomenon impedes therapy. This may well be explained by the temporal effect of the dosing regimen controlling the symptoms and underlying cause of disease such that the impact of a single dose and its pharmacokinetics are mitigated. Steroid therapy of asthma, for example, takes days or weeks to control the disease and the performance of a single dose is not likely to influence the outcome. Nevertheless, dissolution rate may well be the cause of some variability in response. Further study is required to establish the extent to which dissolution is a valuable measure of quality, safety, and efficacy.

Disease

Clearly, factors that influence the anatomy of physiology of the lungs will affect lung deposition and potentially therapeutic outcome (see Chapters 2 and 25). The common considerations are age and gender. However, the most significant influence derives from the disease and its influence on the normal lung structure. The disease influences the deposition of the aerosol but, more significantly, it may change the nature of the drug target. For example, where microorganisms are located in granulomas or bronchiectatic regions, the nature of the final step in drug delivery following deposition remains unknown since these are not ventilated parts of the lungs and require an extra transport step through tissue. At the cellular level, certain infectious organisms are capable of producing biofilms that present another barrier to the delivery of the drug for which specific strategies may be required if therapy is to be achieved. The influence of disease, whether it is airway narrowing and hyperplasia in asthma and chronic obstructive pulmonary disease (COPD), or more complex airway, cellular, or molecular barriers for *Pseudomonas aeruginosa* and nontuberculous mycobacterial infections in cystic fibrosis, cannot be understated. The inability to generalize the factors influencing the anatomy and physiology of diseased airways may require a complete change in the approach to therapy if the intention is to predict the response from first principles. It may be possible to predict outcomes of drug delivery only from specific pharmaceutical aerosol dosage forms by acquiring data on individual airway structure and function. Therapy would then be approached as personalized medicine designed to match the performance of high-quality, controlled drug delivery systems to the unique biological conditions of the individual patient (11,12).

The intent of this text is to be foundational when it comes to the translation of inhaled aerosol therapy to specific clinical applications. The initial summary of the fundamentals of inhaled aerosols will be useful to those who are not immersed in the field. The majority of the text addresses the prominent clinical applications and the optimal approaches to aerosol treatment. Finally, lessons are drawn from the experience of therapy to generalize on dosage form design and the best approaches to overcoming particular disease barriers as a guide to first step when considering the most valuable approach for a specific application.

All of these observations should be considered in the context of the requirements for accuracy and reproducibility of manufacturing and dose delivery required to ensure quality, safety, and efficacy. It is important to recognize the limitations to drug delivery and to acknowledge areas that require further investigation if a truly predictive approach can ever be contemplated.

Inhalation aerosols have saved many lives and improved the quality of life for millions of patients with a variety of diseases around the world. The knowledge gained and technology developed in the last two decades has allowed further therapeutic application. In the information age, with the exponential increase in scientific discovery, the future of these important drug delivery systems is ensured, and the next generation of exciting new devices and targeted therapies are already appearing on the horizon.

REFERENCES

1. Cryan S-A, Sivadas N, Garcia-Contreras L. In vivo animal models for drug delivery across the lung mucosal barrier. *Advanced Drug Delivery Reviews.* 2007;59:1133–1151.
2. Hickey A. Methods of aerosol particle size characterization. In: Hickey A, ed., *Pharmaceutical Inhalation Aerosol Technology*, 2nd ed. New York: Marcel Dekker, 2004, pp. 345–384.

3. Hinds W. *Aerosol Technology, Properties Behavior and Measurement of Airborne Particles*, 2nd ed. New York: John Wiley & Sons, 1999, pp. 250–251.

4. Sbirlea-Apiou G, Newman S, Fleming J, Seikmeier R, Ehrmann S, Scheuch G, Hochhaus G, Hickey A. Bioequivalence of inhaled drugs: Fundamentals, challenges and perspectives. *Therapeutic Delivery*. 2013;4:343–367.

5. Hastedt J, Backman P, Clark A, Doub W, Hickey A, Hochhaus G, Kuehl P, et al. Scope and relevance of a pulmonary biopharmaceutical classification system AAPS/FDA/USP Workshop March 16–17, 2015, in Baltimore, MD. *AAPS Open*. 2016;2:1.

6. Ziffels S, Durham P, Bemelmans N, Hickey A. In vitro dry powder inhaler formulation performance considerations. *Journal of Controlled Release*. 2015;199:45–52.

7. Hickey A. Controlled delivery of inhaled therapeutic agents. *Journal of Controlled Release*. 2014;190:182–188.

8. Davies N, Feddah M. A novel method for assessing dissolution of inhaler products. *International Journal of Pharmaceutics*. 2003;255:175–187.

9. Son Y-J, McConville J. Development of a standardized dissolution test method for inhaled pharmaceutical formulations. *International Journal of Pharmaceutics*. 2009;382:15–22.

10. Gray V, Hickey A, Balmer P, Davies N, Dunbar C, Foster T, Olsson B, et al. The Inhalation ad hoc advisory panel for the USP performance tests of inhalation dosage forms. *Pharmacetuical Forum*. 2008;34:1068–1074.

11. Kopsch T, Murnane D, Symons D. A personalized medicine approach to the design of dry powder inhalers: Selecting the optimal amount of bypass. *International Journal of Pharmaceutics*. 2017;529:589–596.

12. Loh C, Ohar J. Personalization of device therapy: Prime time for peak inspiratory flow rate. *Chronic Obstructive Pulmonary Disease*. 2017;4:172–176.

Index

Note: Page numbers in italic and bold refer to figures and tables, respectively.

AAD (adaptive aerosol delivery) 279
AATD (alpha-1 antitrypsin deficiency) 308
AAV (adeno-associated virus) 260–1
ABC family *see* ATP-binding cassette family
ABC transporters 59
ABPA (allergic bronchopulmonary aspergillosis) 168–9
absorption mechanisms 58, *59*; ABC transporters 59; BCRP/*ABCG2* 61; factors influencing 63–4; immune cells, particulate matters/macromolecules by 63; MRP/*ABCC* 60–1; passive diffusion 58; PEPTs/*SLC15* 62; P-gp/*ABCB1* 60; *SLC22* subfamily 61–2; SLC transporters 61; transporter-mediated absorption and efflux 58–9; vesicle-mediated endocytosis/transcytosis 62–3
Achromobacter xylosoxidans 226
ACI (Andersen Cascade Impactor) 79–80
acquired resistances 229
activation energy 16
active DPI devices 380
active pharmaceutical ingredients (APIs) 3, 49; acceleration 126; delivery efficiency 124; excipients 128–9; pMDIs 127
active targeting approach 191
active transporters 58–9
acute exacerbation 294
acute respiratory distress syndrome (ARDS) 327–8; heliox utility in 337; prevalence and pathophysiology 329–30, *330*; surfactant delivery for 336
adaptive aerosol delivery (AAD) 279
adaptive barrier, AM: antibody-mediated trapping 262–3; IgA in 261, *261*; IgG in *261*, 261–2

adaptive resistances 228–9
ADASUVE™ product 137
adeno-associated virus (AAV) 260–1
adenocarcinoma 187–8
adenosine triphosphate (ATP) 59
adverse effects, inhaled chemotherapy 201–2, **202**
aerodynamic diameter 5–6
aerodynamic particle dispersion model 9
aerodynamic particle size distribution (APSD) 5, 401, 406
aerodynamic stress 10–11
AeroEclipse® Nebulizer 173
Aerolizer® device 135
Aeroneb Pro® 133
aerosol 398; cloud 381; concentration and particle size 331; deposition 189–90; droplets/particles, deposition 78; drugs 369; exposure systems 116; mechanism 400; momentum 46; particle in lungs *58*; penetrance 217; treatments 370; vaccines 369–70
aerosol delivery: devices 173, 194; device selection 150; DPIs 149–50; invasive mechanical ventilation *152*, 152–4; nebulizers 148–9; NIV 147, 151, *151*; pMDIs 149; rate 407; soft mist inhalers 149; tracheostomies 151–2; transnasal 150–1
aerosol device technology: atomization devices 127–34; evaporation–condensation devices 136–7; particle redispersion devices 134–6
aerosol generation, physical principles of: atomization and nebulization 123–4; evaporation–condensation 126–7; particle redispersion 124–6
aerosolized BCG 364

Aerosurf® 137
AERx® 133
AFM (atomic force microscopy) 9
agglomerate-based DPI 136
aggregate strength *7*, 7–9
airflow: CFD modeling 45–6; simulation 42; turbulent characteristics 45
air-liquid interface (ALI) 107, 109, 111, 113, 115–16
air-liquid interface exposure (ALICE) system 116
AIR® pulmonary delivery system 136
airway: caliber 162–3; deposition of drugs 190–1; epithelium host defense *239*, 240; mucosa *225*; pharmacology 216
airway mucus (AM) 257; adaptive barrier properties 261–3; barrier 257–9; in disease 263–4; IgA in 261, *261*; IgG in *261*, 261–2; immune response, anatomy 264–5; immunomodulation in lung 265–6; innate barrier properties 259–61; mucus clearance 263
airway surface liquid (ASL) *225*, 240
alginate 231
ALI *see* air-liquid interface
ALICE (air-liquid interface exposure) system 116
allergic bronchopulmonary aspergillosis (ABPA) 168–9, *169*
alpha-lactose monohydrate crystals 19
alpha-1 antitrypsin deficiency (AATD) 308
α-relaxations 16–17
alveolar-capillary model 113, *114*
alveolar cell lines 80
alveolar macrophages 63–4
AM *see* airway mucus
AMB *see* amphotericin B
American Type Culture Collection (ATCC) 108

aminoglycosides 295
amorphous materials 15–18
amorphous systems 18
amphotericin B (AMB): aerosol delivery devices 173; aerosolized AMBd and ABLC 174; commercial formulations 173; definition 172; DPI 172–3; injectable formulations 172; macrophage targeting system 172; mortality rate and incidence, IPA 174; murine model 173; nebulized liposomal 173–4; NP delivery system 172; polymeric micelles 172; prophylaxis 173–4
amplifiers 243
AMPs (antimicrobial peptides) 229–30
anatomical differences, infants and children 148
Andersen Cascade Impactor (ACI) 79–80
animal models 109–10
anti-asthmatic compounds 81–2
antibiotics 148; regimens 362, **363**; resistance, biofilm 228–9; therapies, CF airway infections 226–7
antibiotic therapy, pulmonary NTM **278**; inhaled antibiotics 278–9; MAC disease 277–8; *Mycobacterium abscessus* 278; *Mycobacterium kansasii* 278
antibody-mediated trapping 262–3
antifungal agents: AMB 172–4; caspofungin 179; ITZ 174–7; VCZ 177–9
antimicrobial peptides (AMPs) 229–30
antisense oligonucleotides (AONs) 244
antisense therapy 200
anti-TB drugs (ATDs) 365
AONs (antisense oligonucleotides) 244
APIs *see* active pharmaceutical ingredients
APSD (aerodynamic particle size distribution) 5, 401, 406
ARDS *see* acute respiratory distress syndrome
ARIA™ pulmonary delivery technology 137
Arrhenius dependence equation 17
ASL (airway surface liquid) *225*, 240
aspergilloma 168, *168*
asperities 8, 20
asthma 71, 74, 110, 115; airway caliber and disease 162–3; breathing maneuver 163; DPIs 164; human factors 163; inhalation

aerosols 161–2; mucus 264, *264*; nebulizers 164; pathology, physiology and pharmacology 162; physicochemical mechanisms 162; pMDIs 163–4; SMIs 164
Ataluren (PTC124, Translarna™) *242*, 242–3
ATCC (American Type Culture Collection) 108
ATDs (anti-TB drugs) 365
atelectasis 323
atomic force microscopy (AFM) 9
atomization devices: defined 123; droplet formation 123–4; liquids, characteristics 124; metered liquid dose inhalers 133–4; nebulizers 131–3; pMDIs 127–31; Weber (*We*) number 124
ATP (adenosine triphosphate) 59
ATP-binding cassette (ABC) family 59

Bacille Calmette-Guérin (BCG) vaccine 363–4
bacteria/cells, inhaled anticancer agents 200–1
bacterial cells 228–9
bacteriophage therapy 230–1
BAL *see* bronchoalveolar lavage
BALF (blood and bronchoalveolar lavage fluid) 366
BA-MDIs (breath-activated pMDIs) 218–19
BCG (Bacille Calmette-Guérin) vaccine 363–4
BCRP (breast cancer resistance protein) 59, 61
BCS (biopharmaceutics classification system) 100
beclomethasone dipropionate (BDP) 24, 383
bedaquiline (BDQ) 281
behavioral differences, children and adults 148
BET (Brunauer–Emmett–Teller) 6
beta-lactam treatment 294
β-relaxations 16–17
bilevel ventilation 147
bioavailability, inhaled compounds: animal models 84; BE 91, **99**, 100; biological samples 87–8; clearance mechanisms 78–9; definition 72–4; dose calculation 85–7; drug release and dissolution 79–80; extravascular route 74; factors 71, *71*; formulation and

delivery devices 77; healthy volunteers 83–4; local action in lungs/airways 90–1, **92–3**, **94–5**, 100; lung diseases **72–3**; mechanisms, drug absorption 81–3, **82–3**; PD parameters 89–90, **90**; permeability 80–1; physicochemical properties 75–7, **76–7**; PK parameters 88–9, 91, **95**; pulmonary route 74, *75*; site of deposition 78; systemic action 91, **96–8**; transporters, lung and substrates 82, **82**
biodegradable polymers 192–3
bioequivalence (BE) studies 91, **99**, 100
biofilm bacteria 228; antibiotic resistance 228–9, *229*; formation, maturation, and propagation stages *228*
biofilm busters: AMPs 229–30; bacteriophage therapy 230–1; chelating agents 231; dispersion compounds 231–2; *in vitro* and *in vivo* investigation **230**; QSIs 232; silver 232
biofilm matrix 229, 231
biomarkers 316
biopharmaceutics classification system (BCS) 100
"black-box" approach 9
blood and bronchoalveolar lavage fluid (BALF) 366
bolus method 32
breakage kernel 10
breast cancer resistance protein (BCRP) 59, 61
breath-activated pMDIs (BA-MDIs) 218–19
breath-actuated/enhanced jet nebulizers 132
breathing frequency and tidal volumes, animal models 84, *84*, 86
breathing maneuver 163
bronchial airways 35
bronchial cells 108; lines 80
bronchial circulation 57
bronchial epithelial cells 82
bronchiectasis 296; pathophysiology 291, *292*
bronchoalveolar lavage (BAL) 87, 196, 240
bronchodilator 149; treatment 36
Brownian diffusion mechanism 3
Brunauer–Emmett–Teller (BET) 6
Burkholderia cepacia complex (Bcc) 226

calcium channel blockers (CCBs) 319
Calu-3 cell line 80–1
capillary aerosol generator (CAG) 334
capsule-based DPI 136, *136*
carbonplatin 199, 201
carrier-based systems, DPI 136
cascade impactor devices 5
caspofungin drug 179
catheters, aerosol delivery 335
cavosonstat (N91115) *246*, 247
central-peripheral (C/P) ratio 32, 36–7
cervicovaginal mucus (CVM) *262*
CF *see* cystic fibrosis
CFCs (chlorofluorocarbons) 24, 128–9, 389
CFD *see* computational fluid dynamics modeling
CF infections, treatments for: antibiotic therapies 226–7; limitations 227–8; mucolytic agents 226
CF respiratory disease: airway epithelium host defense 240; CF lung disease 240; CFTR dysfunctioning 240; lung disease pathophysiology 239–40
CFTR *see* cystic fibrosis transmembrane conductance regulator
CFTR anion channel: mutations and functional defects 241–2; structure and function 241, *241*
CFTR-modulating compounds: AONs 244; class II defects 243–4; F508del-CFTR 244–5, 248; nonsense mutations (class I) 242–3; potentiators 245–7; protein synthesis 247; read-through agent *242*, 242–3
CFTR protein *241*, 246–7; potentiator 246–7; stabilizing 247
chelating agents 231
chemotherapy *see* inhaled chemotherapy
ChiSys® 351
chitosan 351
chlorofluorocarbons (CFCs) 24, 128–9, 389
chronic necrotizing aspergillosis (CNA) 169, *169*, *170*
chronic obstructive pulmonary disease (COPD) 35, 60, 63, 71, 114–15, 303, 379, 383; aerosol penetrance, disease effects 217; airway pharmacology 216; definition 215; drug classes 217–18; inhaled devices and implications 218–19; pathophysiology 215–16

ciliary-mediated clearance 263
Circulaire® 132
cisplatin 196, 199
class II defects, CFTR 243–4
clinical and radiographic criteria, NTM 277
clinical bronchiectasis 291
CNA (chronic necrotizing aspergillosis) 169, *169*, *170*
Cole's vicious cycle model 291
colistin 295
computational fluid dynamics (CFD) modeling 5, 41; deposition modeling 42–3; literature searches on *43*; lung airway models 47; -particle transport modeling 43–7; predictions 46; in 3D 41; whole-lung deposition models 47–8
computed tomography (CT) 42, 49, 382–3
computer-aided design 47
cone-beam technologies 49
continuous positive airway pressure (CPAP) 147, 151
COPD *see* chronic obstructive pulmonary disease
correctors 244
corticosteroid-glucocorticoid receptor (CS-GR) 216
cough-driven clearance 263
CPAP (continuous positive airway pressure) 147, 151
CriticalSorb™ (Critical Pharmaceuticals Ltd.) 351
crystalline materials 15–18
crystallization time 16–17
CT (computed tomography) 42, 49, 382–3
cystic fibrosis (CF) 31, 36–7, *37*, 71, 74, 78, 110, 114–15, 223, 291, 379; airway pathogens 224–6, *225*, *226*; bacterial biofilms in *see* biofilm busters; impaired airway epithelial host defense *239*; lung disease 240; mucus 263–4, *264*; NIV 151; and pulmonary infections 223–4, *225*; treatments 226–8
cystic fibrosis transmembrane conductance regulator (CFTR) 115, 223, 304; anion channel 241–2; corrector 245; dysfunctioning 240; modulators 242–7; mutations and functional defects 241–2; respiratory disease 239–40; therapeutics 247–8

cytochrome P450 enzymes 345
cytokine IFNγ 367

decellularized (DC) tissue 111, 114–15
delayed-type hypersensitivity (DTH) 362
dendritic cells 63
design of experiments (DoE) 5
device-patient interface aerosol losses 333
device resistance, DPI 135
diffusion mechanism 31
diffusive deposition 31
dimeric IgA (dIgA) *261*
dipalmitoyl phosphatidylcholine (DPPC) 20
diphenyleneiodonium chloride (DPIC) 281
direct oral anticoagulants (DOACs) 319
disodium cromoglycate (DSCG) 20
dispersion compounds 231–2
dispersion stresses 10–11
dissolution 407
DissolvIt® device 80
distearoyl phosphatidylcholine (DSPC) 20
DNA gyrase inhibitors 281
dose 405–6, *406*
dose calculation: absorbed dose 86; aerosol administration 86, **86**; capreomycin plasma concentration *versus* time curves 87, *87*; deposited dose 86; dose delivered 86; FDA definition 85; size of doses 85, *85*
dose-metering systems, DPIs 136
doxorubicin (DOX) 197
DPIs *see* dry powder inhalers
droplets, atomization 13–14
drug: carriers 324–5; discovery pipeline, NTM *280*, 280–1; dissolution rate 15; release and dissolution 79–80; resistance, NTM 279–80; solubility 14–15; toxicity and side effects, NTM 280
drug classes, COPD therapy: ICS 218; LABA 217–18; LAMA 217–18
drug–drug interaction, NTM 280
drug-loaded/antibody-containing NPs 193
drug manufacturing files (DMFs) 399
dry powder: dispersion modeling 9–13, *13*; formulations 24; inhaled anticancer agents 191–2

dry powder inhalers (DPIs) 4, 24,
        45, 149–50, 380, 389, 406;
        aggregate dispersion in *12*;
        AMB 173; asthma 164;
        bioavailability *see*
        bioavailability, inhaled
        compounds; COPD 218;
        device resistance, role 135;
        dose administration 134;
        dose-metering systems 136;
        formulations 135–6; ITZ
        176–7; particle fluidization
        and redispersion 134; powder
        redispersion 134–5; VCZ 177–9
Dry Powder Insufflator™ 86
DTH (delayed-type hypersensitivity) 362

ECACC (European Collection
        of Authenticated Cell
        Cultures) 108
ECM (extracellular matrix) 107, 109,
        114, 115
EGFR (epidermal growth factor
        receptor) 188
electronic cigarettes (e-cigarettes) 137
electronic devices 393
ENaC (epithelial sodium transporter
        channel) 240
endocytosis 62
endoscopic visualization 49
endothelial cells (ECs) 315
endothelin A (ETA) 315
endothelin B (ETB) 315
endothelin receptor antagonists
        (ERAs) 316
endotracheal surfactant bolus
        instillation 334
engineered solid particles 19–23, **21**
enhanced permeability and retention
        (EPR) effect 190–1
environmental contamination 202
Envoy/Sidestream, jet nebulizer
        systems 173
epidermal growth factor receptor
        (EGFR) 188
epithelial sodium transporter channel
        (ENaC) 240
EPR (enhanced permeability and
        retention) effect 190–1
EPS (extracellular polymeric substance)
        matrix 228, 231
eradication therapy 294
European Collection of Authenticated
        Cell Cultures (ECACC) 108
European Union Reference Laboratory
        for Alternatives to animal
        testing (EURL-ECVAM) 116

evaporation–condensation devices
        126–7, 136–7
EVLP (*ex vivo* lung perfusion) model 109,
        112, 116
excipients, pMDIs 128–9
expansion chamber, pMDI 129–30, *130*
expectorant agents 296
extracellular matrix (ECM) 107, 109,
        114, 115
extracellular polymeric substance (EPS)
        matrix 228, 231
extrathoracic airways, deposition in 33
Exubera® (Pfizer) inhaler 135
ex vivo lung perfusion (EVLP) model
        109, 112, 116

F508del-CFTR: folding defect
        244–5; restoration 247–8;
        small molecule CFTR
        modulation 248
facilitated transporters 58
FDKP (fumaryl diketopiperazine) 20
FF (formoterol fumarate) 383
fibrosis 303
fine particle dose 406
fine particle fraction (FPF) 3, 5, 20, 380
Fisoneb® nebulizer 173
fluorocarbon 20
fluoroquinolones 295
force-controlled agents 19
formoterol fumarate (FF) 383
formulations, inhaled anticancer
        agents: dry powders 191–2;
        inorganic nanocarriers 193–4;
        liposomes 192; micelles 193;
        microparticles 192–3; NPs
        193; solutions 191; swellable
        hydrogels 193
Fortical® 348
FORWARD study 383
Fourier decomposition (FD-MRI)
        methods 383
FPF (fine particle fraction) 3, 5, 20, 380
Franz diffusion cell 79–80
fumaryl diketopiperazine (FDKP) 20
functional respiratory imaging
        (FRI) 383
FUTURE study 383

gallium (Ga) 281
GANTT charts 398
gene therapy 199–201
genotypic *versus* phenotypic 405
GlaxoSmithKline (GSK) 365–7
glycopeptidolipids (GLP) 281
goblet cells 258, *259*
Goprelto® 350, **351**

GSK (GlaxoSmithKline) 365–7

Haemophilus influenzae 291
HCA (high content analysis) 116
HDT (host-directed immunotherapy)
        367
heated high flow nasal cannula
        (HHFNC) 147, 150–1
heliox 337
herpes simplex virus (HSV) 262, *262*
herpes simplex virus 1 thymidine kinase
        (HSVtk) gene 200
HFA (hydrofluoroalkane) 24, 128–9,
        129, 149
HHFNC (heated high flow nasal
        cannula) 147, 150–1
HIF-1 (hypoxia inducible factor-1) 315
high content analysis (HCA) 116
hollow particles 20
host-directed immunotherapy (HDT) 367
HPβCD-ITZ (2-hydroxypropyl-
        cyclodextrin) 175–6
human immunodeficiency virus (HIV)
        361
human tissue models 109
hydrofluoroalkane (HFA) 24, 128–9, *129*,
        149
hydrogels 111, 115
2-hydroxypropyl-cyclodextrin (HPβCD-
        ITZ) 175–6
hyperinflation 379
hyperpolarized helium (^{3}He) 383
hypertonic saline 296
hypoxia inducible factor-1 (HIF-1) 315

ICSs (inhaled corticosteroids) therapy 80,
        218, 296
idiopathic pulmonary fibrosis (IPF)
        114–15, 303, *305*, 384
iDMS (Insulin Diabetes Management
        System) 133
IgA in AM 261, *261*
IGC (inverse gas chromatography) 9
IgG in AM *261*, 261–2
image charge force 333
Imitrex® (GlaxoSmithKline) 350, **351**
immune cells, particulate matters/
        macromolecules by 63
immune response, anatomy of 264–5
immunohistological analysis 315
immunologics/cytokines 194–5, 201
immunomodulation in lung 265–6
immunotherapy 367
impaction mechanism 31
inhalation therapy 293, *293*, 390
inhaled 5-fluorouracil (5-FU) 197, 201
inhaled antibiotics 278–9

inhaled anticancer agents: aerosol delivery devices 194; aerosol deposition 189–90; anti-sense therapy 200; bacteria/cells 200–1; chemotherapy 196–9, **198**; clinical use 201; formulations 191–4; gene therapy 199–200; immunologics/cytokines 194–5; limitations 202–3; monoclonal antibodies 195–6; targeting approaches, airway deposition 190–1

inhaled chemotherapy: adverse effects 201–2, **202**; clinical studies **198**, 201; doxorubicin 197; L-9NC 197, 199; nucleoside analogs 197; paclitaxel 199; pharmacokinetics 196–7; platinum agents 199; preclinical efficacy 197

inhaled corticosteroids (ICSs) therapy 80, 218, 296

inhaled devices and implications 218; technology-based clinical outcomes 219

inhaled pharmaceutical products 398, 398–9

inhaled therapeutics against TB: antibiotic regimens 362, **363**; antibiotic-resistant MTB 362–3; clinical pathology of infection 362; resurgence of old epidemic 361–2; stalled progress 362–4

inhaler devices clinical use, challenges 392

inhaler performance 3–5

inhalers in real life 385, **385**

innate barrier, AM: adhesive interactions 259–61; mucin mesh 259

INOmax® nitric oxide gas inhalation 318

inorganic nanocarriers 193–4

Insulin Diabetes Management System (iDMS) 133

interferons (IFNs) 195

interleukin 2 (IL-2) 195

interleukin 12 (IL-12) 195

interstitial fluid pressure (IFP) 190

interstitial lung disease (ILD) 303

intracellular tight junctions (TJs) 81–2

intranasal drug delivery: in clinical trials **350**; to CNS 348, 350; peptides and proteins 348; therapies using 347–8

intrinsic resistances 228

invasive pulmonary aspergillosis (IPA) 170–1, *171*

inverse gas chromatography (IGC) 9

in vitro cell culture models and *ex vivo* models **108**, 108–9

in vitro–in vivo correlation (IVIVC) 107

in vivo/in vitro dissolution 14

IPA (invasive pulmonary aspergillosis) 170–1, *171*

IPF *see* idiopathic pulmonary fibrosis

Ishikawa diagrams 397

itraconazole (ITZ) 174; adverse effects 174; amorphous and aerosolized nanostructured 177; concentrations 174; DPI 176; drug–drug interaction 174; HPβCD-ITZ 175–6; lipid NP 175–6; nano-size reduction 175; pharmacokinetics 177; polymeric micelles 176; SFL formulation 177; solid dispersion 174–5

ivacaftor (Kalydeco®, VX-770) 246, *246*

IVIVC (*in vitro–in vivo* correlation) 107

jet milling process 307

jet nebulizers 164, 381; breath-actuated 132; breath-enhanced 132; bronchopulmonary dysplasia 152; collection bag 131–2; invasive mechanical ventilation 152–4; NIV 151; principle 131; reservoir tube 131; tracheostomy delivery 152

Johari-Goldstein relaxations 16

Johnson-Kendall-Roberts (JKR) model 8

LABA (long-acting beta agonist) 216–18

lactose carriers and adhesive blends 18–19

LAMAs (long-acting muscarinic antagonists) 217–18

latent TB 362

LC–MS/MS (liquid chromatography–mass spectrometry/mass spectrometry) 60–2

lipid-coated NPs 193

Lipinski rule of five 75

liposomal-9-nitro camptothecin (L-9NC) 197, 199

liposomes 23–4, 192

liquid-based delivery systems 353

liquid chromatography–mass spectrometry/mass spectrometry (LC–MS/MS) 60–2

liquid formulations 24

L-9NC (liposomal-9-nitro camptothecin) 197, 199

London–van der Waals forces 125

long-acting beta agonist (LABA) 216–18

long-acting muscarinic antagonists (LAMAs) 217–18

low-Reynolds-number (LRN) k-$f\omega$ turbulence model 46

lumacaftor (VX-809) 244–5, *245*

lung: CFD-particle transport modeling 46–7; disease pathophysiology 239–40; interstitium 57; periphery, intra-airway deposition to 331–2; transplantation 319

lung cancer **188**, 188–9; adverse effects 201–2; inhaled anticancer agents *see* inhaled anticancer agents

lung-on-a-chip technology 112–13, *114*

lung surfactant 323; replacement therapeutics **324**, 324–5

lymphatic vessels network 57

macrophages *265*; *see also* alveolar macrophages; targeting system 172

magnetic resonance imaging (MRI) 42, 49, 383

mannitol 19, 296

mass median aerodynamic diameter (MMAD) 6, 9, 24, 148, 150, 152–3, 392

matrix metalloprotease-9 (MMP-9) 353

MDIs (metered-dose inhalers) 33, 45, 365

MDR *see* multidrug resistance

MDSCs (myeloid-derived suppressor cells) 195

mean absorption time (MAT) 89

melatonin 346

mesoporous silica NPs (MSN) 194, *194*

metabolic enzymes 79

metabolic modulators 318

metastasis 188, 199–200

metered-dose inhalers (MDIs) 33, 45, 365

metered liquid dose inhalers 133–4

MIC (minimum inhibitory concentration) 227

micellar delivery system 172, 176

micelles 23, 193

MicroAir® Ultrasonic Model 132

microbiologic laboratory diagnosis 277

microdialysis 88

microfluidic chips 112–13, *114*

microparticles 192–3

MicroSprayer® 86, 194

Migranal® 350, **351**
mild-moderate asthmatics 36, *36*
minimally invasive surfactant bolus instillation 334
minimally invasive surfactant therapy (MIST) 334
minimum inhibitory concentration (MIC) 227
MIST (minimally invasive surfactant therapy) 334
mitochondria reactive oxygen species (mROS) 315
MMAD *see* mass median aerodynamic diameter
monoclonal antibodies 195–6
mouth/throat (MT) region 45; CFD-particle transport modeling 45–6; geometries 45–7
MPPD (multiple-path particle dosimetry) model 48
MRI (magnetic resonance imaging) 42, 49, 383
mROS (mitochondria reactive oxygen species) 315
MRP/*ABCC* (multidrug resistance-related proteins) 60–1
MSN (mesoporous silica NPs) 194, *194*
MTB (mycobacterium tuberculosis) 362
MT region *see* mouth/throat region
MUC5AC 258–9, *259*
MUC5B 258–9, *259*
mucin mesh 259
mucin monomers *258*
mucoactive agents 296
mucociliary clearance 293, 344; mechanism 189; respiratory epithelium *345*
mucokinetic agents 296–7
mucolytic agents 226
mucus barrier: composition and characteristics 257–8; mucin properties and structure 258–9; mucins into mucus 259; nonmucin components 259
mucus clearance 263
mucus in disease *264*; asthma 264, *264*; CF 263–4
multidrug resistance (MDR) 59, 226; -TB 362
multidrug resistance-related proteins (MRP/*ABCC*) 60–1
multiple-path particle dosimetry (MPPD) model 48
multi-scale approaches 41
multivariate statistical design 398
muscarinic receptors 216
Mycobacterium bovis 363

mycobacterium tuberculosis (MTB) 362
myeloid-derived suppressor cells (MDSCs) 195

N-acetylcysteine (NAC) therapy 307
nanoaggregates 22
nanoparticles (NPs) 8; -based drug delivery 191; delivery system 172; lipid 175–6; SLNs 23, 193
nanostructured lipid carrier (NLC) 176
Narcan® 350, **351**
nasal CFD-particle transport modeling: applications 44; experimental data to 45; literature 43; models and application 43–5; reviews **44**
nasal clearance 344–5
nasal drug delivery 343; administration, technologies for 353; anatomy and physical barriers to 343; disease effect on 345; drug absorption 350–3; enzyme metabolism in 345–6; FDA-approved indications for **348**; *in vitro* models to 346–7; using intranasal administration 347, *347*
nasal non-protein/non-peptide drugs *352*
nasal protein/peptide drugs *349*, **349**
Navier-Stokes equations 42
NCA (noncompartmental analysis) method 88
NDSD (non-dimensional specific dissipation) 9
nebulization 123–4
nebulized saline 296
nebulizers 191; asthma 164; COPD 218–19; endotracheal tube, placement 152; infants 148–9; jet 131–2, 153; pMDIs 150; SMIs and 381; ultrasonic 132, 153; vibrating mesh 132–3, 150–1, 153
neonatal-pediatric drug delivery: aerosol delivery devices, children 148–50; animal models 147; children and adults 148; neonatal population 147; pediatric population 148; respiratory support 150–4; surfactant replacement therapy 154
neonatal respiratory distress syndrome (nRDS) 327–8; heliox utility in 337; prevalence and pathophysiology *328*, 328–9
neovascularization 315

neutrophils 224
New Generation Impactor (NGI) 79–80
NEXThaler® 380
NF-E2-related factor 2 (Nrf2) activators 318
Nicotrol® 350, **351**
nintedanib 304–5, *306*
nitric oxide synthase (NOS) 314
NIV (noninvasive ventilation) 147, 151, *151*
NLC (nanostructured lipid carrier) 176
noncompartmental analysis (NCA) method 88
non-dimensional specific dissipation (NDSD) 9
noninvasive routes 348
noninvasive ventilation (NIV) 147, 151, *151*
nonmucin components 259
nonsense mutations (class I) 242–3
non-small cell lung cancer (NSCLC) 187–9; tissue 61
non-Stokesian flow regimes 6
nontuberculous mycobacteria (NTM) 226, 275, 364; clinical studies 281, **282–3**; in lung disease 276–7; pulmonary disease 276–7; treatment 277–81, **278**
normal human bronchial epithelial cells (NHBECs) 60
novel oral anticoagulants (NOACs) 319
novel organic cation transporters (OCTN1 and 2) 61–2
Noyes-Whitney diffusion equation 14–15
NPs *see* nanoparticles
nRDS *see* neonatal respiratory distress syndrome
NSCLC *see* non-small cell lung cancer
NTM *see* nontuberculous mycobacteria

OCT1-3 (organic cation transporters) 61
Ohnesorge number 14
OIDPs (orally inhaled drug products) 400
olfactory region 344, 353
Omron MicroAir 133
ONZETRA® Xsail® 353
Optinose, Inc. 353
oral anticoagulants 318–19
orally inhaled delivery, milestones *390*
orally inhaled drug products (OIDPs) 400
organic cation transporters (OCT1-3) 61
ORKAMBI® (Vertex Pharmaceuticals) 246–8
Oswald ripening 14

paclitaxel 196, 199
PADDOCC (Pharmaceutical Deposition
　　　　Device on Cell Culture)
　　　　system 116
parametric response mapping (PRM)
　　　　382–3
parenteral route 348
Pari eFlow system 133, 308
particle: dissolution mechanism 14–15;
　　　　engineering techniques 24;
　　　　inertial deposition 3; transport
　　　　simulation 42–3
particle aerosolization, factors affecting:
　　　　aerodynamic diameter and
　　　　Stokes number 5–7; droplets,
　　　　atomization 13–14; dry powder
　　　　dispersion modeling 9–13, 13;
　　　　particle aggregate strength 7, 7–9
particle deposition mechanisms 31–2, 48;
　　　　in COPD and asthma 35;
　　　　in respiratory tract 31
particle image velocimetry (PIV) 45
particle-particle interaction forces
　　　　124–5, **126**
particle redispersion devices: DPIs
　　　　134–6; mechanisms 125–6;
　　　　particle-particle interaction
　　　　forces 124–5, **126**
particle replication in nonwetting
　　　　templates (PRINT)
　　　　technology 192
particle size distribution (PSD) 3
passive diffusion 58
passive targeting approach 190
passive transporters 58
pattern recognition receptors (PRRs) 265
PBPK (physiologically based
　　　　pharmacokinetic) modeling
　　　　41, 49
PD (pharmacodynamic) parameters 89–90
pediatric population 148
penetration volume (Vp) 32
peptide transporters (PEPTs)/*SLC15* 62
periciliary liquid (PCL) *224*
permeability 80–1
PET *see* polyethylene terephthalate;
　　　　positron emission
　　　　tomography
P-glycoprotein (P-gp) 59–60
PH (pulmonary hypertension) 313,
　　　　317, **317**
phagocytosis 63–4
Pharmaceutical Deposition Device on
　　　　Cell Culture (PADDOCC)
　　　　system 116
pharmacodynamic (PD) parameters
　　　　89–90, **90**

pharmacokinetic (PK) parameters 88–9,
　　　　91, **96**
phosphatidylcholines (PC) 20, 23
phospholipid-protein complex 323
physicochemical properties: inhaled
　　　　compounds 75–7, **76–7**;
　　　　particles 3–5, **4**
physiological differences, infants and
　　　　children 148
physiologically based pharmacokinetic
　　　　(PBPK) modeling 41, 49
pirfenidone 307
PIV (particle image velocimetry) 45
PK (pharmacokinetic) parameters 88–9,
　　　　91, **96**
pMDIs *see* pressurized metered-dose
　　　　inhalers
polycarbonate (PC) 109
polyethylene terephthalate (PET) 109
porous particles 20, 178, 191
porous scaffolds, DC tissue 111
positron emission tomography (PET) 32,
　　　　60, 381–2
potentiators 245–6
powder-based delivery systems 353
powder redispersion, factors 125, **126**
PreciseInhale® system 80, 86–7
predisposing factors, NTM disease: age
　　　　276; chronic lung diseases 276;
　　　　immunocompromised patients
　　　　277; race 277; sex 277
pressurized metered-dose inhalers
　　　　(pMDIs) 4, 24, 63, 380, 406;
　　　　aerosol formation 129–30;
　　　　asthma 163–4; CFCs 128; COPD
　　　　218–19; dose counters and
　　　　electronic monitoring devices
　　　　130–1; excipients 128–9; HFA
　　　　128–9, *129*; liquid propellants
　　　　128, **128**; lung diseases 127;
　　　　metered valves, actuators design,
　　　　and nozzle 127–8; solutions and
　　　　suspensions 24–5; spacers 149;
　　　　tracheostomies 151–2; VHC *see*
　　　　valve-holding chambers
prevention of infection (POI) 365
prevention of recurrence (POR) 365
PRM (parametric response mapping)
　　　　382–3
process analytical technology 399
product development: QbD 399–400; risk
　　　　management *398*, 400; TPP 399
product quality 397–8, *398*
Proneb Ultra/Pari LC Star 173, 179
propellant atomization 24
prophylactic post-exposure vaccines 365
prophylactic pre-exposure vaccines 365

prostacyclin 316; analog 384
prostanoids 316
proteins/peptides 393
PRRs (pattern recognition receptors) 265
PS (pulmonary surfactant) 323–4
PSD (particle size distribution) 3
Pseudomonas aeruginosa 224, 226–7, 384
PTI-428 243
Pulmicort Turbuhaler® (AstraZeneca) 136
Pulmo-Aide/Micromist, jet nebulizer
　　　　systems 173
pulmonary arterial hypertension
　　　　(PAH) 313
pulmonary arterial smooth muscle cells
　　　　(PASMCs) 315
pulmonary aspergillosis: ABPA 168–9,
　　　　169; antifungal agents 172–9;
　　　　aspergilloma 168, *168*; clinical
　　　　syndromes 168; CNA 169–70;
　　　　definition 167; IPA 171, *171*;
　　　　pathogen and severity 167, *168*;
　　　　treatment of 171, **171**
pulmonary circulation 57
pulmonary drugs/vaccines 365,
　　　　366, 369; antibiotics 367;
　　　　immunotherapy 367; TBVI/
　　　　GSK 365–7
pulmonary hypertension (PH) 313,
　　　　317, **317**
pulmonary infections and CF: PCL *224*;
　　　　progression and prevalence
　　　　225, *226*
pulmonary NTM disease: classification
　　　　276; epidemiology 276;
　　　　pathogenesis 276; predisposing
　　　　factors 276–7; prevalence 276
pulmonary surfactant (PS) 323–4
pulmonary therapeutics in TB 368;
　　　　aerosol drugs 369; aerosol
　　　　treatments 370; aerosol
　　　　vaccines 369–70; challenges
　　　　368; pulmonary drug delivery
　　　　368; regulatory approval 369
pulmonary *versus* parenteral route
　　　　delivery, TB: alveolar
　　　　macrophages 365; devices
　　　　available 365; rationale for *364*,
　　　　364–5
PulmoSphere® process 20, 25, 136, 380

quality by design (QbD) 397, 399;
　　　　IPAC-RS 398; principles 397;
　　　　process analytical technology
　　　　399; statistical experimental
　　　　design 399; statistical process
　　　　control 399–400, *400*
quorum sensing inhibitors (QSIs) 232

Raman spectroscopy 80
RANS (Reynolds-averaged Navier-Stokes) turbulence models 45–6
read-through agents, CFTR *242*, 242–3
recombinant human DNase (rhDNase) therapy 297
regional deposition 33–4, *34*
regional particle deposition 31
reservoir tube, jet nebulizers 131
Respimat® device 381
Respimat® SoftMist™ Inhaler 133
respirable dose 406
respiratory cell culture models, epithelial cells **108**, 108–9
respiratory diseases: asthma and IPF 115; CF 114; COPD 114
respiratory distress syndrome (RDS) 323
respiratory dosimetry modeling 49
respiratory drug delivery 3–4; crystalline and amorphous materials 15–18; engineered solid particles 19–23, **21**; lactose carriers and adhesive blends 18–19; liposomes 23–4; pMDI solutions and suspensions 24–5; polymers for 23
respiratory region 344, 353
respiratory tract: anatomy 3; geometry 42; needs and directions for 48–9; particle deposition in 31; total and regional deposition in 32–7
Reynolds-averaged Navier-Stokes (RANS) turbulence models 45–6
Reynolds number (Re) 5
rhDNase (recombinant human DNase) therapy 297
rhodamine 123 (Rh123) 60
Rho-kinase inhibitors 318
risk management *398*, 400

scaffold biomaterials 111, *111*
scanning electron microscopy *22*
SCF (supercritical fluid) methods 20–1
scintigraphy 381–2, *382*
SCLC (small cell lung cancer) 187, 189
secretory IgA (sIgA) *261*
sedimentation mechanism 31
segmentation process 42
selective precision deuterium substitution 246
selective serotonin reuptake inhibitors (SSRIs) 318

septum 343
"shortcourse" anti-TB therapy 362
silver, biofilm busters 232
simulated lung fluid (SLF) 79
single-path models 48
single-photon emission computed tomography (SPECT) 32, 381–2
16HBE14o-cell line 80–1
SLC *see* solute carrier family
SLF (simulated lung fluid) 79
SLNs (solid lipid NPs) 23, 193
small cell lung cancer (SCLC) 187, 189
smooth muscle cells (SMCs) 315
soft mist 389
soft mist inhalers (SMIs) 149, 164, 379, 381; COPD 218
solid lipid NPs (SLNs) 23, 193
solute carrier (SLC) family 59; *SLC22* subfamily 61–2; transporters 61
space-charge force 333
SP-A, lung surfactant proteins 323
specific surface area (SSA) 6
SPECT (single-photon emission computed tomography) 32, 381–2
spheroids 112, *113*, 115
Spiriva® Handihaler® *136*
spray drying 191
SSRIs (selective serotonin reuptake inhibitors) 318
Staccato inhaler 380
standard operating procedures (SOPs) 399
statistical experimental design 399
statistical process control 399–400, *400*
stem cell therapies 319
Stimate® 348
stochastic whole-lung models 48
Stokesian flow regime 6
Stokes number 5–7
supercritical fluid (SCF) methods 20–1
supplementary oxygen (O_2) therapy 319
surface-to-volume shape factor 6
surfactant aerosol 331; delivery and noninvasive ventilation 335–6; generation 334; technological advances in 336–7; wet and dry 332–3
surfactant formulations 330–1
surfactant replacement therapy 154
suspension formulations 24
swellable hydrogels 193
Synarel® 348
systemic delivery 393

targeting approach, airway deposition 190–1
target inhalation mode (TIM) 190
target product profile (TPP) 399
TB (tuberculosis) 74, 361
TB region *see* tracheobronchial region
TBVI (tuberculosis vaccine initiative) 365–7
T-cells 265–6
TEER (transepithelial electrical resistance) value 81
tensile strength 9
terbutaline 297
tetradecyl maltoside (TDM) 351
tezacaftor (VX-661) 245, *245*
TH (thyroid hormone) 308
therapeutic vaccines 365
thiopeptide antibiotics 281
3D CFD models 49; respiratory tract geometry for 42; upper TB airways 47
3D culture platforms, respiratory drug development: microfluidic chips 112–13, *114*; scaffold biomaterials 111, *112*; spheroids 112, *113*; types 110, *110*
three-dimensional (3D) culture models, inhaled drug development: animal models 109–10; *in vitro* cell and *ex vivo* models **108**, 108–9; opportunities and challenges 115–16; platforms 110–14; respiratory diseases 114–15
thyroid hormone (TH) 308
TLRs (toll-like receptors) 195, 265
TNM staging system 188
TOBI® Podhaler 134
tocopherol polyethylene glycol 1000 succinate (TPGS) 176
toll-like receptors (TLRs) 195, 265
total deposition 33, *33*
TPGS (tocopherol polyethylene glycol 1000 succinate) 176
TPP (target product profile) 399
tracheobronchial (TB) region 33, 401; deposition in 34; tree 47
tracheostomies 151–2
transcytosis 62–3
transepithelial electrical resistance (TEER) value 81
translational read-through process 242
transmission electron micrographs *23*

transnasal aerosol delivery 150–1
Transwell® system 80
Treatment Action Group (TAG) 365
treatment, NTM infections **278**;
   antibiotic therapy 277–9;
   clinical studies 281, **282–3**;
   drug discovery pipeline *280*,
   280–1; limitations 279–80;
   surgery 279
treprostinil 316, 318
triboelectrification 125
TRILOGY study 384
tuberculosis (TB) 74, 361
tuberculosis vaccine initiative (TBVI)
   365–7
tumor-associated macrophages 195
turbulent fluctuation 9–10
2D gamma scintigraphy *32*
TYVASO® (treprostinil) inhalation
   solution 318

UIP (usual interstitial pneumonia) 303
ultra-rapid freezing (URF) 175
ultrasonic nebulizers 132, 153, 164, 173

ultra-spray freezing (USF) 175
ultra-Stokesian flow regime 6
URF (ultra-rapid freezing) 175
usual interstitial pneumonia
   (UIP) 303

vaccine 363–4
valve-holding chambers (VHCs) 91, 164;
   albuterol HFA 149; nebulizers
   150; soft mist inhalers
   149; tracheostomy 151–2;
   vibrating mesh and ultrasonic
   nebulizers 153
van der Waals force 125
vasoconstriction 314
VCZ *see* voriconazole
VENTAVIS® (iloprost) inhalation
   solution 318
ventilation images 381
very long-acting beta agonists (VLABAs)
   217–18
vesicle-mediated endocytosis/
   transcytosis 62–3
VHCs *see* valve-holding chambers

vibrating mesh nebulizers 132–3, 334,
   334; invasive mechanical
   ventilation 153–4; NIV 151;
   tracheostomy 152; transnasal
   aerosol delivery 150
vibrating mesh technology (VMT) 279
vicious cycle 292
viscous stresses 11
VLABAs (very long-acting beta agonists)
   217–18
VMT (vibrating mesh technology) 279
voriconazole (VCZ): adverse effects 177;
   Aspergillus fumigatus 178; DPI
   177–8; nebulized formulations
   177; pharmacokinetics 177

wet and dry surfactant aerosol 332–3
whole-lung deposition models 47–8
World Health Organization (WHO)
   313, 361

XHANCE™ 353

Zomig® 350, **351**

T - #0560 - 071024 - C436 - 280/208/19 - PB - 9780367731489 - Gloss Lamination